About the Authors

Lawrence D. Shriberg, Ph.D., is Professor Emeritus of Communicative Disorders and a principal investigator in the Communicative and Cognitive Sciences Group, Waisman Center, University of Wisconsin-Madison. His research is centered on genetic and other origins of pediatric speech sound disorders of known and unknown bases.

Raymond D. Kent, Ph.D., is Professor Emeritus of Communicative Disorders at the University of Wisconsin-Madison. His research has been primarily in the acoustics and physiology of speech, typical and atypical development of speech in children, and neurogenic communication disorders in children and adults with an emphasis on acoustic analysis and the assessment of intelligibility.

Clinical Phonetics

Fourth Edition

Clinical Phonetics

Lawrence D. Shriberg
University of Wisconsin–Madison

Raymond D. Kent
University of Wisconsin–Madison

PEARSON

Boston Columbus Indianapolis New York San Francisco Upper Saddle River
Amsterdam Cape Town Dubai London Madrid Milan Munich Paris Montreal Toronto
Delhi Mexico City São Paulo Sydney Hong Kong Seoul Singapore Taipei Tokyo

Executive Editor and Publisher: Stephen D. Dragin
Vice President, Director of Marketing: Margaret Waples
Editorial Assistant: Michelle Hochberg
Marketing Manager: Joanna Sabella
Production Editor: Mary Beth Finch
Editorial Production Service: Walsh & Associates, Inc.
Manufacturing Buyer: Megan Cochran
Electronic Composition: Jouve India
Cover Designer: Jennifer Hart

Credits and acknowledgments borrowed from other sources and reproduced, with permission, in this textbook appear on appropriate page within text.

Library of Congress Cataloging-in-Publication Date

Shriberg, Lawrence D.
Clinical phonetics / Lawrence D. Shriberg, Raymond D. Kent,. — 4th ed.
p. cm.
Includes bibliographical references and index.
ISBN-13: 978-0-13-702106-2
ISBN-10: 0-13-702106-2
1. Speech therapy. 2. Phonetics. 3. English language—Phonetics. I. Kent, Raymond D. II. Title.
RC423.S515 2013
616.85'506—dc23

2012001124

10 9 8 7 6 5

PEARSON

ISBN-10: 0-13-702106-2
ISBN-13: 978-0-13-702106-2

To our wives, Linda and Jane

What's New in This Edition?

Every chapter has been updated and revised according to reviewer suggestions.

The major changes are:

1. Information on dialects, multicultural, and cross-linguistic aspects of phonetics has been significantly expanded in a new chapter, Chapter 10. In the last edition, dialects were discussed in an appendix. In addition, recordings for dialect transcription are now included on the companion website.
2. Acoustic properties of speech sounds are now discussed at the end of relevant chapters. In the previous edition, materials on acoustics were placed in the final chapter and were not well integrated with the earlier chapters. Several new illustrations have been added to clarify acoustic aspects of speech sounds. The discussion of speech acoustics assumes minimal background in acoustics and is designed to introduce students to this aspect of phonetics.
3. Boxes of supplementary information or items of special interest have been added to most chapters.
4. At the request of numerous instructors, the book has been reformatted into two sections: a text section and a skills practice section. The latter is distinguished by a stripe on the page edges, so that readers can readily find the transcription training materials.
5. Samples of childhood apraxia of speech have been placed on the companion website. These samples give students valuable transcription experience with this type of speech disorder.
6. The glossaries that had been placed at the end of individual chapters are now consolidated at the end of the book for easy reference and review.
7. Several of the appendices have been moved to the companion website where they are easily accessible and can be updated.

NEW! COURSESMART eTEXTBOOK AVAILABLE

CourseSmart is an exciting new choice for students looking to save money. As an alternative to purchasing the printed textbook, students can purchase an electronic version of the same content. With a CourseSmart eTextbook, students can search the text, make notes online, print out reading assignments that incorporate lecture notes, and bookmark important passages for later review. For more information, or to purchase access to the CourseSmart eTextbook, visit www.coursesmart.com.

SUPPLEMENTARY MATERIALS: RESOURCES FOR PROFESSORS AND STUDENTS

Companion Website

Located at www.pearsonhigher.com/shriberg4e, the Companion Website for this text includes a wealth of resources such as Learning Objectives, Practice Questions, Flash Cards, and Useful Websites that will help ensure student mastery.

Contents

Foreword

For almost three decades the first three editions of *Clinical Phonetics* have provided exemplary materials for learning about phonetic transcriptions of normal and disordered speech. Quite remarkably, these texts have melded information from the basic and applied sciences underlying the discipline of Clinical Phonetics. The goal has been the practical application of phonetic transcriptions for evaluation, diagnosis, and monitoring of progress in a wide range of communication disorders. The Forewords to the first three editions were written by Thomas J. Hixon, an admired speech scientist, editor, and former Dean of the Graduate School and Vice President for Research at the University of Arizona. With each edition he accurately chronicled the thoughtful evolution of the content of *Clinical Phonetics* and the continuing enhancement of the stimulus materials and teaching examples used in the book. Hixon extolled the impressive teaching skills of Shriberg and Kent as demonstrated through their selection of material for coverage of linguistic phonetics; speech physiology; speech acoustics; production of vowels, diphthongs, and consonants; phonetic transcription; diacritics for narrow transcription; suprasegmental features; and the rich array of audio examples used for transcription training and practice. Hixon believed that the standard of excellence created by *Clinical Phonetics* through its first three editions deserved the applause of the discipline of Communication Sciences and Disorders. Tom Hixon loved this book and was "spot on" when he said that he couldn't imagine teaching a course in Clinical Phonetics without using this text.

With Tom Hixon's untimely death, I was asked to carry on the tradition of preparing a Foreword for the fourth edition. I am excited by the sensitivity the authors have devoted to providing accurate transcriptions of speech disorders. This commitment is accomplished through transcription practice on vowels, diphthongs, and consonants using time-tested clinical recordings of children's responses to articulation tests and a detailed system of diacritics to accurately transcribe disordered speech. A new excellent chapter by Benjamin Munson provides clinically useful information on dialects and multicultural and cross-linguistic aspects of phonetics. The fourth edition now includes acoustic information at the end of relevant chapters rather then at the end of the book. This change makes it easier for students to understand the acoustic characteristics of various classes of sounds. I was pleased to see that the discussions of speech acoustics assume no technical background and are designed to introduce students to this aspect of phonetics.

In summary, I share Tom Hixon's enthusiasm for this text. This new edition of *Clinical Phonetics* will continue to provide the requisite knowledge and skills in phonetics in academic institutions educating students in Communication Sciences and Disorders and to speech-language pathologists in clinical practice. I am proud to have it on my desk. I only wish *Clinical Phonetics* was available when I taught phonetics in the 1960s and 1970s.

Fred D. Minifie
Professor Emeritus
University of Washington

Preface

When the first edition of *Clinical Phonetics* was published in 1982, we did not foresee that 30 years later we would publish a fourth edition. We are gratified that our book has been adopted by many instructors as a vehicle to introduce students to the special problems in the clinical application of phonetics. Each new edition—and this one is no exception—has attempted to retain the strengths of previous editions while seeking to improve the work as a whole. This fourth edition differs from its predecessors in several ways, some of which are relatively minor, such as wording changes to improve clarity, and some of which are major and substantive, such as the addition or revision of major parts of the book. We are grateful to the reviewers of the previous edition. Their suggestions and comments were most helpful to us as we developed a revision plan for this new edition.

New in this edition is a thoroughly reworked discussion of suprasegmentals, a different approach to the discussion of acoustics, an expanded treatment of dialects, and a new set of materials available on a website. We also endeavored to make the text more streamlined, more efficient, and more friendly to the reader. But those who are familiar with the earlier editions will quickly recognize that we have not neglected the raison d'etre for this book—the conviction that the clinical application of phonetics requires specialized discussion and training and is not simply an uncritical extension of ideas from conventional phonetics texts. We also retain the use of illustrations that are derived from imaging methods such as cinefluorography and computed tomography. We believe that this approach grounds our book in anatomic and physiologic reality. The specialty of clinical phonetics is no longer a neophyte. This text, like the field itself, has matured and advanced. Let's take a closer look at seven of the major changes that led to the fourth edition:

1. In this edition, the acoustic properties of speech are integrated with the discussion of major topics such as vowels and diphthongs, consonants, and suprasegmentals. In the third edition, acoustic information was presented in a final chapter, nearly disconnected from the earlier information on phonetics. We believe that it is appropriate to consider acoustic characteristics within the major chapters of the book. But instructors who choose not to teach the acoustic information can simply assign the earlier pages of the relevant chapters, as the discussion of acoustics appears mostly at the end of the chapters.
2. Suprasegmental properties of speech are especially challenging, owing in part to the lack of a generally accepted transcription system. Moreover, there are disagreements in the literature about definitions of terms and the relationships among various suprasegmental features. The fourth edition offers a completely revised discussion of this intriguing but difficult topic. We have tried to make the discussion of this topic coherent and easy to follow.
3. In previous editions, information on dialects appeared in an appendix. In this new edition, this topic is given its own chapter, written by Benjamin Munson, who is highly regarded for his exceptional scholarship. The new chapter gives readers a thoughtful and contemporary coverage of dialects.
4. Beginning with its first edition, *Clinical Phonetics* was designed to teach phonetics by the printed word and auditory samples for transcription practice. The fourth edition continues this pattern and makes available on the book website an additional set of recorded samples for dialects and childhood apraxia of speech. This expanded set of transcription materials enriches the text and provides students with valuable skills training.
5. The appendixes have been reduced to two, so as to keep the length (and cost) of the book to an effective minimum. The fourth edition retains Appendix A (Phonetic Symbols and Terms) and Appendix B (Distributional, Structural, and Proportional Occurrence Data for American English Sounds, Syllables, and Words). Instructors have told us that this information is a valuable complement to the text. Two appendices in all prior editions—former Appendix D: Procedures to Calculate Transcription Reliability and Research Findings, and Appendix E: Procedures for Audio Recording and Speech Sampling—have been moved to the website for instructors who continue to find this information useful, including an updated list of references for former Appendix E.
6. We have added blocks of supplementary information to most chapters. These boxes, set off from the text, are intended to highlight topics and issues.
7. In this new edition, the transcription training materials have been consolidated at the end of the book, rather than appearing at the end of the chapters, as in earlier editions.

Instructors have suggested that this arrangement would be more convenient.

Nurturing *Clinical Phonetics* through four editions has been a privilege. We hope you find this text to be a reliable and useful guide through some admittedly difficult territory. Putting sounds to paper is a challenging task, all the more so when the sounds do not conform to the standard production of a speech community. Accepting the challenge is a first step in overcoming it. We welcome you to the world of clinical phonetics.

ACKNOWLEDGMENTS

Every edition of *Clinical Phonetics* has included a grateful salute to many people who helped to bring the book to fruition. This fourth edition continues the tradition. We give our sincere thanks to:

Benjamin Munson, University of Minnesota, for crafting a scholarly and lucid chapter on phonetic variation, and for developing an excellent dialect resource that has been placed on the book's companion website.

Peter Flipsen Jr., Idaho State University, for carefully and insightfully preparing website quiz questions that help students review each chapter.

Jane McSweeny, Waisman Center, University of Wisconsin–Madison, for expertly assembling the audio samples of persons with apraxia of speech that are placed on the book website.

Steve Dragin, Executive Editor and Publisher, Pearson Higher Education, for his constant support and sage advice.

Linda Bayma, Jamie Bushell, and Mary Beth Finch, of Pearson Higher Education, who oversaw the assembly of various pieces of the book into a cohesive whole, solving problems along the way.

Kathy Whittier, of Walsh & Associates, Inc., for refining our words, tying up loose ends, and seeing both the forest and the trees.

The following reviewers of this edition for their time and insightful comments: Susan Abbott, Stephen F. Austin State University; Elizabeth Barnes, North Carolina State University; Robert Hull, Valdosta State University; Thomas Linares, Minot State University; and Deborah Weiss, Southern Connecticut State University.

Preface to the Third Edition

Welcome to the third edition of *Clinical Phonetics*. Like the peripatetic pink bunny, *CP* seems to have kept on trucking into the next millennium. A special thanks to those instructors who have been with us since the second or perhaps even the first edition! Thanks too, for your continued positive comments and specific suggestions for this revision.

The most frequent request during the past few years was to try to expand the teaching examples and to make them readily accessible. We have tried to do both. Although the fundamentals of phonetic transcription have not changed since the first edition, media options for skills acquisition have increased significantly. We hope the features described below enhance both the teaching and the learning experience for students and instructors as you complete a course of study in clinical phonetics.

WHAT'S NEW

This third edition of *Clinical Phonetics* retains the ten chapters designed for a semester-length course. We have also kept the appendixes that provide reference materials and other information for additional reading and applied needs in the clinic and laboratory. The "What's Old" section of the Preface to the Second Edition includes useful information on the transcription system taught in this textbook. Instructors using this book for the first time should also read Notes to Instructors, which includes class-tested suggestions for alternative ways to use the book and the audio examples. We have also updated references wherever possible throughout the text. Clearly, however, many of the classic papers in phonetics stand as the best and, for many topics, as the only available sources of information or data. The following are the major text and media enhancements in *Clinical Phonetics*, 2003:

- Chapter 4, Vowels and Diphthongs, has additional information on vowels in languages other than American English, including a section on the difficulties in learning vowels in a second language.
- Chapter 5, Consonants, has new information on consonants that occur in other languages, with a section on trills, clicks, ejectives, and voiced implosives.
- Chapter 6, Diacritics and Sounds in Context, includes an expanded discussion of coarticulation.
- Chapter 10, Acoustic Phonetics, provides a discussion of formant frequencies for vowels in different languages (with implications for second-language learning) and expanded coverage of the suprasegmental features of loudness, vocal effort, and boundary effects.
- Appendix E, Procedures for Speech Sampling and Audio Recording, has been expanded to include technical information on the selection and use of alternative microphones and recorders for analog and digital recording.
- A new appendix, Appendix F, Dialect: Language Variations across Cultures, written by Linda Carpenter (University of Wisconsin–Eau Claire), focuses on concepts and skills needed for phonetic transcription of regional, social, and foreign dialects; it also includes new audio examples.
- A new appendix, Appendix G, Infant Vocalizations, describes contemporary systems for the transcription of babbling and other vocalizations produced by infants.
- A new appendix, Appendix H, Anatomic Bases of Developmental Phonetics, provides basic summaries of the anatomic development of the respiratory, laryngeal, and articulatory systems of speech production.
- A new set of four CDs has been made available for the transcription skills modules, including the new Appendix F audio samples. Both the CDs and a comparable set of audiocassette tape recordings may be obtained by contacting a bookstore, your local Allyn & Bacon sales representative, or the Allyn & Bacon order department, (800) 852-8024, for instructors, or (800) 278-3525 for student purchases.
- A *Clinical Phonetics* Web site (http://www.ablongman.com/shriberg) provides a number of instructional resources for instructors and students. The Web site includes instructions on how to download the PEPPER font, which is available at no cost at http://www.waisman.wisc.edu/phonology/. The PEPPER font includes all of the main character and diacritic symbols used in *Clinical Phonetics*. Instructors and students should find this font useful for quizzes and for other manuscript needs requiring electronic entry of phonetic symbols. The *Clinical Phonetics* Web site also includes additional transcription practice samples from persons with a variety of speech disorders, sample quizzes for each of the ten chapters and

eight appendixes, technical support information for the PEPPER font, and links to other sites that have interesting audio examples and other information on phonetics transcription.

ACKNOWLEDGMENTS

In addition to the dozens of people whom we have thanked for their significant contributions to the prior editions of *Clinical Phonetics,* we are very grateful to the following colleagues for their expert assistance and guidance with this revision. Our sincere thanks to:

Katherina Hauner, Waisman Center, University of Wisconsin–Madison, for her thorough, thoughtful, and cheerful editorial assistance with every aspect of this revision.

Linda Carpenter, University of Wisconsin–Eau Claire, for her well-articulated discussion of dialects and the unique challenges they pose in contemporary clinical phonetics.

Jane McSweeny, Waisman Center, University of Wisconsin–Madison, for her assistance with a variety of tasks reflecting her expertise in phonetic transcription of child speech-sound disorders, including selection and authorship of supplementary audio examples for the *Clinical Phonetics* Web site.

Peter Flipsen, Jr., University of Tennessee, Knoxville, for his significant contributions to the CD samples and authorship of supplementary practice material for the *Clinic Phonetics* Web site.

Martin Ball, John Esling, Ben Maassen, and Thomas Powell for their gracious assistance in providing phonetics materials and resources for the appendixes.

Connie Nadler and Steve Pittelko, Waisman Center, University of Wisconsin–Madison, and Ron Holder, University of Tennessee, Knoxville, for their expert mastering of the CDs and supplementary audiocassette samples.

We would also like to thank the following reviewers: Anna Marie Schmidt of Kent State University and Alice T. Dyson of the University of Florida.

Steve Dragin, Executive Editor and Publisher, Allyn & Bacon, for his consistent support of *Clinical Phonetics* over the years and his congenial guidance with all aspects of the current revision.

Barbara Strickland, Editorial Assistant, Allyn & Bacon, for her valued editorial assistance and contributions at every step of the publication process.

Larry Shriberg
Ray Kent

Preface to the Second Edition

It has been over a decade since the first edition of *Clinical Phonetics*. Many words of encouragement from colleagues who have used this text over the years suggested that it was time for a revision. We have it on good authority that the most important need was to "get a new binding—one that doesn't self-destruct!" Sorry about that. Many thanks to all instructors who developed ingenious ways to keep intact their well-annotated, but ever disintegrating, desk copies.

WHAT'S NEW?

Content

Revisions in the content of this second edition focus primarily on updating and expansion. Because each section of the book is used in one phonetics course or another, we have not deleted any of the original chapters. Thus, instructors will find everything pretty much in the same place. The only deletion is the former Appendix F, which provided references for phonological analysis—these procedures are now taught routinely in courses in developmental phonological disorders.

We hope we have added some nice treats throughout the text. We have updated references throughout the book. Students should know that many older references in phonetics remain the classic or perhaps only source of information on some topics. Expansions in the text include information on the assessment of prosody and an overview of microcomputer systems for acoustic analysis. Expanded and new appendixes include the following:

Appendix D: research findings on the reliability of phonetic transcription.

Appendix E: guidelines for speech sampling and audiotape recording.

Appendix F: multicultural and multilingual considerations in phonetic transcription.

Appendix G: systems to transcribe infant vocalizations.

Format

Revisions in the format of the text (e.g., two-column text) should enhance readability and ease of use and reference. The graphics and subheadings now include color for emphasis. Frequently used tables have been placed in the inside cover pages for ready reference. The index has been redone too.

Audiotapes and Clinical Phonetics Font

The audiotapes that accompany the text may be obtained by contacting your local sales representative or bookstore.

A font that produces all of the symbols and diacritics in *Clinical Phonetics* is available for several platforms. Instructors and researchers should find the font, termed the PEPPER Font, useful to insert phonetic symbols in quizzes and manuscripts requiring broad and narrow phonetic transcription characters. Students and clinicians should find it useful for papers and clinical reports.

WHAT'S OLD?

A Note on the *Clinical Phonetics* Transcription System

Our primary motivation when we wrote the first edition of *Clinical Phonetics* was to offer students in communicative disorders a phonetics book that was directly relevant to clinical application. This is not to say that traditional courses in phonetics are not worthwhile to students in communicative disorders, but simply to reflect our experience that students who took traditional phonetics instruction were often at a loss when faced with clients who had speech disorders. Surely not everyone believes as we do. However, our opinion is shared by many; so many, in fact, that the International Phonetic Alphabet (IPA) was revised in 1989 to include symbols for the transcription of disordered speech. These additions were termed the "Extensions to the International Phonetic Alphabet" and were sanctioned by the International Phonetic Association. In describing the rationale for these additions, Duckworth, Allen, Hardcastle, and Ball wrote, "People working with individuals who have speech which is not the same as that of the adult community in which they live, have long recognized the limitations of the International Phonetic Alphabet (IPA) for transcribing such speech" (*Clinical Linguistics and Phonetics,* Volume 4, p. 273). We believe that the limitations are significant and therefore welcome the Extensions to the IPA, which are included in Appendix A, Table A-6 of this edition.

Some readers may wonder why we did not simply accept the Extensions to the IPA as a solution to the transcription of disordered speech. There were two reasons. The first was a practical one—it was easier to retain the special symbols introduced in the first edition. These symbols were used in the text and in the answer keys for the transcription exercises. The second—and major—reason was that we preferred the simplicity of the original system to the IPA Extensions. The original system established conventions for the placement of the special "diacritic" symbols. In our teaching experience, the arbitrary placement of diacritic symbols was a stumbling point for students who not only had to remember the symbol for a particular sound modification but also where to place that special symbol in the transcription. We believed, and continue to believe, that life could be easier. Therefore, we continue to use the original system with only minor modification. The modification is designed to make things even easier by enhancing the consistency of symbol location.

Another innovation in the first edition was a system of stress marking based on numbers rather than on the stress symbols used in the IPA. We have retained the number system because it has served us well in clinical transcription and because it overcomes some difficulties with the stress-marking conventions of the IPA. One of these difficulties is that, in complex transcriptions, the stress marks of the IPA tend to be hard to distinguish from other phonetic symbols. The IPA stress marks are easily lost in the symbol-rich world of clinical transcription. The number-based system we favor separates stress marks from the other symbols used in phonetic transcription. This physical separation makes it much easier to scan a transcription for information on stress because the stress marks are always located in the top line of the transcription. Of course, we teach our own students both the IPA system and our number-based system. Ultimately, the students can select the system they prefer. And that is our advice to all readers of this book: Use the system that is most convenient and most useful to you.

ACKNOWLEDGMENTS

The Preface to the First Edition included a hefty list of persons whose efforts and talents made possible the first edition of *Clinical Phonetics.* To each of you—these many years later—thanks once again. *Thanks also to:*

The many friends and colleagues who have taken the time to express kind words about the value of *Clinical Phonetics* in their training programs. In the blur of professional activities within one's discipline, this positive feedback has really meant a lot to us.

Mary Anne Reeves, a former student and later phonetics instructor at the University of Wisconsin–Madison, who provided a detailed list of typographic errors in the first edition and thoughtful suggestions for changes in form and content.

Karen Carlson, a clinical instructor at the University of Wisconsin–Madison. Drawing on her broad experience with nonnative-English-speaking persons, Karen has authored a unique set of transcription guidelines for clinical transcription in multicultural and multilingual environments.

Jamie Murray-Branch, a clinical instructor at the University of Wisconsin–Madison, and her lovely daughter Charmaine, for illustrating the process of speech sampling, transcription, and analysis.

Shirley Hunsaker, photographer at the Waisman Center for Mental Retardation and Human Development, for the excellent photographs.

Darlene Davies, San Diego State University; Michael Moran, Auburn University; Susan Moss-Logan, University of Central Arkansas; and Roberta Wacker-Mundy, SUNY-Plattsburgh, whose thoughtful reviews of the first edition of *Clinical Phonetics* helped us formulate our approach to this edition.

David Wilson, Senior Systems Programmer at the University of Wisconsin–Madison, for creative collaboration in the design, coding, and documentation of the PEPPER Font.

Jane McSweeney, Program Assistant at the University of Wisconsin–Madison, for competent editorial assistance at many phases of this project.

Diane Austin, Research Specialist at the University of Wisconsin–Madison, for remarkable excellence in coauthoring the PEPPER Font and associated graphics, and for thorough and congenial copyediting of this busy manuscript.

Thomas Hixon, University of Arizona, a long-time friend and colleague whose gracious and supportive Forewords have launched both editions of *Clinical Phonetics.*

Larry Shriberg
Ray Kent

Preface to the First Edition

A preface allows authors an "up front" opportunity to express their hopes, regrets, and thanks. Here are ours.

We hope that this book does the job it was intended to do. Several years ago we recognized that something was missing in phonetics textbooks. The existing textbooks lacked materials that taught the specific information and perceptual skills needed by speech-language clinicians. This book and the companion audiotapes are our attempt to meet this need. Our goal has been to assemble information and teach the discrimination skills that are relevant for the use of phonetics in the practice of clinical speech-language pathology. We won't retrace here our lengthy journey toward that end. Moreover, we will spare the reader a list of the features that we believe make our effort unique among available phonetics texts. We hope that instructors will find these materials to be as effective with their students as we have found them to be with ours. And for students, clinicians, and others who will progress through this series, we hope you will find it to be an efficient and enjoyable learning experience.

Regrets about what couldn't be included in the scope of this book would require another lengthy list—a list we also will not present here. Instructors will quickly discern for themselves what could not be accommodated within our goals for this text. Phonetics is taught in a variety of course structures within programs that cover communication disorders. We believe that this textbook has the flexibility to be used successfully, with supplementary readings and assignments provided as needed by course instructors.

One list we very much do want to present includes the names of the many persons who assisted us in developing both the text and the audio materials.

Our deepest thanks to:

Wayne Swisher, for co-authoring a 1972 paper on an articulation scoring system that was to become the prototype for the audiotape modules used in this text.

Kathleen Gruenewald and Joan Kwiatkowski, who are the excellent clinician-examiners on several of the lengthier tape segments.

Carol Caldwell, Catherine Jackson, Julie Baran Peterson, and Linda Wurzman, who each provided effective and efficient research assistance in culling, dubbing, and transcribing tape segments for possible inclusion in the series.

Shelly Bezack, Jill Brooks, Denise Dinan, Michele Goodman, Constance Kemper, and Sylvia Thompson, who each volunteered to participate in several pilot studies of phonetic transcription in audio versus video modes.

The several classes of undergraduate students who provided detailed feedback and suggestions for discrimination training.

Frederick Baecker, Stanley Ewanowski, Robert Nellis, and Francesca Spinelli, who each lent time and expertise to provide audio and visual materials used throughout the text.

William Horne, for his tireless, thorough guidance in preparation of the audiotapes.

Helen Goodluck, who provided expert counsel on source materials for Appendix F.

Anne J. Smith, whose scholarly research assistance is reflected throughout the text, particularly in the appendix materials dealing with phonetics systems and statistical summaries.

Thomas Klee and Christine Dollaghan for their thorough and efficient assistance with final stages of manuscript preparation, including the Index.

Mary Louise Edwards, Mary Elbert, and Elaine Paden, our expert listeners, who provided phonetic transcriptions of all audio materials and extremely useful suggestions on program content.

John Bernthal, Raphael Haller, and David Kuehn, for their productive editorial reviews of the manuscript.

Thomas Hixon, for his usual insightful review of the manuscript and his assistance with other phases of the project.

Carole Dugan, for a remarkable effort and performance in typing the manuscript.

The administrative and secretarial staffs at the Department of Communicative Disorders, University of Wisconsin–Madison, and at the Boys Town Institute for Communication Disorders in Children for their consistent support.

L. D. Shriberg
R. D. Kent

Notes to Instructors

We are mindful of the problems instructors face in becoming familiar with a new textbook. These notes bring together facts, impressions, and suggestions collected during field tests of this book with undergraduate students. Many of these observations concern the audiotaped discrimination modules. We hope both new and experienced instructors will find these comments relevant to their teaching task.

TECHNICAL NOTES

The audio materials were selected from a library of over 350 tapes originally made in public schools and speech-language clinics. Approximately 1500 individual sound and word segments were isolated for reproduction. The intensity of the most intense sound on each tape segment was balanced to peak within ± 1 dB of the calibration tone setting. The four compact discs that accompany the text were reproduced from these master tapes and supplementary samples.

Field tests have been conducted with first-generation cassette dubs to ensure that they contain sufficient signal information for discrimination purposes. Their quality and fidelity have been endorsed by consultants and by the panel of five expert judges who contributed to the keys that accompany the tapes. We strongly discourage dubbing copies of the audio examples. Aside from violating copyright, important signal components might be lost from second-generation dubs.

CONTENT NOTES

Three particular content areas of this book warrant brief comment here.

We have found that intuition and verbal descriptions do not always help students to understand how sounds are produced. In writing this book, we have relied almost exclusively on tracings from imaging films to illustrate the articulatory configurations of English sounds. Accordingly, the student can learn how sounds are produced from factual illustrations rather than contrived drawings. Only a few simplifications have been made in adapting the original imaging tracings to published illustrations. We intentionally have oriented the imaging tracings to face both left and right, because we believe it is important that the student be able to imagine vocal tract shapes no matter which way a speaker is facing. In our experience, students benefit from drawing vocal tract shapes for different sounds, and we recommend this exercise as a useful part of phonetics education.

The diacritic system presented in Chapter 6 and used in the transcription modules departs in some ways from other diacritic systems we have seen. The primary innovation in the system used in this book is the spatial orientation or location of the diacritic marks: All marks denoting a general class of sound modification, such as tongue articulation, laryngeal function, or velopharyngeal function, are placed in the same position relative to the phonetic symbol that is being modified. Thus, the various modifications of tongue articulation—such as dentalization, lateralization, palatalization, and rhotacization (a term we favor over retroflexion)—are all marked by placing the appropriate diacritic mark *below* the phonetic symbol that represents the sound segment. We have tried as much as possible to use the conventional characters for the diacritic marks, but we have changed their transcription positions. One benefit of this innovation is that it becomes easier for the student to remember the diacritic marks—because all marks of a particular class go in the same place. Another benefit is that the spatial position of a diacritic can carry some clinical meaning. For example, because the diacritics pertaining to velopharyngeal function are placed above the phonetic symbol being modified, the clinician can determine from a quick scan of a transcription the number and variety of modifications in velopharyngeal function.

Instructors also should note the material in the appendixes. Appendix B, in particular, is a consolidation of data that is useful for many types of class assignments, including preclinical exercises in the rationale for assembling stimulus materials. Beginning students are especially motivated to learn statistical information about English linguistic forms if this information is made "relevant" for their upcoming clinical practice. The materials in each of the other appendixes are also designed for use in clinical transcription in communicative disorders.

TRAINING NOTES

The key to the acquisition of discrimination skills is clearly *practice.* Questionnaire-discussion sessions with our students have yielded the following comments and suggestions about discrimination practice.

Time

Students should not be asked to do "too much, too soon." Of all comments about the program, this one was made most often by students. In the press of other coursework, students need to schedule time each day and each week to practice on the audio modules. Many students like to go over each module several times, returning later to certain modules as needed. Quizzes must be scheduled carefully to allow for adequately spaced practice throughout the semester.

Assistance

Some form of assistance should be available on a regular basis throughout the program, particularly for beginning students. Such help may be provided by the instructor, a teaching assistant, another student, or some other way to students when they simply "don't get it." Some approaches to group and individually guided assistance are listed as follows (see also Chapter 7).

- Classroom demonstrations using acoustic displays can be helpful in contrasting visually the target sound or sound errors with other sounds in question.
- Students can accomplish production-perception practice in pairs or in small groups. One person can produce (simulate) predetermined errors from a laboratory workshop, for example, while others transcribe what they hear on paper or at the blackboard. Differences in production and perception should then be discussed, with corrective feedback provided by the instructor and other students as necessary.
- The instructor can make recordings in which the same word is used in contrast drills; for example, "see" [s i], [s̪̚ i], [s̪̑ i], [s̢̪ i]. Students practice saying the same word with the different speech errors, gradually increasing their rate of production. Word forms can proceed from simple ("see") to more complex ("Mississippi").
- Students can generate their own lists of helpful comments, in addition to those provided in the text, describing how they have learned to make a particular sound change. As the text stresses, students must become able to produce each sound change readily before learning to discriminate it from other sound changes.
- Students can make their own recordings of particular sound changes. Students can trade recordings, score them, and discuss differences in conjunction with the instructor or within their own student sessions.

Grading

Instructors have several alternatives in grading the skills development portion of any academic coursework. In the ideal situation, instructors would use criterion-referenced grading of phonetics skill acquisition, assigning each student a grade based on the level of skill demonstrated at the conclusion of a period of training. This approach seems most ethical from the perspective of the consumer; that is, it will provide information about students' skill levels as they enter clinical practicum. However, a number of other grading practices are also defensible. Such matters are ultimately left to instructors to arrange within the context of their curricula in communication disorders. However, three issues related to any grading system are important to note here.

First, instructors will need to provide audio materials for quizzes. We have found it useful to use a combination of instructor stimuli (normal speech and error simulations) and audio samples from children (normal speech and errored speech) to test students' acquisition of discrimination skills. Such materials are initially challenging to construct. Over time, the instructor will accumulate a large pool of reliable recorded items, much like the accumulation of a set of useful objective test questions.

Second, the instructor needs to establish clearly the criteria used for determining grades based on the percentage of agreement between students' responses and the keys for quizzes. The companion website describes three bases for calculating agreement—exact agreement, functional equivalence, and near functional equivalence. We have used each of these criteria, our choice depending on the difficulty level of the discrimination task. What is important is that students know exactly which criteria will be used to convert their quiz performance into grades. When considering grading criteria, the instructor should keep in mind that published studies involving speech errors (for example, /r/, /s/ distortions) routinely report interjudge agreement percentages no higher than 75 to 80 percent (see also Chapter 7).

Especially in the early stages of a phonetics course, we have found it beneficial to use a rather lax criterion in grading transcription quizzes. One particular device that we have used is to give students a second-choice selection in transcription. That is, students are allowed to enter a second-choice symbol above their first-choice symbol. For example, in transcribing the word *dog*, a student who is unsure whether the vowel is /ɔ/ or /ɑ/ can write

ɑ
/dɔg/

Although this option runs a certain risk of abuse (such as second-choice symbols for every element in a transcription), we never encounter such overuse. In fact, few students use the option as often as we might expect. However, students appreciate having a second choice, particularly for more subtle auditory discriminations. Some phonetic decisions are difficult to make, and not all errors in transcription are equal. As experiments have shown, not even the experts agree exactly in their phonetic transcriptions of the same utterance.

Third, as noted previously, it is important to gauge carefully the frequency and timing of quizzes throughout a period of training. We have found frequent quizzes covering small amounts of material to work well. Students need time to assimilate and consolidate their developing phonetics skills.

If they feel rushed, fears and frustrations develop. Ideally, students should be allowed to schedule each quiz as they are ready, rather than scheduling the perceptual quizzes in large groups. Students especially appreciate efforts to allow for individual differences in level of entrance skills and in rates of learning throughout the training period.

PROGRAM NOTES

Students have indicated that there are benefits from the experience of progressing through the text and the audio modules beyond the informational content and skills acquisition. Instructors may wish to include lecture or discussion materials to augment the following observations made by students.

- They enjoy the opportunity to hear examples of children talking, an experience that for most beginning students is both educational and entertaining.
- They appreciate the opportunity to hear clinicians talking to children with speech errors, particularly to learn how competent clinicians talk to children who have severe intelligibility deficits.
- They profit from the exposure to several procedures for obtaining speech samples from children, including standard articulation tests and continuous speech sampling procedures.
- They learn to respect the variety of spoken forms of languages and individual differences across cultures and among speakers.
- They develop the discipline needed for learning independently, including learning to arrange their own listening schedule and study group sessions with other students.
- They experience the pride of accomplishment—with reference to the clinical phonetics component of speech pathology, they feel prepared to meet the challenge of their first clinical practicum assignment.

L. D. S.
R. D. K.

Contents of the Audio Samples

CD	TRACK	EXERCISE	TIME
1	1 (Tape 1A)	Transcription List A	6:22
1	2 (Tape 1A)	Transcription List B	6:03
1	3 (Tape 1A)	Transcription List C	5:51
1	4 (Tape 1A)	Transcription List D	9:29
1	5 (Tape 1B)	Transcription List E	5:00
1	6 (Tape 1B)	Transcription List F	2:34
1	7 (Tape 1B)	Vowels and Diphthongs Quiz	5:53
1	8 (Tape 1B)	Transcription Quiz	7:28
1	9 (Tape 1B)	Diacritics Examples	7:05
2	1 (Tape 2A)	Vowels and Diphthongs Module 1: Vowel and Diphthong Substitutions	3:14
2	2 (Tape 2A)	Vowels and Diphthongs Module 2: Vowels and Diphthong Modifications	5:07
2	3 (Tape 2A)	Vowels and Diphthongs Module 3: Central Vowels	1:46
2	4 (Tape 2A)	Vowels and Diphthongs Module 4 Vowel-Diphthong Substitutions, Modifications, and Central Vowels.	3:44
2	5 (Tape 2A)	Vowels and Diphthongs Module 5: Multiple Element Changes	4:09
2	6 (Tape 2A)	Vowels and Diphthongs Module 6: Vowels and Diphthong Lengthening	3:28
2	7 (Tape 2A)	Vowels and Diphthongs Module 7: Vowels and Diphthong Nasalization	3:37
2	8 (Tape 2A)	Vowels and Diphthongs Module 8: Summary Quiz	4:18
2	9 (Tape 2B)	Stops Module 1: Stop Substitutions	2:54
2	10 (Tape 2B)	Stops Module 2: Voicing of Voiceless Stops	1:57
2	11 (Tape 2B)	Stops Module 3: Devoicing of Voiced Stops	3:19
2	12 (Tape 2B)	Stops Module 4: Glottal Stop Substitutions	1:49
2	13 (Tape 2B)	Stops Module 5: Stop Deletions	4:12
2	14 (Tape 2B)	Stops Module 6: Frictionalized Stops	1:36
2	15 (Tape 2B)	Stops Module 7: Summary Quiz	5:02
2	16 (Tape 2B)	Fricatives and Affricates Module 1: / f /and / v / Changes	5:35
2	17 (Tape 2B)	Fricatives and Affricates Module 2: / h / deletions	1:48
3	1 (Tape 3A)	Fricatives and Afficates Module 3: Voiceless and Voiced *th* Changes	6:32
3	2 (Tape 3A)	Fricatives and Affricates Module 4: Fricative and Affricate Voicing Changes	5:53
3	3 (Tape 3A)	Fricatives and Affricates Module 5: Fricative and Affricate Substitutions	5:49
3	4 (Tape 3A)	Fricatives and Affricates Module 6: Dentalized Sibilants	5:16
3	5 (Tape 3A)	Fricatives and Affricates Module 7: Lateralized Sibilants	2:39
3	6 (Tape 3A)	Fricatives and Affricates Module 8: Retroflexed Sibilants	2:51
3	7 (Tape 3B)	Fricatives and Affricates Module 9: Sibilants Quiz	2:54

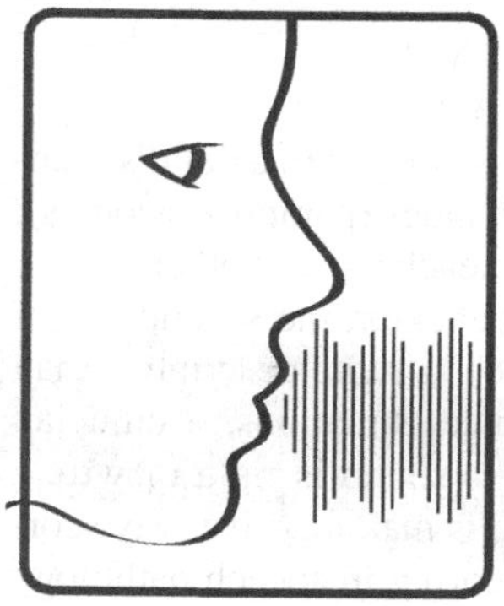

CHAPTER 1

Overview of Clinical Phonetics

Welcome

Beginning a new course of study is exciting. If this is one of your first courses in a program leading to a degree in communication disorders, we welcome you to a dynamic and challenging field. We hope that your interests and needs in phonetics will be met by this text. This opening overview is intended to help you get the "big picture" before you begin a chapter-by-chapter progression through this series.

What is **clinical phonetics,** and what role does it play in the training of a speech-language clinician?

Clinical Phonetics

Phonetics is the study of the perception and production of speech sounds. Subdisciplines within phonetics, such as articulatory phonetics and acoustic phonetics, date back several centuries. In coining the term *clinical* phonetics for the first edition of this book, we wanted to acknowledge that the application of phonetics is a legitimate area of study in its own right. In the past three decades this discipline has seen extensive growth, including an active research base and several journals that publish papers that are of direct relevance to clinical practice. We divide your pursuit of competence in using clinical phonetics in speech-language pathology into two major domains: informational and perceptual.

The Informational Domain of Clinical Phonetics

Clinical phonetics includes a wealth of descriptive information about speech sounds. Students often have difficulty understanding how such information is relevant to clinical practice. We hope you will perceive in this text the importance of phonetic knowledge to your skills in assessing and managing people with communication disorders. A personal anecdote might illustrate this point.

A student once asked one of the authors for an opinion on therapy materials she was preparing. Although this student was *not* a major in communication disorders, she was called upon in her student teaching practicum to help a child who had trouble "pronouncing his *s*'s." She had constructed a word list for working on the *s* sound in the word-final position; here are some of the items on her list:

base
face
hose

What's wrong here? Without the benefit of the most basic information in phonetics, this well-meaning student was going to ask the child to say the *z* sound, not the *s* sound, in the word *hose.*

The point of this example is that knowledge about speech sounds is basic to efficient and effective clinical practice. Clinicians who are well grounded in phonetics will possess the tools to assess and manage people with communication disorders. Knowledge of facts such as how often speech sounds occur in running speech is essential when dealing with a child or adult who is not making sounds correctly, for whatever reason.

We have presented descriptive information about sound production verbally and pictorially. Because it is difficult to understand how sounds are produced from verbal descriptions alone, many illustrations accompany the text. Virtually all of the illustrations of speech sound formation are based on imaging materials collected by author Raymond D. Kent. We believe that many phonetics texts rely on impressionistic drawings that often mislead the reader about how sounds really are formed. Therefore, we decided at the outset to use, as much as possible, illustrations that relate directly to anatomical reality. Careful study of these illustrations should give the student the ability to visualize the positions and motions of the speech structures. This ability is invaluable to the specialist in communication disorders.

As previewed in the front matter of this text, your knowledge of clinical phonetics from multicultural perspectives has become an increasingly important component of clinical competence. Chapter 10 includes a wide-ranging discussion of relevant concepts and terms for contemporary practice as a speech-language pathologist.

The Perceptual Domain of Clinical Phonetics

In addition to acquiring knowledge in the informational domain of clinical phonetics, a person who wishes to become competent in clinical phonetics must also acquire adequate skill in making perceptual discriminations. Figure 1.1 depicts 24 situations in which discrimination skill is needed in clinical speech pathology. The 24 blocks in this figure embrace levels of increasing skill, from those that can be learned fairly rapidly to those that require considerable training to acquire. That is, each sequentially numbered block requires more skill than the numbered blocks that precede it. You will have the opportunity to acquire discrimination skill in each of the 24 clinical situations depicted in Figure 1.1. Here we describe each of the axes on this three-dimensional representation of the perceptual domain of clinical phonetics.

System Complexity. The vertical axis in Figure 1.1 includes the three systems used in clinical phonetics. Each of these systems is appropriate in certain situations in assessing and managing people with communication disorders.

In the lowest row, blocks 1 to 8, **two-way scoring** refers to dichotomous decision making about speech behavior. A clinician must decide if a target behavior is "correct" or "incorrect," "right" or "wrong," "socially acceptable" or "socially unacceptable," or some other binary decision. In Chapter 7 more will be said about such decisions. The points to be made here are that a dichotomous decision about behavior, termed two-way scoring, is the easiest of the three systems in terms of complexity; and, of the three systems, it is most often used. Two-way scoring is done not only by clinicians but also by people who may be assisting with a child's management program, such as speech aides (paraprofessionals); the child's parents, caregivers, or teachers; and others.

Five-way scoring of speech behavior, the second tier of blocks in Figure 1.1 (cells 9 to 16), is more descriptive than two-way scoring. For some clinical situations, a clinician needs to know not only whether a sound is right or wrong but also what type of error a child is making. Five-way scoring is the traditional system of scoring in speech pathology that provides such information. In addition to the "correct" category, four "wrong" categories specify the type of error. A sound can be deleted altogether (**deletion** or **omission**), replaced by another sound (**substitution**), not said quite correctly (**distortion**), or said correctly but preceded or followed by an intrusive sound (**addition**). These five categories—"correct," "deletion," "substitution," "distortion," and "addition"—constitute the five-way system of scoring. Again, practical information on matters pertaining to five-way scoring will be presented in Chapter 7.

Finally, at the highest level of the model presented in Figure 1.1 is **phonetic transcription**. There is a fundamental distinction between the two scoring systems (two-way scoring and five-way scoring) and phonetic transcription. Whereas each of the scoring systems involves judgments about speech—they require the clinician to "score" a behavior—phonetic transcription is concerned only with *description* of behavior. The task in phonetic transcription is to represent what the child says rather than to score or judge it by some arbitrary standard. The degree of precision required in transcription depends on the clinician's purpose, as discussed in detail in Chapter 7. Depending on the number and type of symbols used, clinicians can do a **broad transcription** or a

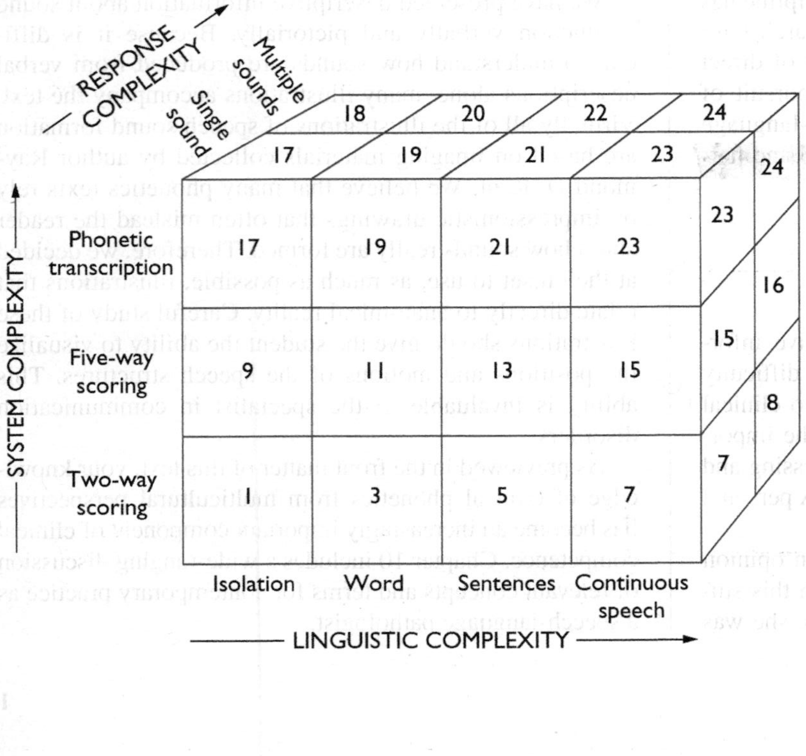

FIGURE 1.1
The perceptual domain of clinical phonetics. A student who wishes to become competent in clinical phonetics must acquire adequate discrimination skills for each of the clinical situations depicted in this representation.

narrow (close) transcription of behavior. Essentially, as you will learn in later chapters, narrow transcription adds phonetic detail to broad transcription, using the set of diacritics shown in the inside back cover. As depicted in Figure 1.1, phonetic transcription requires the highest level of skill from a clinician. Whereas speech aides, parents, caregivers, teachers, and others may be trained for two-way and even five-way scoring, broad and narrow phonetic transcription typically is done only by clinicians.

Linguistic Complexity. The horizontal axis in Figure 1.1 divides speech into four linguistic contexts of increasing **linguistic complexity,** as indicated by higher numbers. The far left blocks require the clinician to score or transcribe speech sounds in *isolation.* For example, a child is asked to say a sound, *s,* or a series of sounds, *s, f, z,* which the clinician scores or transcribes. When a sound is embedded in a *word, sentence,* or *continuous speech,* the task of discriminating one or more sounds is more difficult. This left-to-right hierarchy also generally parallels a child's progress in a management program. Clinicians and others who work to help a child carry over skills to new situations must be competent in making perceptual discriminations within all four linguistic contexts.

Response Complexity. The third dimension in the model, **response complexity,** captures an important situational difference between scoring and transcribing. For some clinical tasks, represented in Figure 1.1 by the odd-numbered blocks, the clinician need only score or transcribe one **target sound** per linguistic unit. For other tasks, represented by the even-numbered blocks, the clinician is required to score or transcribe two or more sounds per word. For example, some tests of a child's articulation proficiency are designed to test only one target sound or target cluster per word (for example, "*p*ig," "cu*p*," "cu*ps*"). Other articulation tests, however, require the clinician to score two or as many as four targets per word (for example, "*pig,*" "*cups,*" "*sits,*" "*squirrel,*" "*bus,*" "*fish*"). Obviously, because of memory constraints and other speech processing variables, the multiple-target tests are more difficult to score or transcribe than the single-sound articulation tests.

Competence in Clinical Phonetics

The perceptual domain of clinical phonetics as portrayed in Figure 1.1 includes 24 discrimination situations. In one situation, a clinician may need to make only correct/incorrect decisions about one isolated target sound (Block 1). In another situation, a clinician may need to transcribe phonetically continuous speech (Block 24). This text will provide you with discrimination training in each of the 24 situations depicted in Figure 1.1. Trends in clinical practice support the need for clinicians to be competent in transcribing samples of continuous conversational speech from speakers who come from diverse linguistic communities.

As you begin your study of clinical phonetics, we hope you will keep in mind two objectives—to acquire a firm knowledge of descriptive information about the phonetics of American English and to acquire discrimination skills for the clinical situations represented in Figure 1.1. In our view, demonstrated competence in each of these areas of clinical phonetics is the ethical responsibility of anyone who tests or attempts to change the articulatory behavior of another person.

EXERCISES

Fill in the information that describes each clinical situation depicted in Figure 1.1. Answers for the first situation are provided. (See "Answers to Exercises" at the back of the book.)

	Linguistic Complexity	*System Complexity*	*Response Complexity*
1. A clinician asks a child to say some words, each of which contains one *r* sound (e.g., *r*ug, *r*abbit, ca*r*). After each word, the clinician records whether the child said the *r* sound correctly.	(word)	(two-way scoring)	(single sound)
2. A clinician is interested in knowing whether an adult client is saying *s* and *sh* correctly at work. The client obtains a 10-minute recording of her speech at the office. The clinician scores all occurring *s* and *sh* sounds as correct or incorrect.	continuous	Two way	Multiple
3. As part of his management program, a boy reads 20 sentences, each of which is composed of several words containing one or more *l* sounds. After each sentence, the clinician scores each *l* sound as correct, distorted, substituted for, added to, or deleted.	sentences	Five way	Single

4. An audio recording is made of a 5-year-old girl with extremely delayed speech who is talking about her favorite television program. The clinician later transcribes the entire speech sample.

Linguistic Complexity	System Complexity	Response Complexity
continuous	phonetic transcription	Multiple

5. A speech-language pathologist administers a word-level articulation test with multiple targets per word (e.g., *tele*vision, u*mbrell*a, *sc*i*ss*o*rs*). Each target sound is scored as correct, distorted, substituted for, added to, or deleted.

Linguistic Complexity	System Complexity	Response Complexity
word	Five way	Multiple

CHAPTER 2

LINGUISTIC PHONETICS

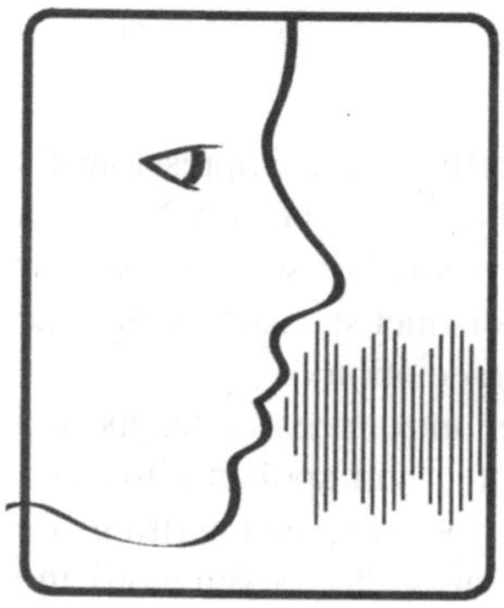

Now the world had one language and a common speech.

—(Genesis 11:1; NIV)

In the biblical story of the tower of Babel, people tried to build on the plain in Shinar a city with a tower that would reach to the heavens. Upon seeing the city and the tower under construction, God said, "If as one people speaking the same language they have begun to do this, then nothing they plan to do will be impossible for them. Come let us go down and confuse their language so they will not understand each other" (Genesis 11:6; NIV). In so doing, God confused the language of the entire world.

LANGUAGE, SPEECH, AND DIALECT

Estimates of the number of languages in the world vary, but we may say conservatively that there are over 3000 and probably closer to 5000. In this book we are concerned with spoken language, that is, a symbolic system in which meanings are communicated by speech. Physically, **speech** is both a pattern of the movements of the speech organs and a pattern of acoustic vibrations. Speech is most conveniently studied in physical terms by observing the movements of the speech structures (tongue, lips, jaw, and so on) and by recording the acoustic signal that the speech structures generate. Therefore, the study of sounds in a spoken language generally includes a description of how individual sounds are formed and information on the acoustic or auditory properties of a sound. For example, we might try to describe the sound represented by the first letter in the word *see* by examining the action of the tongue and by talking about the "noise" that we hear when this sound is uttered.

Spoken language is rooted deeply in human cultures and in the human race itself. Sapir comments on the antiquity of language as follows:

> *The universality and the diversity of speech leads to a significant inference. We are forced to believe that language is an immensely ancient heritage of the human race, whether or not all forms of speech are the outgrowth of a single pristine form. It is doubtful if any other cultural asset of man, be it the art of drilling for fire or of chipping stone, may lay claim to a greater age. I am inclined to believe that it antedated even the lowliest developments of material cultures, that these developments, in fact, were not strictly possible until language, the tool of significant expression, had itself taken shape.* (Sapir, 1921, pp. 22–23)

All of us, except for people with severe vocal or hearing impairment, learn speech as the primary and first modality of language. The parent gauges a child's progress in learning language by the child's utterance of sounds that resemble words in the adult's spoken language. Parents eagerly await their child's first crude attempts at saying "mama" or "dada." As the child matures in linguistic ability, the parents may marvel as the child utters sentence-length expressions, sometimes containing words that the parents had not heard the child say before. Gradually, the child learns to name objects, to express needs and desires, and to remark on attitudes and emotions. Speech becomes a unique and powerful bond by which one person communicates ideas to another. An American visitor in a foreign land who needs directions or advice anxiously asks the persons he or she encounters, "Do you speak English?" in expectation of the simple "Yes" that will open the door to spoken language.

Nations or cultures often are identified by their language. People speaking the same language share not only a communication system but also usually a cultural heritage. Naturally, people who live close together in the same geographic area and who need to communicate with one another will use a common language. These people constitute a **speech community** (a group of people who live within the same geographical boundaries and use the same language). The United States may be called an American-English speech community because most of its citizens speak the same language, American English. However, we can identify smaller speech communities within the United States. For example, the city of Los Angeles has a Mexican American speech community composed of people who share the Spanish language.

Within a country such as the United States, we encounter speakers who use American English but differ from other speakers of that language in pronunciation, vocabulary, or grammatical construction. These different usage patterns within a language are called **dialects.** Many dialects are **regional dialects** because they are characteristic of people who live in a certain region.

Chapter 10 provides a detailed examination of regional, social, and international dialects and includes procedural suggestions for phonetic transcription. The following are some introductory perspectives.

For most purposes in this book, we will assume the dialect of General American English (GAE). But do not be concerned if your pronunciation departs on occasion from that described in this text. We do not use GAE because it is "better" than any other dialect but simply because it is the most commonly used in the United States. We think of dialects as descriptive, not prescriptive. Prescriptive comments are evaluative judgments and state, implicitly or explicitly, preferences for one dialect over another. Descriptive comments simply describe dialectal variations without evaluative judgments.

Because a speaker of New England dialect uses the same language as a speaker of Southern American dialect, they communicate with little difficulty, aside from relatively minor differences in pronunciation and vocabulary. The distinction between language and dialect is one of degree. If two dialects of the same language diverge more and more in pronunciation, vocabulary, and grammatical structure, they may become recognized as different languages as communicative interaction diminishes.

Each of us belongs to a speech community and uses a certain dialect. The authors of this book share American English as a language but differ in dialect, one being a native of the Boston area and the other being a native of Montana. Thus, the authors share a language but not a dialect. Because the written form of language usually does not vary appreciably across dialects, our dialectal differences did not interfere with the writing of this book. However, in preparing the audio samples that accompany the book, dialectal differences were immediately apparent. The author from Boston "dropped" his *r*'s (*car* became *caw* or *cah* to the other author's ears), and the author from Montana used the same vowel for the words *cot* and *caught.* The authors also differ in other aspects of pronunciation because of dialectal differences. For example, the author from Montana occasionally pronounces words like *palm* and *calm* with an *l* because his parents pronounce them that way. The author from Boston pronounces them without an *l.* Despite the many differences in pronunciation, the two authors wrote a book in the same language (although our writing styles may differ somewhat). In written language many dialectal differences disappear. The two authors spell *car, caught,* and *palm* the same way, despite their differences in pronouncing each of these words.

In addition to a dialect, each person has a unique form of spoken language that is called an **idiolect** (*idio-* meaning personal or distinct; *-lect* apparently borrowed from *dialect*). The idiolect is determined by our membership in a speech community, by our regional background, by our social class, and by various individual factors and experiences. Thus, the idiolect is the speech pattern that distinguishes us as individuals. When the impressionist impersonates a famous personality, the success of the act depends partly on the impressionist's ability to recreate the idiolect of the famous person. Whereas dialects may associate us with a regional or social class, our idiolects mark us as separate and distinct speakers within the broader groups of our linguistic association.

The remainder of this chapter introduces concepts and terms useful in the study of written and spoken language. Keep in mind as you read that speaking and writing are modes of language expression. That is, the spoken word and the printed word are not language per se but expressions of language. The **sign language,** or manual communication, used by people who are deaf or hard of hearing is another mode of language expression. We know of a young man born deaf and blind who communicates by still another mode—he uses a tactile coding device that allows him to "feel" language through his fingers and to type his message on a keyboard.

Speech can be understood even though it may not be heard. Expert speechreaders can understand much of what a speaker says by observing the visible movements that accompany speech. Finally, the user of a special method called Tadoma "feels" speech by placing a hand against a speaker's face. All this is simply to underscore the point that speech is a popular, but not a necessary, mode of language.

Now let us consider some basic units of linguistic analysis, beginning with the morpheme and the phoneme. Our examination will include both written and spoken language.

The Morpheme

The **morpheme** is the minimal unit of meaning, or, more formally, the morpheme is the smallest unit of language that carries a semantic interpretation. The list of morphemes in a language is called the **lexicon** of that language. Individual morphemes may be stems, endings for plurals and verb tenses, and other suffixes and prefixes. Thus, the word *cat* is a single morpheme, whereas the words *cats* and *catlike* each consist of two morphemes.

cats = cat + s (the plural ending or suffix is a morpheme)

catlike = cat + like

Each word in a language is made up of one or more morphemes, but an individual morpheme is not necessarily a word. As shown above, the plural ending *s* in the word *cats* is a morpheme even though *s* is not a word in the English language. Any word in the **dictionary** of our language is composed of stems, suffixes, prefixes, and endings for tense, possession, and pluralization, and these constituent parts of words are the morphemes of the language. *Words make up the dictionary of the language, and morphemes make up the lexicon of the language.*

Sometimes a morpheme of the English language does not look familiar when it is taken out of a word and placed in isolation. Consider the words *desist, consist, resist, insist,* and *persist.* Notice that each of these words is composed of a stem (*sist*) and a prefix (*de, con, re, in,* or *per*). Now, the stem *sist* probably does not look like an English word to you. And, in fact, it is not a word but rather a morpheme that is derived from the Latin word *sistere,* meaning "to stand (set)" or "to cause to stand." The Latin word survives in our language as a part of some of our words even though the morpheme *sist* does not occur by itself as a word in our dictionary. The derivation of English words like *desist* is revealed by morphemic analysis, as illustrated below.

desist = de (from) + sist = "to stand from" or "to stop"
consist = con (together) + sist = "to stand together" or "to be formed of"
resist = re (back) + sist = "to stand back" or "to oppose"
insist = in (in, on) + sist = "to stand on" or "to demand"
persist = per (through) + sist = "to stand through" or "to persevere"

Here are some additional examples of morphemic decomposition.

relentless = re + lent + less
morpheme = morph + eme
subnormal = sub + norm + al
feather = feather
cupboards = cup + board + s
transmittal = trans + mit + al
permitting = per + mit + ing
teeth = tooth + plural

The study of morphemes is called **morphemics** or **morphology,** and it embraces issues even more complicated than those hinted at in the examples given above. Languages differ greatly in their morphology, and these differences contribute to part of the complexity in this area of linguistic study. For the purposes of this text, a **morphemic transcription** is a written record of the morphemic content of an utterance. Such a transcription might be made if a clinician wants to analyze a language sample from a child. It should be emphasized that such a transcription has as its goal the recognition of meaningful elements rather than individual speech sounds.

The Phoneme

Just as a word has one or more constituent morphemes, a morpheme has one or more constituent phonemes. A **phoneme** is a basic sound segment that has the linguistic function of distinguishing morphemes. For example, consider the words in the following list:

cat mat fat rat bat pat vat hat

First, notice that each of these words is a single morpheme because each is a meaningful unit that cannot be broken down further into two or more meaningful units.[1] Notice further that any two of these words differ only in the initial sound. In other words, the morphemes are distinguished by the sound segments denoted in these words by the alphabet letters (or **graphemes**) *c, m, f, r, b, p, v, h.* The sounds represented by these letters are phonemes of the English language, and they are identified by their role in morphemic contrasts. In fact, the linguist discovers the phonemes in a language by examining **minimal contrasts,** or contrasts between two morphemes that differ in only one sound segment. The linguist knows that *p* and *b* are distinct phonemes in English because of their roles in contrasting pairs like *pay–bay* and *cup–cub.*

It is important to recognize that phonemic contrasts are linguistic contrasts and therefore have the potential to produce entirely different morphemes and words. Changing, say, the *p* in *mop* to a *b* yields a new word that has no semantic similarity to *mop* (that is, there is no similarity in meaning). Is there ever sound change that does not result in a linguistic change? Yes. Consider the initial consonant sound in *key* and the initial consonant sound in *coo.* Despite the difference in spelling (*k* versus *c*), you probably will agree that both words *key* and *coo* begin with the same sound (call it a *k* sound). Yet, as you can verify yourself by touching your finger to your tongue as you say each word, the initial *k* sounds are not made in exactly the same way. Actually, the sound in *coo* is produced farther back in the mouth than the *k* sound in *key.* To most speakers of English, these two *k* sounds sound alike, in fact, identical. But to a speaker of Arabic, they sound quite different. In Arabic, the frontal *k* sound is a different phoneme than the back *k* sound, so to the Arabic speaker, these two sounds seem as different as a *p* and *b* seem to us. This difference, which to an English speaker is barely detectable because it is a nonphonemic difference, is very obvious to the speaker of Arabic (in which the difference is phonemic). Children learn to produce these two different kinds of *k* sounds in English; but, because the difference is nonphonemic, they grow up with little appreciation of the difference between them. Another example of a nonphonemic sound change can be demonstrated with the second *n* in *nine* and *ninth.* If you hold your finger just behind your upper front teeth so that your fingertip touches the gum line, you should notice that as you say the two words, your tongue comes farther forward for the *n* in *ninth* than for the *n* in *nine.*

To sum up, a phonemic difference between two sound segments means not only that they sound different but that the difference can be linguistically significant insofar as it yields two different morphemes or words. Of course, not every sound change in a given word will produce another word in our language. If we substitute a *w* for the *v* in *vat,* we do not get a new English word. But we know that *w* and

[1] Although *at* is a morpheme, the isolated consonants *c, m, f,* etc., are not morphemes. Therefore, *at* is not a base form in these words.

v are different phonemes because some pairs of contrasting morphemes (like *vine–wine*) do exist. The study of such differences is called phonemics.

The International Phonetic Alphabet (IPA)

Sounds come in great variety in the world's languages, but speakers of all languages have in common an anatomical system of speech production. This anatomical system is the mechanism of sound production that places limits on possible sound types and is a basis for their description. Recognizing that a standardized system of notation could be highly useful for transcribing speech sounds, the International Phonetics Association, which was established in Paris in 1886, worked toward the goal of providing the world with a notational standard for the phonetic representation of all languages. This standard is the International Phonetic Alphabet (IPA). Since its introduction in the late 1800s, the IPA was revised and expanded in 1900, 1932, 1989, 1993, and 2005. In 1994, the International Clinical Phonetics and Linguistics Association adopted a set of symbols designed to improve the applicability of the IPA to disordered speech. These are known as the "Extensions to the IPA."

The IPA currently includes 107 symbols to represent consonants and vowels. These are supplemented with 31 diacritics (special marks that indicate modifications of a sound) and 19 signs that indicate variations in suprasegmental qualities such as length, tone, stress, and intonation. A copy of the IPA table of symbols is included in Appendix A.

The IPA is an arbitrary alphabet insofar as the symbols do not have any representational significance. Any given symbol, such as /b/, does not signify anything other than an arbitrary association with the designated sound. One feature of the IPA that is helpful to speakers of English is that many of the symbols are similar to the alphabet characters often associated with a particular sound in the English language. For example, /b/ is the first sound in *bay* and /p/ is the first sound in *pay*. This comes about because the IPA is based largely on Latin. The general principle of the IPA is to assign one symbol for each distinctive sound or speech segment. This principle is very important and underlies the universal application of the IPA (that is, to all natural languages).

Alphabets do not have to be arbitrary, and some have been designed as organic systems in which the symbols represent features of sound production. We consider two examples here—Visible Speech and the Korean alphabet. Visible Speech was invented in 1867 by Alexander Melville Bell, father of Alexander Graham Bell, the inventor of the telephone. Melville Bell was a teacher of the deaf and developed his writing system as an aid to deaf students learning spoken language. Visible Speech was an organic system in that the symbols were designed to give visual representations of the articulatory positions for individual sounds. Visible Speech was the first notation system for the speech sounds not tied to a particular language or dialect. It was therefore universal in its application and was also known as the Physiological Alphabet. The Korean alphabet (known in Korea as *Hangul*) was the inspiration of King Se-jong (1397–1450) who assigned a team of scholars to advise him in creating an alphabet that is now regarded as the most recently invented and most scientifically designed alphabet in the world. Symbols for the consonants are graphical representations of the underlying articulation, so that each symbol depicts the way in which a sound is formed. The symbols for the vowels are based on three elements: man (a vertical line), earth (a horizontal line) and heaven (a dot). The consonants and vowels are arranged in syllable units, so the system can be considered an alphabetic syllabary.

This book follows the IPA with one major exception—the special marks called diacritics, which designate modifications in the production of a particular sound. Diacritics are discussed in Chapter 6, where it will be explained that the diacritic marks used in this book have a systematic rather than arbitrary placement.

The symbols that are used to represent phonemes of a language are placed between virgules, or slashes (/ /), to distinguish them from graphemes and other kinds of symbols. Some symbols are like those in the alphabet of written (or printed) English. The phonemic symbols /p/, /b/, /f/, /v/, /t/, /d/, /k/, /g/, /s/, /z/, /m/, /n/, /l/, /r/, and /h/ represent the same sound segments that ordinarily are conveyed by these letters in printed words. However, the student who studies phonemes also has to learn some symbols that may not be familiar at all, such as /ŋ/, /ʒ/, /ð/, and /ɝ/. The phonemes of English number about 42 to 44, depending on which phonetician does the counting. This number is only a fraction of the total number of phonemes used in the 3000 or so languages of the world; but, even at that, the number of phonemes used in all the different languages is very small compared to the total number of morphemes in these languages.

The relationships between morphemic and phonemic composition are shown for the word *cats* in Figure 2.1. As indicated previously, the word *cats* is composed of two morphemes, *cat* + *s*. The morpheme *cat,* in turn, is composed of the three phonemes /k/ + /æ/ + /t/, or initial consonant + vowel + final consonant. Note that /s/ is only one phonemic realization of the plural morpheme: In a word like *dogs,* /z/ is the phonemic realization.

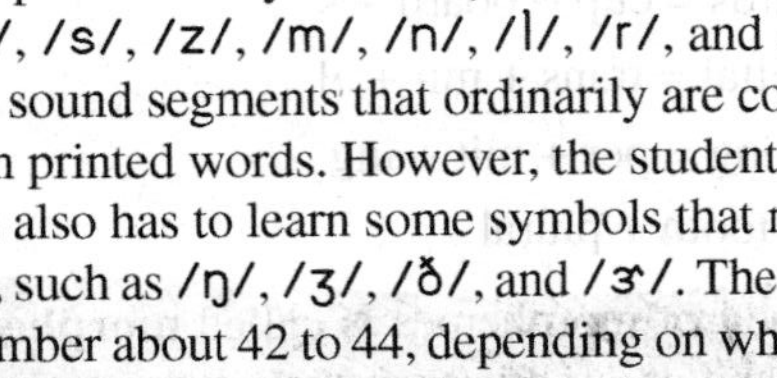

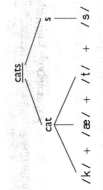

FIGURE 2.1
Morphemic and phonemic analyses of the word *cats*.

Phonology and Phonetics

Phonology is the study of sound systems of language, that is, the structure and function of sounds in languages. Phonetics is the study of how speech sounds are produced and what their acoustic properties are. Thus, two major areas of study in phonetics are **articulatory phonetics** (concerned with how sounds are formed) and **acoustic phonetics** (concerned with the acoustic properties of sounds). Phonetics is closely related to phonology but differs in the sense that two languages could have the same inventory of phonetic units, with exactly the same articulatory and acoustic descriptions, but use this inventory differently to convey meaning. That is, the two languages could have a different phonology. We entitled this chapter "Linguistic Phonetics" to draw attention to its linguistic focus and to show how the study of phonetics is related to the general study of language structure and function. This book is entitled *Clinical Phonetics* because we are concerned ultimately with the study of speech sounds that depart from the phonetic system of the speech community. Whereas phonetics is generally concerned with the study of sounds in normal adult speech, the branch of **clinical phonetics** focuses on the sounds that become the professional concern of the speech-language pathologist. Several years of teaching phonetics to aspiring speech-language clinicians have convinced us that the standard course in phonetics, dealing primarily, if not entirely, with the correct sound productions of adult speakers, does not satisfy the needs of clinical application. We have seen many students trained this way throw up their hands in frustration when they first encounter a child with multiple misarticulations, many of which defy description by the methods that work so well with the normal adult talker.

The Allophone

Although each phoneme in a language is identified by what the linguist calls minimal pairs of contrasting morphemes (*pill* versus *bill,* for example) and is represented by a single symbol from the IPA (/p/ or /b/, for example), the phoneme is not a single, invariant sound. In fact, a phoneme is really a class or family of sounds, and the members of the family are called **allophones.** An allophone may be defined as a phonetic variant of a phoneme, that is, as one of the members of the phoneme family. Two allophones of the same phoneme never contrast to produce two different morphemes; only phonemes have this linguistic function. We already have discussed two examples of allophonic variation in connection with the word pairs *key–coo,* and *nine–ninth.* Recall that in the words *key* and *coo* the initial consonant is produced differently even though we hear the two versions (or allophones) as being the same phoneme. Such phonetic differences between allophones do not produce different morphemes or words, but they are important nonetheless. The allophonic variations in speech are significant in the sound patterns of a language, and failure to use them correctly can sometimes result in striking deviations, as we will discuss later in this book.

The conditions under which a given allophone occurs are described as being either **free variation** or **complementary distribution.** Allophones are said to be in free variation when they can be exchanged for one another in a given phonetic context (or neighborhood of other sounds). For example, the final sound in the word *pop* has two primary allophones: a released allophone for which a burst of air can be heard when the lips abruptly open and an unreleased allophone for which the lips do not open with an audible burst. As you can demonstrate for yourself, either the released or unreleased allophone can be used in producing the final sound of the word *pop.* Therefore, the two allophones are said to be in free variation for this phonetic context.

Allophones are said to be in complementary distribution when they are not normally exchanged for one another in a certain phonetic context. For example, we described earlier two major allophones of the *k* sound, one produced with a relatively fronted tongue position (as in the word *key*) and one with a relatively backed tongue position (as in the word *coo*). The fronted allophone occurs in the context of vowel sounds that have a tongue position near the front of the mouth, and the backed allophone occurs in the context of vowel sounds that have a tongue position near the back of the mouth. Hence, the fronted allophone occurs in the words *key, kit, cape, ken,* and *cat* but not in the words *coo, cook, coat,* or *cot.* Because the fronted and backed allophones do not occur in the same context, they are said to be in complementary distribution. This term indicates that the conditions of occurrence of one allophone complement the conditions of occurrence of another allophone.

Phonemic symbols are placed within virgules, for example /k/. **Phonetic symbols,** that is, symbols used to represent allophones or phonetic variants of phonemes, are placed within brackets, for example [k]. Because a given phoneme may have a large number of allophonic variants, phonetic symbols may be modified by special marks called **diacritic marks.** For instance, if we wish to transcribe phonetically the initial consonant in *key,* we could write [k̟], where the diacritic mark under the *k* denotes a tongue position toward the front of the mouth. Similarly, we can characterize the difference between the second *n* in *nine* and in *ninth* by transcribing the latter as [n̪], where the diacritic mark symbolizes a dental (toward the teeth) modification of the tongue position during the consonant production. Such small changes in sound production will be considered in detail in the course of this text.

The relationships among morphemic, phonemic, and allophonic analyses of the word *cats* are illustrated in Figure 2.2. This illustration is like that in Figure 2.1 except that the appropriate allophonic variants have been added to indicate the phonetic realization of the phonemes /k/, /æ/, /t/, and /s/. Hence, this illustration demonstrates three levels of

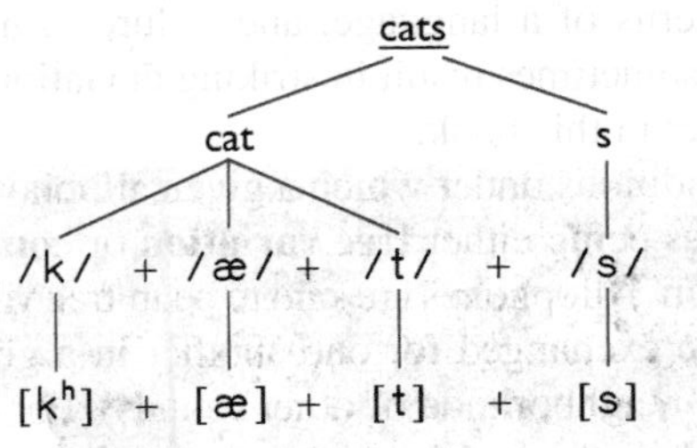

FIGURE 2.2
Morphemic, phonemic, and allophonic (phonetic) analyses of the word *cats.*

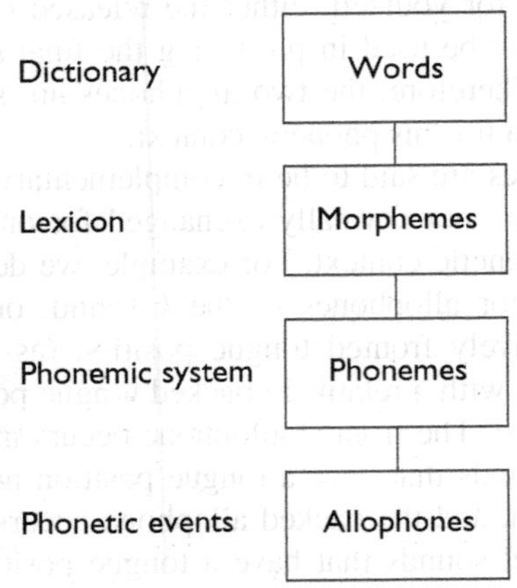

FIGURE 2.3
Some units of linguistic analysis pertinent to the study of phonetics. Higher-level units, such as phrases and sentences, are not shown in this drawing, but they also figure in the study of phonetics.

analysis: morphemic, phonemic, and allophonic. Similarly, we can speak of three kinds of transcription:

- *morphemic transcription,* or the identification of meaningful units
- *phonemic transcription,* or the identification of sound segments that have linguistic significance in the speaker's language
- *phonetic transcription,* or the identification of the allophonic variants in a speaker's pattern of sounds

A pictorial summary of the terms introduced in this chapter is given in Figure 2.3.

DIGRAPH VERSUS CLUSTER

Written or printed forms of English often make use of **digraphs**, or sequences of two or more alphabetic characters that represent a single sound. Some examples are ***pa*th**, ***ph*one**, ***gh*ost**, and ***sh*y**. Note that the two-character sequences printed in bold type represent single phonemes in each word. These combinations are quite different from consonant clusters that appear in a phonetic transcription, where the elements of the cluster are individual phonemes. Consider, for example, the clusters in the words *street, thrive, flat,* and *break.* The digraphs used in written or printed English can lead us astray when we do phonetic transcriptions. It is important to rely on our ears and not only our eyes.

THE MORPH AND THE PHONE

A few more fundamental terms are needed to complete this brief introduction to linguistic phonetics. Individual morphemelike shapes encountered in a language sample are called **morphs**. Most morphs indeed turn out to be morphemes, but some may not. The *o* in *drunkometer* is a morph but not a morpheme, because it is not a minimal unit of meaning. Some linguists refer to the *o* as a meaningless morph. Hence, the individual morphs discovered in a linguistic analysis are shapes that may or may not be morphemes. Of course, the vast majority of morphs in any natural language are morphemes. Until a given unit has been confidently established as being a morpheme, it may be called a morph.

Any particular occurrence of a sound segment of speech is a **phone**. Thus, phonemes and allophones are identified by examining phones. Just as morphs are the raw material for morphemic analysis, so are phones the raw material for phonemic and phonetic analysis.

Neologisms, or newly coined words, sometimes introduce some strange twists in word derivations; for example, the word *workaholic,* which is used to describe someone who works to excess. Thus, the legendary hard-driving executive who neglects his or her family might be called a workaholic. This word was formed as a parallel to alcoholic, or someone who drinks to excess. However, if we attempt to break *workaholic* into its morphemic subparts, we discover that we have the three apparent units *work* + *ahol* + *ic.* Both *work* and *ic* are in fact legitimate morphemes of the English language, but *ahol* does not have morphemic status, being rather like the meaningless morph *o* in *drunkometer.* No doubt some etymologists (those who study word derivations) deplore such coinages as *workaholic,* but if this principle is extended to other forms, such as jogaholic, sexaholic, and footballaholic, it may become a fixture of the English language.

THE ALPHABET AND THE ALLOGRAPH

An **alphabet** (from the Greek *alpha* + *beta*) is a set of letters or other characters used for the writing of a language. The elements of an alphabet are not always directly related to the way the language is pronounced. The same letter in English may be associated with several different sounds. For example, the alphabet letter *g* represents very different sounds in the words *go, gist,* and *weigh.* Similarly, the same sound can be represented by many different alphabet letters (singly or in combination). For example, the sound that is most commonly represented by the letter combination *sh,* as in *ship,* also is represented by *s* as in *sugar, ss* as in *tissue, ch* as in *machine, ti* as in *creation, ci* as in *precious,* and *x* as in *anxious.* Such sound–letter confusions are a source of difficulty to children (or non-English-speaking persons) learning to read the English language.

Different letters or combinations of letters that represent the same phoneme are called **allographs.** Thus, for the *sh* sound, as in *ship,* a partial listing of allographs is: *sh, s, ss, ch, ti, ci, x.* Note that any one of these allographs may itself represent different phonemes. The combination *ch* also represents the sounds in the words *chasm* and *chair.* In this book, the allographs for the vowels and consonants of English are listed at the ends of the chapters for these two major sound classes.

Some letters are occasionally silent. Examples are the *e* in *came*, the second *b* in *bomb*, *h* as in *honor*, *gh* as in *weigh*, *n* as in *damn,* and *g* as in *paradigm.* Interestingly, the phonetic significance of these "silent" letters sometimes is revealed through affixing (adding prefixes or suffixes). Consider the following pairs: *bomb–bombastic; damn–damnation; paradigm–paradigmatic.* Thus, silent letters are not always useless accidents in the development of a written language. Some letters can be either pronounced or silent in the same position in a word: Compare *hour, honest,* and *honor* with *humble, hat,* and *hospital.* Moreover, a letter in a word may be either silent or not depending on who says it. Some people pronounce the words *human, humor,* and *humid* with the same initial sound as that in *happy,* but other people drop the *h.* This ambiguity with *h* may reflect the influence of spelling. As Kerek (1976) observed, words like *hospital, heritage,* and *humble* were not produced with an *h* sound as late as the eighteenth century, but the fact that these words are spelled with *h* has reestablished their pronunciation with an *h* sound. Perhaps the same fate will come to *hour, honor,* and *honest,* which are now pronounced without an *h* sound.

Positional and Contextual Terminology for Phonetic Descriptions

Certain terms are widely used to describe the position of a sound with respect to a linguistic unit or to describe the context within which a sound occurs. The terms **initial, medial,** and **final** are used to denote sound locations at the beginning, middle, or end of a word, respectively. For example, the *t* sound is both word-initial and syllable-initial in the word *turn* but only syllable-initial in the word *return.* Syllable-initial and syllable-final sounds also are called **releasing** and **arresting** sounds, respectively. That is, a sound at the beginning of a syllable is said to release the syllable, whereas a sound at the end of a syllable is said to arrest the syllable. Medial sounds occur somewhere within a word or syllable, not at the beginning or end of it. However, the medial position can occur in quite different phonetic contexts in different words; consider the sound *b* in the words ru*bb*er, tooth*b*rush, and a*b*ove.

With some exceptions to be discussed later, all syllables contain a vowel. Therefore, it is often convenient and useful to describe consonant positions relative to the location of a vowel. The term **prevocalic** notes that a sound (usually a consonant) occurs before a given vowel, and the term **postvocalic** denotes that a sound occurs after a given vowel. In the word *tub,* the *t* sound is prevocalic and the *b* sound is postvocalic.

Geminate (from the Latin *geminus,* meaning "twin") sounds occur together as a pair, that is, two adjacent sounds are the same. For example, the two *k* sounds are geminates in the word *bookkeeper* (the double letters *oo* and *ee* are not truly geminates because these pairs each represent a single sound). Geminate sounds occur word-medially (as in *bookkeeper*) or across word boundaries (as in *sad day*).

THE SYLLABLE

A syllable is a unit of spoken language that in its most general form is comprised of a syllable nucleus (typically a vowel but occasionally a consonant) with optional initial and final margins (typically consonants). The general form of a syllable can be schematized as [initial margin] + [nucleus] + [final margin]. Both the initial and final margins have three main possibilities: null (no consonant), a single consonant, or a sequence of consonants (a consonant cluster). The initial margin is also referred to as a releasing consonant or as an **onset.** The final margin is also known as an arresting consonant or as a **coda.** Syllables are very useful in accounting for the phonological patterns of words. More will be said about syllables in following chapters.

The two major types of syllables are **open** and **closed.** An open syllable is one that does not end in a consonant, whereas a closed syllable does end in a consonant. *Law, see, throw,* and *spry* are open syllables (note that the *w* in *throw* is not pronounced as a consonant). *Lot, seep, throat,* and *sprite* are closed syllables. What then is a syllable? Actually the syllable is difficult to define. We prefer to think of syllables as highly adaptive units for the articulatory organization of speech. A syllable is a grouping of speech movements, usually linked together with other syllables in a rhythmic pattern.

The difficulty of giving a physical definition of syllable can be demonstrated by editing some digitized sound files. If you create a sound file of certain two-syllable words like *wrestling, tussling,* or *nestling* and then cut off the segment of the recorded words that contains the *-ing* portion of the word, you will now hear the words as *wrestle, tussle,* and *nestle.* Notice that the vowel of the second syllable of the original two-syllable word has been discarded, yet we still hear two-syllable words. This experiment shows us that syllables are relational units, that is, units that are defined with respect to their function in an utterance. Furthermore, it is not always easy to break up a word into syllables. Where does the first syllable end and the final syllable begin in the word *cupboard?*

Some phonetics books mention syllables without ever defining what a syllable is. Of the definitions we have seen, none is satisfactory. It is instructive to look at a couple of examples. Calvert (1980) defines a syllable as "a cluster of coarticulated sounds with a single vowel or diphthong[2] nucleus, with or without surrounding consonants" (p. 179). Aside from the inherent contradiction of allowing some "clusters" to consist of one element (like the first syllable *o-* of *obey*), this definition is not totally satisfactory because it does not allow for syllabic consonants. These consonants, to be discussed in more detail later, are like vowels in serving as the nucleus of a syllable. For example, the word *button* typically is pronounced with only one vowel (represented by the alphabet letter *u*), yet it seems to contain two syllables. The second syllable is formed by the syllabic consonant *n,* that is, a consonant that acts like a vowel. In addition the term *coarticulated* doesn't help much. This term (which also will be discussed in more detail later) means that the movements for adjacent sounds overlap one another. Such overlapping of movements or articulations has been thought to be a useful way of defining syllables because the overlapping indicates a cohesiveness or "belonging together." However, studies of speech production have made it clear that overlapping commonly occurs across word boundaries and across what almost anybody would call a syllable boundary. Certain kinds of overlapping occur even between adjacent vowels (which can be in different words). In short, coarticulation, or overlapping of movements, is not restricted to any one kind of unit.

Kantner and West (1941) define a syllable as a "unit of speech containing a peak of sonority [loudness or carrying power] and divided from other such peaks by a hiatus or a weakening of sonority" (p. 62). But the sonority criterion is difficult to apply consistently. In words such as *piano, chaos,* and *trio,* the syllable divisions marked by / in the syllabifications pi/an/o, cha/os, and tri/o are not necessarily associated with a change in sonority so much as with a change in vowel quality. In fact, if we look at the actual physical power in these words, it is not always easy to identify distinct peaks that correspond to the number of syllables we hear.

The difficulty in defining the syllable does not mean that it is an unimportant unit in the study of phonetics. The syllable is a useful construct and plays a role in the explanation of many phonetic phenomena. It is well to study Malmberg's comments on the syllable:

> *It [the syllable] is one of the fundamental notions of phonetics. If phoneticians are not always in agreement about defining a syllable, it is partly because different points of view have been chosen for its definition (acoustics, articulatory, functional), partly because the apparatus which has been used up to now has not enabled phoneticians to locate the boundaries of syllables on the graphs or tracings obtained. But it would be an error to conclude that the syllable as a phonetic phenomenon does not exist and that the grouping of phonemes in syllables is a mere convention without any objective reality.... Even a person without any linguistic training usually has a very clear idea of the number of syllables in a spoken chain.* (Malmberg, 1963, p. 65)

A formal definition of *syllable* will be postponed until Chapter 6.

Syllabaries

A **syllabary** is a phonetic writing system that uses symbols to represent syllables rather than individual sounds. Typically, the syllables are composed of a single vowel (V) or a consonant plus a vowel (CV). Syllabaries have been used especially in linguistic studies of Japanese languages and some Native American languages.

But the concept of syllabary may have a more general use that is fundamental to the way we talk. An influential model of language production proposes that we access a "mental syllabary" to produce spoken language (Levelt, Roelofs, & Meyer, 1999). The most frequently used syllables suffice for the production of most of the verbal productions in a language. These syllables are stored in a mental syllabary as motor programs (basically sets of instructions to the muscles) that can be quickly retrieved as the need arises. These hard-working syllables are prepackaged and ready to go. What about less frequently used syllables? The model proposes that these are not stored in the syllabary but rather are constructed for motor execution as they are encountered. As can be seen in Appendix Table B.12, only 16 frequently occurring syllables account for more than 40 percent of the speech content of American English. These 16 syllables are good candidates for a mental syllabary of American English and would go a long way to meet the needs of communication. This is one example of the importance of data on frequency of occurrence, as tabulated in Appendix B. Syllabaries can be defined for other languages as well. For example, the 27 most frequently occurring syllables in Spanish account for about half of all syllable occurrences (Guirao & Jurado, 1990).

[2] A diphthong is a sequence of vowel sounds that behaves phonemically as a single vowel.

CONCLUSION

An extraordinary number of languages are spoken on this planet, but all of them can be described and analyzed using the basic tools of linguistics. Spoken language involves several different levels of organization. This is true even for a single word, which we can analyze to identify its morphemes, phonemes, and allophones. A competent speaker has knowledge—whether implicit or explicit—about each of these levels. This chapter has introduced basic concepts that are fundamental to the succeeding chapters.

EXERCISES

1. Morphemic analysis. Count the number of morphemes contained in each of the following words.

   Example: The word *stairways* contains three morphemes (*stair* + *way* + *s*)

Word	*Number of Morphemes*
(a) lightened	3
(b) table	1
(c) morphemic	3
(d) recruitment	3
(e) dismissed	3
(f) television	3
(g) finger	1
(h) singers	3
(i) revealing	3
(j) imposition	4

2. By adding prefixes and suffixes to the stem *pose,* create as many words as you can. For example, the word *imposition* (j above) is formed by adding the prefix *im* and the suffixes *it* and *ion* to the stem *pose.*

3. Phonemic analysis. Count the number of phonemes contained in each of the following words.

   Example: The word *chair* contains three phonemes: the initial consonant, the vowel, and the final consonant.

Word	*Number of Phonemes*
(a) daughter	4
(b) laughter	5
(c) phone	3
(d) cupboard	5
(e) cellophane	7
(f) knead	3
(g) Chicago	6
(h) finger	5
(i) singer	4
(j) six	4

4. Sequential phonemic constraints. In this list of 12 "words," only half of them are really words in the English language. The other six are words that have been made up for this exercise. Separate this list of words into two groups—one group for words that you think could be found in an English dictionary, and the other group for words that you would not expect to find in an English dictionary. The "real" words are sufficiently rare that you probably have never heard of them. After you have made up the two lists of words, explain the factors that you used in making your decisions.

   (a) fsew
   (b) grith
   (c) srin
   (d) scute
   (e) trave
   (f) ktun
   (g) skeg
   (h) dlut
   (i) shlar
   (j) gvise
   (k) spile
   (l) knar

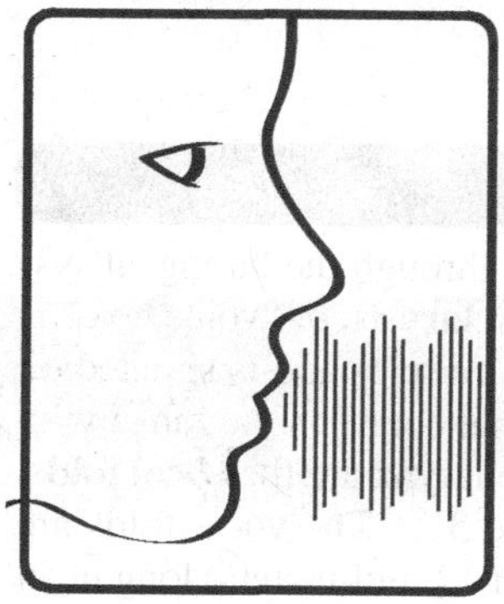

CHAPTER 3

The Three Systems of Speech Production

The human vocal tract may be described as an apparatus for the conversion of muscular energy into acoustic energy.

—(*J. C. Catford, 1968, p. 310*)

Speech is easy to take for granted, but it is really a remarkable human capability. Here are four properties of speech that reveal how exceptional it is:

1. Conversational speech is produced at rates of up to six to nine syllables per second (20 to 30 phonetic segments per second)—faster than any other discrete human motor performance, including typing and texting.
2. The production of speech involves more than 100 muscles.
3. Speech movements meet some of the most exacting coordination demands of any human muscular system.
4. Speech production relies on more motor fibers than any other human mechanical activity.

Speech is produced by the carefully controlled action of over 100 muscles in the chest, abdomen, neck, and head. We can simplify the description of speech production by considering three major functional systems—**respiratory, laryngeal,** and **supralaryngeal** (or pharyngeal-oral-nasal). These three systems are illustrated in Figure 3.1.

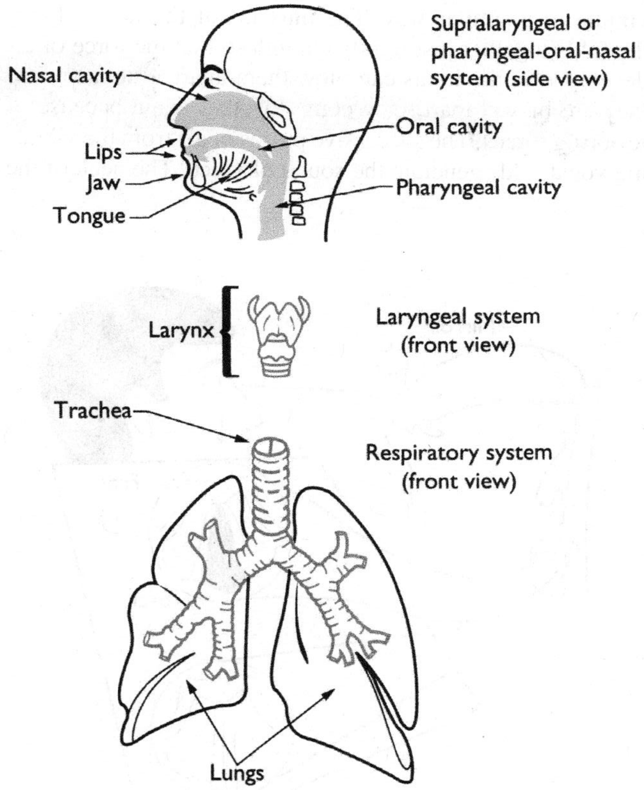

FIGURE 3.1
The three systems of speech production: respiratory, laryngeal, and supralaryngeal. Some parts of the respiratory system are not shown in the drawing, for example, the rib cage.

The Respiratory System

The respiratory system, consisting primarily of the lungs, rib cage, abdomen, and associated muscles, acts like a pump to provide the movement of air needed for speech production. All sounds in the English language normally are **egressive,** meaning that they are produced with a flow of air that moves outward from the lungs. Kantner and West (1941) wrote, "All English sounds normally produced have one factor in common: they are based upon the utilization of the moving column of air furnished by the expiratory phase of the process of respiration" (p. 39). Some languages include **ingressive** sounds, or sounds produced with an inward flow of air. The respiratory system supplies the forces of air that are used to generate most sounds. For egressive sounds, air that has been drawn into the lungs during inspiration is then forced outward through the mouth or nose. As one speech scientist, the late Thomas Hixon, put it, speaking is a process of making oneself gradually smaller. That is, after we make ourselves larger by taking in air through inspiration, the air is driven out in small pulses that are formed into sounds.

The role of the respiratory system in speech can be summarized as follows:

1. During inspiration, air is drawn into the lungs as the result of muscle contractions that increase the volume of the **thoracic,** or chest, **cavity.**
2. The muscles of the respiratory system release air into the larynx and supralaryngeal system for the purpose of generating speech.
3. In situations when an unusually strong burst of air is required—as when special emphasis or loudness is desired—the respiratory muscles can act to provide this additional pulse of energy by a forceful squeezing of the thoracic cavity.

Speech that is continued for more than a few seconds necessarily takes on the rhythm of respiration—cycles of inspiration and expiration. This pattern gives rise to a unit called the **breath group,** which is simply the sequence of words or syllables produced on a single expiration. The breath group is distinctive of speech and is not necessarily well defined in other types of communication, such as manual signing or typing. That is, a person who uses manual signs, such as in American Sign Language, does not need to pause the flow of signs to take in a breath. In ordinary conversation, we typically speak for no more than 10 seconds on a single breath. Normally, we interrupt for inspiration at syntactically appropriate places, such as phrase or clause boundaries. Therefore, breath groups often coincide with syntactic units.

The Laryngeal System

The air from the lungs travels up through the laryngeal system, where voice is produced. The **larynx,** or "voice box," is made up largely of cartilage and muscles and is situated on top of the **trachea,** the air pipe that connects the lungs with the larynx (Figure 3.1). Inside the larynx are the **vocal folds,** small cushions of muscle (Figure 3.2). The vocal folds are about three-quarters of an inch (or 17 millimeters) long in an adult male. Their length is shorter in women and in children. At the front, they attach close to the "Adam's apple." If you put your finger on your throat, you should be able to feel a small notch at the top of your larynx. The vocal folds attach just below this notch and have their other place of attachment on tiny cartilages located at the back of the larynx. A physician or speech pathologist can examine the vocal folds by using a special mirror, as shown in Figure 3.2.

During breathing, the vocal folds are kept apart so that air can move freely into and out of the lungs. When voice is required, the vocal folds are brought together so that air escaping from the lungs can set them into vibration. This process is like the production of a sound that results when a person suddenly releases an inflated balloon. The vocal folds vibrate in a similar way. The muscles of the larynx bring the folds together just tightly enough so that the force of air developed in the lungs can blow them apart. But each time they are blown apart, they come together again because of restoring forces. The successive pulses of air from the vibrating vocal folds generate the sound of voice. The neck of the

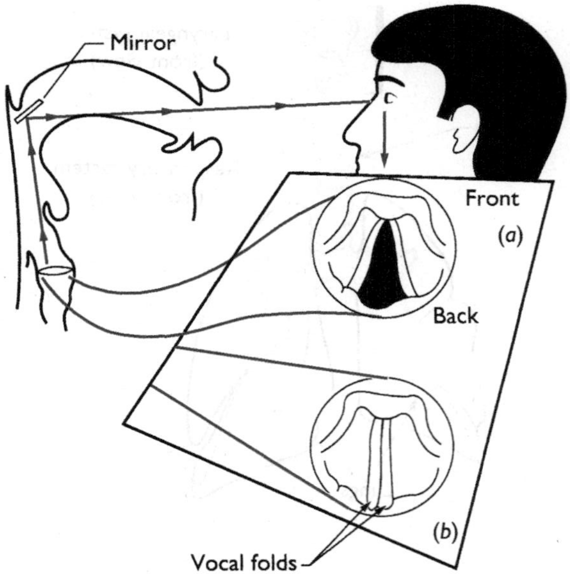

FIGURE 3.2
Viewing the vocal folds with a laryngeal mirror. In *(a)* the vocal folds are shown in their abducted (open) state. In *(b)* the vocal folds are in their adducted (drawn together) state.

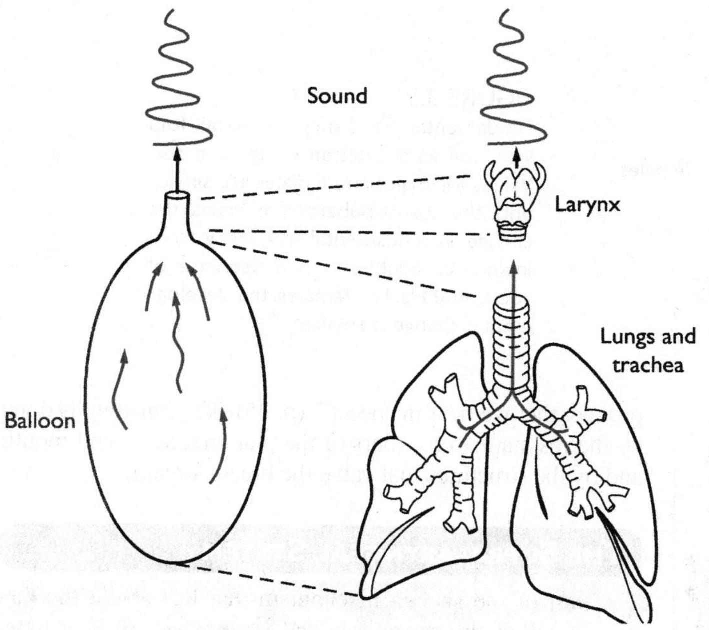

FIGURE 3.3
Balloon analogy of respiratory-laryngeal action in voice production. Air escaping from the deflating balloon causes neck of balloon to vibrate with a fluttering sound. Similarly, the air driven outward from lungs causes vocal folds to vibrate.

rapidly deflating balloon does the same thing, first opening as a burst of air escapes and then closing again. Curious as it seems, the escaping air itself is one reason why the vocal folds (and the balloon mouthpiece) can close again. The rapidly moving air momentarily creates a lower pressure between the vocal folds (or the lips of the balloon mouthpiece), and this force helps to restore closure.

The deflating balloon is a crude analogy of the respiratory-laryngeal action in voice production (Figure 3.3). Inflation of the balloon is similar to the inspiration of air that precedes voice production. As the neck of the balloon is released, air escapes—just as air is driven from the lungs once the vocal folds are separated. Then, as just explained, the vocal folds, or the lips of the balloon mouthpiece, are forced to vibrate as the air rushes through them. And, of course, the balloon, like a person's thoracic cavity, gradually gets smaller as the air flows out of it. As you can demonstrate very easily yourself, the vocal folds can be set into vibration both by air that flows *out* of the lungs and by air that flows *into* the lungs. That is, we can phonate, or produce voice, during either expiration (the usual way) or inspiration, so long as the vocal folds are positioned properly. If the folds are not closed sufficiently, voice will not be produced because the air will move through them like air through a straw.

As a consequence of the alternating opening and closing motions of the vocal folds, small pulses of air enter the chambers of the mouth and nose. Figure 3.4 shows the sequence of events in vocal fold vibration. In the words of Denes and Pinson (1973/1963), "The vibrating vocal cords [folds] rhythmically open and close the air passage between the lungs and mouth." The rate of vocal fold vibration, or the number of opening–closing cycles in a unit of time, is about

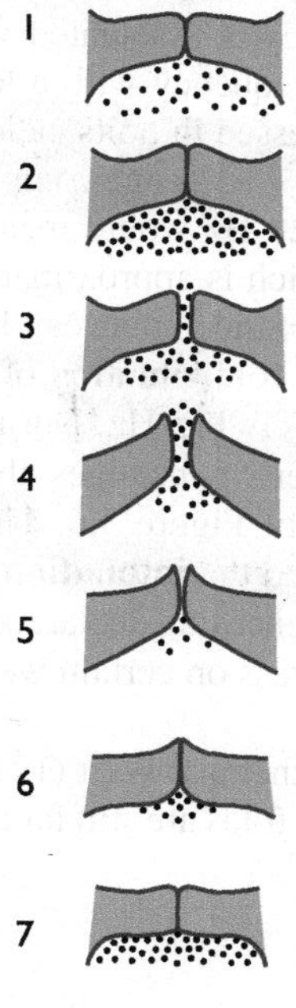

FIGURE 3.4
Series of events in vocal fold vibration. (1) Folds are closed and air pressure builds up beneath them. (2) Folds just before they burst apart in response to air pressure. (3) Folds burst apart, and air flows through them. (4) Folds are maximally open. (5) Folds begin to close. (6) Folds are closed. (7) Cycle begins again.

125 per second for an adult male. In an adult female, the rate is higher, averaging about 250 per second. Higher rates of vibration occur for young children; for example, the cry of a newborn baby has an average rate of vocal fold vibration

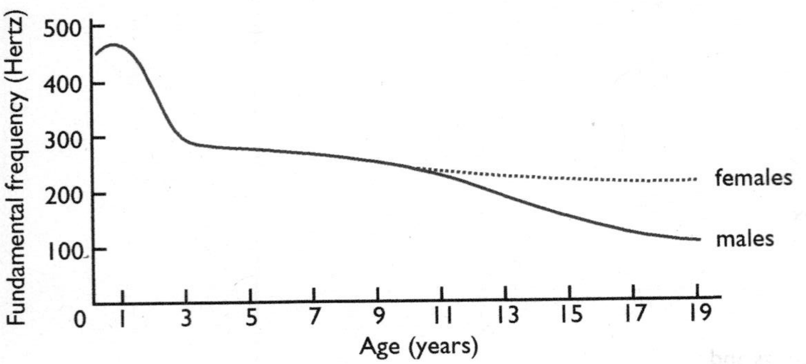

FIGURE 3.5
Fundamental frequency of vocal fold vibration as a function of age and sex. Values for males and females are similar until the age of puberty. For males, the change in fundamental frequency from infancy to adulthood is a decrease of about 400 Hz. For females, the developmental change is smaller.

of about 500 per second. The developmental variation in rate of vibration is graphed in Figure 3.5. It is because of these differences in the rate of vibration that voices have different pitches. A man's voice sounds lower in pitch than a woman's or a child's because his vocal folds vibrate at a slower average rate. When we change the pitch of our voices during speaking or singing, the vocal folds vibrate at different rates. For example, we sing up a musical scale by making our vocal folds thinner and more tense so they vibrate at higher rates. The rate of vocal fold vibration is commonly called the **fundamental frequency of the voice,** symbolized as f_0. A high fundamental frequency is associated with a high pitch and a low fundamental frequency with a low pitch. Fundamental frequency is expressed in units called Hertz (abbreviated Hz). One **Hertz** is defined as one complete cycle of vibration per second. Hence, 20 Hz would mean 20 complete vibrations per second, which is approximately the lower limit of the frequency range of the human ear. If an adult male has an average rate of vocal fold vibration of 125 per second, then we can say that his f_0 is 125 Hz. During ordinary conversational speech, a talker's f_0 changes almost continuously, as shown in the graph of Figure 3.6. These changes underlie much of what is called the **intonation** of speech. Intonation is used to mark sentences as declarative or interrogative, to place emphasis or stress on certain words, or to signal emotions and attitudes.

But, to quote Kantner and West (1941), "The sound waves produced at the vocal folds are still far from being the finished product that we hear in speech" (p. 45). The finishing is done by the resonating chambers of the pharynx, nose, and mouth and by the structures that valve the breath stream.

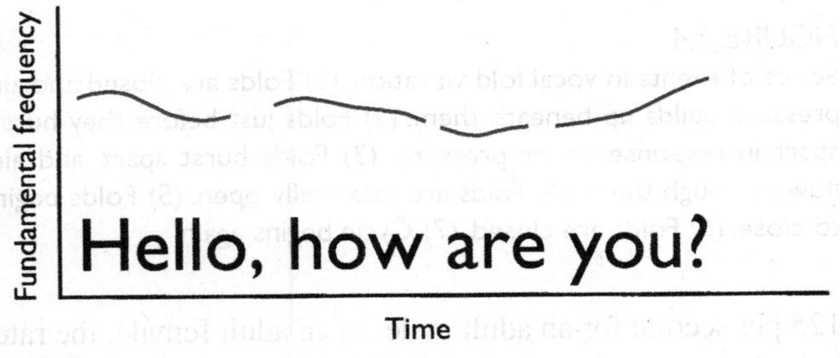

FIGURE 3.6
Variation in fundamental frequency of the voice during the utterance "Hello, how are you?"

The Supralaryngeal System

The part of the speech mechanism that lies above the larynx is called the supralaryngeal system (*supra* is a morpheme that means "above"). This system also may be called the pharyngeal-oral-nasal system because it consists of three major air cavities or chambers, the pharyngeal, oral, and nasal (Figure 3.7). Lying directly above the larynx is the pharynx, or pharyngeal cavity, which is essentially a muscular tube. The pharynx divides into two other cavities, the oral (or mouth) and the nasal (or nose). Sound energy from the larynx travels up through the pharynx and then enters the oral cavity, the nasal cavity, or both. The direction of sound travel is determined by the position of the **velum,** or **soft palate.** The velum is rather like a hanging door. When the door is raised, it presses against the back and side walls of the pharynx to close off the nasal cavity from the pharynx and oral cavity so that sound is directed into the oral cavity. On the other hand, when the velum is lowered, sound energy may enter the nasal cavity and escape through the nose. In a word like *fast,* the velum is raised throughout so that all of the sound energy travels through the oral cavity. This is called **oral radiation of sound** energy. For a word like *man,* the sound energy travels through the nose for the nasal consonants *m* and *n* and through *both* mouth and nose for the intervening vowel. You can demonstrate the importance of the nasal cavity for these nasal consonants by pinching your nose tightly as you say the word *man.* The speech of a person with a severe cold gives a similar lesson: Because of the stopped-up nasal passages, *man* may sound like *bad.* An even more effective demonstration is to attempt to produce a sustained *m* sound with your nostrils closed. How long can you make the sound?

Most of the sounds in English are formed by modifying the **pharyngeal, oral,** and **nasal cavities.** These modifications are accomplished by activation of the muscles of the head and neck, which work to move the velum, jaw, tongue, lips, and pharyngeal walls. The process of articulation is one

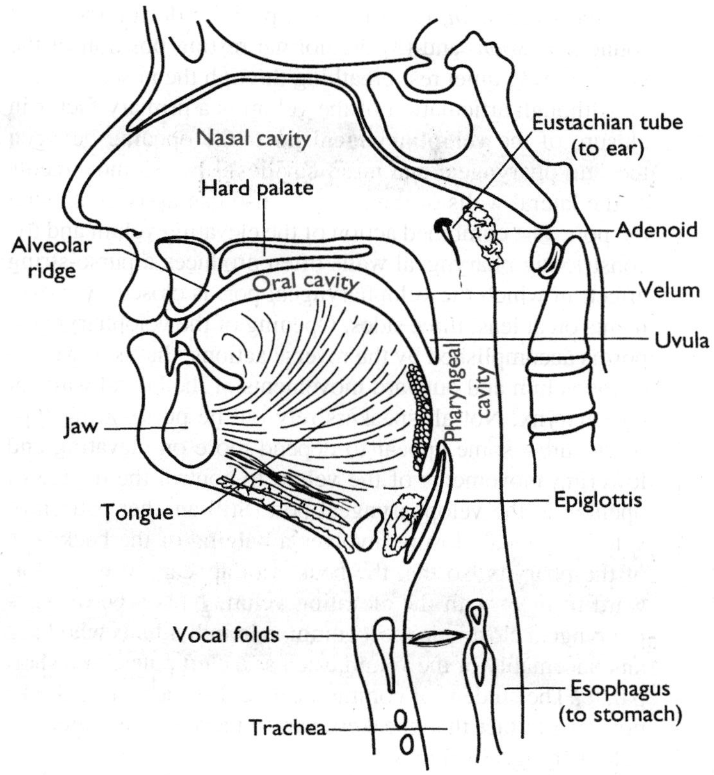

FIGURE 3.7
Structures of the supralaryngeal (pharyngeal-oral-nasal) system. The larynx also is shown.

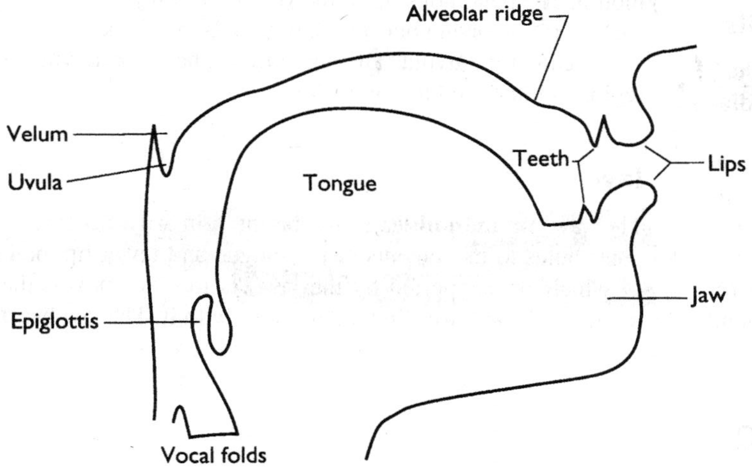

FIGURE 3.8
Tracing of an X-ray photograph of the articulators.

of movement, and the moving structures are called **articulators.** For example, the tongue is an articulator. A tracing of an X-ray view of the articulators is shown in Figure 3.8. Some articulators, like the tongue, change in both shape and position, whereas others, like the jaw, change only in position.

It is customary to view the articulatory organs in the midsagittal plane, which bisects the head into left and right halves. This view shows the principal organs of speech production in the same plane. An image of a young woman's head is shown in Figure 3.9, with major anatomic structures labeled. The oral, nasal, and pharyngeal cavities appear as dark spaces surrounded by other tissues. Figure 3.10 illustrates the arrangement of these cavities within the head (part a), isolated (part b), and schematized (part c). Figure 3.11 is an image of the head of a 1-year-old girl. Comparison of Figures 3.9 and 3.11 gives an idea as to how the structures of speech change in their relative position during the process

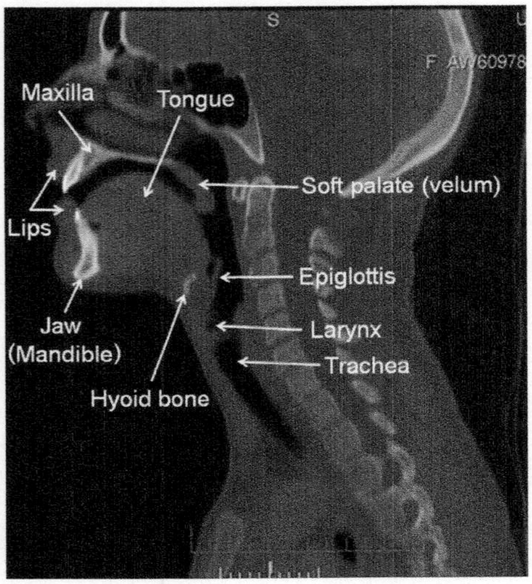

FIGURE 3.9
Computerized tomography (CT) image of the head of a young woman, with major structures of the vocal tract labeled. CT image courtesy of Dr. Houri K. Vorperian, Vocal Tract Development Laboratory, Waisman Center, University of Wisconsin-Madison.

of development and maturation. Note, for example, how the larynx and hyoid bone have lower positions in the woman compared to the child.

Velopharynx: Velum and Pharyngeal Walls

The velum, or soft palate, operates as a valve to open or close the entrance to the nasal cavity, thus permitting **nasal radiation of sound** energy. As just discussed, during respiration and during the production of nasal sounds, the velum is lowered. During oral (nonnasal) sounds or during such activities as sucking or blowing, it is raised. Articulation of the velum is illustrated in Figure 3.12, which was derived from X-ray pictures of a person talking. Velar positions are shown for three events: (1) an elevated position during the oral sound *s* in the word *soon,* (2) a lowered position during the nasal sound *n* in *soon,* and (3) the normal resting position of the velum during quiet rest breathing through the nose.

Although articulation of the velum is a primary factor in closure of the **velopharyngeal port** (the opening between the oral-pharyngeal and nasal cavities), inward movements of the lateral walls of the pharynx also can assist in closing the port. The combined action of the elevating velum and the constricting pharyngeal walls often produces a purse-string effect, in which the velopharyngeal port is closed by movements on at least three sides. Opening of the velopharyngeal port is accomplished by the reverse actions, that is, lowering of the velum and outward movements of the lateral walls of the pharynx. Not all speakers rely on the purse-string type of closure—some appear to depend more on elevating and lowering movements of the velum to control the degree of opening at the velopharyngeal port. Still another pattern of velopharyngeal closure involves a bulging of the back wall of the pharynx, so that the back wall appears to move forward to meet with the elevating velum. This type of velopharyngeal closure is most common in individuals who have an abnormality of the velum, such as a cleft palate or a short palate. The student of communicative disorders should take note of the fact that speakers vary widely in the pattern of velopharyngeal valving.

The velum might be regarded as a muscle-and-flesh extension of the bony hard palate that forms the roof of the mouth. The pendulous tip of the velum, which you probably can see if you open your mouth widely as you look in a mirror, is called the uvula. The anatomy of the velopharyngeal region is illustrated in Figure 3.7.

Jaw

The jaw, or **mandible,** is important primarily because it contributes to movements of the tongue and lower lip, both of which are supported by the jaw. As the jaw moves, the tongue and the lower lip tend to move with it. The jaw has a

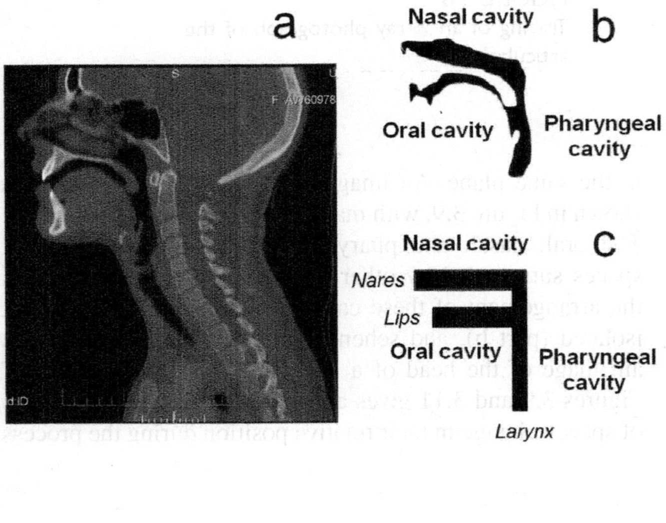

FIGURE 3.10
(a) CT image of the vocal tract. (b) Oral, nasal, and pharyngeal cavities derived from the image in (a). (c) Schematized vocal tract corresponding to (b). CT image courtesy of Dr. Houri K. Vorperian, Vocal Tract Development Laboratory, Waisman Center, University of Wisconsin-Madison.

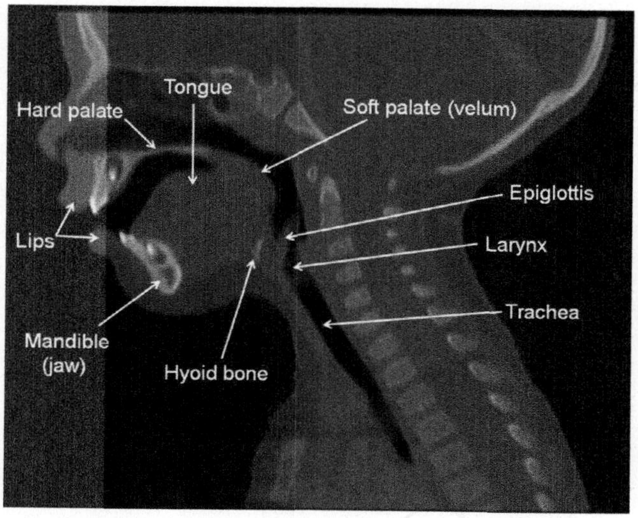

FIGURE 3.11
CT image of the head of a 1-year-old girl, with major structures of the vocal tract labeled. CT image courtesy of Dr. Houri K. Vorperian, Vocal Tract Development Laboratory, Waisman Center, University of Wisconsin-Madison.

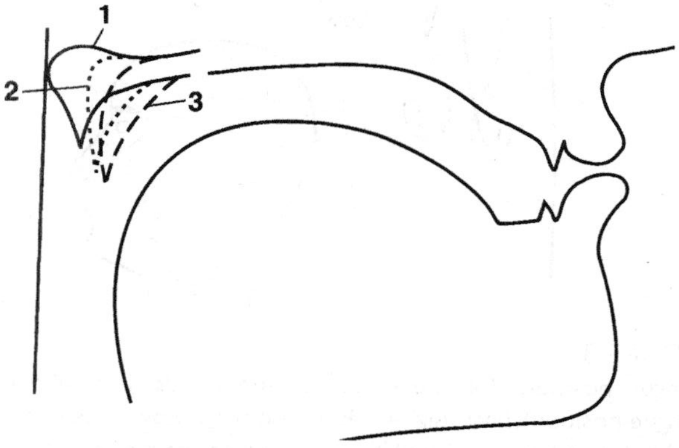

FIGURE 3.12
Articulation of velum, represented by positions for (1) *s* sound in *soon,* (2) *n* sound in *soon,* and (3) normal rest breathing. Velopharyngeal port is open for positions (2) and (3).

hingelike motion made possible by a joint located close to the ear on either side of the head. The hinge is formed at a place called the **temporomandibular joint,** where the jaw (mandible) inserts into the temporal bone of the skull. Because of this hinge joint, the jaw rotates along an arc of opening and closing. However, the joint is constructed so that the jaw can move slightly forward and backward as well, so that some degree of mandibular protrusion and retrusion is possible. The shape of the jaw is illustrated in Figure 3.13. Jaw motion during speech is shown in Figure 3.14. The jaw positions shown here were obtained from X-ray pictures of the word *saw.* For the *s* sound, the jaw assumes a relatively closed

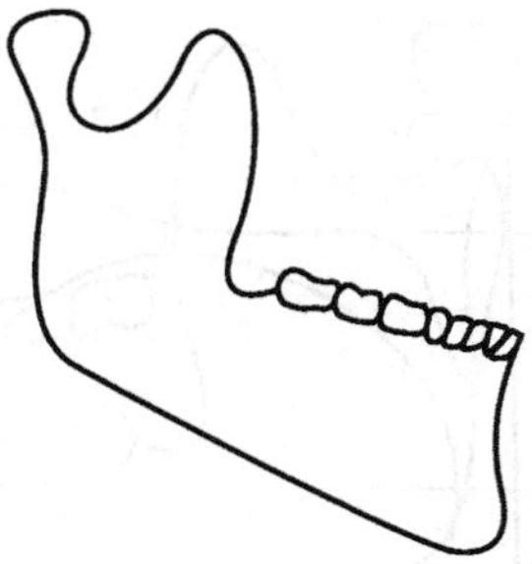

FIGURE 3.13
Shape of jaw, seen in lateral view.

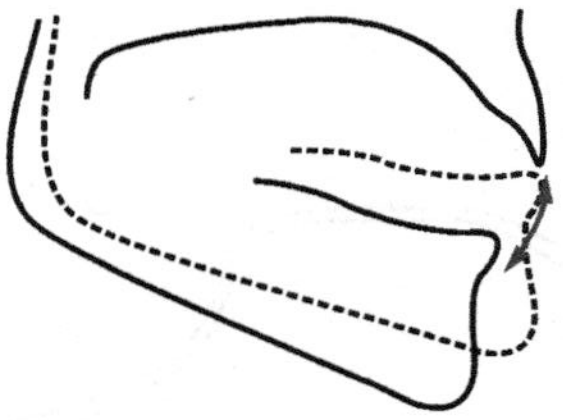

FIGURE 3.14
Jaw motion during speech. The closed position is for *s* in *saw,* and the open position is for the vowel.

(or elevated) position, whereas for the following vowel, it assumes a relatively open (or lowered) position.

Tongue

The tongue is a muscular organ that has no internal skeleton but derives skeletal support from the jaw and the hyoid bone (these bony structures and the tongue are illustrated in Figure 3.15). In addition, various muscles attach the tongue to the skull, the palate, the pharynx, and the epiglottis. Partly because of the variety of its attachments and partly because of its own versatile musculature, the tongue is capable of complicated movements. To describe these movements, it is convenient to divide the tongue into five functional parts, as shown in Figure 3.16.

The **body of the tongue** refers to its primary bulk or mass. The overall position of the tongue in the mouth is described by specifying the location of the body. Vowel articulation, in particular, is described with reference to the tongue body. For example, the four vowels in the words *heat, hoot, hot,* and *hat* have tongue body positions described as high-front, high-back, low-back, and low-front, respectively. These tongue positions are illustrated in Figure 3.17. Note, for example, that the vowel in *heat* has a tongue position that is high and in the front part of the mouth. Hence, the description "high-front" refers to the relative location of the bulk of the tongue.

The **tip of the tongue,** also called its apex, is the part that is visible when the tongue is protruded between the lips.

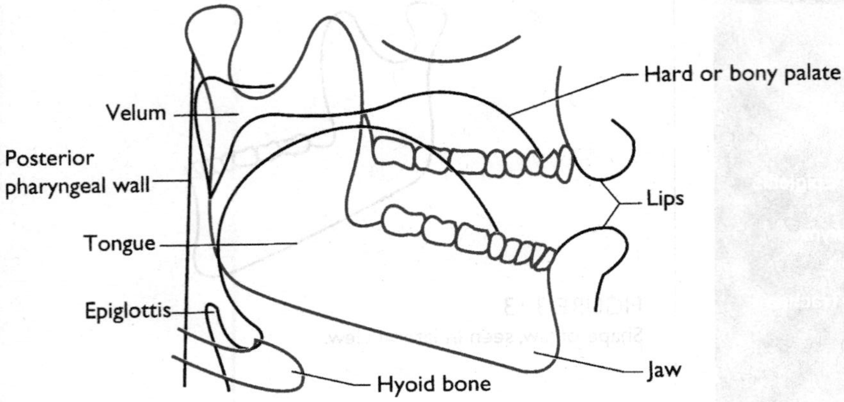

FIGURE 3.15
Skeletal or bony structures of the articulatory system shown by blue lines. Tongue and lips are also shown (compare with X-ray tracing in Figure 3.12).

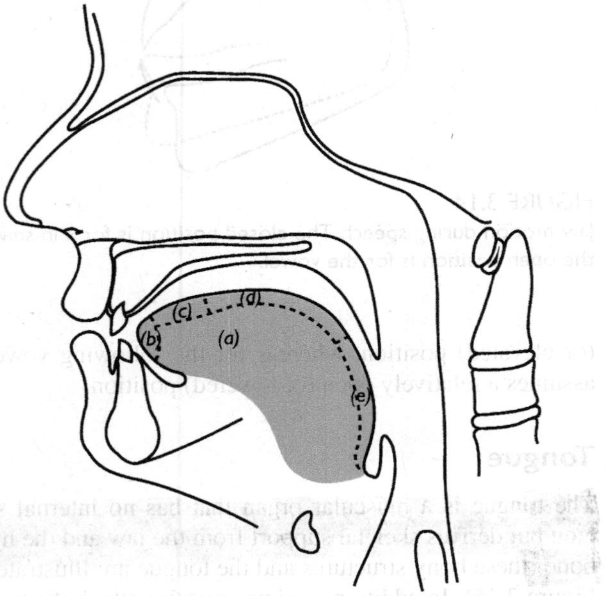

FIGURE 3.16
Functional divisions of tongue: *(a)* body, *(b)* tip or apex, *(c)* blade, *(d)* dorsum, and *(e)* root.

The tip is very important in speech articulation and accounts for over 50 percent of the consonant contacts made in an average sample of English conversation. If you have ever accidentally bitten the tip of your tongue, you probably became well aware of how often it is used in making English speech sounds. The underlined letters in this sentence are produced with the tip of the tongue making contact somewhere in the mouth. Obviously, the tip is kept very busy in the task of speaking.

The **blade of the tongue,** located just behind the tip, is the part that makes the constriction for the *sh* sound in *sheep.* The blade is used in making constrictions for only a small number of sounds, but it also plays a role in shaping the tongue for other speech sounds.

The **dorsum of the tongue** (also known as the back) is the portion used in making the first sounds in the words *key*

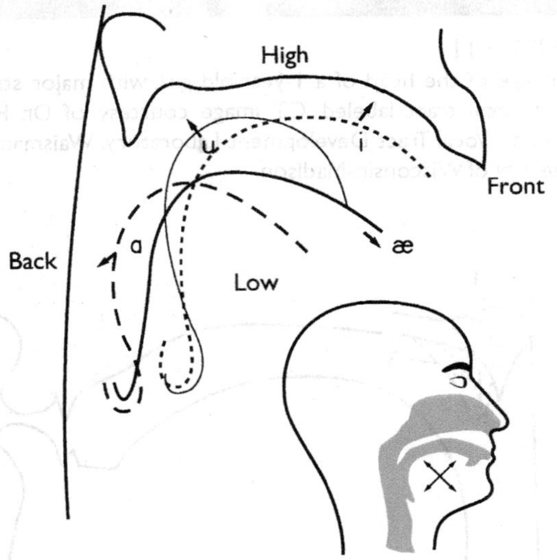

FIGURE 3.17
Tongue positions for the vowels in the words *heat* (high-front tongue position), *hoot* (high-back position), *hot* (low-back position), and *hat* (low-front position) Tongue outlines are labeled with phonetic symbols.

and *go* and the last sound in *thing.* This rather large segment contacts the roof of the mouth. As you might be able to determine from saying the three words given, the actual point of closure varies along the ceiling of the oral cavity. Indeed, the dorsum makes its articulations with both the hard palate and the soft palate.

The **root of the tongue** is the long segment that forms the front wall of the pharynx. The root does not actually make contacts or closures for English consonants, but it is important in shaping the vocal tract for vowel and consonant sounds.

Lips

The upper and lower lips contribute to speech articulation primarily by opening and closing, as in production of the

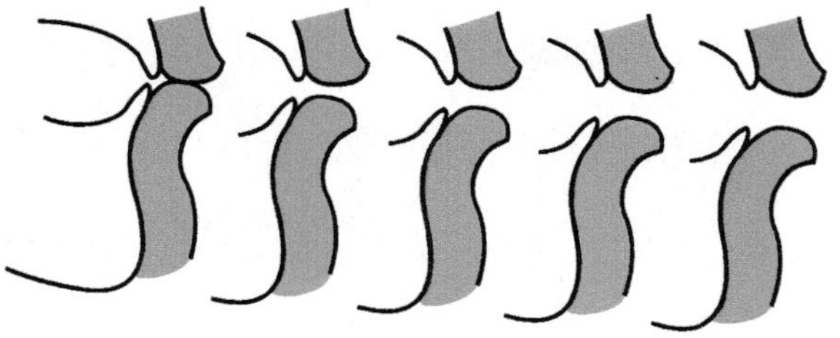

FIGURE 3.18
Lip opening for *p* sound as in *pa*. Lip and jaw positions are shown at intervals of 6.7 milliseconds (0.0067 second).

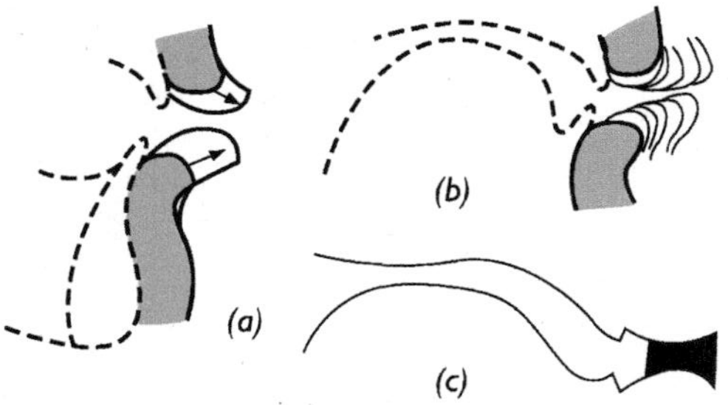

FIGURE 3.19
Articulation of lip rounding or protrusion. Drawing *(a)* shows unrounded and rounded lips. Drawing *(b)* shows successive lip positions as seen in intervals of 20 milliseconds (0.02 second) in an X-ray motion picture. Drawing *(c)* shows lengthening of vocal tract (shaded portion) caused by lip rounding.

word *pop,* and by rounding, or protruding, as for the vowel in *you.* Like the tongue, the lower lip is supported by the jaw, so that jaw movement usually moves the lower lip as well. In most people, the lower lip moves more than the upper lip. The two basic lip articulations are shown in Figures 3.18 and 3.19. Figure 3.18 illustrates the opening of the lips for a release of a *p* sound. Successive positions of lips and jaw are shown at intervals of 6.7 ms (*ms* is an abbreviation for milliseconds, or divisions of 1/1000 of a second). The separation of the lips is accomplished in about 35 ms or one-thirtieth of a second. Figure 3.19 depicts progressive lip positions during an articulation of protrusion. The positions are shown at intervals of 20 ms, in part *(b)* of the figure. The lengthening of the vocal tract caused by lip protrusion is illustrated by the blackened segment in part *(c)* of the figure.

CONCLUSION

It should be emphasized that the three systems described in this chapter interact strongly with each other in the production of speech and that each system is complicated enough to require a book for a reasonably complete description. We have simplified matters greatly by comparing the respiratory system to an air pump or balloon, by likening the vibrating vocal folds to the flapping mouthpiece of a deflating balloon, and by describing the pharyngeal-oral-nasal system as a set of articulators that are a critical part of the conversion of muscular energy to sound energy.

Anatomy and physiology have not been discussed in detail in this book because it is assumed that students of communicative disorders will receive this information from courses on anatomy and physiology. However, the basic concepts presented in this chapter are sufficient for the introductory study of phonetics.

EXERCISES

1. Draw an outline of the vocal tract and label the following: tongue body, root, dorsum, blade, and tip; lips, velum, jaw, alveolar ridge, velopharyngeal port, and pharynx.
2. Discuss the following and check your answers with the material in the text.
   (a) The difference between nasal and oral (nonnasal) consonants.
   (b) The meaning of the term *articulator.*
   (c) The function of the respiratory system in speech.
   (d) The interaction between tongue and jaw and lip and jaw in speech production.
   (e) The time pattern of vocal fold vibration.
3. Say the following words and name the oral articulators used for the sounds represented by the italicized letters.
   *Example: sh*oe—blade of tongue
   (a) *p*ay ______
   (b) gee*s*e ______
   (c) *f*irm ______
   (d) *l*ike ______
   (e) *th*ing ______
   (f) *ch*air*s* ______
   (g) *c*i*ph*er ______
   (h) ba*th*e ______
4. Read aloud the following passage and, as you do so, circle the italicized letters that represent sounds made with the lips and place a check (✓) over the italicized letters that represent sounds made with the tongue.

   Al*th*ough the to*ng*ue is *v*ery i*mp*orta*nt* in spee*ch* ar*t*iculatio*n*, *th*ere are *s*everal re*p*orts of *p*erso*ns* who produ*c*e intelligible *s*peech e*v*en a*f*ter *m*o*s*t of *th*e to*ng*ue has *b*een surgically remo*v*ed (often because of *c*ancer). I*nd*i*v*iduals so*m*etimes co*mp*e*ns*ate *s*urprisi*ng*ly well for da*m*age to the arti*c*u*l*ators.

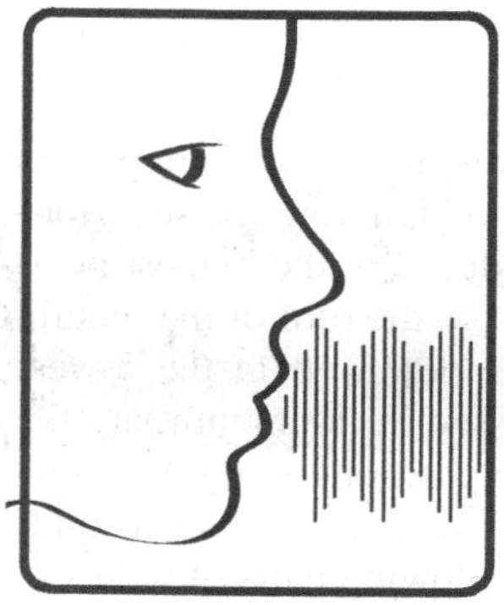

CHAPTER 4

Vowels and Diphthongs

What is a **vowel**? This seemingly innocent question creates more difficulties than the beginning student of phonetics might imagine. The famous phonetician, Kenneth L. Pike, wrote about vowels and consonants as follows:

> *The most basic, characteristic, and universal division made in phonetic classification is that of consonant and vowel. Its delineation is one of the least satisfactory.... Frequently for descriptions of single languages the division is assumed, with no attempt to define it. The distinction is often presented as if it were clear-cut, with every sound belonging to one or the other of the groups. Jones [another famous phonetician], for example, says, "Every speech-sound belongs to one or the other of the two main classes known as Vowels and Consonants." Later, however, various sounds are mentioned by him which have to be discussed separately under different rules, or with various kinds of reservation, because they do not neatly catalog themselves. Occasionally, in contrast to this, a writer frankly admits that his definition either of vowels or of consonants is unsatisfactory.* (Pike, 1943, p. 66)

Wise, in his book *Applied Phonetics,* also was highly cautious in defining consonant and vowel.

> *For consonant and vowel, at least, the student has had serviceable, if unformulated, definitions already in mind from ordinary school experience, which have been sufficient for the time. Actually, the formulation of exact definitions, even of consonant and vowel, is a difficult matter, and a very controversial one. The student must understand that the definitions in this book will not necessarily be approved by critics and other writers of phonetics texts.* (Wise, 1957a, pp. 65–66)

Given this introduction, the reader may appreciate the need for this rather involved definition: *A vowel is a speech sound that is formed without a significant constriction of the oral and pharyngeal cavities and that serves as a syllable nucleus.* By "significant constriction" we mean that the cavities are never narrowed to the degree observed for consonants, such as the underlined sounds in <u>y</u>es, kee<u>p</u>, ro<u>p</u>e. Vowels are associated with a relatively open tract from the larynx through the lips. By "syllable nucleus" we mean that only one vowel sound can occur within the boundaries of a syllable unit and that, therefore, individual vowels can be identified with individual syllables. When the doctor asks you to open your mouth and say "ah," he or she is asking you to produce a vowel. This sound is convenient for the physician's purposes because it keeps the tongue low in the mouth (hence out of the way) and because the patient can sustain this sound for a long time if necessary (hence affording considerable time for observation). Vowels usually are voiced (produced with vibrating vocal folds), but not always. Whispered speech contains vowels that are not associated with vibrating vocal folds. The definition given here (to which occasional reservations might be added as we progress through the phonetic swamp) stresses three aspects of vowel production: (1) a spatial one—the articulators are positioned so as not to constrict the oral and pharyngeal cavities; (2) a temporal one—the sound of interest can be sustained indefinitely; and (3) a functional one—a syllable (with some exceptions) must include a vowel as its nucleus.

A pure vowel, that is, a vowel having a single, unchanging sound quality, is sometimes called a **monophthong** (from the Greek *mono,* meaning "one" and *phthongos,* meaning "voice" or "sound"). The IPA represents these sounds with single symbols, such as /u/ (who), /ɪ/ (hid), or /æ/ (had). But sometimes vowel-like sounds are produced with a gradually changing articulation and hence with a complex, dynamic sound quality. For example, consider the vowel-like sounds in the words *how, eye,* and *hoy.* If you place your finger or a pencil on the top of your tongue as you say these words, you should be able to detect a slow motion. This movement may be very small in the case of *how,* but much larger for *eye* and *hoy.* In addition, for both *how* and *hoy,* you should be able to see (or feel) a change in the shape of the lips. The vowel-like sounds in these words are called **diphthongs** (*di* meaning "two" and *phthongos* meaning "sound"). In the IPA, diphthongs are represented by a digraph, or pair of symbols such as /aɪ/ for the sound of *eye.* That is, the sound is presumed to begin with an /a/-like vowel and to end with an /ɪ/-like vowel. The tongue gradually changes its position from /a/ to /ɪ/, and the slowness of the articulatory motion helps to distinguish the diphthongs from certain "gliding" consonants, such as the *y* in *you* and the *w* in *we.*

Vowel Articulation

The position of the tongue distinguishes among almost all of the vowels in the English language. Tongue position can be described according to two dimensions: a dimension of high–low (superior–inferior) and a dimension of front–back (anterior–posterior).

These two dimensions define a quadrilateral or four-sided figure in which the vowels of all languages can be represented. The corners of this quadrilateral are vowels with the following articulatory descriptors of tongue position: high-front, low-front, high-back, and low-back. These vowels fix the extreme points of vowel articulation, rather like survey posts that establish the boundaries of a piece of property. If you say the vowels in the following words, you will put your tongue body through the limits of its positioning for speech: *heat, hat, hoot, hot.* Now as you repeat each word a few times, try to confirm the following: the vowel in *heat* has a high-front tongue position, the vowel in *hat* has a low-front tongue position, the vowel in *hoot* has a high-back tongue position, and the vowel in *hot* has a low-back position. The phonetic symbols for the corner vowels are /i/ (high-front), /æ/ (low-front), /u/ (high-back) and /ɑ/ (low-back). These vowels are discussed in more detail in following sections where they will be highly useful in introducing other vowels.

As further practice in sensing the tongue position for these corner vowels, try to describe how your tongue changes position as you say the following pairs of words: (a) *he–who,* (b) *who–ha,* (c) *map–mop,* (d) *heap–hop.* The changes are as follows: (a) front to back, with the tongue held in a high position; (b) high to low, with the tongue held in a back position; (c) front to back, with the tongue held in a low position; and (d) high-front to low-back. Each of these articulatory movements is relatively large, covering as they do the corner points of vowel articulation.

Now that we have explored the boundaries of vowel articulation, we can begin to study how other vowels fit into the vowel quadrilateral.

Tongue Height (the High–Low Dimension of Tongue Position)

The term **tongue height** is used here to refer to the relative vertical position of the tongue body. In some cases, tongue height can be determined as the position of the highest point on the tongue, but this procedure has shortcomings. Difficulties with existing phonetic feature systems for vowels are reviewed later in this chapter, and the reader is forewarned that the features used here are not exact descriptions of vowel articulation. The features conform to general articulatory properties of vowels and are motivated largely by the requirements of simplicity and convenience.

In English and most other languages, the tongue has a range of vowel positions in the high–low (or superior–inferior) dimension. Vowels produced in the highest position, in which the tongue is close to the roof of the mouth, are called **high vowels.** Vowels produced in the lowest position, with the tongue depressed in the mouth, are the **low vowels.** Intermediate tongue positions along the high–low dimension are specified with such descriptors as mid-high, mid, or mid-low. Say the following pairs of words to yourself as you try to describe the height of the tongue for each vowel as either *high* or *low.*

heat–hat	*hoot–hot*
Pete–Pat	*soup–sop*
meat–mat	*mood–mod*
leak–lack	*Luke–lock*
ease–as	*you–yaw*

In each pair, the first word contains a high vowel, and the second word contains a low vowel. You can verify the difference in tongue height by touching your finger or a pencil to your tongue as you say the vowel sounds in the words *heat–hat–hoot–hop.* The vowels in *heat* (and in *he* and *ease*) and in *hoot* (and *who* and *you*) are the high vowels. We must emphasize that *high* is a relative term and does not necessarily mean that /i/ (*he*) and /u/ (*who*)[1] can be measured to have exactly the same elevation of the tongue. For some speakers, the tongue position for /u/ (*who*) is lower than that for /i/ (*he*), but the /u/ is the highest of the vowels produced in the back of the oral cavity. Similarly, /i/ is the highest of the vowels produced in the front of the oral cavity. Remember that the virgules or diagonals are placed around phonemic symbols to distinguish them from other symbols, such as letters of the ordinary alphabet.

The vowels in *hat* and *hop* are the low vowels and are given the phonemic symbols /æ/ (*hat*) and /ɑ/ (*hop*). The latter key word is not pronounced exactly the same way by all speakers of American English, so you should be very careful to compare your production of this word with the words on the CD that accompanies this text. Other frequently used key words for vowel /ɑ/ are *father, pot, calm, ah,* and *psalm.* This vowel often is confused with other vowels to be discussed later, so we want to give advance warning that /ɑ/ (*hop*) is another hazard of the phonetic swamp. Special attention to the recorded sample vowels is highly recommended.

---

[1]Note: In the first part of this book, we will always follow a phonetic symbol with a parenthesized key word to help you remember the sound that is represented. For example, the phonemic symbols and key words for the high vowels mentioned above are

/i/ (*he*)
/u/ (*who*)

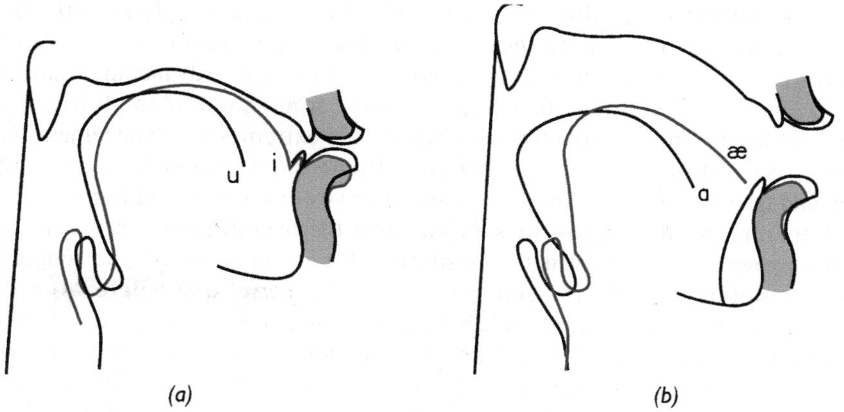

FIGURE 4.1
X-ray tracings of the corner or point vowels. *(a)* Black line shows high-back /u/ *(who)*, and blue line shows high-front /i/ *(he)*; *(b)* black line shows low-back /ɑ/ *(hop)*, and blue line shows low-front /æ/ *(hat)*.

X-ray pictures of the vocal tract are helpful in visualizing the differences between the high and low vowels. The line drawings in Figure 4.1 were derived from X-ray films of vowel production. Composite drawings of two vowels are shown to illustrate the differences between /i/ (*he*) and /u/ (*who*) and between /æ/ (*hat*) and /ɑ/ (*hop*). Note that for both /i/ (*he*) and /u/ (*who*), the tongue is high in the mouth and the jaw is in a nearly closed (or elevated) position, whereas for /æ/ (*hat*) and /ɑ/ (*hop*), the tongue is low in the mouth and the jaw is relatively open (or lowered). Because the tongue is supported by the jaw, it is natural to produce the low vowels /æ/ (*hat*) and /ɑ/ (*hop*) by dropping the jaw, which causes the tongue to assume a low position.

It should be recognized that although tongue and jaw work together in vowel articulation (for example, vowels with a high tongue position are also produced with a closed jaw position), the tongue can move independently of the jaw. Figure 4.2 shows how the high tongue position for vowel /i/ can be accomplished with jaw positions ranging from closed to open (over an inch of opening, in fact). Of course, in order for the tongue to reach a high position when the jaw is open, the tongue must push up very high relative to the jaw, as shown at the bottom of Figure 4.2.

Other vowels assume intermediate positions along the high–low continuum of tongue positions. These sounds will be described in detail after the front–back dimension of tongue positioning has been discussed. But, in the meantime, the reader can get some idea of the variations in tongue height by saying the words (or even better, just the vowel sounds) in this list: *meat, mit, mate, met, mat.* These words are arranged roughly in descending order of tongue height for the vowel, so you should be able to feel the tongue assuming progressively lower positions as you read through the list. We say "roughly" because individual speakers vary somewhat in the tongue height feature of vowel articulation. Read the list forwards and backwards to get a feeling of changes in tongue height.

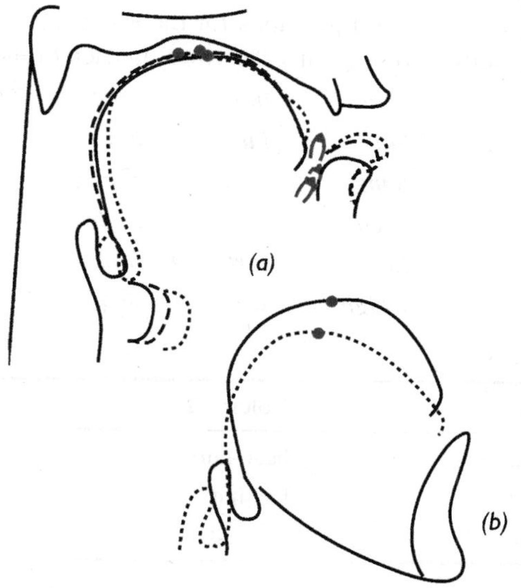

FIGURE 4.2
X-ray tracings showing high-front vowel /i/ produced with various degrees of jaw opening. The filled circle on the dorsum of the tongue is the location of a small marker attached to the tongue surface. *(a)* Articulatory configurations of /i/ with normal closed jaw position (dotted line), large jaw opening (dashed line), and very large jaw opening (solid line); *(b)* the stretching of tongue relative to jaw is shown by this composite of tongue shapes for normal (dotted line) and very large (solid line) jaw openings.

Tongue Advancement (the Front–Back Dimension of Tongue Position)

In any given language, the vowels may vary along a dimension of front–back (anterior–posterior). We will refer to this dimension as **tongue advancement,** although it might just as well be called tongue retraction. Ladefoged (1971) uses the term "backness" to label a similar dimension of tongue position. For the vowels of English, we will use three descriptors of tongue advancement: front, central, and back. There are fewer variations for tongue advancement than for tongue height. As you say the pairs of words in Table 4.1, try to describe the position of the tongue for each vowel, using the choices of front, central, and back.

In Column 1, the first word in each pair contains a front vowel, and the second word contains a back vowel. In Column 2, the first word contains a front vowel, and the second word a central vowel. Finally, in Column 3, the first word has a central vowel, and the second word a back vowel.

Examples of vowels for each of the three places of front–back tongue position are given in Table 4.2. Say the words in each list and try to verify the descriptions of front, central, and back. It may help if you say only the vowel in each word.

One more exercise that helps to give the feel of tongue advancement is to say the following word triads. The three words in each row are arranged in order of front–central–back, so you should be able to feel the tongue assuming progressively backward positions for the words in each group. It may help if you say only the vowel in each of the words.

heat	*hurt*	*hoot*
hat	*hut*	*hot*
Sam	*sum*	*psalm*
deed	*dud*	*dude*
lick	*lurk*	*look*
weigh	*were*	*woe*

TABLE 4.1

Column 1	Column 2	Column 3
heat–hoot	heat–hurt	hurt–hoot
hat–hot	hat–hut	hut–hot
pit–put	pit–putt	putt–put

TABLE 4.2

Front Vowels	Central Vowels	Back Vowels
seat	but	call
that	bird	tune
wet	luck	load
guess	supper (both vowels)	log
did	once	push
late	firm	took

We can fix endpoints or extremes on the front–back dimension by using the vowels /i/ (*heat*), /u/ (*hoot*), /æ/ (*hat*), and /ɑ/ (*hop* or *ah*). That is, for a high tongue position, the extremes in tongue advancement are given by the vowels /i/ (high-front) and /u/ (high-back). For a low tongue position, the extremes in advancement are the vowels /æ/ (low-front) and /ɑ/ (low-back). Figure 4.3 shows how these four vowels compare in terms of tongue positions. Notice that the overall tongue positions, often even the positions of a given point on the tongue, are arranged in the form of a **vowel quadrilateral** or vowel trapezoid, having the vowel corners /i/, /u/, /æ/, and /ɑ/ and the corresponding articulatory descriptions of high-front, high-back, low-front, and low-back. We will return to this quadrilateral description of vowels in a moment, but first we must consider two other features of vowel production.

Tenseness or Length

The terms **tense** and **lax,** representing extremes along a continuum of tenseness, are occasionally used in phonetic descriptions of vowels. Although these terms are very difficult to define, they are used to represent aspects of vowel articulation not covered by the other features. Basically, the feature or dimension of tenseness refers to the degree of muscle activity involved in the vowel articulation and to the duration of the vowel. Tense vowels have greater muscle activity and longer duration than lax vowels. For example, /i/ in *heat* is tense and /ɪ/ in *hit* is lax; /u/ in *Luke* is tense and /ʊ/ in *look* is lax.

As will be discussed later in this chapter, experimental confirmation of the tense–lax distinction has been difficult. However, if this distinction is considered to be primarily one of length rather than one of degree of muscular tension, experimental confirmation is much easier. In fact, it is clear from several acoustic studies that vowels vary in their intrinsic duration. Some vowels are almost always long, whereas others are almost always short. Therefore, the tense–lax distinction might be more satisfactorily considered as a long–short distinction.

To a degree, the vowels traditionally described as tense can be distinguished from those described as lax by examining their distributional properties, that is, the different phonetic conditions of their occurrence. Interestingly, none of the vowels described as lax can appear in stressed open

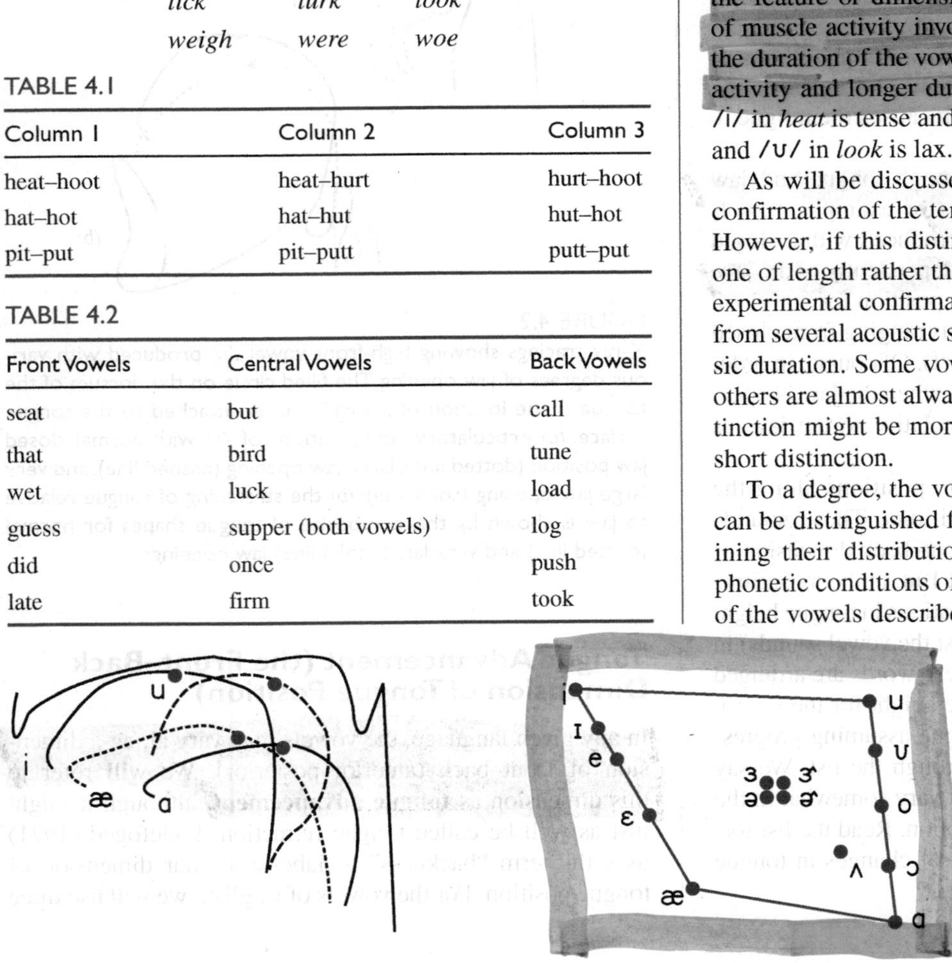

FIGURE 4.3 Vowel quadrilateral formed with vowels /i/, /u/, /ɑ/, and /æ/ as its corners. Tongue positions for vowels are specified as points falling on the sides of, or within, the quadrilateral diagram.

syllables, which is simply to say that lax vowels cannot terminate a stressed syllable. The lax vowels do occur in stressed closed syllables, for example, *hit, book, nut, get.* Tense vowels occur in both types of syllables: closed—*heat, boot, caught;* open—*he, blue, law.* Hence, tense and lax vowels are treated differently in the phonology of English, and this fact alone is sufficient reason to divide vowels into tense and lax groups for phonetic purposes.

Lip Configuration (Rounding)

Lip configuration can be described by a variety of terms (such as rounding, protrusion, retraction, spreading, eversion, and narrowing), but we will consider for the most part only two states of the lips—rounded or unrounded. **Rounded vowels** are produced with the lips in a pursed and protruded state, so that they form a letter O when viewed from the front. **Unrounded vowels** are formed without such pursing or protrusion. See the examples in Figures 4.4 and 4.5. Occasional reference to these figures will be made as individual vowels are described in this chapter.

The best example of a rounded English vowel is the vowel /u/ (*who*), but even with this vowel we must be cautious because not all speakers produce a rounded /u/. Vowels /i/ (*he*) and /æ/ (*had*) are examples of unrounded vowels. As mentioned earlier, lip rounding lengthens the vocal tract, and such lengthening can produce a significant acoustic change in the vowel sound. In English, only some of the back and central vowels are typically rounded. Included among the rounded back vowels are /u/ (*pool*), /ʊ/ (*pull*), /o/ (*pole*), and /ɔ/ (*pawl*). The best example of a rounded central vowel is /ɝ/ (*bird*). No front vowel in English is rounded, although many other languages contain rounded front vowels, as you may know if you have studied French, German, or Swedish.

Vowel Description: Tongue Height, Tongue Advancement, Tenseness, and Lip Rounding

English vowels can be described by considering three series or groupings: the **front series,** the **central series,** and the **back series.** The front and back series correspond to two sides of the vowel quadrilateral, as discussed previously. The vowels in each series are differentiated on the basis of tongue height, tenseness, and rounding. The three series are divisions according to tongue advancement, and the vowels within a series are distinguished by the other three features. Some cautions in the use of these terms are given at the end of the chapter.

The Front Series

The front series includes the following vowels: /i ɪ e ɛ æ/, all of which are unrounded. The articulatory configurations for selected front vowels, as determined from X-ray studies, are shown in Figure 4.6. Note that the tongue is carried near the *front* of the mouth and that the lips are in an *unrounded* state. According to Dewey (1923), who determined the relative frequencies of occurrence of phonemes in standard English prose, the front vowels as a group made up about 20 percent of all sounds recorded. Within the class of vowels and diphthongs, the front vowels accounted for about half of the tokens. Thus, the front vowels have a rather high frequency of occurrence in the English language. Other data on frequency of occurrence are given in Appendix B.

Vowel /i/ (He)

Articulatory Description: High-Front, Tense, and Unrounded Vowel (Figures 4.7 and 4.5). This vowel is produced with the tongue in the extreme front and high position and therefore qualifies as a **point,** or **corner, vowel** on the vowel quadrilateral. The articulation is described as tense because the tongue musculature has a relatively tensed state and the duration is long (compared to /ɪ/, for example). You might be able to verify the difference in tension or overall muscle activity by placing your fingers under the fleshy part of your chin as you say the vowels /i/ (*heed*) and /ɪ/ (*hid*). Many speakers feel a greater tension for /i/ than for /ɪ/. Because /i/ is a high vowel, the jaw usually is held in a closed position to assist the tongue in arching to its high position in the mouth. The velopharynx normally is closed for /i/, but it may be open if the vowel is in a nasal context (for example in the words *me* or *mean*). When the velopharynx is closed, the velum tends to be held in a high position because velar elevation usually is higher for high vowels than for mid or low vowels. For all English vowels, the possibility of nasalization exists for production in nasal contexts. Although we will not repeat this fact in each description that follows, this possibility should be kept in mind. Lip rounding is not tolerated well for /i/, as it causes a marked change in phonetic quality.

Articulatory Summary

Lips:	Unrounded, possibly everted or retracted.
Jaw:	Closed or elevated position.
Tongue:	Tongue body held in high-front position, so that maximal constriction occurs in the palatal region; pharynx is widely opened, with advancement of tongue root.
Velopharynx:	Normally closed unless sound is in nasal context; velum tends to be quite high.

Special Considerations and Allophonic Variations. Although the IPA treats /i/ as a monophthong, some linguists regard it as being diphthongized (/i y/). Vowel /i/ rarely is used before *r* within the same syllable. Vowel /ɪ/ (described next) is used in this position. Other allophonic variations of /i/ are described in the discussion of nasalized vowels in this chapter.

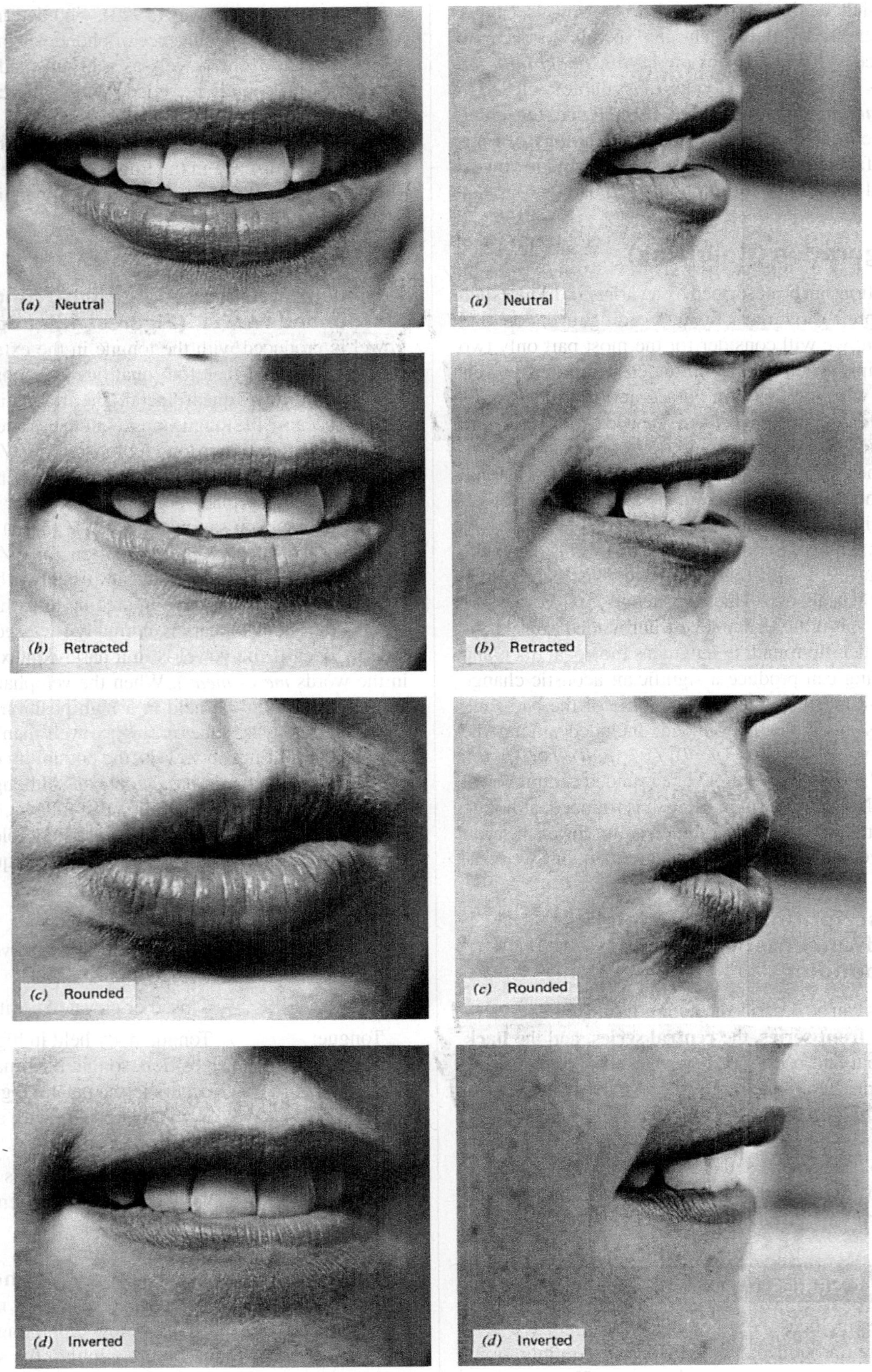

FIGURE 4.4
Major shapes of mouth opening or lip configuration, shown in side and front views: *(a)* neutral, *(b)* retracted, *(c)* rounded, and *(d)* inverted.

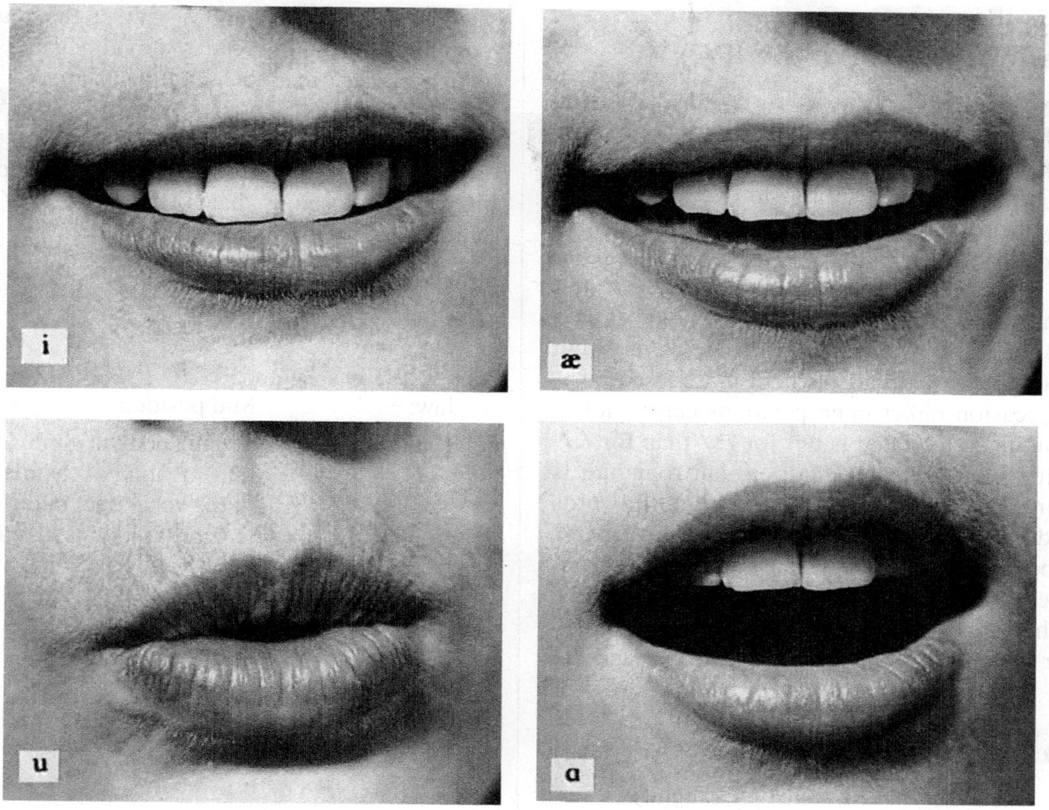

FIGURE 4.5
Photographs of the mouth opening for the vowels in the words *he, who, had,* and *palm*. The phonemic symbols for these vowels are /i/, /u/, /æ/ and /ɑ/, respectively.

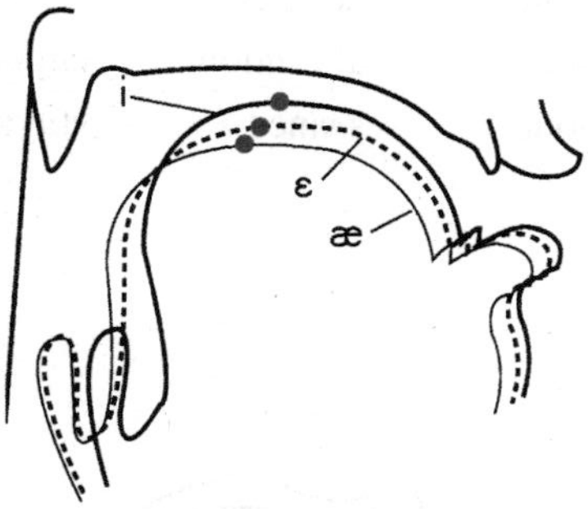

FIGURE 4.6
Composite of X-ray tracings for the front vowels /i/ *(heed)*, /ɛ/ *(head)*, and /æ/ *(had)*. For all three vowels, the tongue is positioned near the front of the oral cavity. The vowels are distinguished primarily by the feature of tongue height. Note that mouth opening varies but lips are unrounded.

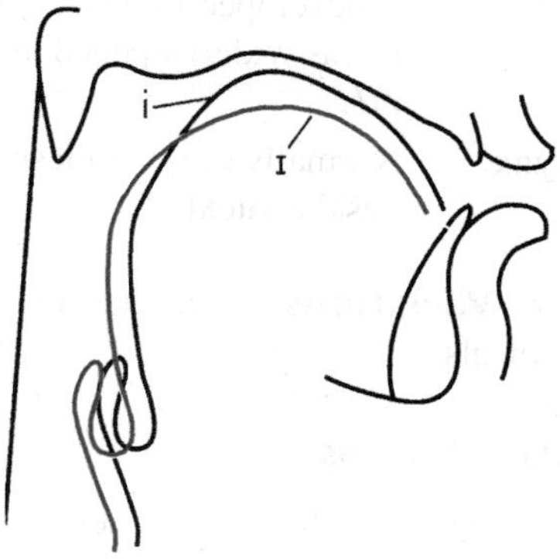

FIGURE 4.7
Comparison X-ray tracings for high-front /i/ *(heed)* and high-mid-front /ɪ/ *(hid)*. Vowel /i/ is shown by black line, /ɪ/ by blue line.

Words for Vowel Recognition or Transcription Practice. Until the student has had some transcription experience with consonants, it is recommended that he or she simply pronounce each word carefully and identify the vowel under consideration. After the student has studied consonants, these words may be used for practice in phonetic transcription.

s*ee*d	C*ae*sar	Ph*oe*nix
rel*ea*se	p*eo*ple	l*ea*p
r*ee*ling	mach*i*ne	est*ee*m
kn*ea*d	bel*ie*ve	c*ei*ling
l*ea*se	pr*e*vious	ben*ea*th
pl*ea*se	an*e*mic	tr*ea*tise

Vowel /ɪ/ (*Hid*) (Also Transcribed /ɩ/ in a Previous Version of the IPA)

Articulatory Description: High-Mid, Front, Lax, and Unrounded Vowel (Figure 4.7). This vowel differs from /i/ in that /ɪ/ is slightly lower (hence, high-mid), relatively lax, and shorter in overall duration. The following word pairs give contrasts of /i/ and /ɪ/: *lead–lid, weak–wick, sheep–ship, team–Tim, seen–sin, heed–hid.* As you say each pair, you should be able to tell that the second vowel, compared to the first, is lower, lax, and shorter. Because /ɪ/ is produced with a relatively high tongue position, the jaw usually is held in a closed position, but on occasion rather open positions can be tolerated. Lip rounding is tolerated better for /ɪ/ than for /i/, especially with reduced vowel duration, but rounding is unusual for either vowel. In word-final position in words like city, muddy, petty, and pity, the choice between /i/ and /ɪ/ can be difficult. However, most phoneticians prefer /ɪ/ in these situations. One practical reason for this preference is the distinction between words such as *warranty–warantee,* for which /ɪ/ is suited for the former and /i/ to the latter.

Articulatory Summary

Lips:	Unrounded, sometimes slightly rounded or retracted.
Jaw:	Closed position, ranging to mid-open.
Tongue:	Tongue body in a high-mid and front posture, so that maximal constriction is developed in palatal region; pharynx not as widely opened as in the case of /i/.
Velopharynx:	Normally closed unless sound is in nasal context.

Allophonic Variations. See nasalized vowels and centralized vowels.

Transcription Words

l*i*mp	d*i*d	c*i*ty
l*i*st	w*o*men	r*i*ch
cyst	tr*i*ck	m*i*ddle
b*i*d	w*i*ck	qu*i*ver
sl*i*d	shr*i*mp	M*i*ck*ey*
t*i*ll	r*i*p	s*i*mple
sw*i*m	W*i*ll*y*	p*i*ck*i*ng

Vowel /e/ (*Chaos*—First Syllable)

Articulatory Description: Mid-Front, Tense, and Unrounded Vowel (Figure 4.8). The vowel /e/ is a monophthongal variant of the sound that more commonly occurs as the diphthongized form /e͡ɪ/, which is described in detail later in this chapter. The monophthong is shorter than the diphthong and does not have the tongue raising that is characteristic of the diphthong. The jaw usually assumes a mid position but may be as closed as that for the vowel /ɪ/. The lips are unrounded.

Articulatory Summary

Lips:	Unrounded.
Jaw:	Mid position.
Tongue:	Tongue body in a mid and front position, creating a maximal constriction of the vocal tract in the palatal region; the constriction is less than that for /ɪ/.
Velopharynx:	Normally closed unless sound is in nasal context.

Allophonic Variations. See nasalized vowels and diphthong /e͡ɪ/.

Transcription Words. Note: The monophthong often occurs in these examples.

ob*e*yance	loc*a*te	incorpor*a*te
oper*a*te	holid*a*y	*e*ighteenth
ball*e*t	alter*a*tion	c*a*pon
ch*a*otic	s*e*ance	st*a*ying

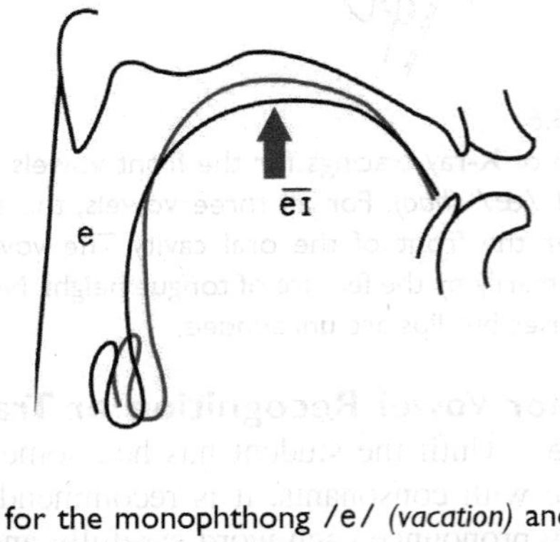

FIGURE 4.8
X-ray tracings for the monophthong /e/ *(vacation)* and the diphthong /e͡ɪ/ *(day)*. The black line shows tongue position for /e/, and the blue line shows the final position assumed after articulation of the diphthong /e͡ɪ/. Hence, the diphthong is produced with a gradual movement in the direction of the arrow.

Vowel /ɛ/ (Head)

Articulatory Description: Low-Mid, Front, Lax, and Unrounded Vowel (Figure 4.9). Vowel /ɛ/ is somewhat lower than /e/ (v*a*cation) and therefore has the articulatory description of low-mid-front (in the lower part of the mid range). This vowel is rather short, and in fact its short duration often distinguishes it from vowel /æ/ (*had*) more than does any other difference. The musculature is in a lax state, as is usually the case for short vowels. The jaw typically is in a mid position, tending to be somewhat more open (lower) than it is for /e/ (ch*a*os). The lips are unrounded.

Articulatory Summary

Lips:	Unrounded.
Jaw:	Mid position.
Tongue:	The tongue body is in a low-mid and front position, so that the constriction of the vocal tract tends to be uniform along its length (that is, there is no region of marked constriction).
Velopharynx:	Normally closed unless sound is in nasal context.

Allophonic Variations. See nasalized vowels. Both /æ/ (described next) and /ɛ/ are used before *r* in words like *chair, care, carry,* and *rare,* but /ɛ/ is more common in general American usage.

Transcription Words

b*e*t	f*e*rry	b*e*rry
ag*ai*n	att*e*mpt	m*e*rry
fr*ie*nd	regr*e*t	*e*xpect
*a*ny	sp*e*ll	rep*e*nt
s*e*nd	t*ea*r	m*e*ssage

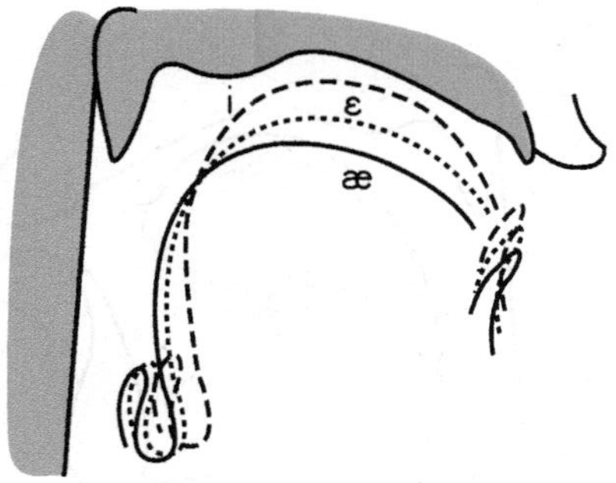

FIGURE 4.9
Composite of X-ray tracings for the vowels /i/ *(heed)*, /ɛ/ *(head)*, and /æ/ *(had)*.

Vowel /æ/ (Had)

Articulatory Description: Low-Front, Lax, and Unrounded Vowel (Figure 4.9). (Note: The IPA describes this sound as high-low-front, to indicate that it has a slightly higher tongue position than the non-English /a/.)

For speakers of General American English, the vowel /æ/ is the lowest front vowel; but for speakers with /a/ in their dialect, /æ/ is slightly higher than /a/. Vowel /æ/ tends to be long in duration but is sometimes described as lax because relatively little muscular tension can be felt under the chin during its articulation (compare /i/ to /æ/). Frequently, however, the major distinction between /æ/ and /ɛ/ is one of duration, and for this reason /æ/ is called long (and sometimes tense). Because /æ/ is quite low, the jaw assumes a low or open position. The lips are unrounded, often even retracted, as shown in Figures 4.4 and 4.5.

Articulatory Summary

Lips:	Unrounded, frequently retracted.
Jaw:	Open position.
Tongue:	Low-front in mouth, nearly the lowest front vowel in the IPA and in fact the lowest front vowel in General American speech.
Velopharynx:	Normally closed unless sound is in a nasal context; velar position during velopharyngeal closure tends to be low compared to other front vowels.

Allophonic Variations. See nasalized vowels. Also, /æ/ often is diphthongized in some dialects and idiolects, for example, /k æ t/ (cat) → /k æ ɪ t/ or /k æ ə t/.

Transcription Words

b*a*d	*a*lab*a*ster	h*a*mmer
s*a*ss	h*a*ng	Alab*a*ma
h*a*nd	h*a*ndsome	S*a*n Diego
*a*nswer	pl*a*ster	pi*a*no
cr*a*ss	*a*nalogous	st*a*ndard
gl*a*ss	*a*lcohol	bl*a*nd

Vowel /a/ (*path*, Eastern dialect)

(Eastern *path* or the initial segment of the diphthongs in *high* and *how;* see diphthong section later in this chapter.)

Articulatory Description: Low-Front, Lax, and Unrounded Vowel (Figure 4.10). This vowel was omitted from the vowel quadrilateral in Figure 4.3 because it rarely appears in isolated production in English. Sometimes it

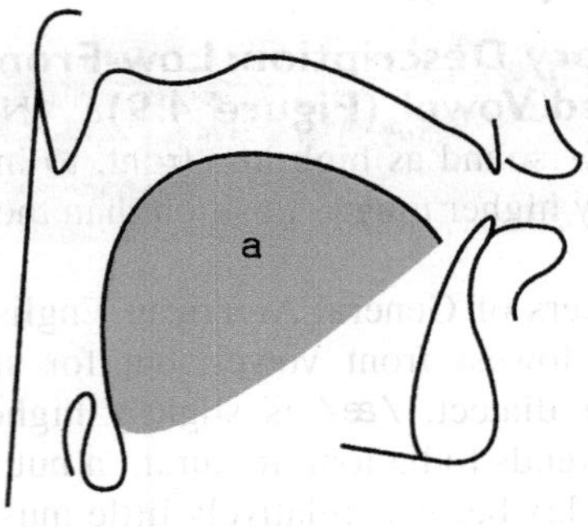

FIGURE 4.10
X-ray tracing of articulatory configuration for vowel /a/ (Eastern *path*).

is used to denote the onglide, or first segment, of the diphthongs in *high* (or *buy, sign, aisle*) and *how* (or *round, house, town*). However, our own observations of vocal tract X-rays indicate that for Midwesterners, these diphthongs often begin with a segment that is very nearly like low-back /ɑ/. Vowel /a/ can be heard in the Eastern speech in words such as *path, park,* or *barn.* Although the IPA lists /a/ as the low-front vowel, many phonetics texts assign this description to /æ/. Because of the infrequent appearance of /a/, we prefer to regard it as an allophone or dialectal variation. For further discussion, see the section on diphthongs later in this chapter.

> **ROUNDED FRONT VOWELS**
>
> If you are a native speaker of English studying certain languages such as French, German, or Swedish, you will learn to produce a rounded front vowel that does not occur in English. This simple exercise gives you an idea of what a rounded front vowel is like. First, produce a sustained vowel /i/ as in *he*. As you phonate this vowel, gradually round your lips in a kissing motion. Your will hear a change in sound quality corresponding to the addition of lip rounding to the front vowel articulation. If you prolong the vowel, keeping your tongue in stable position for /i/, and vary your lip articulation between rounded and spread, you should be able to hear a marked difference in vowel quality.

THE CENTRAL SERIES

The central vowels are /ɝ ɜ ɚ ə ʌ/, which are produced with a tongue body position roughly in the center of the mouth. Tongue height varies little among these vowels except that /ʌ/ is both lower and farther back than the other central vowels. The two vowels /ɝ ɜ/ often are rounded, but the degree of rounding varies considerably with speaker and dialect. The vowels /ə ʌ/ usually are not rounded. The weak or unstressed /ɚ/ is variable in rounding. Some speakers round it most of the time, whereas other speakers do not round it at all. Estimates of the relative frequencies of these vowels are uncertain because of problems in phonetic transcription and dialectal variation, but Dewey (1923) gives the relative frequency of occurrence of /ʌ/ and /ə/ as 2.33 and 4.63 percent, respectively. Within the group of vowels and diphthongs in Dewey's study, these two vowels make up almost one-fifth of the total usage.

The central vowels cannot be described without reference to stress. Whether good or bad, it is a characteristic of the IPA that both segmental and suprasegmental properties can influence phonemic transcription. That is, sometimes one symbol is selected over another because of a perceived difference in stress (the emphasis or prominence given to a syllable). For example, each of the two vowels in the word *further* has *r* coloring, but the vowels differ in stress. The first vowel receives more stress than the second. This difference is represented phonetically by transcribing the first vowel as /ɝ/ and the second vowel as /ɚ/. Therefore, the phonemic transcription of *further* is /f ɝ ð ɚ/. The vowels /ə/ and /ʌ/ also are described as having different stress, with /ʌ/ being more stressed than /ə/. For example, in the words *amuck* and *abut,* the first vowel is produced with less stress than the second. Therefore, the words are transcribed /ə m ʌ k/ and /ə b ʌ t/. The importance of stress in transcribing the central vowels often is underestimated by the beginner, and we have found that many students stumble in this area.

Vowel /ɝ/ (Her)

Articulatory Description: Mid-Central, Tense, and Rounded Vowel (Figure 4.11). Vowel /ɝ/ has a mid-central position and usually is produced with some degree of rounding. The degree of rounding varies across speakers. As noted in the introductory comments on central vowels, /ɝ/ may be regarded as the stressed counterpart to /ɚ/ (which is unstressed). Vowel /ɝ/ is sometimes described as **r-colored, retroflex,** or **rhotacized.** Some vowels followed by consonantal /r/ occasionally are confused with /ɝ/ (see the description of /r/ in the chapter on consonants). Note the distinction between /ɝ/ in *burr* and the vowel + /r/ combination in *bar, bore, bear,* and *beer.*

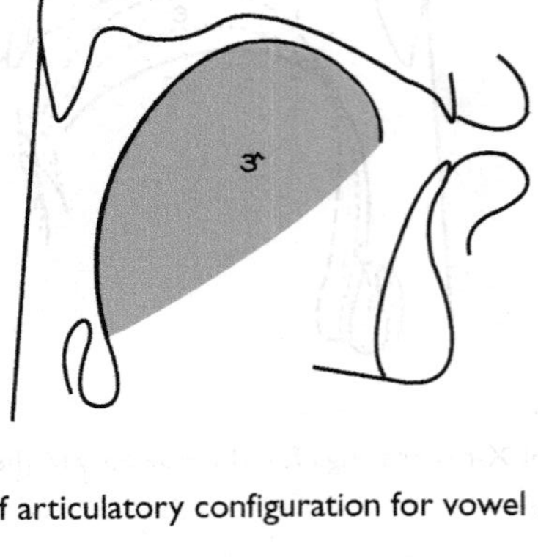

FIGURE 4.11
X-ray tracing of articulatory configuration for vowel /ɝ/ *(her)*.

Articulatory Summary

Lips:	Usually rounded.
Jaw:	Mid-open position.
Tongue:	Tongue body in mid-central position, often bunched in the palatal region.
Velopharynx:	Normally closed except for nasal contexts.

Allophonic Variations. See nasalized vowels, vowels /ɜ/ and /ɚ/, and consonant /r/.

Transcription Words

s*ir*	ret*ur*n	perv*er*se
l*ear*n	b*ur*ner	t*ur*pentine
ch*ur*ch	ass*er*t	s*er*pent
*ir*k	w*or*ker	st*irr*up
w*or*thy	p*ur*ged	k*er*nel
w*or*k	div*er*t	in*er*t

Vowel /ɜ/ (British or Southern *Her*)

Articulatory Description: Mid-Central, Tense, and Rounded Vowel. Vowel /ɜ/ is similar to /ɝ/ and replaces it as a dialectal variant in British, Southern, and occasionally Eastern speech. Perhaps the best description of /ɜ/ is "/ɝ/ without the *r* coloring." /ɜ/ does not normally occur in General American speech, but it does occur in some dialects and in developing speech. Some children who have difficulty with /ɝ/ will substitute /ɜ/ for it.

Vowel /ɚ/ (*Further*, Sometimes Called Schwar)

Articulatory Description: Mid-Central, Lax, and Rounded Vowel (Figure 4.12). Vowel /ɚ/ is the unstressed counterpart to /ɝ/ and shares with /ɝ/ a mid-central tongue position and *r* coloring. Generally, we will restrict /ɚ/ to unstressed (low-level stress) conditions. Thus, /ɚ/ does not occur in isolated single-syllables. For such words, /ɝ/ is the preferred symbol, for example, *word* /wɝd/. Although /ɚ/ generally is described as rounded, it may be produced as unrounded by some speakers. That is, lip rounding is not an invariant characteristic.

Articulatory Summary

Lips:	Rounded, but not necessarily so.
Jaw:	Usually closed to mid position.
Tongue:	Mid-central tongue body, with a bunching toward the palatal area (Figure 4.12).
Velopharynx:	Normally closed except in nasal contexts.

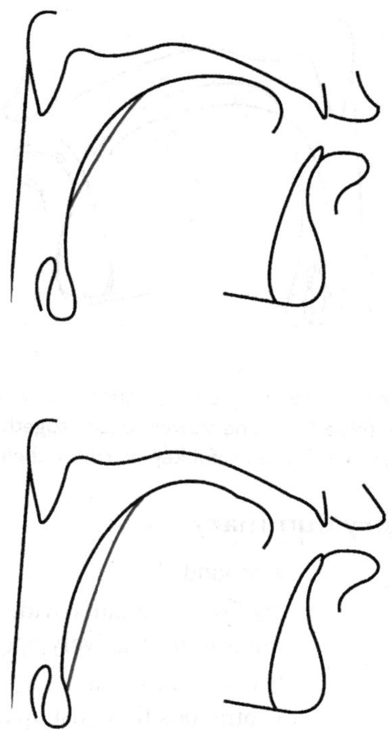

FIGURE 4.12
X-ray tracings of articulatory configurations for vowel /ɚ/ (*further*). The blue line is the lingual midline, which is indented because of grooving of the tongue. Because the two tracings are from different words (*honor* and *polar*), the configurations vary slightly.

Allophonic Variations. See nasalized vowels and vowel /ɝ/. In some dialects (particularly Eastern) and some individual usage, /ɚ/ may be produced as /ə/, for example, the final /ɚ/ in *brother, sister, butter.*

Transcription Words

north*er*n	stup*or*	murd*erer*
upp*er*	laqu*er*	murm*ur*ing
rul*er*	surg*ery*	earn*er*
stirr*er*	loit*er*ing	high*er*
merg*er*	work*er*	barb*er*

Vowel /ʌ/ (Hub)

Articulatory Description: Low-Mid, Back-Central, Lax, and Unrounded Vowel (Figure 4.13). This vowel is produced with a tongue body position that is shifted somewhat toward /ɑ/ from the mid-central position. It may be regarded as lying about midway along an axis between the central position and the position for /ɑ/ (to be described). In addition, /ʌ/ is shorter in duration than /ɑ/. The lips are not rounded, and the jaw usually is quite open but ranges from relatively open to relatively closed, depending upon phonetic context, stress, and other factors.

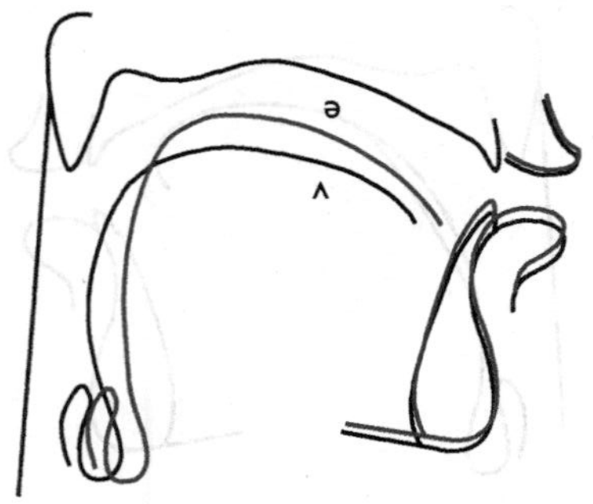

FIGURE 4.13
X-ray tracings of articulatory configurations for vowels /ʌ/ (black line) and /ə/ (blue line). The vowels occur together in the word *abut* /ə b ʌ t/, which is a useful key word for their contrast.

Articulatory Summary

Lips:	Unrounded.
Jaw:	Varies over a fairly wide range but tends to be relatively open.
Tongue:	Tongue body is in a low-mid, back-central position, just up and forward from that for /ɑ/.
Velopharynx:	Normally closed except for nasal contexts.

Allophonic Variations. See nasalized vowels and vowel /ə/.

Transcription Words

r*ou*gh	cl*u*tter	s*u*pper
n*u*t	t*u*mble	n*u*mber
ab*u*t	some*o*ne	*u*pset
en*ou*gh	r*u*ckus	p*u*ppet
s*u*n	l*u*strous	*o*nce
tr*u*st	c*u*stomer	b*u*cket

Vowel /ə/ (*Above*, Sometimes Called Schwa)

Articulatory Description: Mid-Central, Lax, and Unrounded Vowel (Figure 4.13). Vowel /ə/, also known as the **schwa** (from the Hebrew *shua*) vowel, is the unstressed counterpart to /ʌ/. As noted earlier, the stress contrast appears in the words *above* and *abut,* where /ə/ is used in the first syllable and /ʌ/ in the second. Vowel /ə/ is produced with the tongue in the mid-central position and with the lips unrounded. However, the mid-central position is rather an idealized description in that X-ray films do not always reveal a stable articulatory position, especially in phonetic context. The tongue does not necessarily stop at a mid-central position but instead passes through it or near it while moving from the sound before /ə/ to the sound following /ə/. For example, in the word *ruckus* the tongue moves almost continuously from the *k* to the *s.* Often, what we hear as the vowel /ə/ is a short duration vocalic segment brought about by continuous tongue movement. The jaw ranges between closed to mid-open position.

Generally speaking, /ə/ does not receive more than tertiary (third-level) stress, although some phoneticians occasionally use it with higher stress levels. One reason to restrict it to the weakest stress level is that its use can be taken as evidence of unstressing, or **reduction.** In normal adult speech, some vowels are reduced greatly in duration compared to others. When the reduction is great enough, almost any vowel can approach /ə/, although this reduction is especially likely for the vowel /ʌ/. A diagram of vowel reduction is shown in Figure 4.14. The arrows indicate the direction of vowel changes as a result of reduction. Normally, the duration of /ə/ is quite short. For example, when adult speakers say the sentence "We saw you hit the cat," the vowel /æ/ in *cat* is five times as long as the vowel in *the.*

Articulatory Summary

Lips:	Unrounded.
Jaw:	Closed to mid-open position.
Tongue:	Ideally mid-central in isolated production, but tongue position is often not stable in connected speech.
Velopharynx:	Normally closed except when in nasal context.

Allophonic Variations. See nasalized vowels and previous discussion. Vowel /ə/, or schwa, is the ultimately unstressed vowel in that it has the shortest duration and the most nearly central tongue position.

Transcription Words. Note: Because we will try in this book to restrict the use of /ə/ to conditions of weak stress, it will not be used in single syllables produced in isolation. Such words necessarily carry first-level or primary stress.

*e*nough	lustr*ou*s	im*i*tate
*a*gain	cust*o*mer	radi*u*m
*a*but	pupp*e*t	purp*o*se
ruck*u*s	*a*wait	religi*o*n
tel*e*phone	*a*mount	rust*e*d

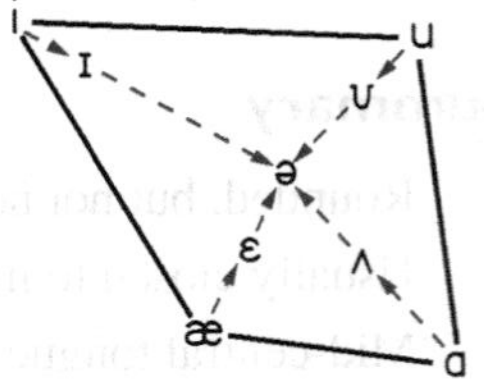

FIGURE 4.14
Diagram of vowel reduction. Reduction occurs along the blue lines; for example, /i/ reduces to /ɪ/, and /ɪ/ reduces to /ə/. Schwa /ə/ is the maximally central, maximally reduced vowel.

The Back Series

This series includes the vowels /u ʊ o ɔ ɑ/, all of which except /ɑ/ tend to be rounded. Figure 4.15 is a composite illustration of the articulatory configurations for some of these vowels. Notice that the tongue is positioned near the back of the mouth for these vowels, but there is some variation in their position along a front–back dimension. The drawings also show lip rounding for three of the vowels. Because the tongue is in the back of the mouth, the region of greatest constriction is in the pharynx or near the velum. In Dewey's (1923) study of frequency of occurrence, these vowels constituted 12 percent of the vowels and diphthongs and about 4 percent of all sounds recorded. However, these figures do not include the diphthongs, three of which involve a back vowel.

Vowel /u/ (*Who*)

Articulatory Description: High-Back, Tense, and Rounded Vowel (Figures 4.5 and 4.15). The tongue is in the extreme high-back position, so that /u/ is one of the point vowels. The articulation constricts the oral cavity in the velar region. The tenseness of the articulation can be sensed by comparison of /u/ with the lax /ʊ/ (book). The tense–lax (or long–short) contrast of /u/–/ʊ/ is analogous with that of /i/–/ɪ/. Like /i/, /u/ usually is produced with a closed jaw position to aid the tongue in reaching its high articulation. Although most speakers produce /u/ with rounding and protrusion of the lips (Figures 4.4 and 4.5), some persons make this sound with a narrowed opening but little protrusion. The acoustic consequences of narrowing and protrusion of the lips are highly similar.

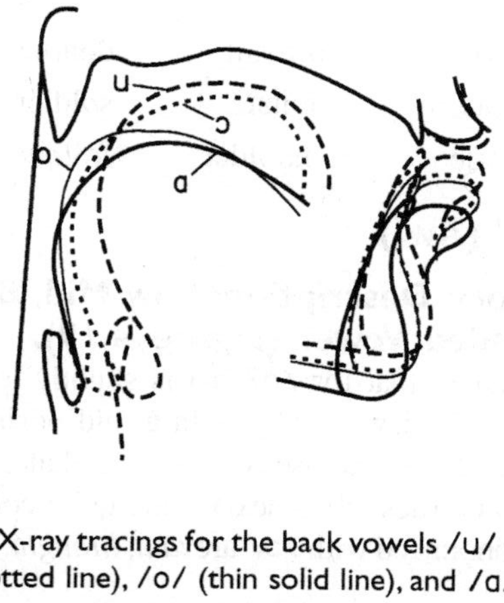

FIGURE 4.15
Composite of X-ray tracings for the back vowels /u/ (dashed line), /ɔ/ in /ɔ r/ (dotted line), /o/ (thin solid line), and /ɑ/ (thick solid line). The tongue is carried toward the back of the oral cavity for all these vowels, but tongue height and mouth opening vary among them. All except /ɑ/ are rounded. The configuration for /ɔ r/ represents a rhotacized modification (to be discussed later) and should not be taken as a typical example of /ɔ/.

Articulatory Summary

Lips:	Rounded and/or narrowed.
Jaw:	Closed position.
Tongue:	Tongue body in high-back position; tongue root is advanced so that lower pharynx is wide; maximal constriction in velar region.
Velopharynx:	Normally closed except when sound is in nasal context; velum tends to be high.

Special Considerations and Allophonic Variations. Some phoneticians regard the /ju/ combination, as in the words *use, you,* and *excuse,* to be a diphthong. Frequently, tongue movements from a consonant to /u/ are gradual, almost glidelike in character. As shown in Figure 4.16, /u/ sometimes has an allophonic variant of a front, rounded vowel in words like *commune.*

Transcription Words

s*ue*	n*oo*dle	st*u*dent
*oo*ze	dil*u*te	ball*oo*n
dr*ew*	poll*u*te	all*u*de
can*oe*	ast*u*te	st*u*pid
cr*ui*se	cr*u*el	*u*seful
n*ew*	r*u*dely	*u*niverse

Vowel /ʊ/ (*Book*, also Transcribed /ɷ/ in a Previous Version of the IPA)

Articulatory Description: High-Mid, Back, Lax, and Rounded Vowel (Figure 4.17). Compared to /u/, /ʊ/ is lax, slightly lower, and shorter in duration. Note the contrast of /u/ and /ʊ/ in these word pairs: *Luke–look, cooed–could, fool–full, wooed–would,* and *stewed–stood.* Jaw position usually is closed for /ʊ/. Lip rounding frequently is not as pronounced as with /u/ and may be neglected altogether.

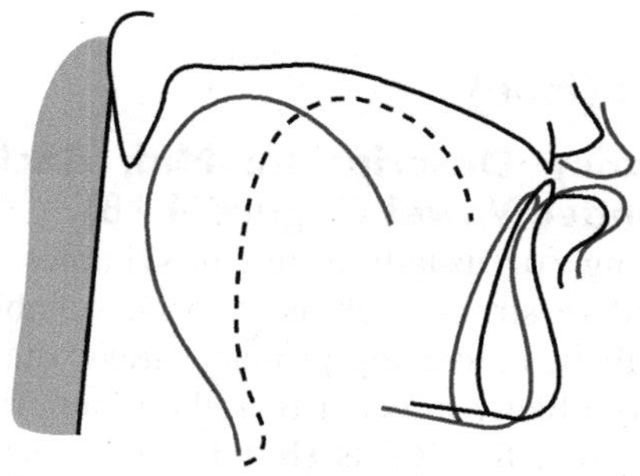

FIGURE 4.16
X-ray tracing for the second vowel in the word *commune* (dashed line) compared to tracing for vowel /u/ (solid line). Note that configuration shown by dashed line resembles a rounded front vowel.

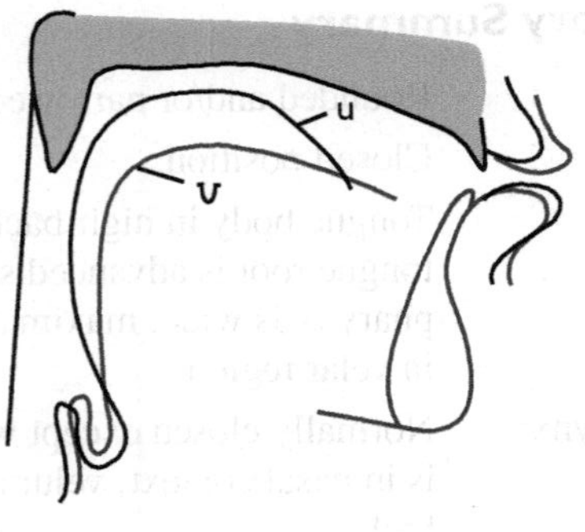

FIGURE 4.17
X-ray tracings of articulatory configurations of vowels /u/ (black line) and /ʊ/ (blue line). Vowel /ʊ/ is essentially a reduced version of /u/, being shorter in duration, more central in tongue position, and less rounded.

Articulatory Summary

Lips:	Rounded in most cases.
Jaw:	Closed position, but ranging to mid-open.
Tongue:	Tongue body in high-mid and back position, with width of pharynx less than for /u/.
Velopharynx:	Open only for nasal contexts.

Allophonic Variations. See nasalized vowels. See /ʌ/, described in the central series. Note that some words can be pronounced with either /ʊ/ or /u/: *hoof, roof, root, broom.*

Transcription Words

w*oo*d	underst*oo*d	br*oo*k
h*oo*f	g*oo*d	f*u*llness
sh*ou*ld	c*oo*k	r*oo*k
n*oo*k	p*u*ll	sh*oo*k
b*u*ll	s*u*gar	f*oo*t

Vowel /o/ (*Hoe*)

Articulatory Description: Mid, Back, Tense, and Rounded Vowel (Figure 4.18). The pure or monophthong /o/ usually occurs in syllables of no more than secondary stress, such as the first syllable in *notation.* In syllables receiving primary stress, the diphthong /o͡ʊ/ is more likely to occur than the monophthong /o/. Tongue position for /o/ is slightly lower than for /ʊ/, and a distinct rounding of the lips usually can be seen. For diphthong /o͡ʊ/, the tongue makes a raising gesture from /o/ roughly to /ʊ/. Jaw position varies from closed to mid, depending upon phonetic context, stress, and other prosodic variables.

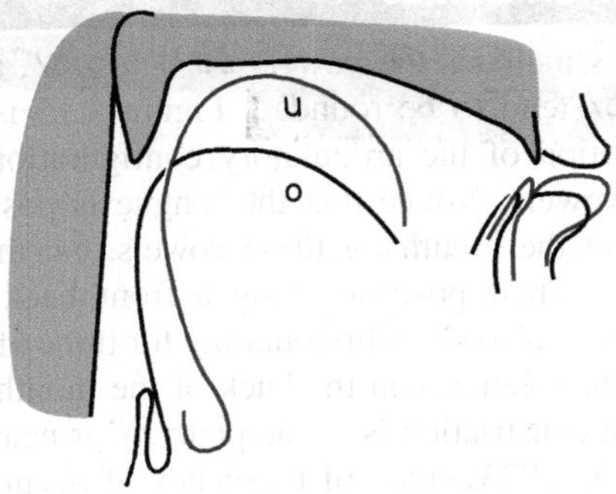

FIGURE 4.18
X-ray tracing of articulatory configuration of vowel /o/ (black line) compared with that of vowel /u/ (blue line).

Articulatory Summary

Lips:	Rounded.
Jaw:	Closed to mid position.
Tongue:	Tongue body is in a back position, not quite as high as for /ʊ/, resulting in a constricted region in the pharynx.
Velopharynx:	Normally closed, except when sound is in nasal context.

Allophonic Variations. See nasalized vowels and diphthong /o͡ʊ/.

Transcription Words. Note: both /o/ and /o͡ʊ/ may occur in some words.

r*o*tate	c*o*llate	rode*o*
l*o*cate	em*o*tion	sol*o*
m*o*de	r*oa*d	R*oa*noke
t*oe*s	r*o*llcall	den*o*te
*o*cean	d*o*nate	s*o*ldier
*o*de	sh*ou*lder	foll*ow*

Vowel /ɔ/ (*Awl*)

Articulatory Description: Low-Mid, Back, Tense, and Rounded Vowel (Figure 4.19). Tongue position is similar to that for /o/ but is slightly lower. The lips are rounded. The jaw usually is in a mid position. Speakers vary considerably in the use of /ɔ/, with dialectal alternation of /ɔ/ and /ɑ/ (described next) being quite common. Words typically pronounced with /ɔ/ are *taut, brought, all,* and *wash.*

Articulatory Summary

Lips:	Rounded, though often not as much as for /u/ or /o/.
Jaw:	Mid position.

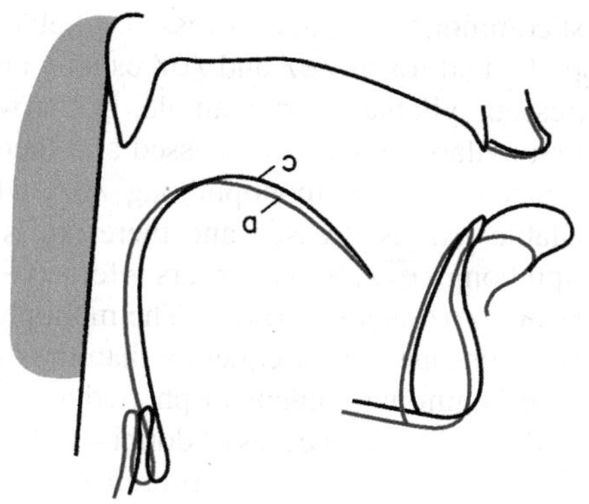

FIGURE 4.19
Comparison X-ray tracings of the articulatory configurations of vowels /ɔ/ (black line) and /ɑ/ (blue line). Vowel /ɔ/ *(awl)* is higher than /ɑ/ and is rounded.

Tongue:	Tongue body is in a low-mid and back position, so that the most constricted region of the vocal tract is in the mid-pharyngeal segment.
Velopharynx:	Normally closed except for nasal contexts.

Allophonic Variations. See nasalized vowels. Either /ɔ/ or /o/ can be used before *r* in words like *tore, port, more,* and *sport.* Vowel /ɔ/ is similar to the British vowel /ɒ/ (Br. *hot*) but tends to be longer. See description of /ɑ/.

Transcription Words

*aw*l	d*o*g	qu*a*rrel
*ou*ght	c*ou*gh	h*au*nt
c*au*ght	*o*ffice	f*o*reign
*o*range	c*o*rd	l*au*rel
l*aw*	*o*rigin	m*o*ral

Vowel /ɑ/ (*Hop*)

Articulatory Description: Low, Back, Tense, and Unrounded Vowel (Figures 4.5, 4.15, and 4.19). The vowel /ɑ/, with its low-back tongue position, completes the vowel quadrilateral. The lips are unrounded and widely open (Figure 4.5). The jaw is in an open position; in fact, for most speakers, this vowel is the most open vowel. The region of greatest constriction of the vocal tract is between the root of the tongue and the mid to lower pharynx. Because the use of this vowel varies widely with dialect, selection of a key word is troublesome. Generally useful key words include *father, calm, hot, barn,* and *ah.* In attempting to say /ɑ/, the speaker should be careful to place the tongue in the extreme low-back position, avoid rounding, and allow ample duration.

Articulatory Summary

Lips:	Unrounded and widely open.
Jaw:	Open.
Tongue:	Tongue body is in the extreme low and back position, so that the pharynx is constricted. The front cavity is larger than for any other vowel.
Velopharynx:	Open only for nasal contexts, but the velum can be lower than for other vowels.

Special Considerations and Allophonic Variations. See nasalized vowels. Depending on dialect, the vowel /ɑ/ may be replaced by /ɒ/ or /ɔ/ or /a/.

Transcription Words

p*o*t	sl*o*t	imp*o*ster
cl*o*d	c*o*mmon	h*o*ller
b*a*lm	c*o*llege	h*o*nor
f*o*lly	d*o*ll	s*o*cket
*o*pera	h*o*lly	adm*o*nish

LOW-BACK VOWEL MERGER

Was your blanket *caught* in the *cot*? Did *Don* see the *dawn*? Say the italicized words carefully and try to determine if you pronounced the vowel sounds in these words differently. If you spent your childhood in Minnesota, southern Missouri, or California, chances are that there is no difference in your pronunciation of *caught* and *cot,* or *Don* and *dawn*. But if your childhood was spent in Wisconsin, Illinois, or Nevada, you probably produce the two vowels differently. This change is a trend in pronunciation called the "Low-Back Vowel Merger" in which the distinction between the vowels /ɔ/ and /ɑ/ is being lost. Chapter 10 discusses in more detail pronunciation patterns of this kind. The pronunciation of English is dynamic, so that the phonetic standard changes gradually over time.

Diphthong Articulation

As mentioned in the introduction to this chapter, diphthongs are vowel-like sounds produced with a gradually changing articulation. These sounds are represented in phonetic transcription by digraph (two-element) symbols that are meant to describe the onglide, or initial segment, and the offglide, or final segment. Thus, the digraph symbol represents in articulatory terms a position of origin and a position of destination.

Actually, the choice of a digraph symbol for the English diphthongs is not easy, and an examination of this problem takes us into another part of the phonetic swamp. Appendix A lists the various symbols that have been proposed for the diphthongs of American English. The reader should be aware of this diversity and not necessarily expect any two phoneticians to use the same diphthong symbols. In this text, with some exceptions, we will use the symbols of the IPA. The two symbol elements are connected with an overhead bar to indicate their phonemic unity.

The phonetic symbols and selected key words for the diphthongs of American English are given in Table 4.3. Notice that three of the diphthongs /a͞ɪ/ (*bye*), /ɔ͞ɪ/ (*boy*), and /a͞ʊ/ (*bough*) are called *phonemic,* whereas the diphthongs /e͞ɪ/ (*bay*) and /o͞ʊ/ (*bow*) are *nonphonemic.* The phonemic diphthongs cannot be reduced to **monophthongs**, but the nonphonemic diphthongs can. This difference can be illustrated with the words in the following columns.

bind	/ba͞ɪnd/	bond	/band/
loin	/lɔ͞ɪn/	lawn	/lɔn/
down	/da͞ʊn/	Don	/dan/

In the column at the left, the phonemic diphthongs occur in common English words. Imagine saying each of these words by producing only the first element in each diphthong and omitting the second element, that is, reducing the diphthong to a monophthong. If you do this, *bind* should sound something like *bond, loin* should sound something like *lawn,* and *down* should sound something like *Don.* In short, reducing the diphthong to a monophthong results in a new morpheme. As was explained in Chapter 2, morphemes are distinguished by phonemic contrasts. Hence, the diphthong in *loin* is phonemically distinct from the monophthong in *lawn.* The phonemic diphthongs /a͞ɪ/ (*bye*), /ɔ͞ɪ/ (*boy*), and /a͞ʊ/ (*bough*) cannot be reduced or simplified to monophthongs.

The nonphonemic diphthongs /e͞ɪ/ (*bay*) and /o͞ʊ/ (*bow*) can be, and often are, reduced to monophthongs without producing different phonemes. The words *bait, state,* and *nape* commonly are produced with the diphthong /e͞ɪ/, but they can be produced with the monophthong /e/ without any change in their morphemic status. Similarly, the words *boat, soap,* and *tote* commonly are produced with the diphthong /o͞ʊ/, but they can be produced with the monophthong /o/. Thus, for these two diphthongs, the diphthongal and monophthongal forms are allophonic variations, not

TABLE 4.3
Diphthongs of American English

	Symbol	Key Words
Phonemic	/a͞ɪ/	bye, eye, aisle
	/ɔ͞ɪ/	boy, toy, oil
	/a͞ʊ/	bough, how, owl
Nonphonemic	/e͞ɪ/	bay, hay, pail
	/o͞ʊ/	bow, hoe, pole

distinct phonemes. The diphthongal forms /e͞ɪ/ and /o͞ʊ/ occur most commonly in heavily stressed syllables, whereas the monophthongal forms /e/ and /o/ usually are found in weakly stressed syllables. For example, in the word *vacation,* the first syllable *va-* is not stressed and therefore usually is produced with the monophthong /e/, whereas the second syllable *-ca-* is stressed and therefore is produced with the diphthong /e͞ɪ/. Some writers refer to the monophthongs /e/ and /o/ as *pure* vowels. The monophthongal or pure forms occur much less frequently than the diphthongal forms, so the beginning student in phonetics is advised to use the diphthongal form in cases of doubt—at least until his or her ear is sharpened to hear the difference.

To familiarize yourself with the diphthongs, look at the words below and write in the blanks the diphthongs that are used.

life	______
Troy	______
Dane	______
bone	______
coy	______
side	______
sewed	______
weighed	______
bound	______
cry	______
cloud	______
home	______
toys	______
cow	______
braid	______
known	______
pout	______
pray	______
Roy	______
Ray	______
town	______
blow	______

As Appendix A shows, there is little agreement among phoneticians as to which vowels should be used to symbolize the English diphthongs. Most phoneticians do agree that two symbols are required, one to represent the **onglide,** or beginning position, and another to represent the **offglide,** or ending position. However, different phoneticians often hear different vowels for both the onglide and offglide segments, so that the diphthong in *bye* is variously transcribed as /aɪ/, /ay/, /ai/, /ɑɪ/, /ɑy/, /ɑi/, /ae/, and so on. Actually, it is not surprising that different sounds are heard because X-ray and acoustic studies have shown that a given diphthong is not always produced with exactly the same onglide and offglide segments. In fact, even an individual speaker may use different onglide and offglide segments from one occasion to another, depending on phonetic context (that is, the influence of surrounding sounds), his or her rate of speaking, and the degree of stress. Figure 4.20 illustrates the variation in onglide and offglide positions for diphthong /a͡ɪ/ uttered at different speaking rates. Notice that different degrees of tongue movement are used. Hence, one production might sound as though it ends with /i/, and another might sound as though it ends with /ɪ/. The student of phonetics should keep this variability in mind and recognize that the phonetic symbols are partly a matter of convenience and best guess. When we produce a diphthong symbolized as /a͡ɪ/, we do not always move the tongue exactly from a position for /ɑ/ to one for /ɪ/. Rather, these vowels serve as the approximate targets for the diphthong's onglide and off-glide segments.

We have examined diphthong articulation in several speakers of General American speech, Midwestern dialect, using both acoustic analysis (spectrograms) and X-ray motion pictures. Onglide and offglide segments obtained from X-ray analyses are illustrated for the five English diphthongs in Figures 4.21, 4.22, 4.23, 4.24, and 4.25. We recommend that the student study these illustrations while making these sounds, attempting to feel the changes in lip, tongue, and jaw positions.

Diphthong /a͡ɪ/ (*Bye*; Figure 4.21)

The IPA symbol /a͡ɪ/ is somewhat misleading as an articulatory description of this sound because, at least in Midwestern speech, the onglide is highly similar to the low-back /ɑ/ (Kent, 1970). The offglide is highly variable and depends on stress, speaking rate, and phonetic context. The variation in the tongue movement for /a͡ɪ/ is illustrated in Figure 4.20. This drawing was obtained from X-ray films of diphthong /a͡ɪ/ uttered at two different speaking rates, slow and fast. For the slow production shown in *(a)*, the tongue movement is much greater than for the fast production shown in *(b)*. Indeed, both acoustic and X-ray studies have shown that diphthongs produced at increasingly faster rates of speech have progressively smaller movements, up to some limiting movement needed for recognition of the sound. Figure 4.20 shows that a diphthong does not have a stable and invariant offglide. In fact, the onglide also varies somewhat with phonetic context and speaking rate (Kent, 1970).

Thus, the diphthong cannot be defined as a movement from one invariant vocal tract configuration to another invariant vocal tract configuration. Neither the configuration of the onglide or offglide nor the amount of articulator movement is constant from one condition to another. The phonetic symbols used to represent diphthongs are thus best approximations and should not be taken literally

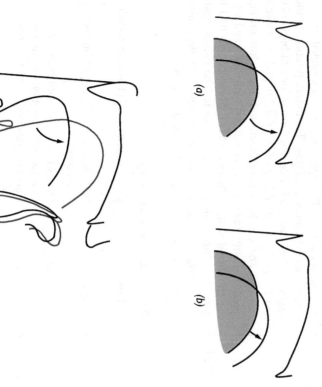

FIGURE 4.20
Articulations of diphthong /a͡ɪ/ *(bye)* at a slow speaking rate *(a)* and a rapid speaking rate *(b)*. Onglide position is shown by shaded region and offglide position by the heavy outline. At the more rapid rate, tongue movement is reduced.

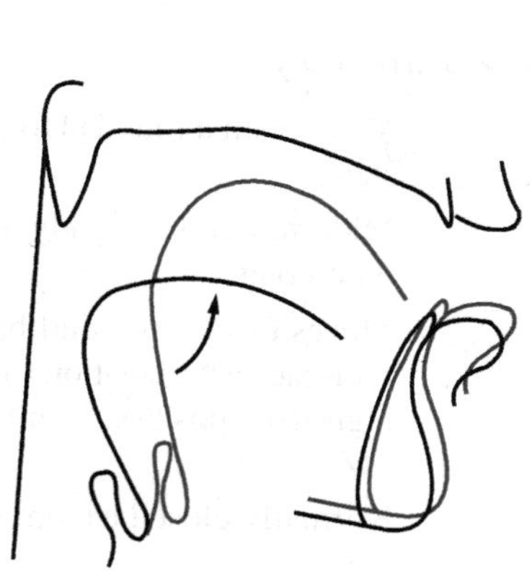

FIGURE 4.21
Articulation of diphthong /a͡ɪ/ *(bye)* shown as onglide (black line) and offglide (blue line) configurations.

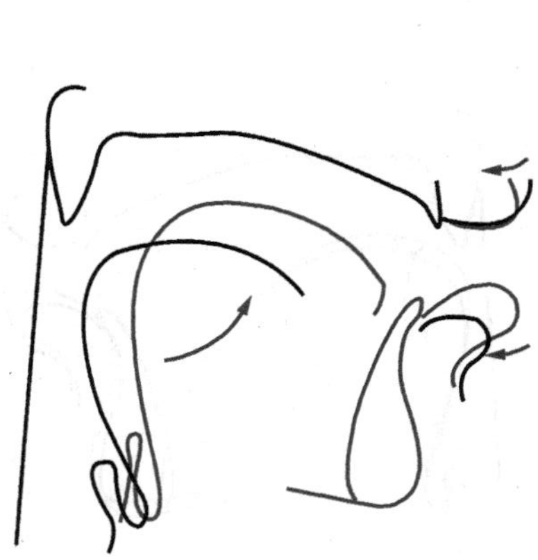

FIGURE 4.22
Articulation of diphthong /ɔ͡ɪ/ *(boy)* shown as onglide (black line) and offglide (blue line) configurations.

as accurate descriptions of the movements that a speaker makes. A given diphthong actually has a range of onglide and offglide configurations.

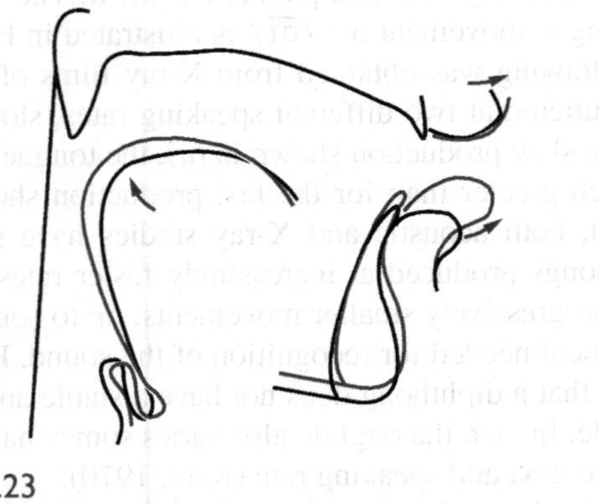

FIGURE 4.23
Articulation of diphthong /a͡ʊ/ *(bough)* shown as onglide (black line) and offglide (blue line) configurations.

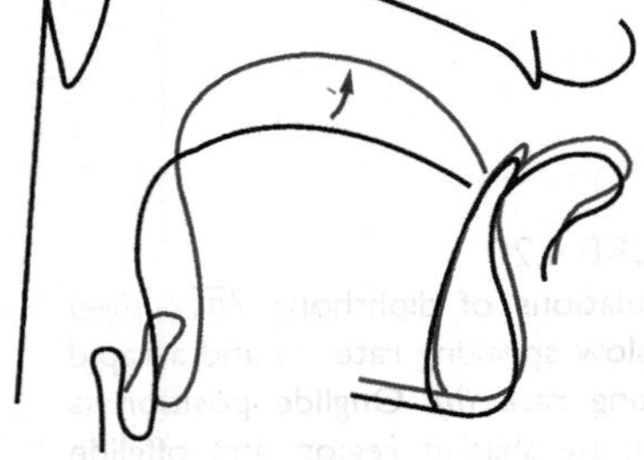

FIGURE 4.24
Articulation of diphthong /e͡ɪ/ *(bay)* shown as onglide (black line) and offglide (blue line) configurations.

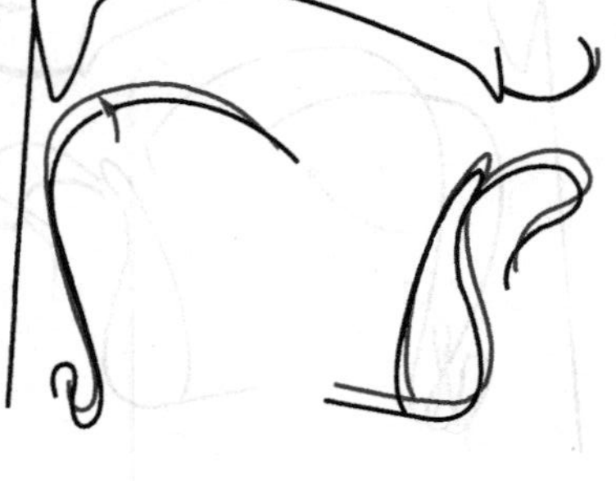

FIGURE 4.25
Articulation of diphthong /o͡ʊ/ *(bow)* shown as onglide (black line) and offglide (blue line) configurations.

Articulatory Summary

Lips:	Unrounded; usually make a slight to moderate closing motion during the diphthong.
Jaw:	Mid-open to open for the onglide, then closes somewhat for the offglide.
Tongue:	Moves from a low-back onglide to a mid-front or high-front offglide. The onglide is similar to /a/ or /ɑ/ and the offglide may be like /e/, /ɪ/, or /i/.
Velopharynx:	Normally closed, except for nasal contexts.

Allophonic Variations. See nasalized vowels and monophthongization.

Transcription Words

sigh	style	n*igh*ttime
*ai*sle	m*igh*t	Fr*i*day
m*i*ne	s*i*lo	W*y*oming
t*y*ke	r*i*ot	*rhy*me
l*i*ke	tr*i*al	*i*ce
br*i*ne	l*igh*tning	b*i*cycle

Diphthong /ɔ͡ɪ/ (Boy; Figure 4.22)

This diphthong is produced with coordinated movements of the lips and tongue. The lips move from a rounded or protruded state to an unrounded state. The tongue position for the onglide is low-mid-back, like that for /ɔ/, or mid-back, like that for /o/. The similarity of the /ɔ͡ɪ/ onglide to vowels /ɔ/ and /o/ can be demonstrated with the words *tawing* (produced with /ɔ/), *toeing* (produced with /o/), and *toying* (produced with diphthong /ɔ͡ɪ/). Some people find it difficult to distinguish these three words. The tongue position for the offglide is mid-front to high-front, depending upon stress, speaking rate, and phonetic context.

Articulatory Summary

Lips:	Move from a rounded to an unrounded state.
Jaw:	Mid; may close slightly during the diphthong.
Tongue:	Moves from a low-mid-back /ɔ/ or mid-back /o/ position to a mid-to-high-front position, similar to /e/, /ɪ/, or /i/.
Velopharynx:	Normally closed except for nasal contexts.

Allophonic Variations. See nasalized vowels and monophthongization.

Transcription Words

pl*oy*	sirl*oi*n	dec*oy*
t*oy*	typh*oi*d	an*oi*nt
R*oy*	cl*oi*ster	f*oy*er
sp*oi*l	all*oy*	destr*oy*
b*oi*l	r*oy*al	ann*oy*
*oi*l	p*oi*nt	turqu*oi*se

Diphthong /ɑ͞ʊ/ (*Bough*; Figure 4.23)

The lips and tongue have coordinated movements of rounding and raising, respectively. As was the case for /ɑ͞ɪ/, the onglide of /ɑ͞ʊ/ in Midwestern speech is highly similar to vowel /ɑ/ and may be described as low-back or low-mid-back. As shown in the illustration, the tongue makes a raising motion of small extent, toward the position for /ʊ/. The lips are unrounded and usually relatively open for the onglide, then they gradually move to a rounded state for the offglide. The IPA symbol /a͞ʊ/ is misleading in that, strictly speaking, it indicates a tongue movement from low-front to high-mid-back. But, as shown in Figure 4.23, the movement is almost entirely one of raising from a low-back or low-mid-back position.

Articulatory Summary

Lips:	Move from a relatively open, unrounded state to a rounded state.
Jaw:	Mid-open to open for the onglide; often closes somewhat for the offglide.
Tongue:	Moves from an onglide position of low-back (similar to /ɑ/) or low-mid-back (similar to /ɔ/) to an offglide position of mid-back (similar to /o/) or high-mid-back (similar to /ʊ/).
Velopharynx:	Normally closed except in nasal contexts.

Allophonic Variations. See nasalized vowels and monophthongization.

Transcription Words

c*ow*	*ou*ster	h*ou*sewife
r*ou*nd	d*ow*nt*ow*n	*ou*tcast
fl*ou*t	t*ow*er	d*ou*btful
cl*ow*n	al*ou*d	d*ow*nsp*ou*t
st*ou*t	ast*ou*nd	tr*au*ma
c*ou*ch	ch*ow*der	*ou*rselves

Diphthong /e͞ɪ/ (*Bay*; Figure 4.24)

Diphthong /e͞ɪ/ is essentially an allophone, alternating with the monophthong /e/. The diphthong is more likely to occur when the syllable is strongly stressed or the speaking rate is slow. The articulatory positions for the onglide are those for vowel /e/, and the positions for the offglide are roughly those for /ɪ/. However, the actual extent of tongue and jaw movement varies with stress, speaking rate, and phonetic context.

Articulatory Summary

Lips:	Mid-open and unrounded.
Jaw:	Mid; may close somewhat during the diphthong.
Tongue:	Moves from a mid-front /e/ to a high-mid-front /ɪ/.
Velopharynx:	Normally closed except in nasal contexts.

Allophonic Variations. See nasalized vowels, monophthongization, and vowel /e/.

Transcription Words

w*ay*	m*ay*be	l*ay*man
p*ai*d	n*ei*ghbor	str*aigh*t
tr*a*de	fianc*ee*	dissu*a*de
*eigh*t	tod*ay*	s*ai*lor
st*ea*k	w*ay*side	h*a*lo
wh*ey*	par*a*de	d*ay*time

Diphthong /o͞ʊ/ (*Bow*; Figure 4.25)

Diphthong /o͞ʊ/ alternates allophonically with /o/. The diphthong is more likely to occur when the syllable is strongly stressed or the speaking rate is slow. The onglide is vowel /o/: mid-back tongue position and rounded lips. The offglide is essentially vowel /ʊ/: high-mid-back tongue position and rounded lips. The diphthong gesture can be characterized as a raising tongue movement and a slight narrowing of the lips.

Articulatory Summary

Lips:	Rounded with progressive narrowing.
Jaw:	Mid-open; often closes slightly during the diphthong.
Tongue:	Moves from a mid-back /o/ position to a high-mid-back /ʊ/.
Velopharynx:	Normally closed except in nasal contexts.

Allophonic Variations. See nasalized vowels, monophthongization, and vowel /o/.

Transcription Words

m*o*de	br*oo*ch	sh*ou*lder
n*o*	y*eo*man	b*o*lder
sl*ow*	m*o*lded	t*oa*ster
b*eau*	sn*ow*man	ab*o*de
h*oe*	*ow*ner	r*oa*ming
s*ew*	l*oa*ned	r*o*lling

Special Notes on the Phonetic Properties of Vowels

Some Cautions about Vowel Features

The terms used in this book to describe vowel articulation were chosen for their simplicity and general relevance to observed patterns of vowel articulation. However, these terms are not entirely accurate for all speakers. For example, it is not exactly true that the vowels within the front, central, or back series are always satisfactorily distinguished by descriptions of tongue height. Ladefoged (1971) commented that the tongue shapes for the back vowels "can be considered as differing simply in terms of the single parameter called tongue height only [by] neglecting large and varied differences in the front–back dimension" (p. 69). Differences in the front–back dimension (advancement) are evident in Figure 4.15. For example, the tongue position for /u/ and /o/ is more fronted than the position for /ɑ/. In view of these difficulties in the description of tongue height, phoneticians have sought other descriptions of vowel articulation.

Ladefoged (1971) concluded that there is no one simple set of parameters that is equally accurate for describing the tongue shapes of different vowels. Similarly, Nearey (1978) remarked in his evaluation of phonetic feature systems for vowels that "It would appear that neither the traditional features nor recent modifications of them stand up to empirical tests.... Indeed, empirical research since the thirties has produced evidence that weighs heavily against the notion of invariant articulatory specification in anything like that implied by traditional phonetic theory" (p. 69).

Even the description of tongue height for the front vowels is not without contradictions. Russell (1928); Ladefoged, DeClerk, Lindau, and Papcun (1972); and Nearey (1978) reported that actual measurements of tongue height show that /e/ and /æ/ can be higher than /ɪ/, in disagreement with traditional phonetic theory.

Matters are even worse for the tense–lax distinction, especially when articulatory correlates for this dimension are sought in studies of tongue shape. Although Perkell (1971) proposed that vowels usually called "tense" have an advanced tongue root and that vowels usually called "lax" have a constricted pharynx, Ladefoged et al. (1972) and Nearey (1978) did not confirm these observations. One study of the electrical activity in contracting muscles (electromyography) provided only modest support for the idea that tense vowels involve greater muscle activity. Raphael and Bell-Berti (1975) reported that, of twelve muscles studied with this method, only two showed consistently greater activity for the tense vowels than for the lax vowels. Generally, the durational difference between tense and lax vowels has fared better than other correlates when tests are made. Tense vowels are longer in duration than lax vowels.

Obviously, systems of articulatory description for vowels are not perfect. The system used in this book should be used with that recognition. It should suffice for general articulatory description and most clinical purposes, but its details should not be accepted uncritically. It is partly because of the inadequacies of phonetic feature systems for vowels that we include many drawings based on X-ray pictures of vowel articulation. Where verbal descriptions fail, these drawings should help to fill the gap. It is recommended that the illustrations be studied closely and compared against the vowel features used in verbal description.

Tongue and Jaw Interaction

It has been proposed that when the tongue positions for different vowels are compared relative to the jaw, the tongue shapes fall into a small number of groups or families (Lindblom & Sundberg, 1969). An illustration of this idea is shown in Figure 4.26 for vowels produced by author Kent. Note that the front vowels /i/, /ɛ/, and /æ/ have fairly similar shapes and might be grouped together as one family. Vowels /o/, /ɑ/, and /ʌ/ might be grouped in another family. Vowel /u/ has a tongue shape unlike that for any other vowel but quite similar to that for the velar consonants (the final sounds in the words *back, dog,* and *ring*). These results may indicate that a talker does not have to make as many adjustments of the tongue as there are vowels in the language. A small number of tongue shapes, combined with various positions of the jaw (and lips) can suffice to produce several different vowels. The three basic tongue shapes for author Kent are shown in Figure 4.27. The shape drawn with a solid line represents the front vowels fairly well; the shape drawn with a dotted line satisfactorily represents low-back to mid-back vowels; and the shape drawn with a dashed line represents the high-back vowel /u/.

Of course, one should bear in mind that a speaker can produce all of the English vowels while clenching a pencil between the teeth or with the jaw propped open (Figure 4.2). Hence, we know that the tongue, without the aid of jaw movement, can make adequate adjustments for the vowels of English. What results like those in Figure 4.26 may tell us is that, when both tongue and jaw are free to vary, the tongue tends to assume a small number of preferred shapes relative to the jaw.

Lip and Jaw Interaction

The general remarks made about tongue and jaw interaction apply as well to the interaction between lip and jaw. Usually,

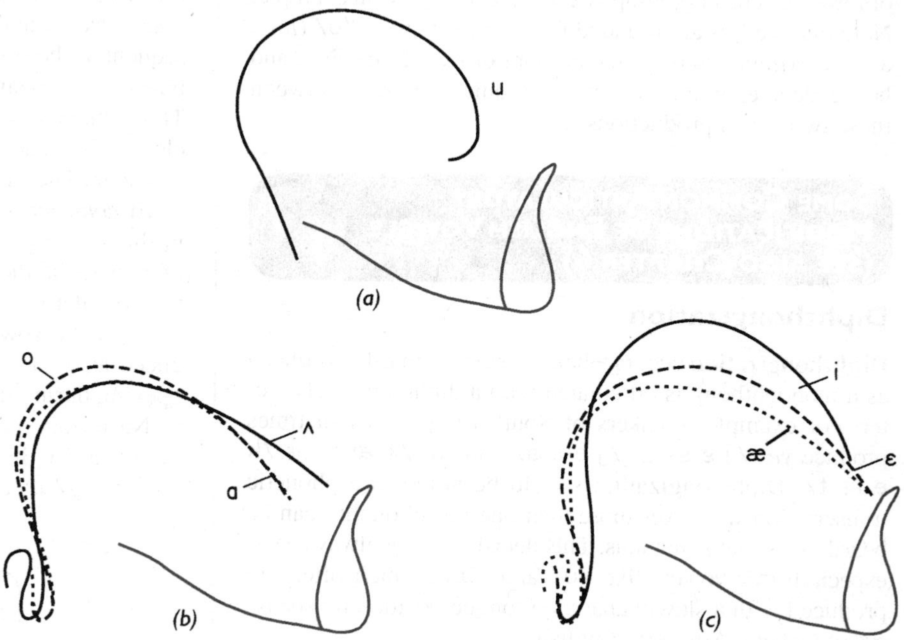

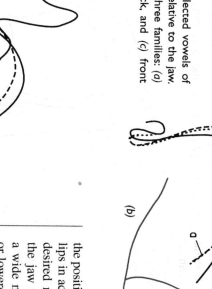

FIGURE 4.26
Tongue shapes for selected vowels of author Kent, shown relative to the jaw. The shapes fall into three families: *(a)* high-back, *(b)* low-back, and *(c)* front vowels.

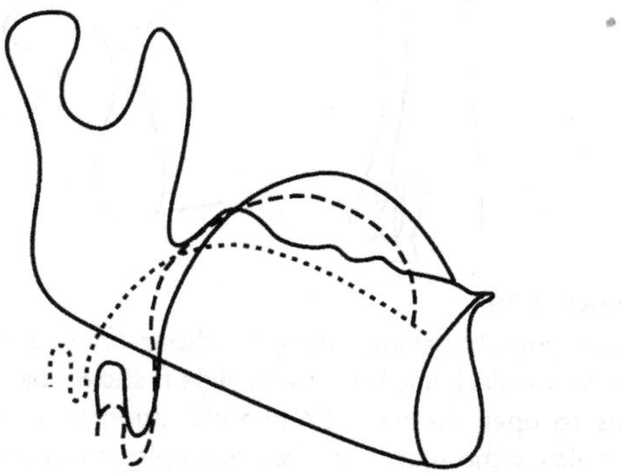

FIGURE 4.27
Three basic tongue shapes for author Kent derived from the shape families illustrated in Figure 4.26.

the position of the jaw during speech is controlled to assist the lips in achieving a desired mouth opening. Hence, when the desired mouth opening is one of narrowing or rounding, the jaw typically is closed or elevated. Conversely, when a wide mouth opening is desired, the jaw usually is open or lowered. However, when the jaw is not free to move, as in the case of a pipe smoker, the lips can function independently to make the appropriate changes in mouth opening. In addition, a given phonetic feature of lip articulation can be accomplished while the jaw satisfies one of two opposing articulatory requirements. Consider, for example, the feature of rounding for the back vowels. Because the rounded back vowels have jaw positions ranging from relatively closed (/u/ in *who*) to relatively open (/ɔ/ in *law*), the feature of rounding must be accomplished whether the jaw is elevated

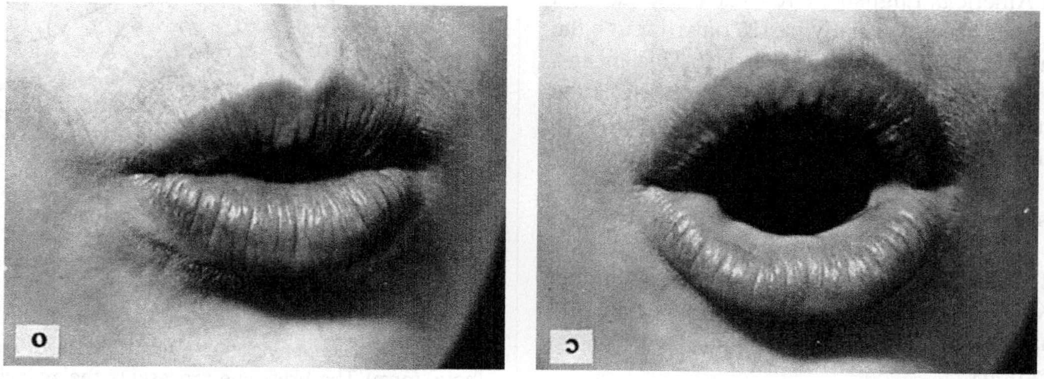

FIGURE 4.28
Photographs of the mouth opening for the vowels /o/ *(low)* and /ɔ/ *(law)*. Notice that the lips can be rounded in association with different degrees of mouth opening (jaw elevation).

or lowered. The photographs in Figure 4.28 give an example. Note that the lips are rounded for both the vowels /o/ (*low*) and /ɔ/ (*law*), although the amount of mouth opening, and hence degree of jaw lowering, is quite different between these two vowel productions.

Some Common Articulatory Modifications of English Vowels (see also Chapter 6)

Diphthongization

Diphthongization occurs when a vowel ordinarily produced as a monophthong is articulated with a diphthongal character. For example, speakers of Southern speech sometimes produce *yes* /j ɛ s/ as /j e ə s/ and *cat* /k æ t/ as /k e æ t/. Diphthongization should be noted in a phonetic transcription whenever more than one vowel quality can be heard in a syllable nucleus. This decision is not always easy, especially for vowels like /u/ and /æ/, which often are produced with a slowly changing tongue position by speakers of General American English.

Monophthongization

Monophthongization means that a diphthong is produced as a monophthong, or single-element vowel. For example, a speaker who says /ɑ/ for /ɑ͡ɪ/, as often happens in Southern speech, is monophthongizing diphthong /ɑ͡ɪ/. This modification is transcribed with the symbol of the single vowel element that replaces the diphthong. As noted in the discussion of diphthongs, /e͡ɪ/ and /o͡ʊ/ tend to be produced as the monophthongs /e/ and /o/, respectively, at rapid rates of speech or when they are not strongly stressed. The diphthongs /ɑ͡ɪ/, /a͡ʊ/, and /ɔ͡ɪ/ do not have monophthong allophones in General American English.

Nasalization

Isolated vowels and diphthongs produced by normal speakers of General American English are resonated and radiated orally; that is, sound energy usually passes only through the oral cavity and not through the nasal cavity. This means, in articulatory terms, that the velopharynx is closed as the vowel is produced. But when English vowels and diphthongs are produced in the context of nasal segments, they usually are **nasalized** to some degree. Velopharyngeal opening for a preceding nasal segment is maintained during the vowel or diphthong, and velopharyngeal opening for a following nasal segment is anticipated during the vowel or diphthong. Of course, a vowel or diphthong that is both preceded and followed by nasal segments, like /i/ in *mean,* is influenced from both directions.

Velopharyngeal opening of the anticipatory kind is illustrated for the articulation of diphthong /ɑ͡ɪ/ in Figure 4.29. The black line represents the diphthong onglide and the blue line, the diphthong offglide. Because this diphthong was followed by a nasal consonant, the velopharynx begins to open during the diphthongal movement of the tongue. Consequently, the diphthong is nasalized. A conspicuous velopharyngeal opening can be seen for the diphthong offglide. Thus, the velopharynx is already open by the time the oral closure is made for the following nasal consonant, in this case /n/. The same pattern can be seen for vowel /ɑ/ in the word *contract* (noun form) in Figure 4.30. The black line in this figure shows the articulatory positions at the instant of release of the consonant /k/, and the blue line shows the articulatory positions assumed during the mid-point (in time) of the vowel /ɑ/. Obviously, the vowel will be produced as a nasalized sound because of the velopharyngeal opening during the vowel articulation.

Nasalization of a vowel rarely, if ever, will alter the meaning of an English word. The word *eye* (or *I*), phonetically diphthong /ɑ͡ɪ/, means the same thing to a listener whether

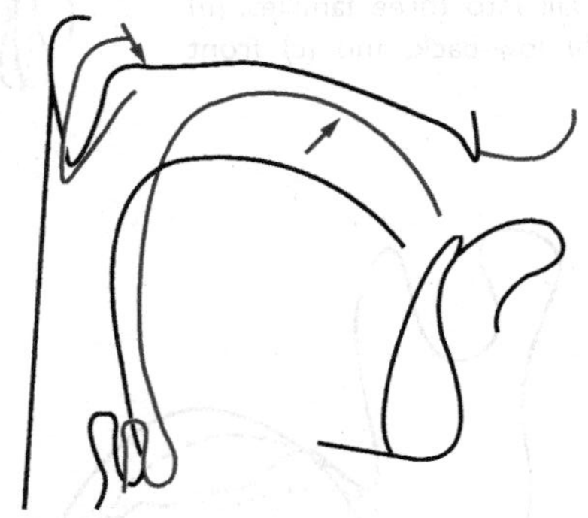

FIGURE 4.29
Velopharyngeal opening during diphthong /ɑ͡ɪ/. Diphthong onglide is shown by black line, and the offglide is shown by blue line. Velum begins to open during /ɑ͡ɪ/ in anticipation of a nasal consonant that follows the diphthong; for example, the phrase *I know* /ɑ͡ɪ n o͡ʊ/.

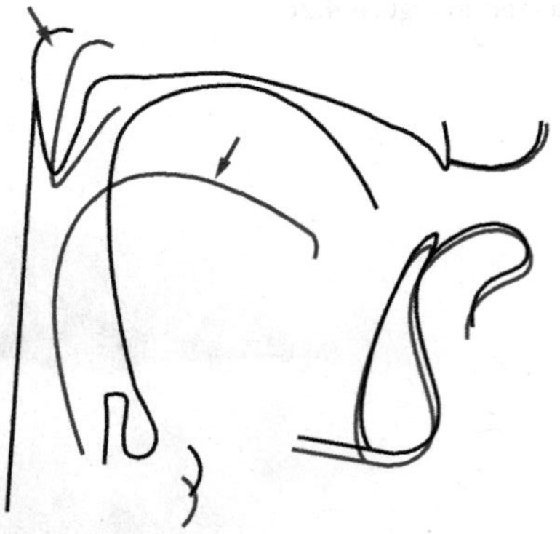

FIGURE 4.30
Velopharyngeal opening in the first syllable of the word *contract* (noun form). The black line represents the articulatory configuration at the beginning of movement from the first consonant (contract) to the following vowel (contract). The blue line represents the configuration for vowel /ɑ/, which is nasalized in anticipation of the following nasal consonant (contract).

the vowel is produced with or without nasal resonance. In other words, vowel nasalization is allophonic in English. Furthermore, the nasalized allophone is in complementary distribution (this term is discussed in Chapter 2) to the oral (nonnasalized) vowel allophone, because the nasal variant normally occurs only in the context of nasal sounds. Because a nasalized vowel is an allophonic member of a family (the vowel phoneme), the feature of nasalization does not change the phoneme symbol. Hence, phoneme /i/ includes both the oral and nasal allophones. The occurrence of nasalization is transcribed by adding a diacritic mark to the phonetic symbol, which is placed within brackets rather than virgules. Diacritic marks are discussed in detail in Chapter 6. For the moment, suffice it to say that the nasal allophone of a vowel phoneme is indicated by the special mark placed over the symbol that identifies the vowel. For example, the nasalized vowel in *mean* is transcribed phonetically as [ĩ].

Reduction

Reduction was discussed in connection with the schwa /ə/, and a general diagram of reduction was shown in Figure 4.14. Reduction occurs as the rate of speaking increases or as the stress on a vowel is decreased. For example, as the stress on the second syllable of the word *educate* is progressively lessened, the vowel tends to change from /u/ to /ʊ/ and from /ʊ/ to /ə/. Reduction can be characterized along the two dimensions of length (duration) and centralization. As a vowel is reduced, its duration decreases, and it is articulated more toward the center of the oral cavity. The schwa vowel /ə/ represents the limit of reduction because it has the shortest duration of all vowels (Klatt [1976] says that unstressed vowels like schwa reach the compression limit of vowel production) and because it is produced with a central tongue position. Generally, centralization can be represented along vectors or lines within the quadrilateral diagram of vowel articulation (Figure 4.14). The vowel changes in the second syllable of *educate* can be represented as articulatory changes along a line that runs from /u/ to /ʊ/ to /ə/. Shortening of vowel duration and centralization of the vowel articulation tend to co-occur because, as the duration of a vowel is decreased, there is less time for the articulators to reach extreme positions (that is, positions near the sides of the quadrilateral diagram). Reduction is a powerful factor in the articulation of vowels in context.

THE ELASTIC VOWEL

Vowels are elastic speech sounds that undergo adjustments in duration because of various factors, both intrinsic and extrinsic. Intrinsic factors are inherent to vowel identity; for example, tense vowels have a longer duration than lax vowels. Children acquire the duration difference between tense and lax vowels relatively early. Ko (2007) showed that this difference is present in children's speech by the age of 2 years. Extrinsic factors are those pertaining to the larger context of vowel production—factors such as:

(a) Speaking rate: Vowels are longer at slower rates than at faster rates.
(b) Stress pattern: Vowels are longer in stressed than unstressed syllables.
(c) The number of syllables in a word: Vowels tend to be longer in words of few syllables,
(d) Characteristics of the listener or communication channel: Mothers lengthen their vowels when speaking to their young children ("motherese," as discussed in Chapter 6), and speakers produce longer vowels when they are trying to be understood over a noisy communication channel.

Dialects of American English can have different vowel durations. Jacewicz, Fox, and Salmons (2007) compared vowel durations in three dialects and discovered that durations were longest in the South, shortest in the Inland North, and intermediate in the Midlands.

Rhotacization and Derhotacization

The vowels /ɝ/ and /ɚ/ (f*ur*th*er*) always carry *r* coloring; other vowels can carry *r* coloring when they occur adjacent to /r/. For example, the /ɔ/ in *morning* [m ɔ r n ɪ ŋ] is colored by, or affected by, the following /r/. Following Ladefoged (1975), we refer to this *r* coloring of a vowel as rhotacization (or rhotacism). Thus, a rhotacized vowel is one with *r* coloring, and it occurs in normal speech adjacent to /r/. The term **derhotacization** (or derhotacism) applies to a situation in which a normally *r*-colored vowel loses all or part of the *r* color. See the discussion of /r/ in Chapter 5 for the articulatory correlates of rhotacization.

Other Modifications

A more complete listing of articulatory modifications of vowels is given in Chapter 6, which also defines diacritic marks for transcription.

ALLOGRAPHS OF THE VOWEL PHONEMES OF ENGLISH

In Chapter 2, *allograph* was defined as any one alphabet letter or combination of letters that represents a particular phoneme. Any one phoneme usually can be spelled in a number of ways, and any one alphabet letter often can be used to represent different sounds. Table 4.4 gives the allographs for the vowel phonemes of English. Each allograph is italicized in a sample word. For example, for phoneme /i/, some allographs are the *e* in *be,* the *ee* in *see,* and the *ea* in *eat.* In each list of allographs, the most common ones are given first.

TABLE 4.4
Allographs of the Vowel Phonemes of English

Phoneme	Allograph (Italicized in Sample Word)
/i/	be, see, eat, marine, key, either, chief, Caesar, people, aeon, debris, Phoenix, quay
/ɪ/	it, pretty, hear, hymn, here (e-e), sheer, weird, been, busy, sieve, women, built, give (i-e)
/e/ or /eɪ/	fate, rain, steak, reign, eight, prey, sachet, gauge, say
/ɛ/	bed, head, there (e-e), care (a-e), air, their, aerial, any, says, heifer, leopard, friend, bury, aesthetic, guest
/æ/	hat, plaid, laugh, have (a-e), meringue
/ɑ/	top, was, palm, heart, guard, knowledge, honest, bazaar, sergeant, ah (and frequently in words containing ar, e.g., bar)
/ɔ/	haunt, yawn, caught, ought, cloth, all, George, abroad (speakers vary in the pronunciation of these words)
/o/ or /oʊ/	bold, home (o-e), sow, hoe, sew, though, boat, brooch, yeoman, beau, chauffeur, soul
/ʊ/	book, put, would, bosom
/u/	hoot, to, true, blew, shoe, you, rule (u-e), fruit, lose (o-e), lieu, Sioux, Sault, through, beauty (as part of a /ju/ combination), two, rheumatic, gnu, queue
/ʌ/	cut, done (o-e), rough, son, does, blood
/ə/	Can be spelled by virtually any of the orthographic vowels of English and by many combinations of these orthographic vowels
/ɝ/	her, burn, bird, learn, worm, purr, journey, Myrtle, restaurant, search, curd
/ɚ/	father, labor, tapir, martyr, murmur, acre
/ɑɪ/	find, ride (i-e), by, aisle, ay, eye, dye, night, die, buy, height, type (y-e)
/ɑʊ/	out, cow, bough, Faust, Macleod
/ɔɪ/	oil, toy

VOWELS IN THE ENGLISH ALPHABET

As we all learned in elementary school, if not even earlier, the English alphabet has only five vowels, A, E, I, O, U (and sometimes Y for words like *city*). But as you have seen in this chapter, the English phonetic system has fourteen or fifteen vowels, depending on dialect, along with five diphthongs. This discrepancy is one example of how the alphabet for the writing of English differs from the phonetics of the language. Because the alphabet is very limited in its notation of vowels, dictionaries give advice on pronunciation by using special characters called *diacritics*. As one example, consider the short and long vowels in words like *apple* (short vowel) and *ape* (long vowel). Dictionaries typically indicate a short vowel with a special symbol called a *breve* (/briv/; from the Latin for *short* or *brief*) that is placed over the alphabet character. Long vowels are marked with another symbol called a *macron*. Notice that the name of the vowels in the English alphabet correspond to the long vowel. Therefore, the name of the letter A is /eɪ/ and the name of the letter E is /i/. As we will discover in Chapter 6, phonetic transcription also makes use of diacritics to mark sound variations.

FREQUENCY OF OCCURRENCE FOR ENGLISH VOWELS

Data on the frequency of occurrence of English vowels are given in Appendix B, and it is a good idea to spend some time examining the tabled data to learn how unequally different vowels are used in our language. Figure 4.31 summarizes one of the major conclusions. This illustration shows the relative frequency of occurrence of front, central, and back vowels as proportionate areas of a quadrilateral. Note that front vowels are used to a much greater degree than either central or back vowels and that the central vowels occur more frequently than the back vowels. As Figure 4.31 shows, the front vowels make

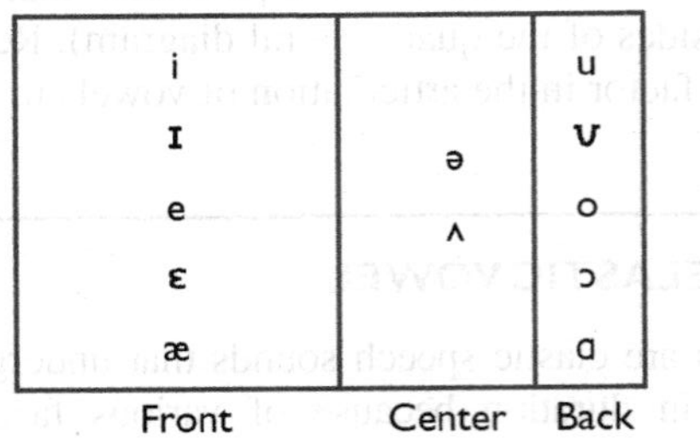

FIGURE 4.31
Relative frequency of occurrence of front, central, and back vowels, shown as proportions of a quadrilateral. Based on the data of Mines, Hanson, and Shoup (1978).

up about 50 percent of the total frequency of occurrence data for English vowels. Because rounded vowels are generally back vowels, it is also implicit from this illustration that lip rounding for vowels is used relatively infrequently compared to neutral or retracted lip shapes. For other breakdowns of the frequency of occurrence data, see Appendix B.

CARDINAL VOWELS

The word *cardinal* is borrowed from the four principal points of the compass—north, south, east and west. In the early 1900s, the phonetician Daniel Jones (1917) sought to define a set of reference points for vowels, specifying the positions of the tongue and lips. The cardinal vowels are described in terms of tongue advancement (either front or back), tongue height (with the four gradations of close, half-close, half-open, and open), and lip position (rounded or spread) (Figure 4.32). Three cardinal vowels, [i], [a] and [u], are defined in articulatory terms. Vowel [i] is made with the tongue in its most forward and high position, and with spread lips. Vowel [u] is made with the tongue in its most back and high position, and with pursed lips. Vowel [a] is made with the tongue in its lowest and most back position. The other vowels are considered to be "auditorily equidistant" between these three corner vowels and are specified with four degrees of aperture or "height": close (high tongue position), close-mid, open-mid, and open (low tongue position).

Jones proposed two systems, primary and secondary. In the primary system, the front vowels are spread and the back vowels are rounded. The secondary system reverses this pattern, so that the front vowels are rounded and the back vowels are spread. Jones believed that any two adjacent cardinal vowels represented the same degree of acoustic separation. Over the years, the cardinal vowel system has had both advocates and detractors. It is associated with the British tradition in phonetics and is not even mentioned in some contemporary textbooks on phonetics. The idea of cardinal vowels is attractive because they would serve as referents for all other vowels. Cardinality rests on the assumption of an invariant tongue position. But, as Wise (1957a) wrote, "Actually only the vowels at the corners of the diagram . . . can properly be called cardinal vowels, for they and they alone can be reproduced invariably with the same tongue position" (p. 86). Other authorities doubt that even the corner vowels have invariant tongue positions.

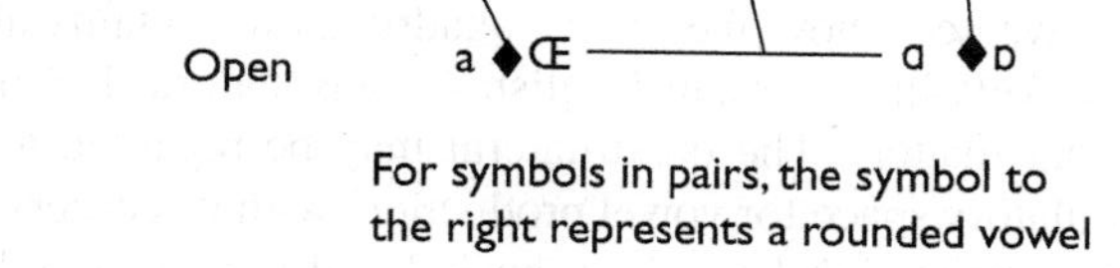

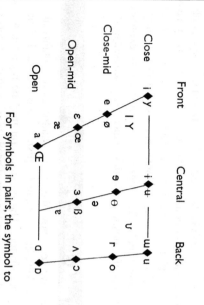

FIGURE 4.32
For symbols in pairs, the symbol to the right represents a rounded vowel.

VOWELS AROUND THE WORLD

American English uses only a fraction of the possible vowels in a natural language. It is not clear exactly how many different vowels are used in all of the languages of the world, but one source of information to answer this question is the UCLA Phonological Segment Inventory Database, abbreviated UPSID (Maddieson, 1984). This database provides valuable information on the phonetic inventories of 317 languages. (A more recent version is based on 451 languages; Maddieson & Precoda, 1990.) Schwartz, Boe, Vallee, and Abry (1997) analyzed UPSID to determine the major patterns in the vowel inventories of the represented languages. Figure 4.33 shows the grid for 37 different vowel symbols in UPSID. Although these 37 vowels may not cover all of the possible vowels in the world's languages, they go a long way toward this goal. Schwartz et al. reached several conclusions about vowel inventories, some of which are summarized here:

1. Languages first select vowels from a primary vowel system of three to nine vowels that have a high frequency of occurrence across languages and for which duration (length) is the typical modification. In this primary system, five to seven vowels are particularly favored. Most languages select the three corner vowels /i/, /a/, and /u/. The triangle formed by these vowels is therefore a basic pattern selected by a large number of languages.

2. For languages that have more than about nine vowels, the additional vowels (from one to seven) are selected from a new dimension. Schwartz and colleagues termed these vowels a secondary system. The favored number of vowels in this system is five.

3. The vowels in both the primary and secondary systems are concentrated at the periphery of the vowel grid (i.e., the sides of the vowel quadrilateral), usually with a balance between front and back vowels. American English is a good example of a balanced front–back system. For languages without such a balance, front vowels generally outnumber back vowels.

4. The preferred nonperipheral (i.e., not located on the sides of the quadrilateral) vowel is the schwa. Because the occurrence of schwa apparently does not interact

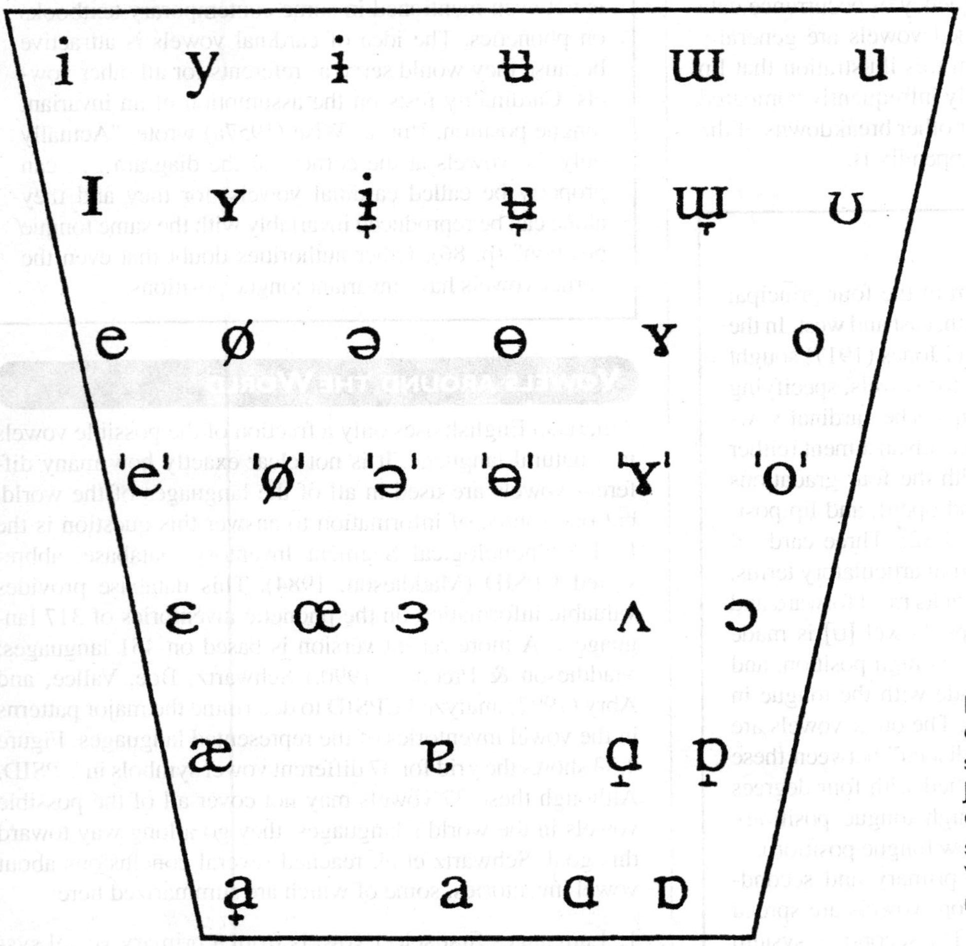

FIGURE 4.33
Grid for representing the 37 vowel symbols in UPSID. Reprinted from J. L. Schwartz, L.-J. Boe, N. Vallee, and C. Abry (1997), "Major trends in vowel system inventories." *Journal of Phonetics*, Volume 25, p. 236. Reprinted with permission of Academic Press. Copyright 1997.

with other vowel selections in a system, it is considered a "parallel" vowel. Selection of schwa may be based on intrinsic principles such as vowel reduction.

The vowel grid in Figure 4.33 is useful for several purposes beyond an inventory of the world's vowels. It can be used to compare different languages and, for example, to understand some of the issues in learning a new language. Consider a child whose first language (L1) is Spanish (a five-vowel system, consisting of the vowels /i e a o u/) but is acquiring American English as a second language (L2). One of the main tasks, then, is to acquire several additional vowels, including some that differ in duration or length from the vowels in the Spanish system. The same general situation would apply to a child whose first language is modern Hebrew or Japanese (both of which are five-vowel systems similar to Spanish). But now consider a child whose L1 is Korean, which has the ten vowels /i ɨ e ɛ ɑ o ø u y ʌ/. In this case, some of the L1 vowels do not carry over to American English as an L2. In particular, the rounded front vowels /ø/ and /y/ do not occur in American English. If we reverse the situation and consider a child whose L1 is American English and who is learning Korean as L2, we see that this child must learn two rounded front vowels.

A general conclusion from studies of L2 vowel acquisition is that the difficulty of learning the new vowels depends on their similarity to vowels in L1. A vowel in L2 is difficult to learn if it is similar, but not identical, to a vowel in L1. Apparently, the similarity creates an interference between the new sound to be learned and a vowel in the original phonetic system. In contrast, a vowel in L2 is relatively easy to learn if it is quite different from any vowel in L1. The new L2 vowel is readily adopted because it does not compete with vowels in L1. The degree of similarity can be expressed in terms of acoustic properties, which are discussed next.

The Acoustic Properties of Vowels

We have seen how the vowel quadrilateral contains all of the vowels in American English (or any natural language, for that matter). The quadrilateral may be regarded as the articulatory space for vowel production, with its corners representing the high-front, high-back, low-front, and low-back articulatory extremes. This articulatory vowel space has an acoustic counterpart, an **acoustic vowel space**. To understand this acoustic space, we need to introduce some concepts on the acoustics of speech.

The Vocal Tract as a Resonator

Recall that a vowel is produced with an open vocal tract. In normal voiced speech, the energy source for vowels is the vibration of the vocal folds. (When we whisper a vowel, the energy source is a noise, but the present discussion centers on normally voiced vowels). The energy source of voicing is very similar for all vowels—so similar, in fact, that we can assume for the moment that it is exactly the same. What makes vowels different (phonetically identifiable) is what happens to the source energy as it passes through the vocal tract. The vocal tract is a **resonator**, meaning that it selectively reinforces certain aspects of sound. For each vowel configuration (combination of tongue height and advancement, along with lip rounding), there is a particular set of resonances, called **formants**. This description corresponds to a major theory of speech production called the **source-filter theory**, which states that energy from the source (vibrating vocal folds in the larynx) is filtered or modified by the resonances of the vocal tract. For vowels, the source energy is a buzzing type of sound that does not sound like any particular vowel. It is rather like a drone. This energy passes through the vocal tract, eventually emanating through the lips, where it is called **radiated acoustic energy**. The radiated energy shaped by the vocal tract reaches our ears, and it is this sound that we can identify as a particular vowel and assign to it a phonetic symbol.

When we hear a given vowel, we detect a particular combination of formants that defines the vowel. Formants can be visualized in an acoustic analysis called a **spectrogram**, which, as schematized in Figure 4.34, is a three-dimensional display of sound. The horizontal dimension is time (proceeding from left to right), the vertical dimension is frequency (low frequencies at the bottom and high frequencies at the top), and the third dimension, expressed as a gray scale or variation in darkness, is energy. These three dimensions suffice to characterize a sound, whether it is human speech, bird call, whale song, or machine noise. At any one point in time, we can see the frequency content of a sound, that is, its energy distribution across frequencies. The basic idea of a spectrogram is that it is a kind of acoustic signature, showing how the **spectrum** (a graph of energy versus frequency; plural **spectra**) changes over time. A spectrogram is like a spectrum with a time dimension, allowing us to visualize how a sound changes over time. When a vowel is prolonged, its spectrogram does not change appreciably over time because there is no change in its articulation and therefore no change in its spectrum. In later chapters, we will examine sounds that have spectra that change markedly over time.

Theoretically, an infinite number of formants are produced in a resonating tube like the vocal tract. However, only the first few formants need to be considered because the higher formants have very little energy and are so high in frequency that they are not transmitted in ordinary telephone conversations. In fact, only three formants are sufficient to make phonetic distinctions among vowels in almost all languages. These are identified as the first formant (F1),

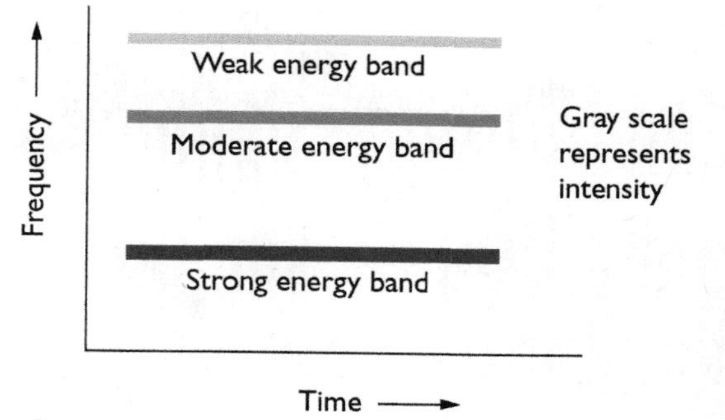

FIGURE 4.34
Basic dimensions of a spectrogram: time, frequency, and energy.

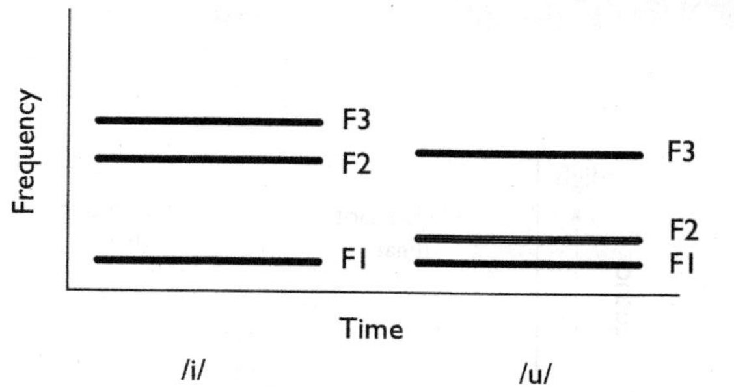

FIGURE 4.35
Stylized spectrograms of the vowels /i/ and /u/, showing the relative locations of the first three formants F1, F2, and F3.

second formant (F2), and third formant (F3). Figure 4.35 is a stylized diagram showing how the three formants appear on a spectrogram for two different vowels. For our purposes, we will consider only one quantitative aspect of formants, the **formant frequency**. This is essentially the frequency at the center or midpoint of the energy band associated with the formant. To be more accurate, then, we can say that each vowel is associated with three frequency values: frequency of F1, frequency of F2, and frequency of F3.

So far, we have looked at highly schematized versions of spectrograms. Let's examine the real thing. Figure 4.36 is a spectrogram of three vowels produced in rapid succession. Notice that all of the vowels are associated with bands of energy that extend horizontally across the spectrogram, rather like caterpillars crawling across the page. These bands, or formants, have a different pattern across the three vowels. When we hear a vowel sound, we are detecting a particular pattern of formants.

We can now return to the idea that there is an acoustic vowel space that corresponds to the articulatory vowel space. To simplify matters, we will consider only two formants, F1 and F2, so that we can depict vowels in a two-dimensional graph. To a first approximation, the frequency of F1 varies inversely with tongue height: the higher the tongue, the lower the frequency of F1. In other words, low vowels have a high F1 frequency, and high vowels have a low F1 frequency. This relationship is shown on the horizontal axis of Figure 4.37. The frequency of F2 varies with the degree of advancement

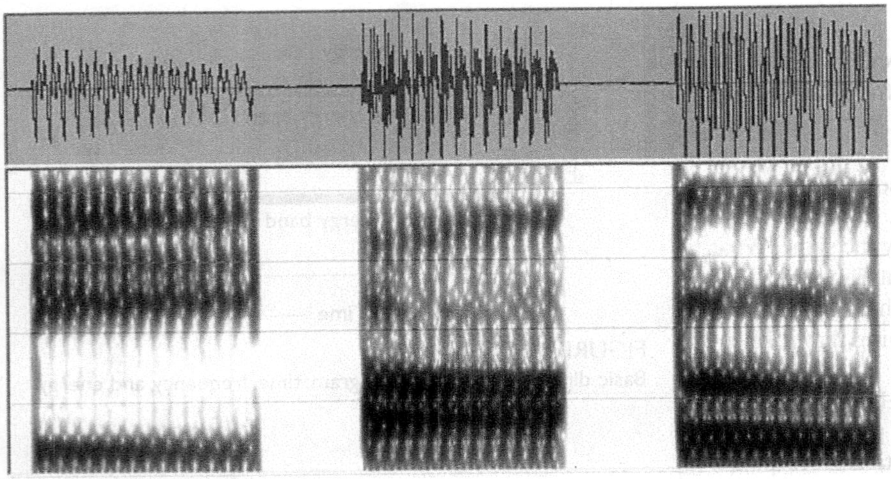

FIGURE 4.36
Spectrogram of three vowels produced in succession. Spectrograms from: http://commons.wikimedia.org/wiki/File:Spectrogram_-iua-.png#file

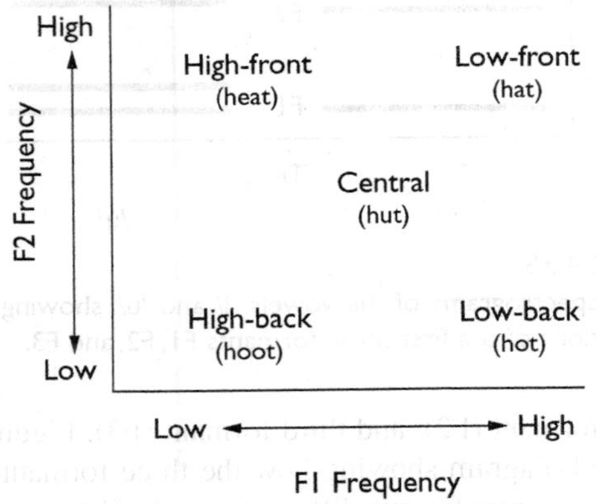

FIGURE 4.37
Acoustic vowel space defined by the F1 and F2 frequencies. The frequency of F1 is plotted on the horizontal axis, and the frequency of F2 is plotted on the vertical axis. The positions of the corner and central vowels (along with a keyword) are shown in the graph. Note the relationships: High vowels have a low F1 frequency, low vowels have a high F1 frequency, front vowels have a high F2 frequency, and back vowels have a low F2 frequency.

of the vowel: The more frontal the tongue, the higher is the frequency of F2. In other words, back vowels have a low F2 frequency, and front vowels have a high F2 frequency. This relationship is shown on the vertical axis of Figure 4.37. So it can be seen in Figure 4.37 that the articulatory vowel space maps onto an acoustic vowel space, sometimes called the **F1-F2 chart** or **F1-F2 graph**. The corners of the acoustic vowel quadrilateral correspond to the corners of the articulatory vowel quadrilateral, with central vowels positioned in the middle of the graph.

One reason why acoustic representation of vowel is important is that acoustic analysis provides a quantitative description of vowels that can be a useful complement to perceptual descriptions such as those used in phonetic transcription. The formant frequencies of vowels vary not only with vowel identity but also with speaker characteristics such as age and sex. The reason for the variation with the last two factors is that formant frequencies depend on the length of the resonator, that is, the vocal tract. Adult males have long vocal tracts and therefore relatively low formant frequencies. Adult females have shorter vocal tracts and therefore relatively higher formant frequencies than adult males. Young children have even shorter vocal tracts than women and therefore have the highest formant frequencies. As a crude analogy, we can think of the different lengths of the vocal tract as being like different lengths of the pipes in a pipe organ—the shorter the pipe, the higher its frequency (corresponding to our perception of pitch).

You may have wondered why the earlier figures in this section on vowel acoustics did not include numerical values on the frequency axis. The reason is that we wanted to emphasize the relative pattern of formant frequencies, which are nearly the same across variations in speaker characteristics such as age and sex. As a first step to attach actual numerical values to vowel formant frequencies, let's look at the frequency changes in F1 and F2 for adult males. As Figure 4.38 shows, the frequency of F1 varies over a range from about 270 Hz to 750 Hz, while the frequency of F2 varies from about 800 Hz to 2200 Hz. Formant frequencies would be higher for women and children. Figure 4.39 illustrates the F1 and F2 frequencies for a mixed group of speakers from a classic study by Peterson and Barney (1952; see box on Peterson and Barney). Note that the F1-F2 points from the group of speakers form ellipses in which the values for men (M) are closest to the origin, the values for women (W) are in about the middle of the long axis of the ellipse, and the values for children (C) are at the far end of this axis.

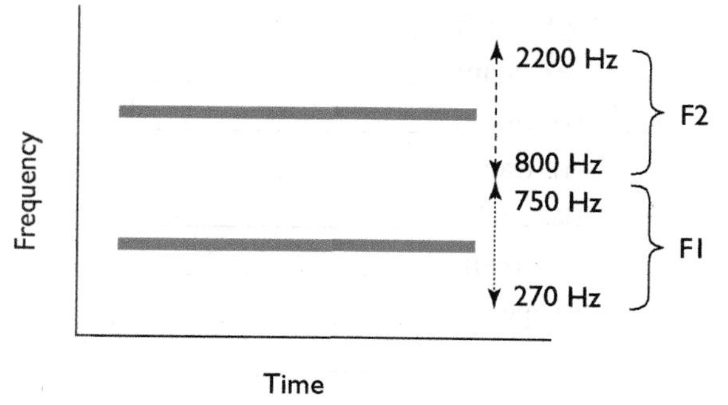

FIGURE 4.38
Stylized spectrogram of a vowel, showing two formants, F1 and F2. The dimensions are frequency (vertical axis), time (horizontal axis), and energy (gray scale or darkness). The frequency variation of F1 and F2 is shown for vowels produced by an adult male (i.e., the frequency of F1 ranges from about 270 to 750 Hz, and the frequency of F2 from about 800 to 2200 Hz).

A RESEARCH CORNERSTONE IN ACOUSTIC PHONETICS

In 1952 Gordon Peterson and Harold Barney published one of the first systematic descriptions of vowel formants in American English. Included in their study were measurements of the frequencies of F1, F2, and F3 for ten vowels produced by seventy-six speakers, including men, women, and children. This classic article is one of the most frequently cited papers in the field of acoustic phonetics. Although acoustic analysis of speech sounds has an earlier history, the article by Peterson and Barney is a milestone that pointed the way to the quantitative investigation of speech sounds. A more recent source on the acoustic properties of vowels in American English is Hillenbrand, Getty, Clark, and Wheeler (1995). If you want to learn more about vowel acoustics, check out James Hillenbrand's website—http://homepages.wmich.edu/~hillenbr. If you want to see a detailed analysis of formant frequencies for speakers of both sexes and various ages, see Vorperian and Kent (2005).

Primary Acoustic Properties of Vowels

Acoustic phonetics, the branch of phonetics that deals with the acoustics of speech, is relevant to describing and explaining a number of phenomena in phonetics. Several properties of vowels introduced in this chapter have acoustic correlates:

1. Vowels are resonant sounds produced with a relatively open vocal tract. The acoustic correlate is that vowels have prominent formant patterns, which appear as horizontally oriented bands of energy.

2. Vowels are perceived to be the loudest of speech sounds. Acoustically, vowels have the greatest energy of all sounds and typically it is the energy in F1, the strongest formant, that determines the perceived loudness of a vowel. Recall that energy is represented as the third dimension in a **spectrogram**—darkness (so-called "gray scale"). Therefore, the most intense sounds have the darkest appearance. Typically, then, vowels are relatively dark on a spectrogram, and F1 of the vowel usually is the darkest formant in a given vowel. Weaker sounds will not be as dark, as we will see later in discussions of consonants, which are generally less intense than vowels.

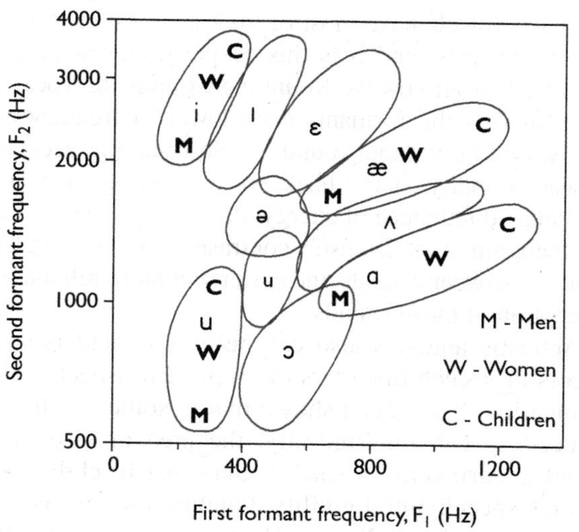

FIGURE 4.39
F1 and F2 frequencies for several vowels produced by men, women, and children, based on the data of Peterson and Barney (1952). For each vowel, identified by the phonetic symbols in the center of the ellipses, the formant-frequency values for men are located toward the origin, the values for women are farther from the origin, and the values for children are farthest from the origin. Approximate values for men, women, and children are shown on some of the ellipses for individual vowels.
Note: Subscripts for formant number are sometimes used in acoustic studies of speech, as in the case of this graph. But the modern convention is use the subscript only for fundamental frequency, f_0.

3. Vowels are perceptually judged to have different durations, especially between the tense and lax vowels. Acoustic measurements are a way of quantifying these durational differences. The briefest vowel (schwa) has a lower limit of about 50 ms (one-twentieth of a second); long vowels in heavily stressed syllables can have durations of 300 ms (one-third of a second) or even longer in exceptional circumstances.

As an example of the insights we can gain from acoustic analysis, we have seen in this chapter that in English only back vowels are rounded. In fact, this is a general tendency across languages, as a minority of languages have rounded front vowels. What is the reason for the affinity between rounding and backness? A likely explanation is that back vowels have most of their acoustic energy in the low frequencies, and it is this property that distinguishes them from front vowels. Rounding extends the vocal tract, which makes the formants even lower in frequency than they would be without rounding. So rounding accentuates a basic property of the back vowels, giving them a low-frequency dominance of energy. Perceiving speech involves the recognition of acoustic contrasts, and the greater the contrast between sounds, the easier and more reliable is our perception of those sounds.

Acoustic analysis also can help us to understand the effects of speech disorders on important aspects of communication. It has been shown that in some children with reduced speech intelligibility, the area or size of their vowel quadrilateral is smaller than that in children with normal speech intelligibility (studies on this issue are reviewed by Kent, Pagan, Hustad, & Wertzner, 2009). Apparently, shrinking the acoustic vowel quadrilateral can have a detrimental effect on a talker's intelligibility. Phonetics is often a study of contrasts—differences in tongue position being one example. Acoustic analysis is a means to quantify the size of contrasts. Acoustic properties of vowels also are mentioned in Chapter 10, with reference to dialectal variations in vowel production. The F1-F2 chart is very useful in describing the differences in vowels across dialects and across languages. No matter how many vowels a language has, the individual vowels can be plotted in the F1-F2 chart. Computer systems for acoustic analysis can be acquired at little or no cost, which makes the capability for acoustically aided transcription very economical.

EXERCISES

1. Draw a quadrilateral figure and label on it the articulatory dimensions of front–back and high–low. Then mark on the quadrilateral the locations of the following vowels: /i ɪ e æ u ʊ o ɔ ɑ ʌ ə ɝ/. Practice this exercise until you can easily and quickly construct the vowel quadrilateral.

2. Relying on the General American pronunciation of the following words, classify the vowel in each word with the appropriate articulatory descriptors: high, high-mid, mid, low-mid, low; front, central, back.

   (a) troop ______
   (b) caught ______
   (c) beg ______
   (d) look ______
   (e) steel ______
   (f) wand ______
   (g) shook ______
   (h) steam ______
   (i) rib ______
   (j) track ______
   (k) cook ______
   (l) roam ______
   (m) pearl ______
   (n) still ______

3. Each of the following words contains two adjacent vowels. Describe in articulatory terms the movements of the tongue and lips (if any) during the transition from the first vowel to the second. For example, in the word *neon* [n i ɑ n] the tongue moves back and down in going from /i/ to /ɑ/, and the mouth (lip) opening increases.

   (a) piano ______
   (b) duo ______
   (c) trio ______
   (d) rayon ______
   (e) coerce ______
   (f) react ______
   (g) nuance ______
   (h) noel ______
   (i) seance ______
   (j) coeval ______
   (k) reiterate ______
   (l) cooperate ______

4. Each time you read through the following passage, do one or more of the following: (a) underline every letter that represents a front vowel, (b) double-underline every letter that represents a central vowel, (c) draw a vertical line through every letter that represents a back vowel, and (d) overline every letter that represents a diphthong.

   Vowels are early sounds to appear in a child's speech. Front vowels tend to predominate in an infant's early vowel usage. It has been suggested that an infant could produce a set of front vowels by holding the tongue near the front of the mouth and varying the amount of jaw opening. A closed jaw position would yield /i/, and an open jaw position would yield /æ/.

5. Assuming General American dialect, center over each vowel alphabet letter(s) in the following words the phoneme symbol that best fits the vowel pronunciation.

(a) mōne̅y̅
(b) fēncepōst
(c) dīplōmāt
(d) lāmpli̅g̅h̅te̅r̅
(e) su̅i̅tcāse
(f) lībrārȳ
(g) ōve̅r̅po̅w̅e̅r̅
(h) la̅u̅ndrōmāt
(i) bo̅o̅kmārk
(j) re̅i̅ntērprēt
(k) kno̅w̅ho̅w̅
(l) mūstārd
(m) mērcīlēss
(n) bo̅i̅le̅r̅plāte
(o) wānde̅r̅lūst
(p) rēctīfȳ
(q) ne̅o̅lōgīsm
(r) ādmīnīstrāte
(s) lūnche̅o̅nētte
(t) ge̅o̅mētrȳ
(u) ūtēnsīl
(v) mīsūnde̅r̅sto̅o̅d

6. Say the following words to yourself, or ask someone to say them for you. As you hear each word, write the phonetic symbol for each vowel. Some words contain only one vowel and others have two.

1. keep
2. hatch
3. father
4. station
5. window
6. eighth
7. nine
8. fifty
9. brawny
10. use
11. token
12. surprise
13. fetch
14. bookish
15. butter

PROCEED TO: Clinical Phonetics CD 1, Tracks 1, 2, 3, 4: Transcription Lists A, B, C, D

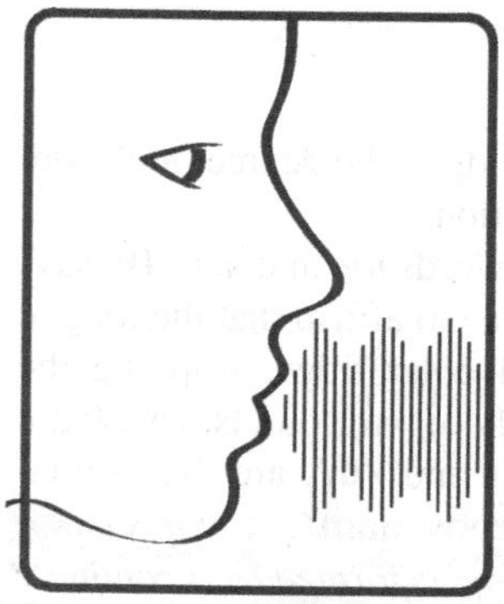

CHAPTER 5

CONSONANTS

The word *consonant* is derived from Latin roots meaning "to sound with" or "to sound together." This meaning reflects the idea that consonants generally occur with a vowel to form spoken syllables. It certainly is possible to produce an isolated consonant (such as a hissing sound made by prolonging the fricative /s/ as in *see*), but it is exceedingly rare for an isolated consonant to have lexical status in natural languages. However, a single consonant can have morphemic status; for example, the final /s/ in the word *cats* is a morpheme signifying plural. But even then, the /s/ must be attached to another morpheme to achieve its morphemic purpose. Consonants pair with vowels to form the syllables and words of our language. The most general feature of consonants is that they are associated with a closure or constriction of the vocal tract. Because vowels are associated with a relatively open vocal tract, consonants and vowels naturally form two opposing sets of sounds. The CV (consonant + vowel) syllable is among the most frequently used syllable structures across the world's languages. It appears to be used in all languages and occasionally is the only syllable type (as in Hawaiian). Although this chapter focuses on consonants, it is well to remember that consonants work with vowels to form syllables and words.

Consonant articulation is described with respect to three basic dimensions: place, manner, and voice. The **place of articulation** tells *where* a sound is formed, the **manner of articulation** tells *how* it is formed, and **voice** tells whether the *vocal folds are vibrating* in association with the consonant segment. English consonants can be described by using a modifier or descriptor for each of these three dimensions, as shown in the following list.

Voicing	*Place*	*Manner*
voiced	bilabial	stop
voiceless	labiodental	nasal
	interdental	fricative
	alveolar	affricate
	palatal	liquid
	palatal-velar	(a) lateral
	glottal	(b) rhotic
		glide

Using all these possible combinations of voicing, place, and manner, we would have a total of almost 100 consonants. However, the English language uses only about one-fourth of this number. The number of *possible* consonant sounds is far larger than 100, because other languages have voicing, place, and manner capabilities in addition to those just listed. For example, some languages incorporate whistles, clicks, and sounds formed at other places in the vocal tract. But it also should be noted that not all combinations of the descriptors given above are possible sounds, for some combinations are not pronounceable.

Consonant phonemes in English, then, can be described by specifying the voicing, place, and manner. For instance, the sound *b,* as in *b*ee, a*b*ove, and ru*b*, is described as a voiced, bilabial, stop consonant. This description tells us that the sound is produced with vibrating vocal folds (voiced), with a constriction at the lips (*bi* meaning "two" and *labia* meaning "lips"), and with a complete closure (stopping) at the place of articulation. Given our earlier definition of phonemes with respect to minimal pairs of words, it should be possible to change the voicing, place, or manner features and thereby create other consonants. For example, if we alter only the voicing, changing it to voiceless instead of voiced, we have the sound *p,* as in *p*ea, a*pp*le, and ri*p*. Notice that *b* and *p* are alike in place of articulation (both involving the lips) and manner of articulation (both involving a complete closure or stopping), but that they differ in activity of the vocal folds. Because changes in the voicing, place, and manner may produce different phonemes, they are called the phonemic features of English. That is, these are the modifications of consonant sound production that can be used to create the morphemes of the English language.

A simple model will be used to explain the general properties of consonant production. This model (Figure 5.1) consists of a lung chamber, pharyngeal cavity, oral cavity, and nasal cavity. The lung is separated from the pharyngeal cavity by the vocal folds, and the oral and nasal cavities are separated by the velopharynx. Each open circle in the model represents a valve or opening. The blue area represents air pressure contained within a chamber, and the lines ending in the open arrowheads represent airflow.

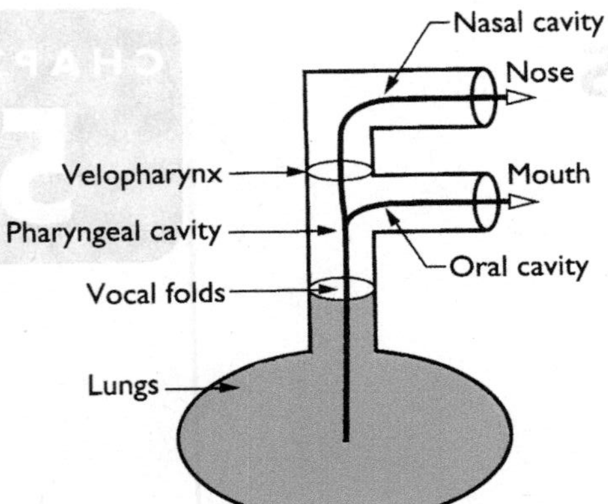

FIGURE 5.1
Simplified model to describe consonant production. The blue area represents heightened air pressure, and lines with open arrowheads represent airflow. This drawing illustrates that airflow resulting from an overpressure in the lungs can escape through both the oral and nasal cavities.

Manner of Articulation

Stops

This class of sounds is known by various names, including *occlusive, plosive, stop-plosive, plosive consonant, stop consonant*, and *stop*. We use the term *stop* for reasons of simplicity and generality. But the variety of names is understandable given that these sounds involve a blockage of the vocal tract and, in many cases, an explosive release of the air pressure built up behind the obstruction.

Although there is no one place of articulation at which all manners of articulation are used in English, there is one place at which *almost all* manners apply, and that is the lingua-alveolar articulation. Therefore, we will use this place of articulation to contrast the basic manner types. **Lingua** means tongue, and **alveolar** refers to the prominent ridge just behind the upper central teeth. This place of articulation normally is used for the initial sounds in the words *too, dew, sue, zoo, Lou*, and *new*. Say these words to yourself and note the similarity in place of articulation for the initial consonants. To produce these sounds, a speaker places the tongue tip close to or in contact with the alveolar ridge. The degree of closure depends on the manner of articulation.

Let us concentrate first on the words *too* and *dew*. By saying these words, you should be able to affirm that the tongue tip presses tightly against the alveolar ridge, stopping the egressive airflow momentarily. These two sounds, which are given the phonemic symbols /t/ and /d/, are the lingua-alveolar (or just alveolar) **stop consonants.** *A stop consonant, regardless of where it is made, is formed by a complete closure of the vocal tract, so that airflow ceases temporarily and air pressure builds up behind the point of closure.* This manner of articulation is illustrated in Figure 5.2(a). Because air is impounded behind the closure, the cavity becomes a pressure chamber. When the impounded air is released, it produces a short burst of noise, called the **stop burst.** Because the release of the stop is associated with an audible burst, some phoneticians call sounds like /t/ a stop plosive or plosive (*plosive* referring to the small explosion of escaping air). However, the plosive phase does not always occur in the production of sounds like /t/. For example, the word *tot* can be produced with an intelligible final /t/ even if the tongue tip remains closed against the alveolar ridge at the completion of the word. Thus, when the stop is in the word-final position, a release burst is not a necessary characteristic of this sound. For that reason, we prefer the term **stop** to *stop plosive* or *plosive.*

Stops—Articulatory Summary

1. The oral cavity is completely closed at some point for a brief interval.
2. The velopharynx is closed (otherwise, the air within the oral pressure chamber would escape through the nose).
3. Upon release of the stop closure, a burst of noise typically is heard.
4. The closing and opening movements for stops tend to be quite fast, usually the fastest movements in speech.

A frequently occurring allophone (phonetic variant) of the /t/ and /d/ phonemes occurs in words such as *city, ladder, latter, butter, writer, rider, patty*, and *laddy.* Speakers of English usually produce these words with the allophonic

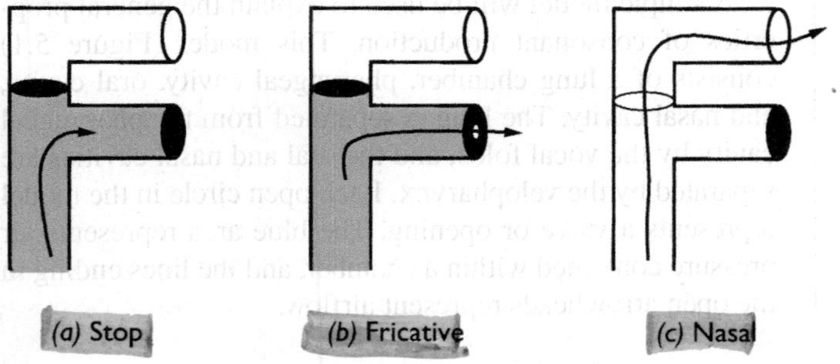

FIGURE 5.2
Simplified model shown in Figure 5.1 adapted for production of *(a)* stops, *(b)* fricatives, and *(c)* nasals. A blackened port indicates closure, and a partially blackened port indicates frication constriction.

lingua-alveolar **flap** /ɾ/ in the intervocalic position. The flap is a modified stop sound, in which a rapid stroking or flapping motion of the tongue tip contacts the alveolar ridge very briefly. The flap also is known by the names **tap** and **one-tap trill.** In a sense, the flap may be regarded as a reduced version of /t/ and /d/, as it can replace both of these phonemes in pairs such as *latter–ladder, writer–rider,* and *knotting–nodding.* Some phoneticians give the flap full phonemic status as a manner of production, but we prefer to view it as a variant or modification of the more general stop category.

The stop phonemes of English are represented by the initial sounds in the words *pill, bill, till, dill, kill, gill.* Say these words to yourself and attempt to verify the similarity in manner, but not place, of production. Note in particular the four features described above: oral closure, velopharyngeal closure, noise burst associated with release, and rapid articulatory movement.

Fricatives

The initial sounds of *sue* and *zoo* are lingua-alveolar **fricatives.** They are produced by bringing the tongue tip up to the alveolar ridge but not pressing tightly against it. Because the closure is incomplete, air escapes with a hissing noise through a narrow central groove in the tongue. All fricatives are made with a continuous noise production (called frication). *Thus, a fricative is defined as a sound that is produced with a narrow constriction through which air escapes with a continuous noise.* The intensity of the noise varies with place of articulation. The lingua-alveolar fricatives are among the most intense. Although both stops (as in *too, due*) and fricatives (as in *sue, zoo*) can have associated noise segments, the noise burst segment for stops (10 to 20 ms) is much briefer than that for fricatives (100 ms or so). The nature of fricative production is illustrated schematically in Figure 5.2(b), which shows the air pressure chamber behind the constriction and the narrow constriction or passageway. Noise energy is generated as air escapes through the passage.

Fricatives—Articulatory Summary

1. The articulators form a narrow constriction through which airflow is channeled. Air pressure increases in the chamber behind the constriction.
2. As the air flows through the narrow opening, a continuous frication noise is generated.
3. Because effective noise production demands that all of the escaping air be directed through the oral constriction, fricatives are produced with a closed velopharynx.

The nine fricatives of English are represented by the final sounds in the words *leaf, leave, teeth, teethe, bus, buzz, rush,* and *rouge* and the initial sound of *he* (this sound does not occur word-finally). Say these sounds and attempt to verify the three articulatory features just listed.

Nasals

The first sound in *new* is a lingua-alveolar nasal consonant. For **nasal** consonants, the sound energy created by pulses of air from the vibrating vocal folds must radiate (pass) through the nasal cavities, with the oral tract usually being completely closed. To demonstrate to yourself that this sound involves the nasal tract, try saying the words *new, no, knee,* and *nay* while pinching your nose tightly with your fingers. The resulting sounds will not be acceptable *n* sounds, although they will bear some similarity to them.

By definition, a nasal consonant is produced with a complete oral closure (like a stop), but with an open velopharynx, so that voicing energy travels out through the nose. In most languages, including English, the characteristic of nasal sound transmission also affects vowel sounds adjacent to nasal consonants. In the words *no* and *on,* the vowels following and preceding the *n* sound tend to be nasalized (sound energy passes through both the nose and mouth). Figure 5.2(c) illustrates the salient features of nasal consonant production.

Nasals—Articulatory Summary

1. The oral tract is completely closed, as it is for a stop.
2. The velopharyngeal port is open to permit sound energy to radiate outward through the nasal cavities.
3. Even if the oral closure is broken, sound may continue to travel through the nose as long as the velopharynx remains open.

The nasals of English are represented by the final consonants in the words *ram, ran,* and *rang.* Verify the nasal manner by saying each word with your nostrils alternately open and closed.

Liquids

There are two types of **liquids: lateral** sounds and **rhotic** sounds. Here we will discuss both only briefly, as a more detailed analysis will be presented later. The lateral sound occurs initially in the words *Lou, Lee, law,* and *low.* The tongue tip makes a midline, or central, closure with the alveolar ridge, but an opening is maintained at the sides of the tongue. Therefore, sound energy generated in the larynx radiates laterally, or around the sides of the tongue. *Hence, a lateral sound has midline closure and lateral opening for sound transmission,* as shown in Figure 5.3.

The rhotic liquid consonant is the *r* consonant, as in *rue, raw,* and *ray.* This is a complex sound, to be considered in depth later in this chapter. *For the present, it is sufficient to note that the common ways of producing the rhotic, or* r, *sound are to (1) hold the tongue tip so it is curled back slightly and not quite touching the alveolar ridge or the adjoining palatal area, and (2) bunch the tongue in the palatal area of the mouth.* (See Figure 5.4.) Sound energy from

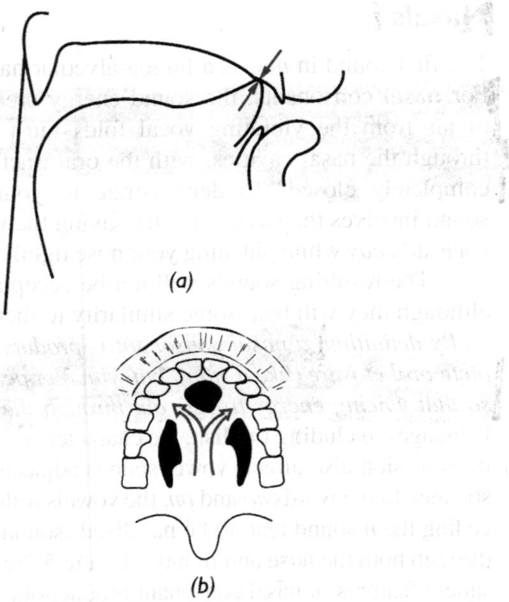

FIGURE 5.3
Articulation of the lateral consonant /l/. A lateral-view articulatory configuration is shown in *(a)*, and an inferior view of the roof of the mouth is shown in *(b)*. Lateral opening around the point of tongue contact shown in *(a)* allows sound energy to pass through the mouth. Regions of tongue contact are shown in *(b)* as dark areas.

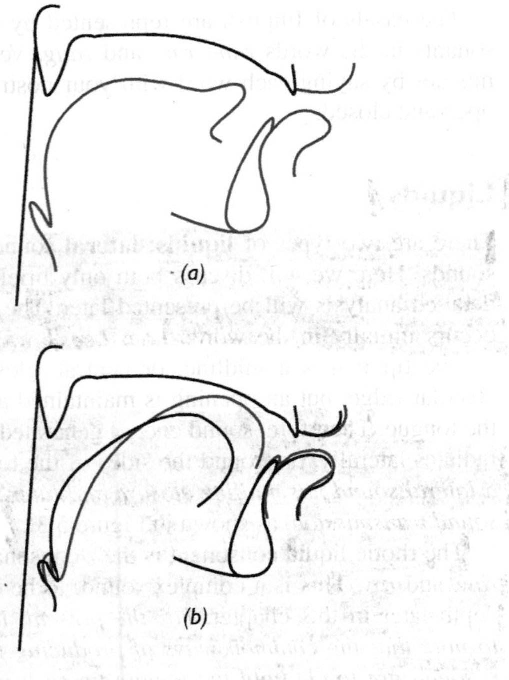

FIGURE 5.4
Articulations of the rhotic /r/. The retroflex articulation is shown in *(a)* and the bunched articulation in *(b)*. The black and blue lines in *(b)* represent the bunched /r/ in two different vowel contexts.

the vibrating vocal folds then passes through the opening between tongue and palatal vault.

Both the lateral sound, as in *Lou,* and the rhotic sound, as in *rue,* are liquids. *A liquid is a vowel-like consonant in which voicing energy passes through a vocal tract that is constricted only somewhat more than for vowels. The shape and location of the constriction is a critical defining property, being distinctive for a given type of liquid.*

Liquids—Articulatory Summary

1. Sound energy from the vocal folds is directed through a distinctively shaped oral passage, one that can be held indefinitely for sustained production of the sound, if required.
2. The velopharynx is always (or at least almost always) closed.
3. The oral passageway is narrower than that for vowels but wider than that for stops, fricatives, and nasals.

The lateral /l/ in *Lou* and the rhotic /r/ in *rue* occur at only one place of articulation in General American English. However, in some dialects and in some speech disorders, lateralized or rhotic modifications occur for other sounds, as discussed in Chapter 6.

Glides

Glide sounds, also known as **semivowels,** are made at two places in English: lingua-palatal and labio-lingua-velar. The lingua-palatal glide (symbolized phonemically as /j/) occurs in the words *you, yes,* and *yawn.* The voiced labio-lingua-velar /w/ occurs in the words *woo, we,* and *one,* and the voiceless labio-lingua-velar /ʍ/ is used by some speakers in the words *why, which,* and *when. A glide sound has a vocal tract constriction somewhat narrower than that for vowels but less severe than that for stops and fricatives and is characterized by a gliding motion of the articulators from a partly constricted state to a more open state for the following vowel.* (A glide is always followed by a vowel.) The gliding motion from the constricted state to the following vowel is the distinguishing and defining property of glides. These gliding movements are slower than the closing and opening movements for stops. An illustration of glide production is given in Figure 5.5.

Glides—Articulatory Summary

1. The constricted state for the glide is narrower than that for a vowel but wider than that for stops and fricatives.
2. The articulators make a gradual gliding motion from the constricted segment to the more open configuration for the following vowel.
3. The velopharynx is generally, if not always, closed.
4. The sound energy from the vocal folds passes through the mouth, in a fashion similar to that for vowels.

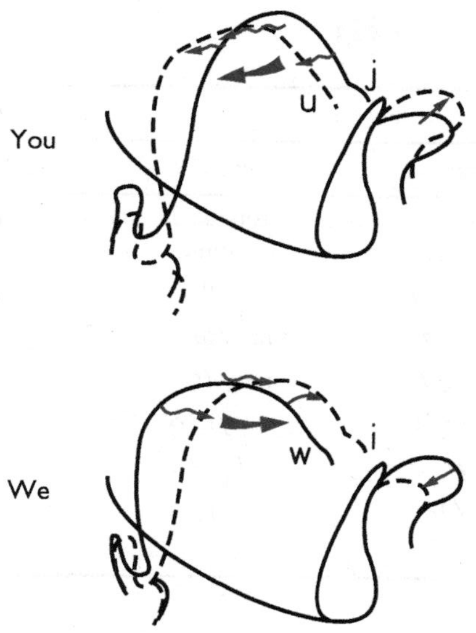

FIGURE 5.5
Articulations for the glide consonants /j/ and /w/ in the words *you* and *we*, respectively. The drawings show lip and tongue movements relative to the jaw. Notice that the glide articulations for *you* are essentially opposite to those for *we*.

There are only three glides in English, represented by the initial sounds in *you* (/j/), *we* (/w/), and *while* (/ʍ/ in some but not all pronunciations).

Affricates

Affricates *are best viewed as combination sounds involving a stop closure followed by a fricative segment.* Air pressure built up during the stop phase is released as a burst of noise, similar in duration to that for fricative sounds. The affricates of English are produced only at the palatal place of production, as in the words *church* and *judge*. In these words, both the initial and final segments are affricates. The basic properties of affricates are illustrated schematically in Figure 5.6.

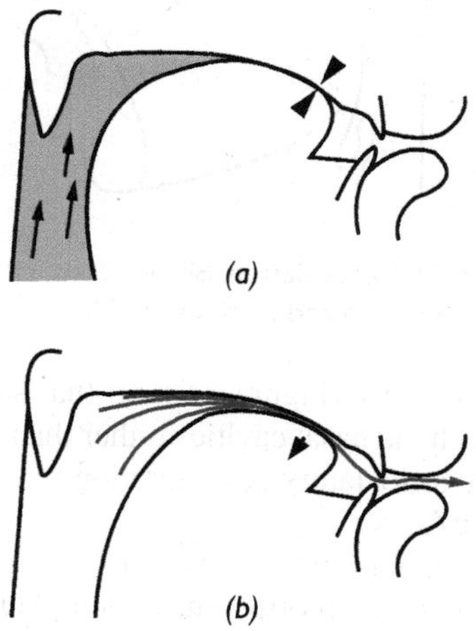

FIGURE 5.6
Schematic illustration of affricate production, showing *(a)* the buildup of air pressure during the stop portion and *(b)* the release of air through a narrow passage during the fricative portion.

Affricates—Articulatory Summary

1. Affricates are a combination of a stop closure and a fricative segment, with the frication noise closely following the stop portion.
2. Affricates are made with complete closure of the velo pharynx.

Place of Articulation

It should be apparent by now that most consonants are formed by completely or nearly closing the vocal tract at some point. Place of articulation describes where the point of closure or constriction is located. An intuitive impression about place of articulation can be gained by reciting the words listed under each place of articulation in Table 5.1 and noting where the italicized sound is produced. The phonetic symbol for each of these sounds is given after the key word. The words *why* and *way* are placed in parentheses to indicate that, for the sound in question, two articulators are involved. The /w/, as in *way* and *wag*, involves constrictions of both lips and tongue, as does the /ʍ/, the voiceless counterpart to /w/.

Bilabials /b/ /p/ /m/ /w/ /ʍ/

Sounds formed at the **bilabial** place of articulation are the voiced and voiceless stops /b/ and /p/, the nasal /m/, and the voiced and voiceless glides /w/ and /ʍ/. The latter two sounds are described as having two places of articulation because they are produced with rounding of the lips and with the tongue in a high-back (/u/-like) position. The tongue-positioning requirement for /w/ and /ʍ/ should be emphasized, because in our experience students sometimes fail to recognize its significance. Notice that no English fricatives or affricates are made at the bilabial place of production.

Two basic lip articulations are needed to produce the five sounds /p b m w ʍ/. The first articulation, lip closure, is required for the bilabial stops /b/ and /p/ and the bilabial nasal /m/. Usually, this articulation consists of a closing phase, a closed phase, and a releasing or opening phase. Both the closing and releasing phases are accomplished in about 50 to 75 ms. These articulations are among the briefest (fastest) in speech. Bilabial closure for /b/ is illustrated in Figure 5.7. Notice that the tongue can take different positions during the bilabial closure; in this illustration, the tongue takes the position for the vowel that follows the /b/. The articulation for /m/ is similar to that for /b/; thus, some

TABLE 5.1
Place of Articulation for English Consonants

			Place of Articulation			
Bilabial	Labiodental	Interdental	Alveolar	Palatal	Velar	Glottal
Both lips	Lips and teeth	Tongue tip and teeth	Tongue tip and ridge behind teeth	Tongue blade and palate	Tongue dorsum and velum	Vocal folds
*p*ie /p/	*f*ear /f/	*th*aw /θ/	*t*wo /t/	ru*sh* /ʃ/	ra*ck* /k/	*h*igh /h/
*b*ye /b/	*v*eer /v/	*th*e /ð/	*d*ue /d/	rou*ge* /ʒ/	ra*g* /g/	
*m*y /m/			*s*ue /s/	ri*ch* /tʃ/	ra*ng* /ŋ/	
(*w*ay) /w/			*z*oo /z/	ri*dge* /ʤ/	(*w*ay) /w/	
(*wh*y) /ʍ/			*n*ew /n/	*r*aw /r/	(*wh*y) /ʍ/	
			*L*ou /l/	*y*aw /j/		
			bu*tt*er /ɾ/			

phoneticians regard /m/ as a "nasalized bilabial stop." The voiced and voiceless /b/ and /p/ have basically the same labial articulation, although some authorities describe /p/ as having a forceful articulation involving greater muscular activity. These authorities describe /p/ as tense and /b/ as lax (see, for example, Chomsky & Halle, 1968). The reality of a tense–lax distinction for voiced and voiceless stops is still a matter of some controversy, but physiologic studies should resolve the issue.

Lower lip articulation (hence, bilabial closure) often is assisted by a closing motion of the jaw. Jaw movement is especially likely when the bilabial consonant is preceded or followed by a low or open vowel, as in the words *bob* and *mop*. However, bilabial closure can be achieved even when the jaw is held in an open or lowered position. Figure 5.8 shows X-ray tracings of bilabial closure for /p/ when the jaw is allowed to close and when the jaw is held open by blocks placed between the teeth. Notice that when the jaw is held open, the lips appear to stretch to make contact with one another.

The stops /b/ and /p/ are oral consonants, produced with velopharyngeal closure to permit the containment of air within the oral cavity. The nasal /m/ is produced with an open velopharynx (Figure 5.9), so that sound energy is radiated through the nasal cavities rather than the oral cavity. Otherwise, the articulatory configuration for /m/ is like that for /b/ and /p/.

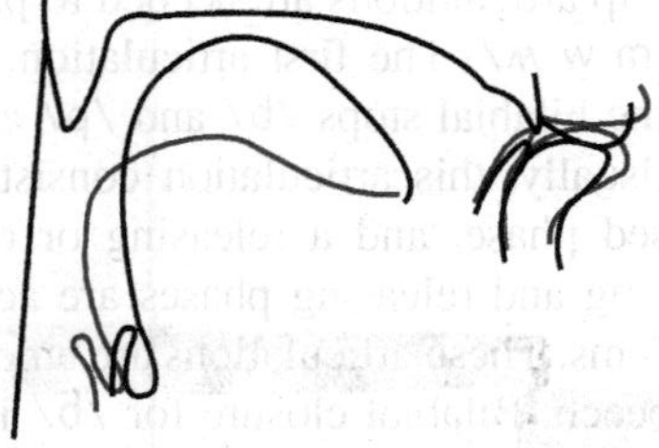

FIGURE 5.7
X-ray tracings of the bilabial closure in /b a/ (black line) and /b u/ (blue line). During the bilabial closure for /b/, the tongue assumes the position for the following vowel.

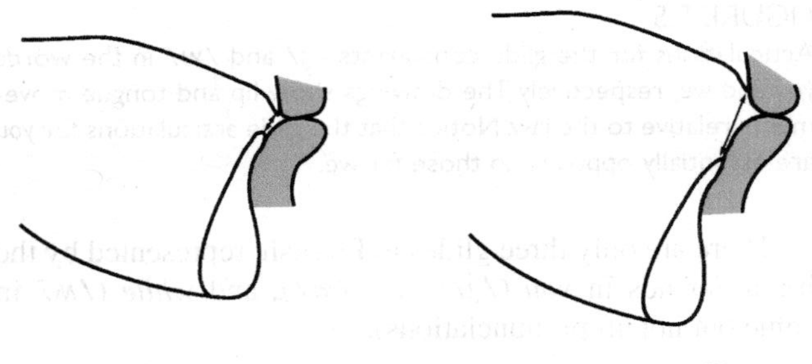

(a) (b)

FIGURE 5.8
Bilabial closure for a closed jaw position in *(a)* and an open jaw position in *(b)*.

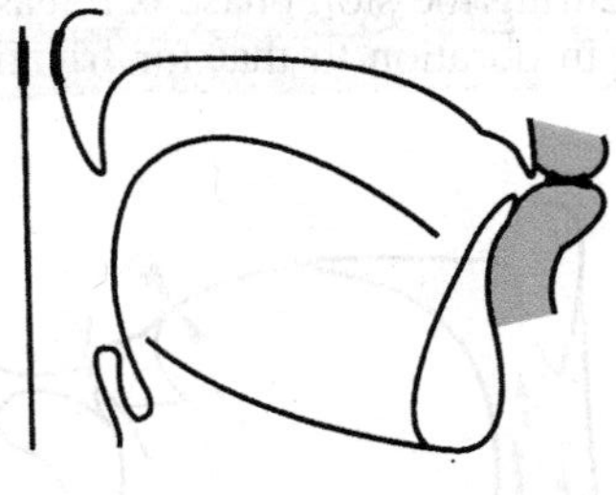

FIGURE 5.9
X-ray tracing of /m/ articulation. Bilabial contact and velopharyngeal opening are emphasized by thickened lines.

The other lip articulation is one variously known as rounding, narrowing, protrusion, or lengthening. Actually, the different names are justified in that different speakers have somewhat different articulations. Whereas some speakers protrude the lips (pushing them forward from the teeth), other speakers have primarily a narrowing movement in which the lips move toward, but do not reach, closure. The

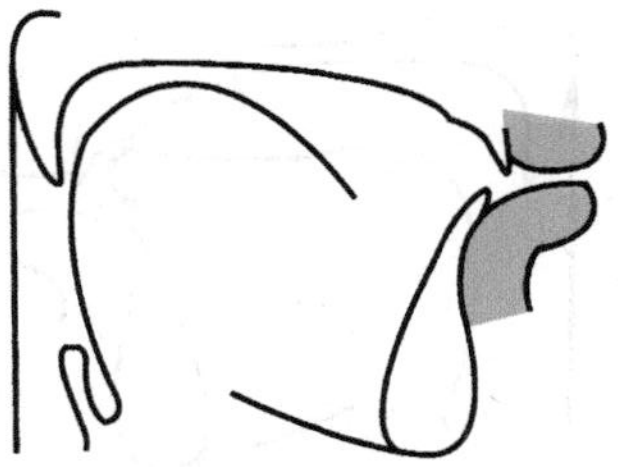

FIGURE 5.10
Lip protrusion, or lip rounding, for the first sound in *we*. Notice the forward extension of lips and the narrow mouth opening.

gesture of rounding or protrusion is shown in Figure 5.10, which is based on X-ray tracings of the /w/ articulation in the word *we*. Photographs of lip rounding are presented in Figure 4.4. The rounding or protrusion articulation is slower than for bilabial closure and generally takes 75 to 100 ms or more.

Labiodentals /f/ /v/

Only the fricatives /f/ (voiceless) as in *fat* and /v/ (voiced) as in *vat* are made as **labiodental** sounds. The basic articulation, shown in Figure 5.11, involves a constriction between the lower lip and the upper teeth (incisors). The fricative energy for /f/ and /v/ is weak compared to that for /s/ and /z/. Because the lower lip is attached to the jaw, the constricting movement of lower lip to upper teeth often is assisted by jaw movement. The lower lip movement for the labiodental constriction is somewhat like that for bilabial closure. The velopharynx is closed, as it is for all consonants except the nasals.

Interdentals (or Dentals) /θ/ /ð/

Only fricatives are formed at the **interdental** (or **dental**) location: the voiceless interdental /θ/ as in *thin* and the voiced interdental /ð/ as in *this*. Figure 5.12 illustrates the articulation, which takes two major forms, interdental and dental. For the interdental, the tongue tip is protruded slightly between the front teeth (incisors), so that a narrow

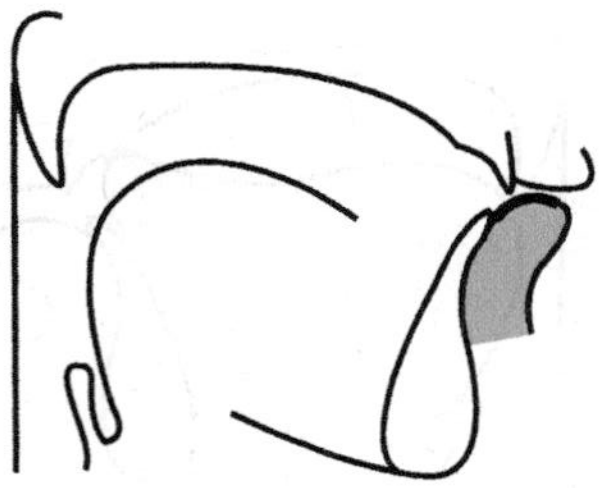

FIGURE 5.11
X-ray tracing of /f/ articulation. Thickened line shows labiodental contact.

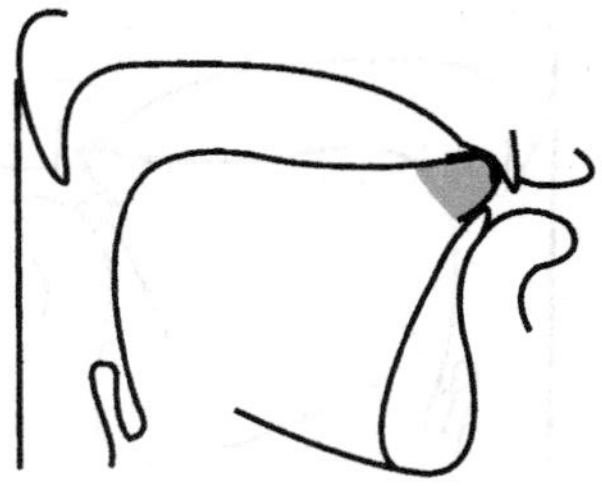

FIGURE 5.12
X-ray tracing of /θ/ articulation. Thickened line shows lingua-dental constriction.

constriction is formed between the tongue and the cutting edge of the teeth. For the dental articulation, the tongue tip contacts the back of the front teeth, so that the constriction is between the tongue and the inside surface of the teeth. The noise energy is weak, comparable to that for /f/ and /v/. In many speakers, the tip of the tongue is visible during /θ ð/ production. Although the jaw often closes somewhat to aid formation of the constriction, it cannot close completely, or there would not be adequate interdental opening for the tongue tip. These sounds tend to be made with a dental, rather than interdental, constriction in rapid speech.

Alveolars /t/ /d/ /s/ /z/ /l/ /n/

Lingua-Alveolar Stops: /t/ and /d/. X-ray tracings of the **lingua-alveolar** consonant closure for /t/ (*two*) and /d/ (*dew*) are shown in Figures 5.13 and 5.14. Note the similarity in articulation. Because both of these sounds are stops and require the development of air pressure behind the point of oral closure, the velopharynx is closed. The jaw often closes partially to aid the lingual contact against the alveolar ridge. The site of lingual contact is nearly identical for /d/ and /t/, but /t/ may have a firmer contact and a more rapid release, both of which are related to the fact that /t/ has a greater air pressure than /d/. In addition, /t/ tends to have a longer duration of closure than /d/. These differences are discussed in the section on voicing later in this chapter.

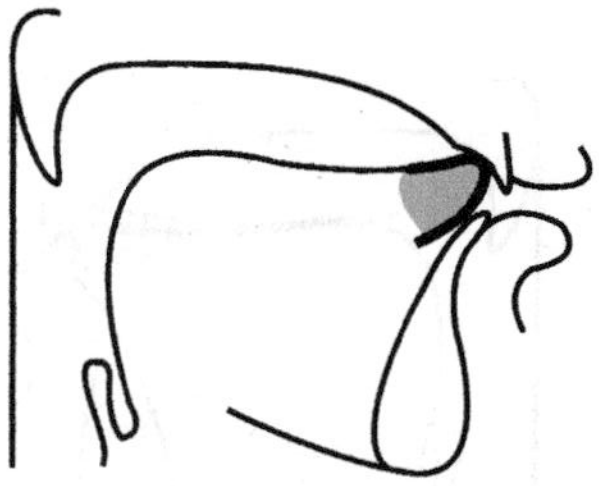

FIGURE 5.13
X-ray tracing of /t/ articulation. Thickened line shows lingua-alveolar contact.

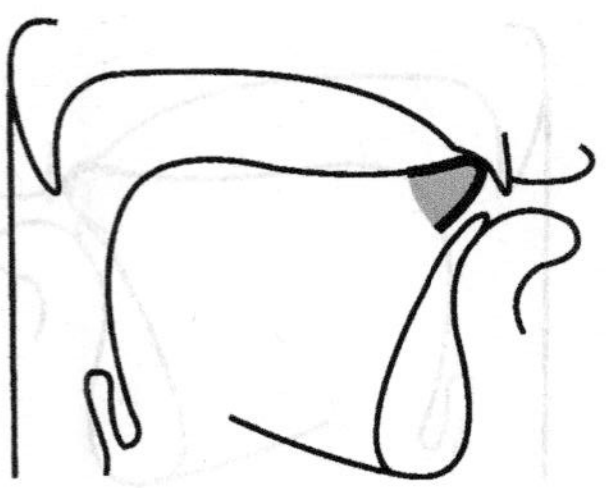

FIGURE 5.14
X-ray tracing of /d/ articulation. Thickened line shows lingua-alveolar contact.

The exact position and shape of the tongue for articulation of /t/ and /d/ varies with phonetic context. One of the most conspicuous contextual effects is that associated with a following dental fricative, as in the words *width* and *eighth.* Because of the influence of the dental fricative, the /d/ and /t/ in these words are made with a dental, rather than alveolar, contact, as illustrated in Figure 5.15. Another fairly frequent modification occurs in the context of palatal sounds, like the /j/ in some pronunciations of *Tuesday* /t j u z d eɪ̄/. The following palatal causes the /t/ to be articulated with the blade of the tongue elevated toward the palate. Other modifications of the alveolar place of articulation are described in the chapter on diacritics. It should be kept in mind that articulatory descriptions such as lingua-alveolar stop express the *typical* formation of the sound and that the actual place of contact varies with the phonetic context of the sound. Speech articulation is flexible and adaptive.

Lingua-Alveolar Fricatives: /s/ and /z/. These sounds are depicted by the X-ray tracing in Figure 5.16. Because /s/ (*sue*) and /z/ (*zoo*) have the same place and manner of articulation, separate X-ray tracings are not shown. For both /s/ and /z/, the velopharynx is closed to allow air pressure to build up in the mouth. The jaw usually assumes a fairly closed position. The /s/ and /z/ are sometimes called groove fricatives, because a midline groove is formed in the tongue as a narrow passageway for escaping air. Some phoneticians describe /s/ and /z/ as having a blade articulation, because the constriction can be made between the alveolar ridge and the part of the tongue just behind the tip.

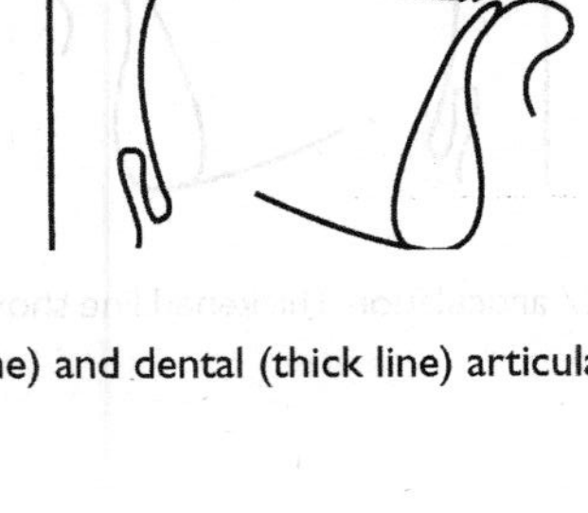

FIGURE 5.15
Alveolar (thin line) and dental (thick line) articulation of /t/.

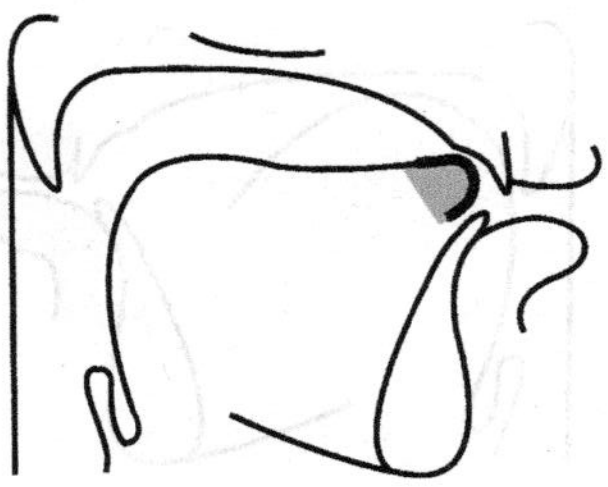

FIGURE 5.16
X-ray tracing of /s/ articulation. Thickened line shows lingua-alveolar constriction.

The lingual articulation for /s/ and /z/ varies somewhat with phonetic context and with speaker. Some speakers consistently use a **dentalized** constriction, in which the tongue makes a constriction with the area just behind the upper front teeth (incisors). These modifications are discussed in detail later in this book.

Lingua-Alveolar Lateral: /l/. The X-ray tracing in Figure 5.17 illustrates the most common articulation of the /l/ (*Lou*) in American English. The tongue tip makes contact with the alveolar ridge, and the dorsum of the tongue assumes a position similar to that for vowel /o/ (*low*). The contact is midline only, so that sound energy radiates through the sides of the mouth, around the midline closure. This sound derives its manner classification from the feature of lateral resonance. The similarity of dorsal tongue position between /l/ and /o/ is shown by the composite X-ray tracings in Figure 5.18. The /l/ might be described as having an /o/-like tongue body and dorsum but a midline contact of the tip. Alveolar contact is not a necessary feature of the sound. Particularly in word-final position, /l/ may be produced without such contact, as shown in Figure 5.19.

Most descriptions of /l/ in phonetics books distinguish between "light *l*" (or "clear *l*") and "dark *l.*" However, there is considerable disagreement about the articulatory differences that underlie the distinction of "light" and "dark." The following quotations are illustrative.

> *When [l] is made with the tongue against the teeth, it is referred to as dental [l], or, more often, as clear [l].*

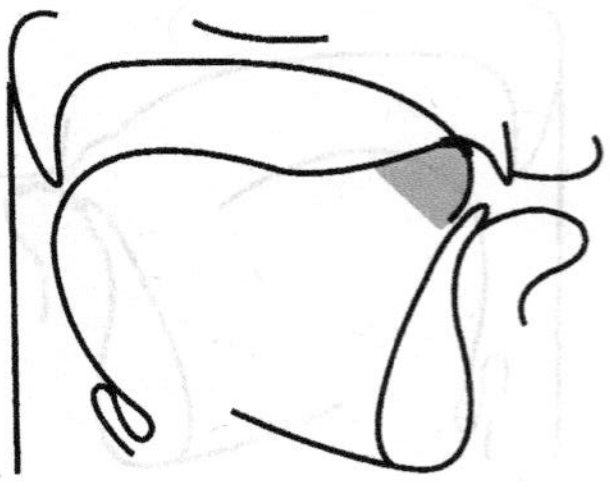

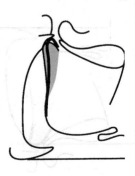

FIGURE 5.17
X-ray tracing of /l/ articulation. Thickened line shows lingua-alveolar contact. (See also Figure 5.3.)

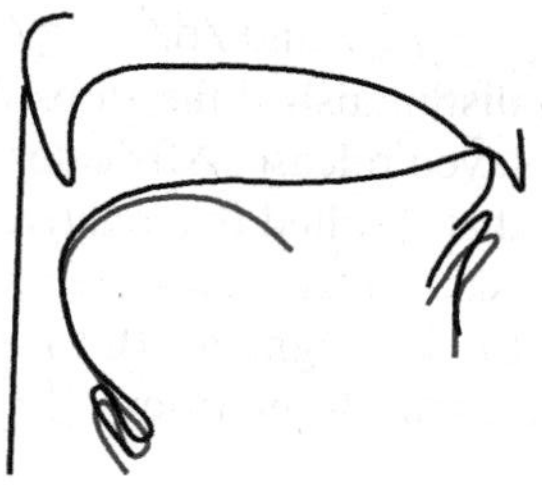

FIGURE 5.18
X-ray tracings of /l/ articulation (black line) and /o/ articulation (red line), showing similarity in root and dorsal positions of the tongue.

> *When it is made alveolarly, it is called "dark l." In Southern, British, and Eastern English, [l] before a front vowel, particularly a high front vowel, is clear. In General American all [l]'s are dark.* (Wise, 1957a, p. 131)
>
> *We should point out here that the so-called "lightness" or "clearness" of an l is not entirely dependent upon the position of the forepart of the tongue. In other words, the terms "front l" and "light l" are not exactly synonymous. A little experimentation will demonstrate that it is possible to keep the tip of the tongue on the upper teeth and produce l's of varying degrees of lightness and darkness.* (Kantner & West, 1941, p. 120)

Kantner and West went on to state that two other factors, besides the point of highest elevation of the tongue, determine the degree of lightness or darkness of /l/. First, increased lip spreading was said to result in a lighter /l/. Second, the back of the tongue was said to be flattened and lowered for a very light /l/ but raised for dark /l/.

Giles (1971) studied /l/ articulation by X-ray motion pictures and concluded that the position of the tongue dorsum distinguishes among three general types of /l/: prevocalic, postvocalic, and syllabic. The postvocalic and syllabic /l/ were quite similar except for the timing of movements for /l/ with respect to the preceding vowel. Postvocalic /l/ differed from the prevocalic variety in having a more posterior (farther back) position of the dorsum. Occasionally, contact of the tongue tip was not made for the postvocalic allophones in words like *Paul* (see Figure 5.19). The only other major variation that was observed in Giles's speech sample was dentalization of /l/ when followed by a dental sound, as in *health* /h ɛ l θ/.

The failure of some normal adult speakers to make tongue tip contact for /l/ in word-final or postvocalic position should be remembered when evaluating /l/ production in children. We frequently hear children produce an /o/-like sound for final /l/ in words like *seal*. Apparently, this "substitution" is not necessarily unusual or deviant, and caution should be observed in evaluating the child's proficiency for /l/ articulation. It is prudent to test /l/ production in more than one context or syllabic position before ascribing the /o/-like sound to an articulatory error.

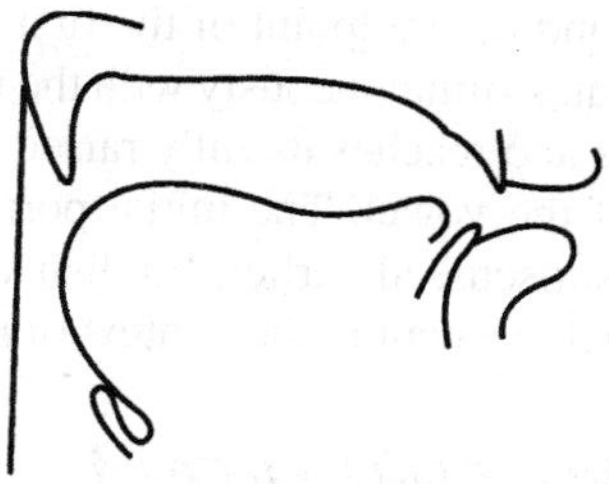

FIGURE 5.19
X-ray tracing of postvocalic /l/ articulated without lingua-alveolar contact.

Lingua-Alveolar Nasal: /n/. As the X-ray tracing in Figure 5.20 shows, /n/ (*new*) is made with a lingua-alveolar contact like that for /t/ and /d/, but with the velopharynx open. Sound energy from the larynx radiates outward through the nasal cavity. Articulatory (allophonic) modifications of the oral closure are similar to those for /t/ and /d/. For example, /n/ is dentalized (made with tongue contact against the upper teeth rather than the alveolar ridge) in words like *ninth,* where it is followed by a dental fricative.

Correct production of /n/ requires that the velopharynx be open during the time of lingua-alveolar closure. Otherwise, it would be heard as a /d/. Therefore, the timing of the velopharyngeal and oral articulations is critical for production of /n/ in running speech. An example of the coordination of velopharyngeal and oral movements is depicted in Figure 5.21, which shows composite tracings for the moment

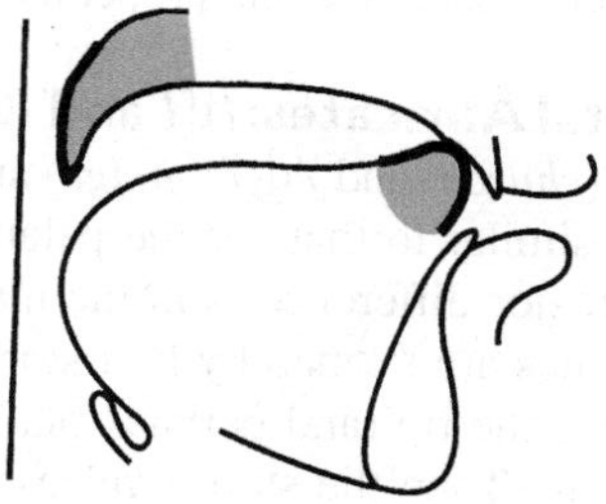

FIGURE 5.20
X-ray tracing of /n/ articulation. Thickened lines show lingua-alveolar contact and velopharyngeal opening.

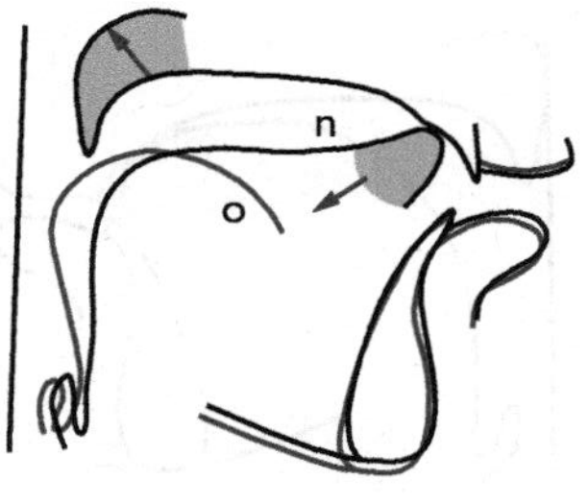

FIGURE 5.21
Articulatory configurations during the word-initial /n/ (black line) and following vowel /o/ in *no one*.

of /n/ release and the midpoint of the first vowel in *no one.* The velum elevates simultaneously with the release of lingua-alveolar closure and reaches its fully raised position at about the midpoint of the vowel. The initial portion of the vowel is nasalized. As discussed earlier, English vowels tend to be nasalized when they occur in the context of nasal consonants.

Palatals /ʃ/ /ʒ/ /tʃ/ /ʤ/ /r/ /j/

Lingua-Palatal Fricatives: /ʃ/ and /ʒ/. As shown by Figure 5.22, /ʃ/ (*shoe*) and /ʒ/ (*rouge*) are produced by elevating the tip and blade of the tongue toward the palate, hence, **palatal.** Fricative noise is generated as air passes through the channel between tongue and palate. The noise is quite intense, similar in total energy to that for /s/ and /z/. Thus, the intense fricatives are /s/, /z/, /ʃ/, and /ʒ/, and the weak fricatives are /f/, /v/, /θ/, /ð/, and /h/. Although /ʃ/ and /ʒ/ can be produced with a variety of lip positions, there is a general tendency for speakers to round the lips for these sounds, especially in isolated production.

Phoneticians describe few allophones of /ʃ/ and /ʒ/. Most articulatory modifications are minor. In addition, some allophones are rarely used. For example, the retroflex or rhotacized [ʃ], /ʃ/ with *r* coloring, normally occurs only when /ʃ/ is surrounded by rhotic or rhotacized sounds, as in the word *harsher* [h ɑ r ʃ ɚ]. Wise (1957) notes in *Applied Phonetics* that /ʒ/ is the least frequently used of all English sounds and that it is not originally an English sound but was introduced "partly from adoption from Norman French and partly by assimilation within the older cluster [zj]" (p. 137). /ʒ/ does not occur word-initially in English, except in proper names.

Lingua-Palatal Affricates: /tʃ/ and /ʤ/. The palatal affricates /tʃ/ (*church*) and /ʤ/ (*judge*) are produced with an articulation similar to that for the palatal fricatives /ʃ/ and /ʒ/. The major difference is in the manner of production. The affricates are formed by first stopping the flow of air by contacting the tip (and perhaps blade) of the tongue against the palate. Then the stop is released gradually into an immediately following fricative. As explained earlier, it is the two-phase articulation that gives rise to the digraph symbols, /t/ + /ʃ/ = /tʃ/ and /d/ + /ʒ/ = /ʤ/. Chomsky and Halle (1968) distinguished the stops from the affricates by a feature of delayed release. Affricates were said to have a delayed release that resulted in a relatively long noise segment. Stops were said to have an instantaneous release that resulted in a short noise segment. But it should be remembered that /t/ and /d/ differ from /tʃ/ and /ʤ/ in *both* place and manner.

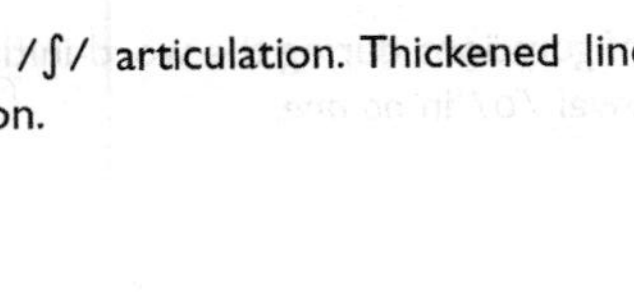

FIGURE 5.22
X-ray tracing of /ʃ/ articulation. Thickened line shows lingua-palatal constriction.

Palatal Rhotic: /r/. Rhotics are a family of sounds usually represented by the letter *r*, as in the word *raw*. The word *rhotic* comes from the seventeenth letter of the Greek alphabet, *rho* (ρ), which is sometimes used as a symbol for a member of the /r/ family of sounds. Rhotics and laterals have some properties in common. They are sonorants and have similar acoustic structure. In addition, they combine with other consonants to form a relatively large number of clusters, (examples for /l/: *blow, plough, fly, slow, clown, glide*; examples for /r/: *bride, prod, fry, thrive, dry, try, shriek, crown, grit*). There is also a degree of articulatory similarity between them, which is sometimes used to clinical advantage for children who misarticulate one of these sounds. For example, for a child who has trouble with /r/, the clinician might ask the child to produce the /l/ sound but to lower the jaw slowly until the position of the /r/ is reached. Alternatively, the child is instructed to say /l/ while the clinician uses a tongue depressor to push the tip of the tongue back in the direction of a normal /r/ articulation. Laterals are notoriously difficult for speakers of Japanese, which does not have lateral sounds. Frequently, they will substitute a rhotic for a lateral.

Despite years of phonetic research, a careful articulatory description of /r/ (*rue*) is still wanting. Examples of /r/ articulation are shown in the X-ray tracings of Figure 5.23, but we stress the word *examples.* This sound can be produced with a number of different tongue and lip articulations by the same speaker. Comparisons across a large number of talkers may reveal an even greater articulatory variability.

Generally, the articulation of /r/ falls into two classes, which we term **retroflex** and **bunched.** Retroflex means "turning or turned back" (the morpheme *retro* means "back" and the morpheme *flex* means "turn") and is intended to describe the action of the tip of the tongue, as shown in Figure 5.23(a). Although the tongue tip does not really "turn backward," the positioning of the tongue is quite striking in an X-ray film, as no other English sound has this type of articulation. The tongue body assumes a mid-central position, and the lips often (but not necessarily) are rounded.

The bunched articulation, shown in Figure 5.23(b), is produced with an elevation of the blade toward the palate but with the tip turned down. The position of the tongue body appears to vary with vowel context, and the lips often are rounded. Sometimes the bunched articulation is accompanied with a bulging of the tongue root in the lower pharynx and with a flattening or depression of the dorsum, as in Figure 5.23(c).

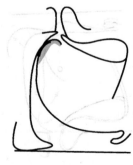

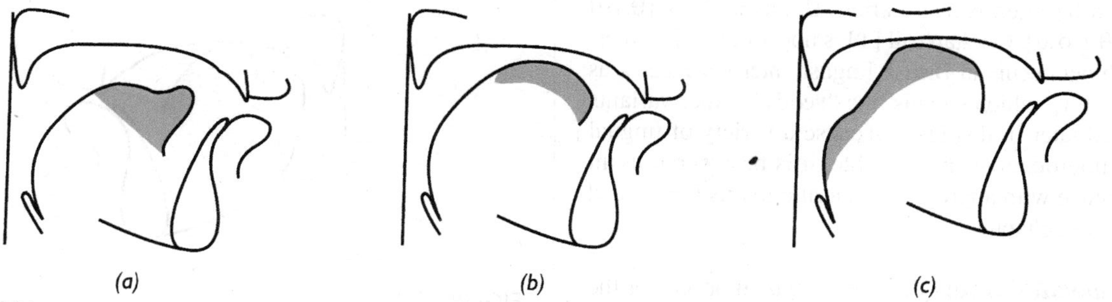

FIGURE 5.23
X-ray tracings of /r/ or rhotic articulations: retroflex articulation in *(a)* and bunched articulations in *(b)* and *(c)*.

It is not clear how these different articulations are associated with phonetic context and syllable position, except that the bunched articulation may be favored postvocalically by some speakers. All the articulations represented in Figure 5.23 are prevocalic. It is clear that /r/ articulation is accommodated to the lingual articulation of the surrounding elements. For example, Figure 5.24 shows how /r/ is produced in the word *true* [t r u]. Upon release of the /t/, the tongue tip is drawn back and downward as the blade is elevated to form a bunched articulation. In the transition from /r/ to /u/, the blade is lowered. The composite drawing illustrates the smooth, flowing motions of the articulators during speech. Because the movements associated with /r/ tend to be slow and glidelike, it can be difficult to determine any one tongue position that represents the /r/. The comments of Kantner and West are instructive:

> r *is a sound that, even more than* t, k, *and* l, *is influenced by neighboring sounds. We will not be far wrong if we think of* r *as being dragged all over the mouth cavity by the various sounds with which it happens to be associated. This means that different sounds that we recognize as* r *are sometimes produced by fundamentally different movements.* (Kantner & West, 1941, pp. 152–153)

In an X-ray study of three speakers, Zawadzki and Kuehn (1980) observed two basic types of /r/: prevocalic /r/ for syllable initiation and postvocalic /r/ for terminating a syllable or for forming a syllabic nucleus. Compared to the postvocalic /r/, the prevocalic allophone was described as having "a greater lip rounding, a more advanced [fronted] tongue position, and less tongue dorsum grooving" (p. 253). Earlier, Delattre and Freeman (1968) identified six different tongue shapes associated with /r/, but most of these six shapes could be classified as bunched articulations. Zawadzki and Kuehn (1980) commented on an important, and often overlooked, feature of the /r/ articulation in the Delattre and Freeman study: All the /r/ allophones had a narrowing of the vocal tract in the pharyngeal region. Some degree of pharyngeal narrowing is evident for most of the /r/ articulations shown in Figures 5.4 and 5.23. It is difficult to determine if this same feature characterizes the /r/ articulations observed by Zawadzki and Kuehn because their X-ray tracings did not include the lower part of the pharyngeal cavity. But pharyngeal narrowing may not be a *necessary* feature of /r/ production, given that one bunched /r/ in Figure 5.4 has an advanced tongue root. In general, /r/ articulations seem to be associated with a narrowing in both the palatal and pharyngeal regions, and the X-ray tracings in Figure 5.23 are good examples of how these two types of narrowing can be accomplished simultaneously. In addition, many speakers produce /r/ with lip rounding, so that the vocal tract configuration may show *three* regions of narrowing: labial, palatal, and pharyngeal.

The complexity of /r/ derives not only from its articulatory constrictions at up to three places in the vocal tract, but also from the timing of its movements, as described by Campbell, Gick, Wilson, and Vatidiotis-Bateson (2010). In syllable-initial position, /r/ has a front-to-back timing pattern: first the lips, then tongue blade, and finally tongue root. In syllable-final position, lip and tongue-root movements are followed by tongue blade. The magnitude of the different movements can vary with syllable position, with tongue-root movement reduced in syllable-initial position and both lip and tongue-blade movements reduced in syllable-final position.

Most phoneticians recognize at least three major manner allophones of /r/ in English: fricative [ɹ] or [ɹ̝]; trilled [r̬]; and one-tap trill [ɾ]. The fricative [ɹ] occurs most frequently after /t/ or /d/, as in *try* [t ɹ a͡ɪ] and *dry* [d ɹ a͡ɪ]. Frication is produced as the tongue breaks contact with the alveolar

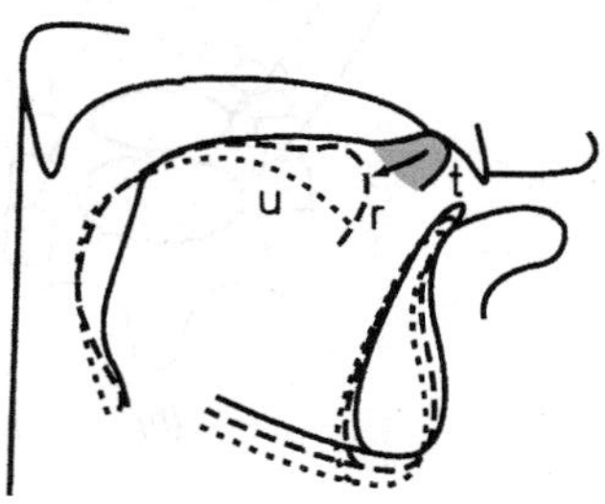

FIGURE 5.24
Composite of articulatory configurations for the three phonetic segments in *true*: /t/—solid lines; /r/—dashed lines; /u/—dotted lines. Because lip positions changed slightly, only one position is shown.

ridge. Trilled [r̬] often is heard after /θ/, as in *three* [θ r̬ i] and *throw* [θ r̬ o ʊ]. One-tap trill [ɾ] is not common in American English but occurs in British English inter vocalically, as in *very* [v ɛ ɾ ɪ], which sounds like "veddy." Other variants are discussed later in this text. Because a variety of lingual and labial modifications are possible, it is best to represent their occurrence with appropriate diacritic marks introduced in the following chapter.

Lingua-Palatal Glide: /j/. The tongue motions for the glide /j/ are depicted in Figure 5.25. The high-front tongue position closely resembles that for vowel /i/ (*he*). The major difference is that the constriction between tongue and palate is more severe for /j/, so that it is described as a consonant articulation. Jaw position also is similar for the two sounds, being relatively closed (elevated).

Glide /j/ in English always precedes a vowel. Therefore, its articulation takes the form of a tongue movement from palatal constriction (high-front tongue body) to the tongue position for the following vowel. The articulatory motion is slower than that observed for stops and fricatives. Because of its resemblance to /i/ and its vowel-like properties, /j/ sometimes is called a semivowel. But /j/ differs from the vowels in that it cannot be used as a nucleus of a syllable and can occur only prevocalically.

A tongue motion similar to that for /j/ occurs in words in which another palatal consonant precedes /u/, for example, *shoe, chew, June*. Usually, the /j/ is not used to transcribe these words: /ʃ u/, not /ʃ j u/. Notice how difficult it is to say a word like *shoe* with a clearly audible /j/ between the /ʃ/ and the /u/.

Velars /k/ /g/ /ŋ/ /w/ /ʍ/

The X-ray tracing in Figure 5.26 shows how the **velar** (or dorsal) stops are made by elevating the lingual dorsum until it contacts the roof of the mouth. The site of articulation varies from the back part of the hard palate to the velum. Vowel context is the major determinant of the exact place of articulation. When /k/ and /g/ are produced in the context of a front vowel, like /i/ (*key*) or /æ/ (*cat*), the articulation is made frontally. But when these sounds are produced in the context of a back vowel, like /u/ (*coo*) or /ɑ/ (*calm*), the articulation is made farther back, near the velum. This variation, illustrated in Figure 5.27, is a good example of the articulatory interaction between sounds.

Jaw position for the velars is quite variable, apparently being determined primarily by the vowel context. Jaw motion does not assist the tongue articulation for velars as much as it does the articulations for dental, alveolar, and palatal sounds. Because the hinge of the jaw is located toward the back of the head, the mechanical advantage that jaw movement gives to lingual consonants declines as the point of articulation moves back in the mouth. Therefore, jaw motion is less helpful in making a velar contact than it is for more frontal contacts. Measurement of the degree of jaw closure for lingual consonants in the same vowel context, that is, /ɑ θ ɑ/, /ɑ s ɑ/, /ɑ ʃ ɑ/, and /ɑ k ɑ/, show that the smallest degree of jaw closing occurs for the velar sound (Kent & Moll, 1972).

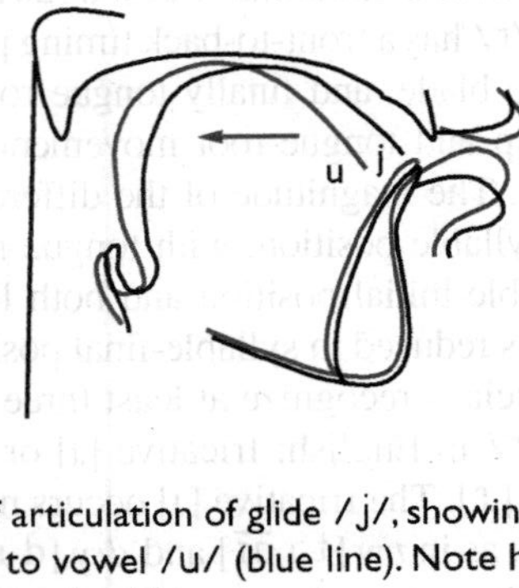

FIGURE 5.25
X-ray tracing of articulation of glide /j/, showing movement from /j/ (black line) to vowel /u/ (blue line). Note high-front, or palatal, tongue position for /j/.

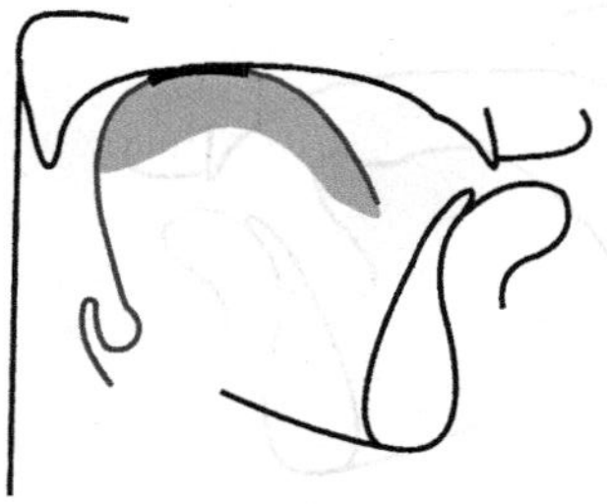

FIGURE 5.26
X-ray tracing of /k/ articulation. Thickened line shows lingua-velar contact.

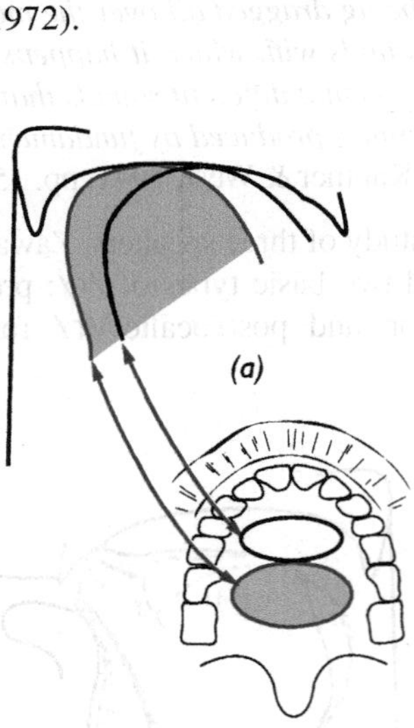

FIGURE 5.27
Variation in place of articulatory contact for the lingua-velar consonants. Contact site varies from front to back over the roof of the mouth. A lateral view is shown in *(a)* and an inferior view of the roof of the mouth is shown in *(b)*.

Although /k/ and /g/ are classified as stops along with /p/, /b/, /t/, and /d/, the velar stops are less stoplike than the bilabial and alveolar stops. /k/ and /g/ frequently are made with a sliding contact of the dorsum against the roof of the mouth. Figure 5.28 illustrates this sliding contact. This figure is based on the movements of small metal markers attached to the surface of the tongue. The movement paths of the markers were observed in an X-ray motion picture. Note that the markers first move upward, then forward during the sliding contact, and finally downward to the positions for the vowel. Because the vowel context was the same on either side of the velar consonant, the beginning and ending points of the movement paths are nearly the same.

Because of the sliding tongue contact and also because the tongue release for /k/ and /g/ is not so abrupt as that for the other stops, the velars tend to generate more noise energy. That is, the noise burst for /k/ and /g/ is longer than that for the other stops. There is little risk that the velar stops will be heard as fricatives because English does not have any velar fricatives.

The velar nasal /ŋ/ (*sing*) has an articulation like that for /k/ and /g/ except that the velopharynx is open (Figure 5.29). The exact site of contact varies with context, especially the surrounding vowels. The tongue elevation for the velars is somewhat higher than that for vowel /u/, as illustrated in Figure 5.30. The overall similarity between the /ŋ/ and /u/ articulations should be kept in mind when evaluating articulatory distinctions

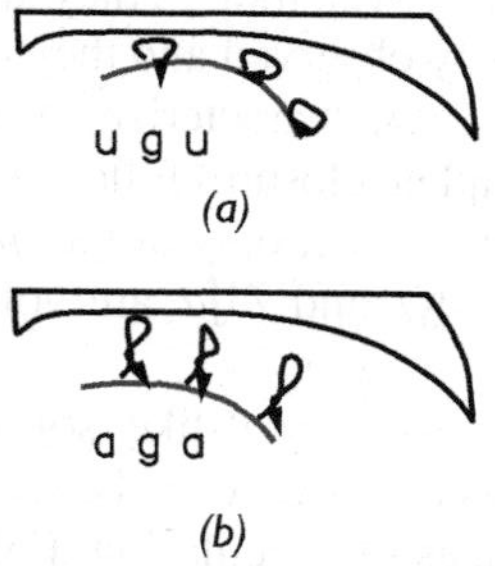

FIGURE 5.28
The lines ending in arrowheads show the motion paths of small pellets attached to the tongue during articulation of /u g u/ in *(a)* and /ɑ g ɑ/ in *(b)*. The motion paths are roughly circular or elliptical because of a sliding motion during articulatory contact for /g/.

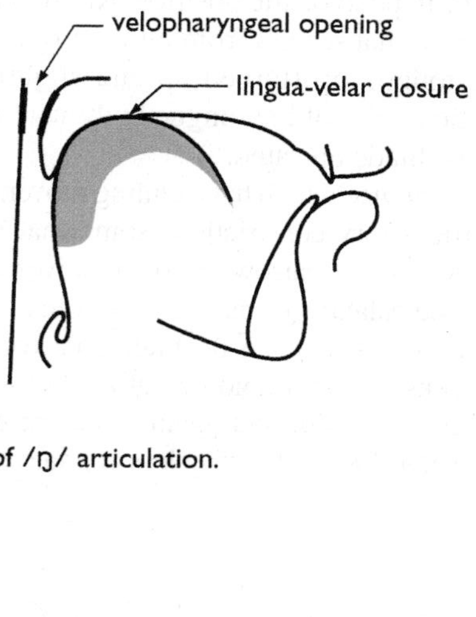

FIGURE 5.29
X-ray tracing of /ŋ/ articulation.

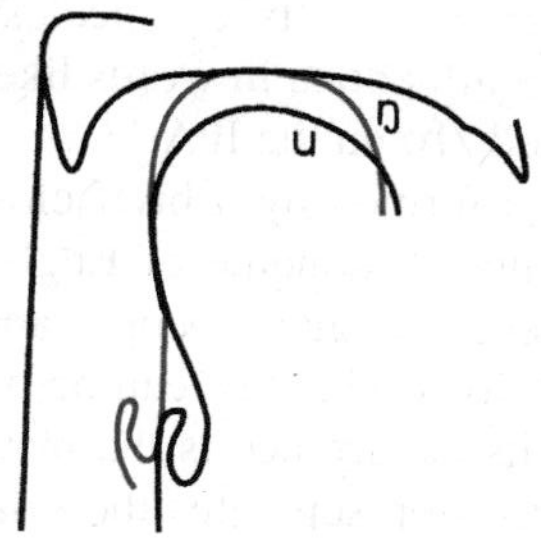

FIGURE 5.30
Composite drawing to show similarity in tongue positions for /ŋ/ (blue line) and /u/ (black line). To simplify the drawing, only the closed velopharyngeal port is shown.

between consonants and vowels. Some authors (e.g., Perkell, 1969), state that consonants and vowels use a different musculature, with the larger muscles being used to position the tongue body for vowels. However, it would appear that these larger muscles also could be used for many consonants, including /w/, /j/, /ʃ/, /r/, /k/, /g/, /ŋ/.

The labio-velar glides /w/ and /ʍ/ (also transcribed /hw/) are produced with a rounding of the lips and an arching of the tongue in the area of the velum. In fact, the articulatory configuration for /w/ (Figures 5.5 and 5.10) closely resembles that for the high-back vowel /u/. Many speakers use the voiceless /ʍ/ rarely, if at all. MacKay (1978) commented that /ʍ/ does not appear in most American dialects, and Tiffany and Carrell (1977) observed that the /w/–/ʍ/ contrast may be in the process of disappearing.

One reason we discuss /w/ and /ʍ/ under the velar place of articulation is to emphasize that these sounds are produced with a high-back tongue position, a fact that quite a few of our students have neglected in quizzes of articulatory description. The participation of both lips and tongue in the articulation of /w/ is particularly important clinically because of the frequent occurrence of /w/ for /r/ substitutions noted in clinical reports. It should be clear from comparisons of the labio-velar articulation in Figures 5.5 and 5.10 with the rhotic (especially bunched allophone) articulation in Figures 5.4 and 5.23 that /w/ and /r/ have at least a general articulatory similarity. At the same time, we suggest that not every /r/ error perceived as a /w/ is in fact produced as a genuine /w/ in the client's phonetic system. We believe that many supposed /w/ for /r/ substitutions are examples of derhotacized /r/ (see Chapter 6).

Glottals /h/ /ʔ/

The **glottals** are sounds formed at the vocal folds and include the glottal fricative /h/ (*who*) and the glottal stop /ʔ/. The /h/ is formed as air passes through a slit between the vocal folds and into the upper airway, thus creating turbulence noise. Because /h/ does not require a supralaryngeal constriction for its formation, the tongue, jaw, and lips are free to assume any positions except those that close off the oral cavity. Although /h/ typically is voiceless, some phoneticians hear a voiced allophone in words like *Ohio*. This allophone is transcribed /ɦ/ in the IPA.

The stop /ʔ/ is formed by a brief closure at the folds. Although /ʔ/ is not a phoneme of English, it occurs frequently in the speech of many people and has allophonic and junctural functions. The /ʔ/ can be hard to hear, but a good example of its occurrence is the phrase *Anna Adams,* in which the glottal stop separates the final vowel of *Anna* from the initial vowel in *Adams*. Thus, *Anna Adams* might be transcribed phonetically as [æ n ə ʔ æ d ə m z].

Summary by Manner of Articulation

The purpose of this review section is to give a unified summary of the information on place of articulation. At the same time, summary comments are made concerning manner of articulation, which is used as the basic outline of discussion.

Stop consonants, which involve a complete blockage of the airstream and an abrupt release of the blockage, are produced at four places: bilabial, alveolar, velar, and glottal. These places of articulation are schematically summarized in Figure 5.31. Voiced and voiceless pairs are produced at the bilabial (/b/–/p/), alveolar (/d/–/t/), and velar (/g/–/k/) sites. The glottal stop /ʔ/ is made by a complete closure of the vocal folds. Although some phoneticians regard /ʔ/ as a voiceless sound because the folds are not vibrating during its production, the requirement that the vocal folds be brought together gives it at least one point of similarity to the voiced sounds. Generally, the stop manner implies that the articulator makes a temporary tight contact that can be released to produce a short burst of noise energy. However, the burst is not a necessary feature of the stops. Furthermore, the velar stops frequently are articulated with a sliding motion of the lingual dorsum against the roof of the mouth; and this property, together with the fact that the articulatory release is somewhat more gradual than that for the bilabial and alveolar stops, causes the velars to be more fricative-like. This difference has perceptual consequences, as listeners confuse velar stops with fricative sounds more often than they confuse the bilabial and alveolar stops with fricatives (Klatt, 1968).

Nasal consonants, produced with complete blockage at some point in the oral cavity but with an open velopharynx, are made at the bilabial (/m/), alveolar (/n/), and velar (/ŋ/) sites of contact. The oral articulation is quite similar to that for the homorganic stop; that is, /m/ resembles /b/, /n/ resembles /d/, and /ŋ/ resembles /g/. The places of oral closure are the same as those shown in Figure 5.31 except that the glottal stop usually is not considered as a nasal because the site of articulation is below that of the oral–nasal division, the velopharynx.

Fricative consonants, produced with an airway constriction sufficiently narrow to generate continuous noise (frication or turbulence noise), are made at the labiodental, dental, alveolar, palatal, and glottal sites of articulation. At

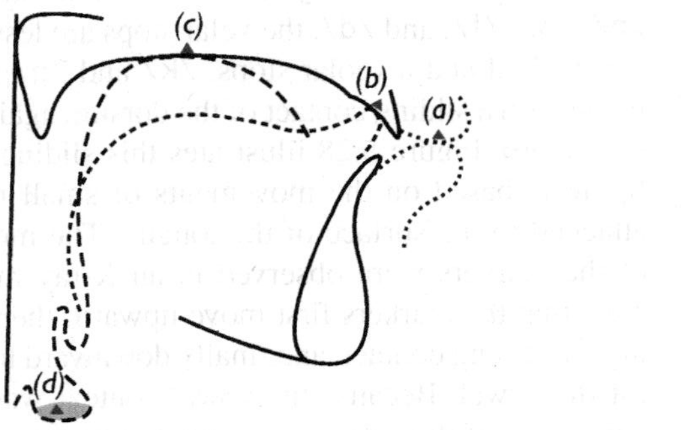

FIGURE 5.31
Places of articulation for stop consonants: *(a)* bilabial, *(b)* alveolar, *(c)* velar, and *(d)* glottal.

each site except the glottal, voiced and voiceless cognates are produced: /v/–/f/, /ð/–/θ/, /z/–/s/, /ʒ/–/ʃ/. For that matter, even the glottal place of articulation has an allophonic voice alternation, for the intervocalic /h/ in words like *Ohio* is sometimes voiced (/ɦ/). The alveolar and palatal fricatives are much more intense than the labiodental, dental, and glottal fricatives. In recognition of this difference, the alveolar and palatal fricatives are called **stridents** or **sibilants.** The weak energy, and hence low audibility, of the labiodental and dental fricatives is offset by their relatively high visibility and low frequency of occurrence (see Appendix B). That is, even though they are not always easily heard, they are easily observed and they occur infrequently.

Affricate consonants, characterized by a two-phase articulation of stop (complete closure) followed by frication (noise segment), occur in English only at the palatal site. The two palatal affricates /ʤ/ and /tʃ/ are voiced and voiceless, respectively.

Liquid consonants, vowel-like sounds that have narrower constrictions than true vowels, are made at the alveolar and palatal places of articulation. Following Ladefoged (1993), we use the term *liquid* as a cover term for the lateral /l/ and the rhotic /r/. The lateral is made with a midline alveolar contact but lateral opening. The tongue dorsum usually assumes an /o/-like position, and this feature may be more constant than the alveolar contact, which does not always occur in postvocalic position. Rhotic /r/ has a palatal constriction that results from either a retroflex articulation of the tongue tip (turned up and slightly back) or a bunched articulation of the tongue body with the tip turned down and the blade elevated.

Glide consonants, which have gliding movements originating from articulatory constrictions somewhat narrower than for vowels but not as narrow as for fricatives and stops, are produced as the palatal /j/ and the labio-velars /w/ and /ʍ/. Palatal /j/ closely resembles the high-front vowel /i/ but has a narrower constriction. Labio-dental /w/ closely resembles the high-back vowel /u/ but again has a narrower constriction. Labio-velar /ʍ/ is the voiceless cognate of /w/.

Summary by Place of Articulation

Obviously, the tongue is used for a number of places of articulation, and these possibilities are shown in Figure 5.32. Part *(a)* of this illustration shows the articulations of the tongue tip: interdental, dental, alveolar, and retroflex. Part *(b)* shows the articulation of blade and palate, and part *(c)* shows the articulation of dorsum and roof of the mouth (velar). Labial articulations are depicted in Figure 5.33, which shows rounding, bilabial closure, and labiodental constriction. Figure 5.34 shows the articulations of the velopharynx, depicted as elevation of the velum for oral consonants and lowering of the velum for nasal consonants. The other structures involved in velopharyngeal closure are not shown, but it should be recalled that the lateral walls of the pharynx can have an important role in velopharyngeal articulation. The larynx serves as an articulator in the production of fricative /h/ and the stop /ʔ/. For the fricative, the folds are separated sufficiently so that frication noise is generated. For the stop, the folds are brought together tightly so that airflow is blocked (and vocal fold vibrations cease) for a period of time. Finally, the jaw is indirectly related to place of articulation in its role as skeletal support for the tongue and lower lip and in its contribution to the movement of these structures.

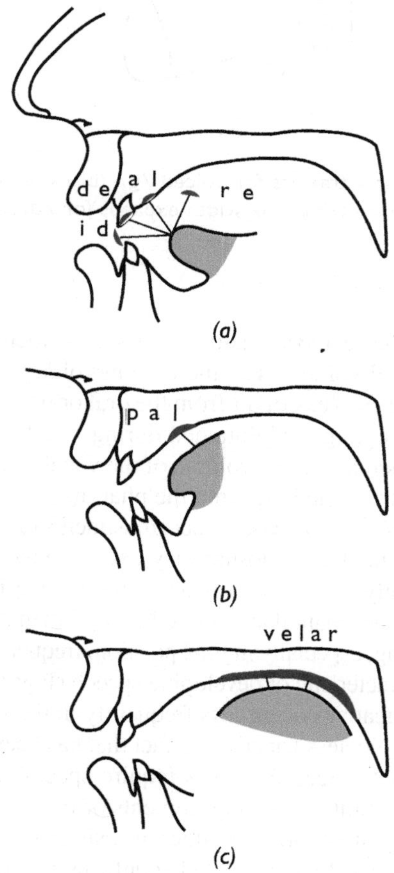

FIGURE 5.32
Places of articulation for lingual consonants: *(a)* interdental (id), dental (de), alveolar (al), and retroflex (re) articulations; *(b)* palatal (pal) articulation; *(c)* major sites (front and back) of velar articulation.

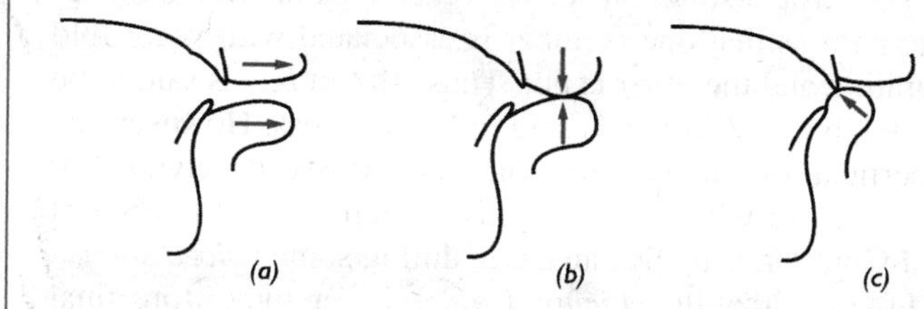

FIGURE 5.33
Lip articulations: *(a)* rounding or protrusion, *(b)* bilabial closure, and *(c)* labiodental constriction.

The Voicing Contrast

The voicing contrast is most easily described for pairs of sounds that share place and manner of articulation but differ in the voicing feature. Such pairs are called **cognates.** The **voiced** and **voiceless** cognate pairs of English are presented in the following list.

	Voiced	Voiceless	Examples
Bilabial stop	/b/	/p/	bay–pay
Labial-velar glide	/w/	/ʍ/	witch–which
Labiodental fricative	/v/	/f/	vat–fat
Interdental fricative	/ð/	/θ/	thy–thigh
Alveolar stop	/d/	/t/	doe–toe
Alveolar fricative	/z/	/s/	zip–sip
Palatal fricative	/ʒ/	/ʃ/	rouge–rush
Palatal affricate	/ʤ/	/tʃ/	gin–chin
Velar stop	/g/	/k/	gap–cap

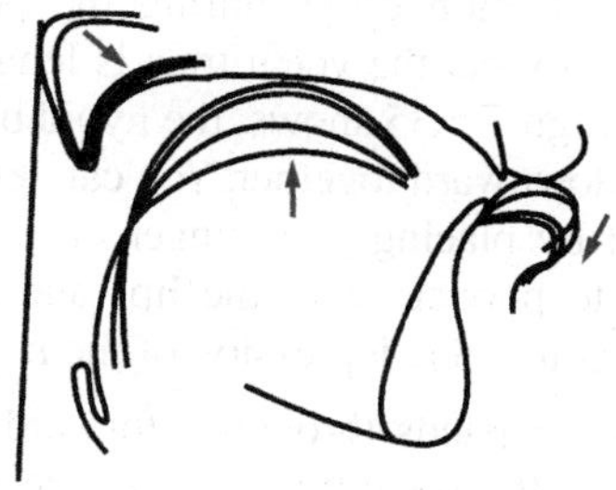

FIGURE 5.34
Composite of X-ray tracings for the [p]–[ɪ]–[ŋ] sequence in the word *camping.* As lips open for [p] release, tongue elevates for [ɪ] and [ŋ], and velopharynx opens.

The basic distinction between each member of these cognate pairs is that one member is associated with vocal fold vibration and the other is not. Thus, /b/ in *bay* is said to be voiced, but /p/ in *pay* is said to be voiceless. However, the superficial simplicity of the voicing contrast is deceiving. For example, we will discuss in this section the fact that vocal fold vibration actually can *cease* during some *voiced sounds* and the fact that the *voicing distinction* for some word-final consonants is carried perceptually by the *length of the vowel* that precedes the consonants. Thus, it is an oversimplification to say that the vocal folds vibrate during voiced sounds and do not vibrate during voiceless sounds.

First, we consider some of the physiological implications of the voicing contrast. It is important to recognize that special adjustments are required to keep the vocal folds vibrating during a period of vocal tract closure. The need for these adjustments can be appreciated by performing a simple experiment: Close your lips tightly, pinch your nostrils closed with your fingers, and try to make a voiced sound, like a sustained /m/. You will notice that phonation is possible only for a short time, and you might puff out your cheeks in an effort to sustain the phonation. Voicing or phonation is difficult under these circumstances because the vocal folds vibrate only if air passes between them. When the vocal tract is closed, airflow eventually ceases (because the air has nowhere to go), and so does voicing. Puffing the cheeks helps to maintain voicing for a short interval because the puffing expands the oral chamber and allows air to pass from the lungs into the mouth. In short, it is difficult to voice sounds when the vocal tract is closed. Voicing is most easily maintained when the vocal tract is open, as in the case of vowels.

How then can a speaker maintain voicing during a period of closure for the italicized sounds in a*b*out, a*bd*icate, a*g*ain, and O*gd*en? There are two general possibilities: (1) Allow a small leakage of air from the vocal tract (for example, through the velopharyngeal port); or (2) increase the volume of the supralaryngeal cavity. Most speakers seem to use the second alternative. The supralaryngeal cavity can be enlarged in several ways, but the two primary means are shown in Figure 5.35, parts *(b)* and *(c)*.

1. The larynx position drops during the period of vocal tract closure so that the vocal tract is lengthened. As the drawing in Figure 5.35 shows, the hyoid bone and larynx may move downward together. You can test this possibility yourself by placing your finger on the larynx while attempting to phonate with the lips and nostrils tightly closed. Do you feel a depression of the larynx?
2. The pharynx expands through a forward motion of the tongue during the vocal tract closure. Pharyngeal expansion is illustrated in Figures 5.35 and 5.36. Figure 5.36 shows X-ray tracings of stop closure for /k/ and /g/. Notice that the size of the pharynx is greater for the voiced stop than it is for the voiceless stop.

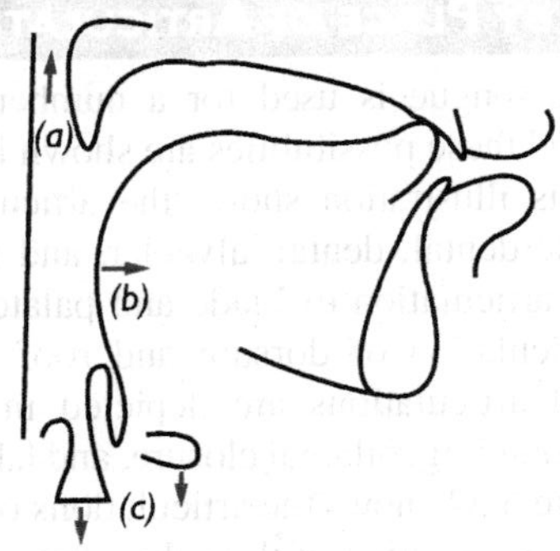

FIGURE 5.35
Possibilities for maintaining voicing during production of voiced stops: *(a)* opening of velopharyngeal port to permit airflow, *(b)* expansion of pharynx, and *(c)* lowering of larynx.

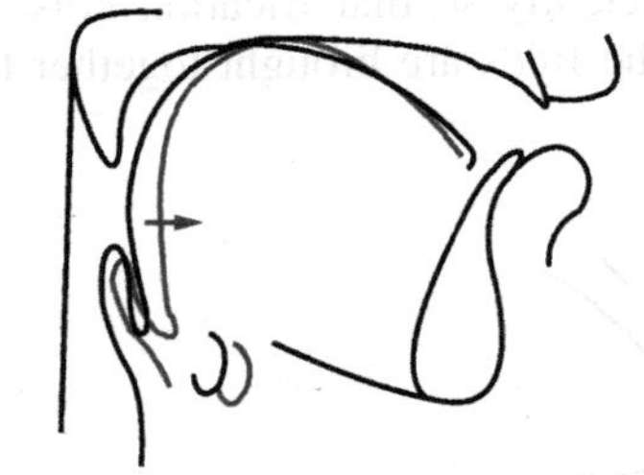

FIGURE 5.36
Composite X-ray tracings for voiced /g/ (black line) and voiceless /k/ (blue line). Pharynx width expands for /g/, as shown by arrow.

Both of these mechanisms result in an increase in the supralaryngeal volume. The increase in volume is functionally the same as a leak of air from the oral or pharyngeal cavity. Hence, voicing is maintained during vocal tract closure by a small increase in the volume of the vocal tract, allowing air to move from the lungs into the pharynx.

The need for special vocal tract adjustments to sustain voicing during articulatory closure may explain why young children frequently devoice consonants; that is, *dog* is produced with a final consonant that is more like /k/ than /g/. Consonant devoicing, especially in final position, frequently has been noted as characteristic of developing speech (Ingram, 1989).

Voiced fricatives occur less frequently in the world's language than voiceless fricatives, a fact that has been explained by noting that voiced fricatives require special adjustments to meet the simultaneous requirements of frication and voicing. A study of fricative production using structural Magnetic Resonance Imaging (MRI) confirms and extends this explanation. Proctor, Shadle, and Iskarous (2010) showed that voiced oral fricatives are produced with a larger pharynx than that observed for their voiceless cognates, apparently to ensure transglottal airflow to maintain voicing. The authors concluded that the production of voiced oral fricatives is complex because a speaker must achieve three goals: (a) form the oral constriction, (b) produce sufficient airflow through the oral constriction to generate frication noise, and (c) maintain vocal fold vibration for voicing though adequate transglottal airflow. It might be expected, then, that voiceless fricatives would be mastered earlier in speech development than their voiced cognates. Some studies of speech development support this conclusion, but the difference in age acquisition is quite small.

Another complication in the phonetic study of voicing is that the sound cues by which we make phonetic judgments of voicing vary with word position and consonant type. For a stop consonant in word-initial position, say, *bat* versus *pat*, the effective difference very often is the **voice onset time** (VOT), which is the time difference between the release of the stop closure and the beginning of the vocal fold vibrations. The timing patterns are illustrated schematically in Figure 5.37. If the vocal fold vibrations begin before the stop is released, the stop is said to be **prevoiced** (or, it has a voicing lead), and the VOT in ms has a negative sign. For example, a VOT of –30 ms means that the voicing began 30 milliseconds before the stop release. If the vocal vibrations begin after the stop release, the stop is said to have a voicing lag, and the VOT in ms is a positive value (for example, VOT = 50 ms). If the vocal vibrations begin simultaneously with the stop release, the VOT is zero. Generally, an initial stop in English is perceived as voiced if (1) voicing precedes articulatory release, as in Figure 5.37*(a)*; (2) voicing begins simultaneously with articulatory release, as in part *(b)*; or (3) voicing begins shortly after, within 25 ms or so, articulatory release, as in part *(c)*. An initial stop is perceived as voiceless if voicing begins significantly later (usually more than 50 ms) than articulatory release, as in part *(d)*. Hence, whether an initial stop is heard as voiced or voiceless depends upon the *relative timing* of vibration in the larynx and articulatory release of the stop.

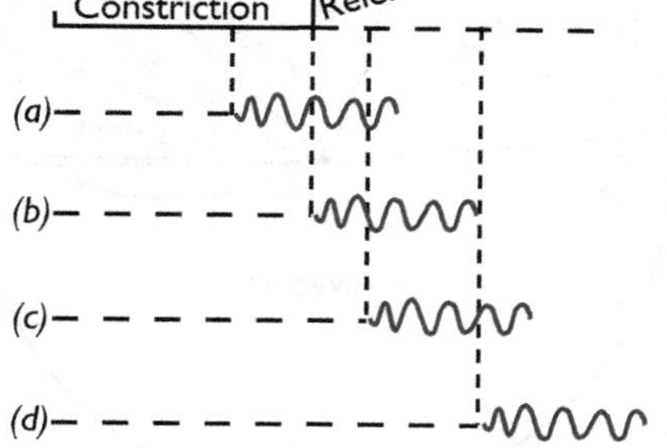

FIGURE 5.37
Timing patterns of supralaryngeal and laryngeal events to explain variations in voice onset time. Onset of voicing (sawtooth line) is described relative to instant of release of consonant articulation.

A feature that is related to voicing for stops is aspiration. **Aspiration** is a friction noise (like that for /h/) generated as air flows through the vocal folds and into the upper cavities. Stops are said to be aspirated if an interval of aspiration, or frication, precedes voicing. Stops are said to be unaspirated if such an interval does not occur. In English, released voiceless stops are aspirated unless they follow /s/. Only when these stops occur after /s/ in the same syllable are they unaspirated. Voiced stops are unaspirated in English. The occurrence of aspiration is controlled by the glottal opening present when the articulatory closure for the stop is released. If the folds are sufficiently separated, aspiration will occur. If the glottal opening is negligible when the stop is released, aspiration will not occur. The occurrence of unaspirated voiceless stops following /s/ seems to be related to the relative timing of vocal fold movement and the oral articulations. That is, if the folds begin to come together during the stop, the glottal opening may be quite small at the moment of stop release.

In the word-medial or intervocalic position, the voicing contrast is associated with a difference in vocal fold vibration and sometimes with a difference in duration of consonant constriction. For example, in the word pair *ribbing–ripping,* the vocal fold vibrations continue throughout the word *ribbing* (all segments being voiced), but they cease for a short time during the bilabial closure for /p/ in *ripping.* In addition, the duration of bilabial closure often is longer for the voiceless consonant, so that the lips may remain closed longer for /p/ than for /b/. Still another possible cue for the word-medial voicing contrast is that the release burst will be stronger for the voiceless stop than for the voiced stop. Finally, it should be noted that the voiced velar stop /g/ sometimes is momentarily devoiced in medial and intervocalic positions. Figure 5.38 shows the envelope of the voicing signal obtained from a contact microphone strapped to the neck tissue over the larynx. The vertical dimension

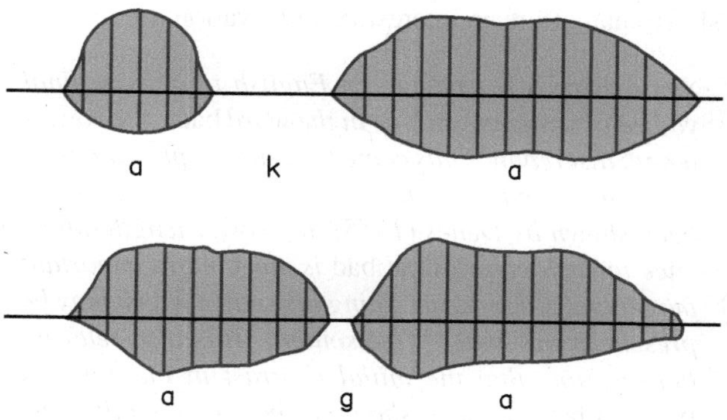

FIGURE 5.38
Envelope of voicing signal recorded by a throat microphone. Voicing signal ceases for a long interval during /k/ (upper trace) and for a brief interval during /g/ (lower trace). Hence, /g/ is not necessarily continuously voiced.

(y-axis) shows the amplitude of voicing, and the horizontal dimension (x-axis) is time. For /ɑ k ɑ/ in the top trace, vocal fold vibration ceases for a considerable period of time, corresponding roughly to the interval of stop closure. But vocal fold vibration also ceases for /ɑ g ɑ/, though for a much shorter time.

Word-finally, the duration of the vowel preceding the consonant is the most important factor in determining whether the consonant will be heard as voiced or voiceless. Vowels preceding voiced consonants are longer than vowels preceding voiceless consonants. For example, it has been shown that the noun and verb forms of the word *use,* /j u s/ and /j u z/, may end in an essentially identical *voiceless* segment. The difference in voicing perceived by a listener depends on the fact that the vowel is longer for the verb form than for the noun form (Denes, 1955).

The tendency for vowels to be longer before voiced than voiceless consonants is common to all languages, but some languages, like English, have capitalized on this difference to make it the voicing contrast for final-position consonants. That is, although all languages have longer vowels before the voiced consonant, English has accentuated this difference in vowel length to make it a reliable cue for voicing of the consonant. Chen (1970) reports the following ratios, calculated as the average length of vowels before voiceless consonants divided by the average length of vowels before voiced consonants (the smaller the ratio, the larger the difference in vowel duration):

English	0.61
French	0.87
Russian	0.82
Korean	0.78
Spanish	0.86
Norwegian	0.82

In view of the peculiarities of the voicing contrast in English, Hyman offers an interesting observation:

> *Since there is a tendency in English to devoice final voiced obstruents (such as in the word* bad*), the vowel-length discrepancy has come to assume a phonological role, and perhaps ultimately a phonemic role. As has been shown by Denes (1955), the vowel-length difference in such pairs as* bat:bad *is much more important perceptually than any voicing difference which may be present in the final C [consonant]. It is also relevant here to note that the initial contrast in the minimal pair* pat:bat *has been shown to be, perceptually, one of aspirated vs. unaspirated, rather than voiceless vs. voiced. It thus appears that English is in the process of losing its voice contrast in consonants (note the loss of the /t/–/d/ contrast in most intervocalic positions): the final voice contrast is being replaced with a length contrast and the initial contrast is being replaced with an aspiration contrast.* (Hyman, 1975, p. 173)

This comment is a good reminder that spoken languages are not dead and fixed. Rather, languages change as they are spoken. A Rip van Winkle who sleeps through a century of change in the language habits of his own country might awake to discover that the people around him speak with a strange dialect.

Allographs of the Consonant Phonemes of English

Recall from Chapter 2 that an *allograph* is any one alphabet letter or combination of letters that represents a given phoneme. The allographs of the consonant phonemes of English are presented in Table 5.2. For each phoneme, the allographs are italicized in a sample word. For example, the allographs for the phoneme /b/ are the *b* in *but,* the *bb* in *rabbit,* and the *pb* in *cupboard.*

Frequency of Occurrence and Place of Articulation

Appendix B summarizes data on the frequency of occurrence of consonants in American English. Obviously, because consonants do not appear with equal frequency, some places of articulation are much more heavily used than others. The unequal use of different places of articulation is represented graphically in Figure 5.39, which is based on data for the 20 most frequently occurring consonants in the study by Mines, Hanson, and Shoup (1978). The sections in the circle graph are sized in proportion to the frequency of use of each place of articulation. The alveolar place of production is used as frequently as all other places combined.

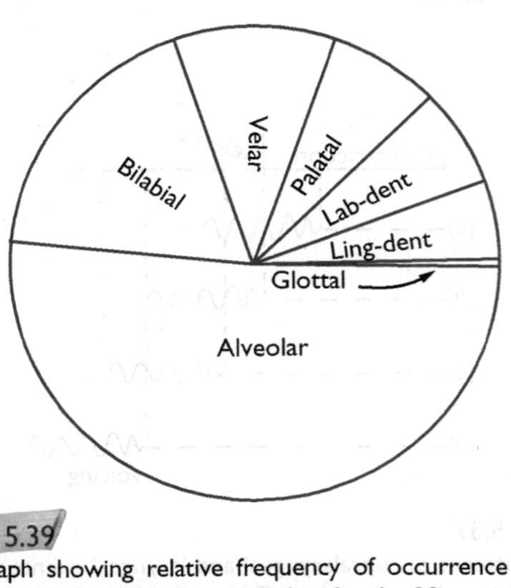

FIGURE 5.39
Circle graph showing relative frequency of occurrence of different places of articulation. Based on data for the 20 most frequently occurring consonants reported by Mines, Hanson, and Shoup (1978).

TABLE 5.2
Allographs of the Consonant Phonemes of English

Phoneme	Allograph (italicized in a sample word)
/b/	*b*ut, ra*bb*it, cu*pb*oard
/p/	*p*ay, su*pp*er, hiccou*gh* (/p/ also may occur as an intrusive in words containing the combinations *mf, mph, mt, mth,* and *ms;* for example, *comfort* may be pronounced [k ʌ m p f ɚ t], and *warmth* may be pronounced [w ɔ r m p θ])
/d/	*d*oll, a*dd,* rais*ed,* cou*ld*
/t/	*t*ail, bu*tt*er, walk*ed,* dou*bt,* recei*pt,* indi*ct,* *Th*omas, *pt*omaine (/t/ also may occur as an intrusive in words containing the combination *nce* or *ns;* for example, *dance* may be pronounced [d æ n t s])
/g/	*g*o, e*gg,* va*gue,* *gu*ess, *gh*ost, e*x*ist (when pronounced with /g z/ rather than /k s/
/k/	ba*ck,* *c*ut, *ch*emical, o*cc*ur, s*q*uall, bouti*que,* *kh*aki, yo*lk,* fi*x* (as part of a /k s/ cluster), *qu*ay (/k/ also may occur as an intrusive in words containing the combination *ngth;* for example, *length* may be pronounced [l ɛ ŋ k θ])
/v/	*v*ine, sa*vv*y, o*f,* Ste*ph*en (some pronunciations)
/f/	*f*an, o*ff,* *ph*one, enou*gh,* ha*lf*
/ð/	*th*is (both /ð/ and /θ/ occur as *th*)
/θ/	*th*in
/z/	*z*oo, bu*zz,* i*s,* sci*ss*ors, di*s*cern, a*sth*ma, *x*ylophone, e*x*ist (when pronounced with /g z rather than /k s/)
/s/	*s*ay, mi*ss,* *c*ity, *sc*ent, *ps*alm, walt*z,* *sc*hism, li*st*en, bo*x* (as part of a /k s/ cluster)
/ʒ/	plea*s*ure, rou*ge,* bi*j*ou, a*z*ure, apha*s*ia, bra*z*ier
/ʃ/	*sh*e, *s*ugar, ac*t*ion, o*c*ean, *ch*ef, pre*c*ious, pa*ss*ion, *sch*ist, fu*chs*ia, con*sc*ious, nau*se*ous, an*x*ious (as part of a /k ʃ/ cluster)
/h/	*h*appy, *wh*o, Mona*gh*an
/m/	*m*an, su*mm*er, wo*mb,* hy*mn,* psa*lm,* diaphra*gm*
/n/	*n*ow, fu*nn*y, *kn*ife, *gn*ome, *pn*eumatic, si*gn,* *mn*emonic
/ŋ/	thi*ng,* thi*n*k, fi*n*ger, si*ng*er, ton*gue,* a*n*xious
/l/	*l*aw, a*ll,* litt*le,* kenn*el,* is*l*and, ki*l*n
/r/	*r*ed, ca*rr*y, *wr*ong, *rh*yme, co*r*ps, mo*r*tgage, cata*rrh*
/ʤ/	*j*am, *g*em, a*dj*acent, bri*dg*e, cor*d*ial, Geor*ge,* gra*d*ual, exa*gg*erate
/tʃ/	*ch*ief, ca*tch,* *c*ello, righ*t*eous, ques*t*ion, na*t*ure, man*s*ion
/w/	*w*on, *o*ne, q*u*een, ch*o*ir
/ʍ/	*wh*ich
/j/	*y*es, on*i*on, hallelu*j*ah, *u*se (as part of a /j u/ combination), poi*g*nant (also occurs in words like *few, fuel, feud* as part of a /j u/ combination)

Recognizing that the front vowels occur more frequently than central or back vowels and that the alveolar place is the most frequently occurring in consonant production, we can represent what should be the most frequently occurring tongue shape and position by a composite of a front vowel (say /ɛ/ for sake of illustration) and an alveolar consonant. This composite is shown in Figure 5.40. Interestingly, the overall shape of the tongue for the front vowel and for the alveolar consonant is highly similar, except of course for the position of the tongue tip. Because alveolar consonants tend to be produced with a fronted tongue body position, the frequently occurring front vowels and the frequently occurring alveolar consonants can be produced with basically the same positioning of the tongue body.

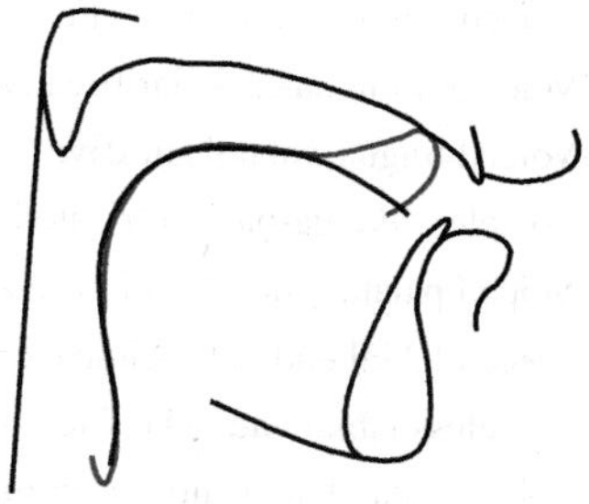

FIGURE 5.40
Composite drawing of articulatory configuration for front vowel /ɛ/ (black line) and alveolar consonant (blue line) produced in isolation. Notice overall similarity of tongue shape.

Summary Classification of Consonants

Table 5.3 summarizes the consonants of American English using the terms introduced in this chapter. Note that each sound is uniquely described by descriptions of voicing, place of articulation, and manner of articulation. When two or more sounds share the same place of articulation, they are called **homorganic.** For example, the initial sounds in the following words are homorganic because they are produced with a common lingua-alveolar articulation: *dip, not, tack.* When two or more sounds share the same manner of articulation, they are called **homotypic.** For example, the initial sounds in the following words are homotypic because they are all fricatives: *four, thick, sour, she.* Sometimes several manners of articulation are grouped into a single category. An **obstruent** is a sound made with a complete or narrow constriction at some point in the vocal tract. The obstruents include the stops, fricatives, and affricates. As mentioned earlier, the class of liquids includes the rhotic and the lateral. Also mentioned earlier, cognates are pairs of sounds that are distinguished by a particular phonetic feature, such as voicing.

TABLE 5.3
Classification of the Consonants of American English

IPA Symbol	Description
[b]	Voiced bilabial stop
[p]	Voiceless bilabial stop
[d]	Voiced lingua-alveolar (apical) stop
[t]	Voiceless lingua-alveolar (apical) stop
[g]	Voiced lingua-velar (dorsal) stop
[k]	Voiceless lingua-velar (dorsal) stop
[m]	Bilabial nasal
[n]	Lingua-alveolar (apical) nasal
[ŋ]	Lingua-velar (dorsal) nasal
[l]	Lingua-alveolar lateral
[ɾ]	Lingua-alveolar flap (one-tap trill)
[r]	Alveolar rhotic or retroflex
[v]	Voiced labiodental fricative
[f]	Voiceless labiodental fricative
[ð]	Voiced lingua-dental fricative
[θ]	Voiceless lingua-dental fricative
[z]	Voiced lingua-alveolar fricative
[s]	Voiceless lingua-alveolar fricative
[ʒ]	Voiced lingua-palatal fricative
[ʃ]	Voiceless lingua-palatal fricative
[j]	Voiced palatal glide (semivowel)
[w]	Voiced labial and velar glide (semivowel)
[h w] or [ʍ]	Voiceless labial and velar fricative/glide
[ʤ]	Voiced palatal affricate; see component sounds
[ʧ]	Voiceless palatal affricate; see component sounds
[ʔ]	Glottal stop
[h]	Voiceless glottal fricative

Consonants Around the World

Compared to other languages, American English is about average in its number of consonants. But as you probably can attest if you have tried to learn other languages, there are many possible consonants that American English does not use.

First, there are manner classes of consonants in other languages that are not used at all in American English. To understand these classes, it is helpful to follow the International Phonetic Association in classifying consonants as pulmonic and nonpulmonic. The pulmonic consonants are produced with a pulmonic (typically egressive) airstream, and the nonpulmonic consonants are not.

The major class of pulmonic consonant not used in American English is the **trill,** defined as a sound made with a supraglottal vibration. The vibration requires a flow of air (hence pulmonic airstream) directed between two articulators that are held together with just enough muscle tension to produce vibration. The mechanism is similar to that used to make the vocal folds vibrate. Many trills involve actions of the lips or tongue, often working with some other part of the vocal tract. The raspberry (or Bronx cheer), often used to express disapproval, is made with the upper lip and tongue. Among the most important trills in different languages are the bilabial trill, the alveolar trill, and the uvular trill (Appendix A.1). Interestingly, infants frequently produce trills in their early sounds even if trills are not used in the ambient language.

The three major classes of nonpulmonic consonants not used in American English are the **clicks, voiced implosives,** and **ejectives** (see Appendix A.1 for IPA symbols). These sounds are made with articulatory (vocal tract) actions that generate sound in the absence of an egressive airstream from the lungs. A click is a stop produced with an ingressive velaric airstream. The back of the tongue closes against the velum simultaneously as another closure is formed at some forward point in the vocal tract. The two closures trap a pocket of air between them. Once this closed space is formed, a downward or backward movement of the tongue enlarges the volume of the space so that a negative air pressure is created. When the articulatory closure is released, air flows to equalize the pressure, and a click is generated.

A voiced implosive (sometimes called ingressive) is a stop made with an ingressive glottalic airstream. To produce this sound, the larynx is pulled rapidly downward while the vocal folds are adducted but not tightly closed. The rapid descent of the larynx causes air to flow ingressively through the glottis, resulting in vocal fold vibration.

An ejective is a stop made with a glottalic egressive airstream. The articulation is a rapid upward movement of the larynx while the vocal folds are closed tightly. In effect, the larynx acts like a piston to produce a positive pressure change in the vocal tract. Ejectives are also known as glottalized or checked, recursives, or abruptives. The IPA diacritic ['] is used to mark an ejective.

American English also does not use all possible places of articulation for the manner categories of stop, nasal, flap, fricative, affricate, and glide. For example, American English does not use retroflex, palatal, or uvular stops; labiodental, retroflex, palatal, or uvular nasals; retroflex, velar, uvular, or pharyngeal fricates; labiodental or velar glides; or retroflex, palatal, or velar laterals. Some of these place variations do occur clinically, especially for individuals who have anatomic abnormalities. Some people with cleft palate may use pharyngeal stops to substitute for the velar stops /k g/ and palatal stops to substitute for the alveolar stops /t d/ and the velar stops /k g/ (Trost, 1981).

Consonant Acoustics

As we saw in Chapter 4, vowels and diphthongs are produced with a relatively open vocal tract, and the primary acoustic appearance of these sounds is a continuous formant pattern. Recall that formants are resonances of the vocal tract that are activated by vibration of the vocal folds (or noise in the case of whispered speech). Formants pretty much tell the story for vowels and diphthongs. Each vowel is associated with a formant pattern that can be sustained indefinitely (as long as a speaker's breath holds out!) Diphthongs are somewhat different in that they involve a gradual change in vocal tract configuration from one vowel to another. But for both vowels and diphthongs, formant structure captures the acoustic essence of the sound, which allows us to represent a monophthongal vowel as a single point in an two-dimensional F1-F2 chart or a three-dimensional F1-F2-F3 space. Formants are fairly continuous bands of energy for these sounds.

The picture changes considerably for consonants. A basic articulatory property of most consonants is that they are produced with a constriction in the oral region of the vocal tract airway. Much of what has been said so far in this chapter pertains to the manner and location of this constriction or narrowing. We have considered constrictions for stops, fricatives, affricates, nasals, and liquids. As Stevens (2000) notes, the narrowing in the oral region for consonants creates particular types of discontinuities in the short-time spectrum of the sound. That is, the acoustic pattern of speech changes abruptly and distinctively—unlike the essentially stable formant pattern for a vowel sound or gradually changing formant pattern for a diphthong. The discontinuities for consonants occur with the formation and release of a constriction. Stevens goes on to state that there are three ways of creating such an acoustic discontinuity.

1. One way is to switch the principal acoustic source from frication (or turbulence noise) generated near a constriction in the oral cavity to the acoustic source at the glottis. An example is the transition from the fricative to the vowel in the word *saw*. The two different acoustic sources modified by the filtering provided by the vocal tract have different acoustic spectra, so that there is a marked discontinuity in the spectrum. This discontinuity is shown in Figure 5.41. Note the marked contrast between the initial

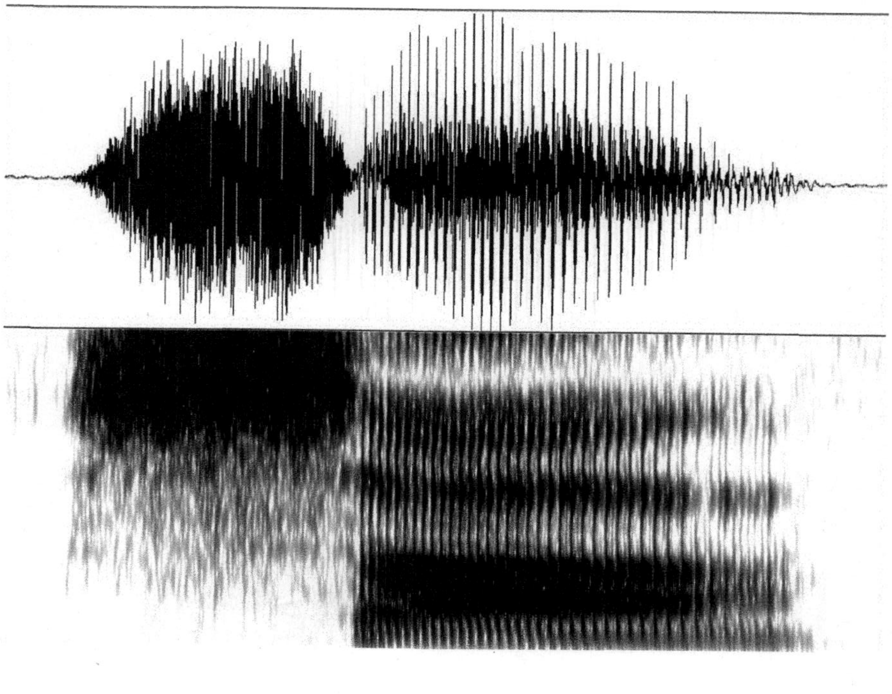

FIGURE 5.41
Waveform (top) and spectrogram (bottom) of the word *saw*.

noise segment and the following resonant segment for the vowel. Because the two sounds are distinctive, you probably can draw an approximate boundary between them.

2. An acoustic discontinuity also can be produced by switching the sound output from the nostrils to the mouth (or vice versa) while a fixed acoustic source (voicing) is maintained at the glottis. In contrast to obstruent consonants, there is no change in the acoustic source at the time this change in the output occurs. In short, voicing continues throughout, but the sound transmission is redirected from nose to mouth, or from mouth to nose. An example is shown in Figure 5.42 for the word *gnaw*. The first sound /n/ involves radiation of sound energy exclusively through the nose, and the second, the diphthong, radiation through the mouth and nose. For both sounds, there is an ongoing resonant pattern, but the pattern for the nasal is distinct from that for the vowel. You should be able to draw an approximate boundary between the nasal consonant and the vowel.

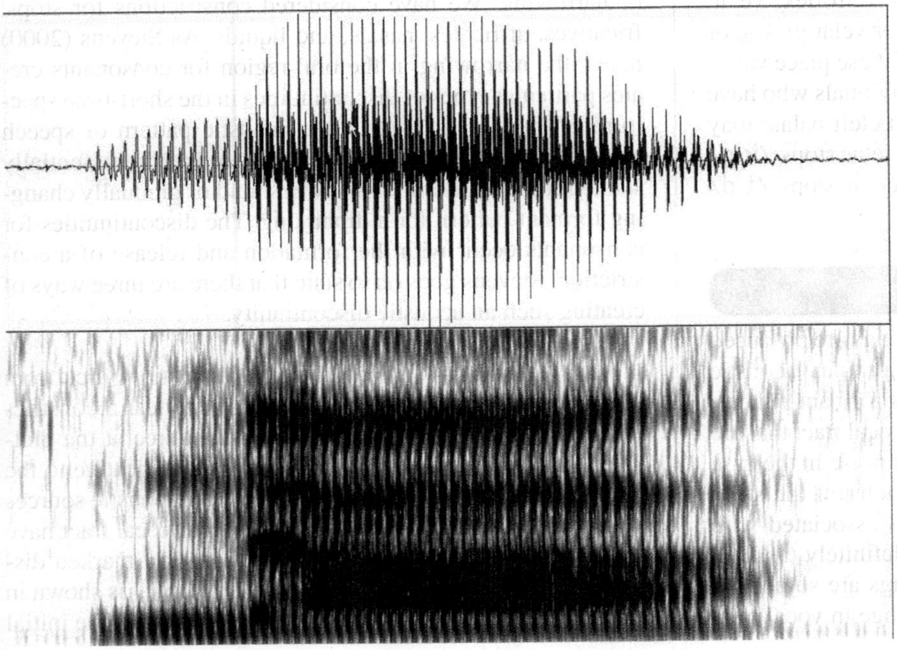

FIGURE 5.42
Waveform (top) and spectrogram (bottom) of the word *gnaw*.

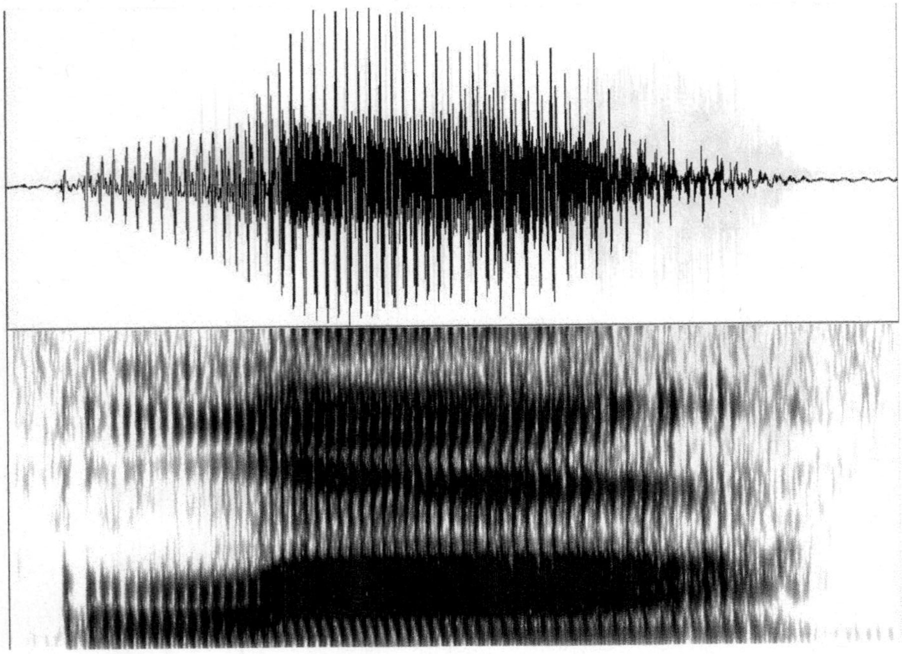

FIGURE 5.43
Waveform (top) and spectrogram (bottom) of the word *law*.

3. An acoustic discontinuity also can be produced when the major acoustic path through the oral cavity switches from a path with a side branch to one in which there is a direct path (no side branch). In English the oral side branch occurs for only one sound, the lateral /l/. As we have seen, this sound involves a midline closure so that sound radiation is directed laterally around the closure. An example is shown in Figure 5.43 for the word *law*, which begins with the lateral consonant and ends with a vowel. Notice that the /l/ segment in this word is rather similar to the /n/ segment in Figure 5.42.

This introduction to consonant acoustics makes the basic point that consonants generally involve the production of acoustic discontinuities that interrupt the smooth formant patterns of vowels and diphthongs. A first step in understanding the acoustic properties of consonants is to see in more detail how they differ from vowels. We now examine these acoustic features in more detail by considering three aspects of consonant production considered earlier in this chapter: (1) the source of energy (voicing, frication noise, burst noise); (2) the manner or degree of vocal tract constriction (for example, complete closure for stops, narrow constriction for fricative, complete oral closure coupled with nasal radiation for nasal consonants, and a vowel-like oral radiation for liquids and glides); and (3) the place of constriction. Our next objective is to identify acoustic cues associated with these three major aspects of consonant articulation.

The acoustics of consonant articulation are complex. Because consonants are of several kinds, some vowel-like, some noiselike, some voiced, some voiceless, some long in duration, and some very brief in duration, a fairly large set of acoustic descriptors is required to discuss the details of consonant acoustics. However, the basic acoustic properties can be discussed broadly with respect to (1) the source of energy (voicing, frication noise, burst noise); (2) the manner or degree of vocal tract constriction (for example, complete closure for stops and affricates, narrow constriction for fricatives, nasal radiation for nasal consonants, or vowel-like oral radiation for liquids and glides); and (3) the place of vocal tract constriction.

Source of Energy

If the vocal folds are vibrating while a sound is produced, the sound is called voiced. A voiced sound has as its acoustic property the quasiperiodic (meaning almost equally spaced in time) pulses of energy created as puffs of air escape through the vibrating vocal folds. Therefore, voiced consonants, like voiced vowels, are associated with vertical striations or voicing pulses on a spectrogram. Notice that, in the wide-band spectrogram of the simple sentence *The sunlight strikes raindrops in the air* in Figure 5.44, voicing pulses continue without interruption from the first vowel /ʌ/ in *sunlight* through the diphthong /ɑ͡ɪ/ in the same word. Because the /n/ and the /l/ are voiced consonants, they show evidence of voicing pulses. However, for voiceless sounds like /t/, /s/, /k/, and /p/, the voicing pulses cease.

The voiceless sounds derive their energy from either frication (continued noise) or burst (brief transient noise). The /s/ sound, which recurs frequently in the spectrogram of Figure 5.44, is an example of a sound with a frication energy source. As air is forced through the narrow groove formed by the tongue tip and the alveolar ridge, noise is generated. A

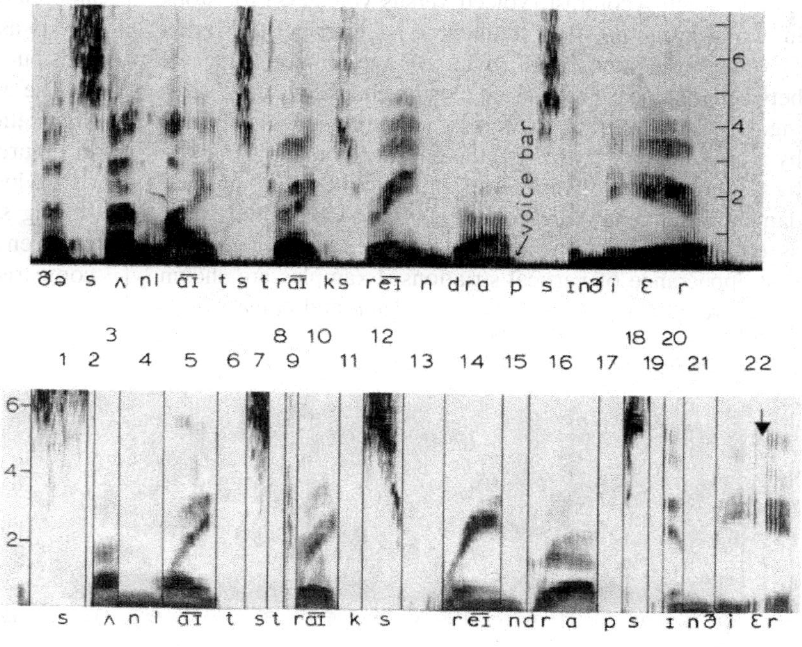

FIGURE 5.44
Spectrogram *(a)* is a man's recitation of the sentence *The sunlight strikes raindrops in the air.* Frequency in kHz is scaled on the vertical axis. The phonetic transcription at the bottom of the spectrogram can be used as a guide to segmentation. Spectrogram *(b)* is a woman's recitation of the sentence. The numbers at the top identify the following vertical slices or segments: 1—frication noise for [s]; 2—brief silent period; 3—vowel [ʌ]; 4—[n] + [l] sequence; 5—diphthong [ɑ͡ɪ]; 6—stop gap for [t]; 7—frication noise for [s]; 8—stop gap for [t]; 9—release burst and voiceless interval for [t]; 10—[r] + [ɑ͡ɪ] sequence; 11—stop gap for [k]; 12—combined noise segment: release burst for [k] and frication for [s]; 13—pause segment showing onset of voicing for following [r]; 14—[r] + [e͡ɪ] sequence; 15—nasal murmur for [n]; 16—[d] + [r] + [ɑ] sequence; 17—stop gap for [p]; 18—frication for [s]; 19—pause or silent interval; 20—vowel [ɪ]; 21—nasal murmur for [n] and weak fricative segment for [ð]; and 22—[i] + [ɛr] sequence (arrow points to glottal stop).

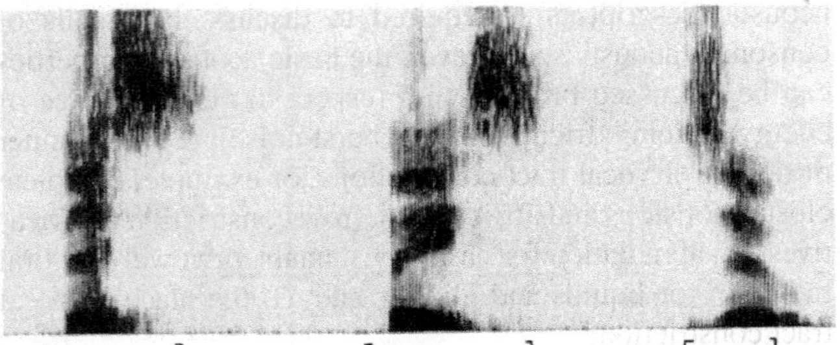

FIGURE 5.45
Spectrograms of words containing the voiced fricatives [ð], [v], and [z]. The noise energy for [ð] and [v] is so weak that it barely appears on the spectrogram.

clear example of burst or transient noise can be seen for the /t/ in *strikes*. This burst noise immediately follows the brief stop gap (silent period) that in turn immediately follows the frication segment for the /s/. The stop gap, which is located just above the /t/ in the phonetic transcription, is a silent interval that results from complete closure of the vocal tract. As the lingua-alveolar closure for the /t/ is released, the air pressure that was contained behind the tongue closure escapes in an explosive burst. The brevity of the noise for the /t/ release contrasts with the much longer frication noise for the /s/.

For voiced fricatives, there are two energy sources: The voicing pulses associated with vocal fold vibration and the frication generated at the site of vocal tract constriction. The appearance of these sounds on a spectrogram is that of noise modulated by voicing (in other words, noise that is regulated in time by the puffs of air from the larynx). Examples of voiced fricatives are shown in Figure 5.45.

The voicing contrast (voiced versus voiceless) for stops in word-initial position frequently is described in terms of voice onset time (VOT), which is the temporal interval between the release of the stop closure and the onset of voicing. On a spectrogram, the release of the closure is signified by a brief burst of noise, and the onset of voicing is marked by the appearance of vertical striations in the voice bar (fundamental frequency) and formants. Thus, VOT is measured as the time separation between the release burst and the first appearance of vertical striations. Examples are shown in Figure 5.46 for the words *tame–dame* and *came–game*. Note that the voiceless stop always has a longer VOT than the voiced stop. Essentially, the difference in VOT between the voiced and voiceless categories means that the voiceless stop has a longer aperiodic (nonvoiced) interval. For voiced stops, voicing begins shortly after release, simultaneously with release, or slightly before release. For voiceless stops, voicing begins an appreciable time after release. The VOT for voiced stops is less than 20 ms, whereas the VOT for voiceless stops usually ranges between 30 and 80 ms, depending on a number of phonetic factors, including speaking rate, stress, and place of articulation.

Manner or Degree of Vocal Tract Constriction

This aspect of consonant production is represented by a number of different spectrographic features, some of which are illustrated in Figure 5.44. Note the spectrographic appearance of the following sounds, arranged roughly *in order of increasing openness of the vocal tract.*

Stops: /t/ and /k/ in *strikes;* /d/ and /p/ in *raindrops.*

Fricatives: the two /s/ sounds in *strikes;* /ð/ in *the.*

Nasals: /n/ in *sunlight, raindrops,* and *in.*

Liquids: /l/ in *sunlight* and /r/ in *strikes* and *raindrops.*

The essential articulatory feature of a stop is articulatory closure, and the corresponding spectrographic feature is a **stop gap,** which is an interval of silence or greatly attenuated (decreased) sound energy. The /t/ in *strikes* has a silent stop gap, but the stop gap for /d/ in *raindrops* contains the low-frequency energy of voicing (the so-called **voice bar** at the extreme low-frequency region of the spectrogram) and, because of the influence of the abutting nasal /n/, a certain amount of nasally radiated energy. The release of a stop usually is associated with a burst of energy, as just discussed. This burst can be seen in the spectrogram of Figure 5.46.

The essential acoustic feature of a fricative is an interval of frication noise, which is conspicuous for the /s/ sounds in Figure 5.44. The intensity of this noise varies with place of production, as will be discussed in more detail in the following section. However, the great difference in intensity between /s/ and /ð/ can be seen from Figure 5.44 in the comparison of the /s/ in *raindrops* with the /ð/ in *the*. The frication noise for the latter is so weak as to be barely visible.

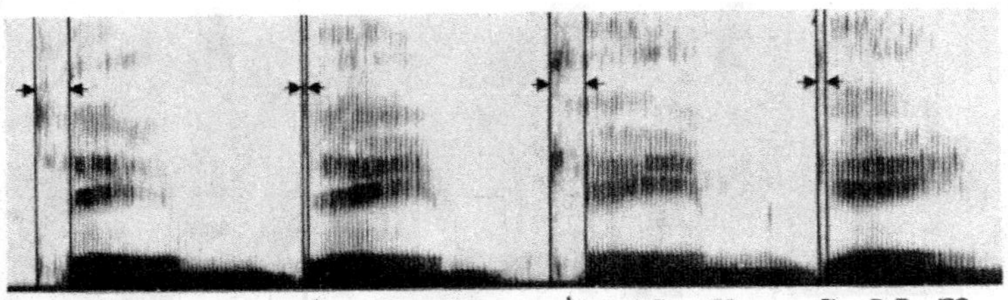

FIGURE 5.46
Spectrograms showing voice onset time (interval marked by arrows) for the initial stop consonants in the words *tame, dame, came,* and *game.*

The nasal consonants /m n ŋ/ are the only phonemes uniquely identified with nasal radiation of the sound energy. Other phonemes are orally radiated. The nasal transmission of acoustic energy has major consequences on the overall intensity of the sound. As can be seen in Figure 5.44, nasal consonants tend to be weaker than surrounding vowels. For example, the /n/ in *sunlight* is markedly less intense (less overall blackness in the spectrogram) than the preceding vowel /ʌ/. Thus, even though the nasal tract is open as a route for radiation of the sound energy, this tract is not as efficient a path as the oral tract. Nasal consonants are weaker than vowel sounds and typically have a region of pronounced low-frequency energy (500 Hz or below).

The lateral /l/ and rhotacized /r/ (sometimes called liquids) are somewhat vowel-like in that they are sounds having a well-defined formant structure. They differ from vowels in that they have less overall energy and a lower frequency F_1. In Figure 5.44, the /l/ in *sunlight* and the /r/ in *strikes* and *raindrops* have bands of energy superimposed on the vertical striations of voicing. The liquids are less intense than surrounding vowels, but they are more intense than most other consonants.

These acoustic features demonstrate that as the vocal tract constriction for a consonant becomes less severe (more open), the consonant looks more like a vowel. In the extreme case of complete closure for a stop, there is little or no radiated acoustic energy during the stop gap. The fricatives have a continuous sound energy, but this energy does not have the well-defined formant structure of the vowels. Liquids and glides are more like vowels and have a distinctive formant pattern.

Place of Constriction

This property has many different acoustic correlates, but two of the most important are **formant transition** and **burst and frication spectra** (noise shaping). Formant transitions are bends or changes in formant structure. Whenever the articulators change position, the formant patterns also change, and transitions simply reflect articulatory movements, such as those between consonants and vowels. Formant transitions for the three CV syllables, /bɑ/, /dɑ/, and /gɑ/ are shown in Figure 5.47. These syllables were produced by a talking computer but are much like human speech and are easy to use for purposes of illustration. The only difference among these syllables lies in the transition for the second and third formants. The first formant, the one lowest in frequency, has the same shape for all three syllables. When we listen to these syllables, it is only the small difference in the transitions for the second and third formants, occurring over an interval of 50 ms, that allows us to distinguish /b/, /d/, and /g/. The pattern of the second and third formants in CV and VC transitions carries information about the place of articulation.

For a given consonant, the formant transition varies with vowel context, as illustrated in Figure 5.48. Notice that for these stylized /d/ + vowel syllables, the direction of the second formant can be either increasing or decreasing in frequency. One way of explaining these various patterns for a given stop is to hypothesize that all second-formant transitions begin at the same characteristic value (the small circle in the illustration) and then move to the second-formant frequency typical for the vowel. The characteristic value for the consonant is called the **second-formant locus,** or **F_2 locus.** As a general principle, the F_2 locus increases in frequency as place of articulation moves back in the mouth.

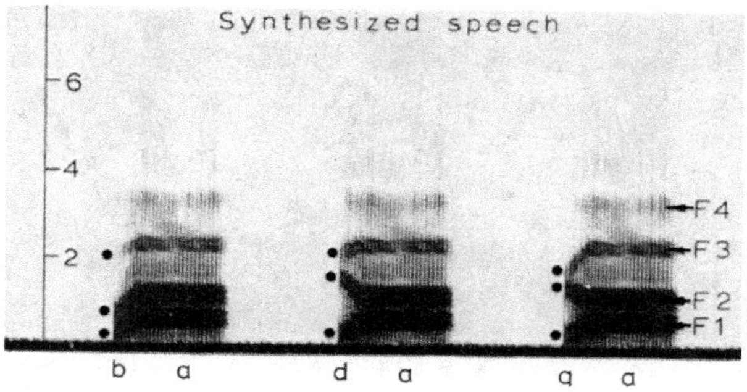

FIGURE 5.47
Spectrograms of the syllables [bɑ], [dɑ], and [gɑ] produced by a talking computer, or speech synthesizer. The small dots show the approximate starting frequencies of the first three formants. Frequency is scaled in kHz.

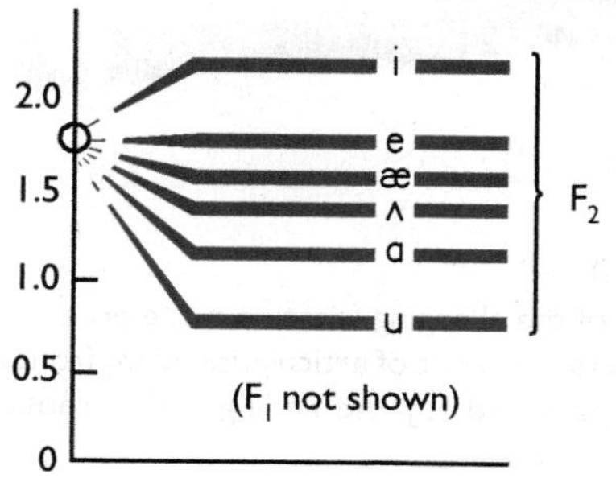

FIGURE 5.48
Composite of the F_2 patterns for [d] + vowel syllables, shown as a stylized spectrogram. Notice that the F_2 transition assumes different shapes depending on the vowel that follows the [d]. Frequency is scaled in kHz.

Other consonants also have formant transitions associated with them; but, because of space limitations, details will not be given here. Some general points of importance are:

- Formant transitions are rapid changes in formant pattern, especially between consonants and vowels.
- These transitions carry information about place (and to some extent manner) of articulation and therefore play a significant role in the intelligibility of speech.
- The exact form of a formant transition depends on both the vowel and consonant involved.

The noise of fricative and stop bursts also has characteristics that vary with place of articulation. Both the overall intensity of noise and the intensity-by-frequency (spectral)

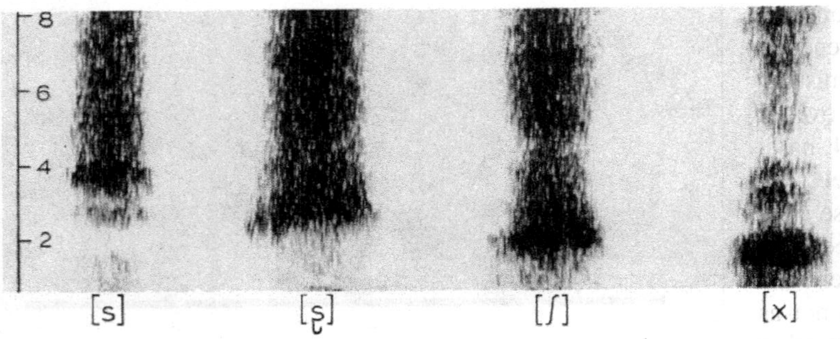

FIGURE 5.49
Spectrograms for the four fricatives [s], [s̺], [ʃ], and [x]. Frequency in kHz is scaled on the vertical axis.

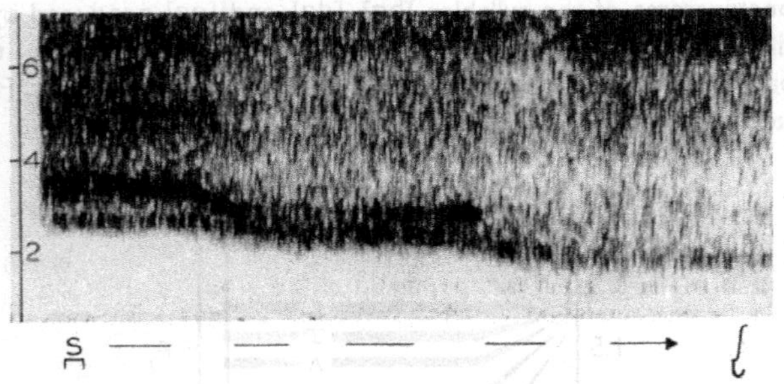

FIGURE 5.50
Spectrogram of the changing frication noise produced as a speaker gradually moves the point of articulation from front to back, beginning with a dentalized [s] and ending with a rhotacized [ʃ]. Frequency is scaled in kHz.

shaping of the noise depend on where the noise is generated. The most frontal fricatives /f v θ ð/ and the glottal fricative /h/ are the weakest. The stronger fricatives /s z ʃ ʒ/ are sometimes called sibilants. The spectral shaping for some lingual fricatives is illustrated in Figure 5.49, which shows spectrograms for a normal lingua-alveolar [s], a rhotacized [s̺] (made with the tongue tip turned up), the lingua-palatal [ʃ], and the lingua-velar [x] (which is not a fricative phoneme in English but occurs in some other languages, such as German). This sequence of fricatives, for which the point of constriction moves progressively backward from /s/ to /x/, illustrates how the noise characteristics of fricatives are influenced by place. Notice in particular that, for this sequence of sounds, the low-frequency limit of the noise is progressively lower, moving from left to right. In part, this difference reflects the length of the resonating cavity in front of the point of constriction. The longer this cavity, the lower in frequency the resonances can be. For /s/, the front cavity is short, so the resonances are relatively high in frequency. For /ʃ/, the front cavity is longer, so the resonances are lower in frequency.

Another illustration of the change in noise spectrum as place of articulation is varied is given by the spectrogram in Figure 5.50. This spectrogram shows the acoustic result as a speaker gradually moves the point of constriction backward in the vocal tract, beginning with a dentalized [s̪] and ending with a rhotacized [ʃ̺].

Figure 5.51 summarizes the articulatory and acoustic properties of the places of articulation for English fricatives (excluding /h/, which is acoustically similar to /f/). The

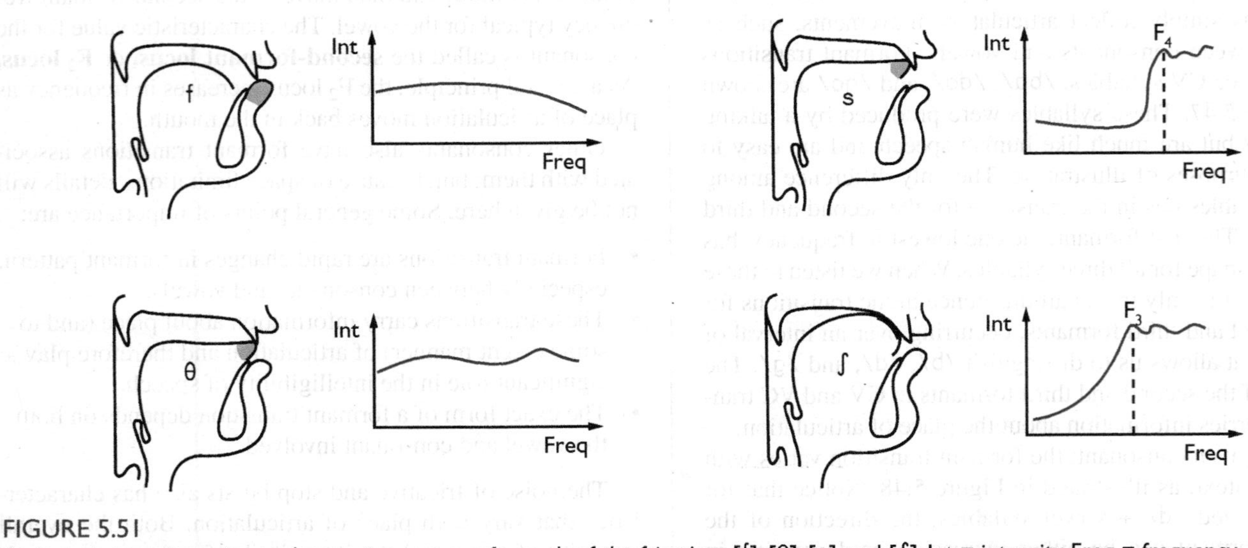

FIGURE 5.51
Articulatory configuration and acoustic spectrum for each of the fricatives [f], [θ], [s], and [ʃ]. Int = intensity, Freq = frequency.

drawings show the vocal tract configuration for each fricative and the general shape of the noise spectrum. The labiodental /f/ is of low intensity and has a "flat" spectrum (that is, with few peaks and valleys). Because the cavity in front of the labiodental constriction is very short, the resonances associated with this cavity are very high in frequency and of little importance to the auditory quality of the sound. Thus, /f/ is weak and flat.

Linguadental /θ/ is similar to /f/ but has a somewhat more important spectral shaping (note the peak at the high-frequency end of the spectrum). Because the anterior cavity, or the cavity in front of the constriction, is longer than that for the /f/, the associated resonances are lower in frequency. Still, like /f/, /θ/ is essentially a weak and flat fricative.

Lingua-alveolar /s/ has a longer front cavity than either /f/ or /θ/, and this factor accounts in part for the prominent spectral shaping of /s/. Most of the energy for /s/ is in the higher frequencies (above 4 kHz for an adult male). As a rule of thumb, the major concentration of acoustic energy for /s/ lies above the frequency value of the fourth formant (F_4) of an adjacent vowel. Both /s/ and lingua-palatal /ʃ/ are sibilants, a term that recognizes their intense noise energy. The /s/ is an intense, high-frequency fricative.

Lingua-palatal /ʃ/ has a longer front cavity than /s/ and has a greater amount of energy in the mid-frequency region. Generally, the major concentration of noise energy lies just above the frequency of the third formant (F_3) for an adjacent vowel (approximately 3 kHz for an adult male). Given these spectral properties, and the fact that /ʃ/ is a sibilant (high-energy fricative), the /ʃ/ may be described as an intense, mid-frequency sound.

Articulatory–Acoustic Relations for Consonants

The consonants are reviewed here by the major classes of obstruents and sonorants. A summary of acoustic information is provided in Table 5.3.

Obstruents. Recall that obstruents include the stops, fricatives, and affricates. Table 5.4 is a summary of the aerodynamic and acoustic properties of obstruent consonants. Aerodynamic variables considered are airflow and air pressure. The acoustic correlates are described for both prevocalic and postvocalic positions.

The individual obstruent types are further discussed as follows.

Stops (/b/, /d/, /g/, /p/, /t/, /k/)

1. **Silence.** A silent interval or stop gap occurs before the release of the stop. This interval is truly silent for voiceless stops, as no energy is radiated from the oral cavity during the obstruction for the stop. However, voiced stops often have a small amount of low-frequency energy attributable to voicing. This energy appears as a low-frequency voice bar on a spectrogram. The duration of the stop gap generally falls in the range of 50 to 100 ms, depending on speaking rate, stress, voicing, and phonetic context.

2. **Voicing.** Vocal fold vibrations occur during most or all of the obstructed interval for voiced stops in medial position. Vocal fold vibrations may not be evident during the closure phase of initial or final stops. Voiced and voiceless stops in initial position are distinguished by voice onset time, or the time that intervenes between the release of the constriction and the beginning of voicing. Voiced stops have short voice onset times, meaning that voicing begins just before, simultaneously with, or just after consonantal release. Voiceless stops have long voice onset times, meaning that voicing begins relatively longer after consonantal release. Frequently, voiced and voiceless stops in final position are distinguished largely by the duration of a preceding vowel. Vowels that precede voiced stops are lengthened relative to vowels that precede voiceless stops. These are not the only cues that signal stop voicing, but they are among the most frequently cited in the literature. One other cue for voicing—aspiration noise for voiceless stops—is discussed in the following paragraph.

3. **Noise.** A burst of noise usually accompanies a stop release, with the duration of the burst varying from about 10 to 30 ms, depending on speaking rate, stress, voicing, and perhaps phonetic context. The noise burst is more prominent for voiceless than for voiced stops, because the former usually have a greater intraoral air pressure and, therefore, a stronger pulse of air upon release. In addition, voiceless stops are often produced with an aspiration noise that immediately follows the burst noise. The two segments of burst noise and aspiration noise usually occur for all voiceless stops except those that follow /s/ or those that are not released. Aspiration noise may be an important cue for voiceless stops. The noise burst for stops has a spectral shape determined by place of articulation. Even a brief noise burst may be sufficient for listeners to categorize place of articulation for stops. A general rule is that bilabials have a spectrum that is flat or gently falling, alveolars have a rising spectrum, and velars have a mid-frequency dominance.

4. **Transitions.** As the vocal tract shape is changed from that for a vowel to one for a consonant (or vice versa), the acoustic resonances also change, so that formant shifts are evident for VC (or CV) articulatory transitions. The duration of the transitions are on the order of about 40 to 60 ms for stops. This interval reflects the major phase of articulatory movement. The first-formant frequency during the vocal obstruction for a stop is nearly zero, so that VC transitions for F_1 are always falling and CV transitions are always rising in frequency. In other words, a very

low F_1 frequency is an acoustic indicator of vocal tract closure. The direction of the second-formant frequency change is slightly more complicated, but the general pattern is shown in Table 5.3. To a first approximation, each place of articulation for stops can be associated with a particular F_2 locus, which specifies the frequency value at which the F_2 transition begins for CV syllables and ends with VC syllables (see Table 5.3). VC transitions tend to have longer durations than CV transitions.

Fricatives (/f/, /v/, /θ/, /ð/, /z/, /s/, /ʒ/, /ʃ/, /h/)

1. **Silence**. Usually none.
2. **Voicing**. Voiced fricatives are characterized by both periodic (or nearly so) vocal fold pulses and turbulence noise. The noise is essentially modulated by the vocal fold vibrations. That is, voiced fricatives have two energy sources—vocal fold vibration at the larynx and noise generated in the vocal tract.
3. **Noise**. Noise energy is the hallmark of the fricative. The noise duration is typically between 50 and 100 ms but can be longer in strongly stressed syllables or very slow speaking rates. Fricatives differ from one another in the intensity of the noise and its spectral shape. The fricatives /s/, /z/, /ʃ/, and /ʒ/ have much more energy than the others. These are sometimes called stridents or sibilants. The palatals /ʃ/ and /ʒ/ have lower-frequency energy than the alveolars /s/ and /z/. Figures 5.52 and 5.53 show the difference between /ʃ/ and /s/. Both the spectrum at the upper left and the spectrogram at the bottom of the illustrations show that the noise energy for /ʃ/ reaches down to about 2 kHz. The /s/ has energy that reaches to a lower limit of about 3.5 kHz. This spectral

TABLE 5.3
Primary Acoustic Cues for Various Consonants Produced in Syllable-Initial, Prevocalic Position[a]

	Bilabial	Labiodental	Linguadental	Lingua-alveolar	Lingua-palatal	Lingua-velar	Glottal
Stops	[b] [p]			[d] [t]		[g] [k]	[ʔ]
	F_1 increases. F_2 increases. Burst has flat or falling spectrum.			F_1 increases. F_2 decreases except for high-front vowels. Burst has rising spectrum.		F_1 increases. F_2 increases or decreases. Wedge-shaped F_2–F_3. Burst has mid-frequency spectrum.	Little formant change.
Nasals	[m]			[n]		[ŋ]	
	F_1 increases. F_2 increases. Nasal murmur			F_1 increases. F_2 decreases except for high-front vowels. Nasal murmur.		F_1 increases. F_2 increases or decreases. Nasal murmur.	
Fricatives		[v] [f]	[ð] [θ]	[z] [s]	[ʒ] [ʃ]		[h]
		F_1 increases. F_2 increases except for some back vowels. Noise segment has weak and flat spectrum.	F_1 increases. F_2 increases except for some back vowels. Noise segment has weak and flat spectrum.	F_1 increases. F_2 decreases except for high-front vowels. Noise segment has intense, high-frequency (above 4 kHz) spectrum.	F_1 increases. F_2 increases or decreases. Noise segment has intense, high-frequency (above 3 kHz) spectrum.		Little formant change. Noise segment has weak and flat spectrum.
Glides	[w]				[j]		
	F_1 increases. F_2 increases.				F_1 increases. F_2 decreases.		

[a]Formant transitions are described as increasing or decreasing in frequency during the consonant-to-vowel transition.

TABLE 5.4
Summary of Aerodynamic and Acoustic Properties for Obstruents

Category	Aerodynamic Properties	Acoustic Properties	
		Prevocalic Position	Postvocalic Position
Voiceless stops	High intraoral air pressure and no oral flow during closure phase, followed by an oral pulse of high airflow upon release.	Stop gap followed by burst and then formant transition; long voice onset time.	Formant transition followed by stop gap and possible burst; short vowel duration.
Voiced stops	Moderate intraoral air pressure and no oral flow during closure phase, followed by an oral pulse of high airflow upon release.	Stop gap followed by burst and then formant transition; short voice onset time.	Formant transition followed by stop gap and possible burst; long vowel duration.
Voiceless fricatives	High intraoral air pressure and high oral airflow.	Noise segment followed by formant transition; voice bar absent.	Formant transition followed by noise segment; short vowel duration.
Voiced fricatives	Moderate intraoral air pressure and high oral airflow.	Noise segment followed by formant transition; voice bar present.	Formant transition followed by noise segment; long vowel duration.
Voiceless affricate	High intraoral air pressure maintained during two phases: (1) no airflow during closure and (2) high oral airflow upon release and frication.	Stop gap followed by noise segment and then formant transition; voice bar absent.	Formant transition followed by stop gap and then noise segment; short vowel duration.
Voiced affricate	Moderate intraoral air pressure maintained during two phases: (1) no airflow during closure and (2) high oral airflow upon release and frication.	Stop gap followed by noise segment and then formant transition; voice bar present.	Formant transition followed by stop gap and then noise segment; long vowel duration.

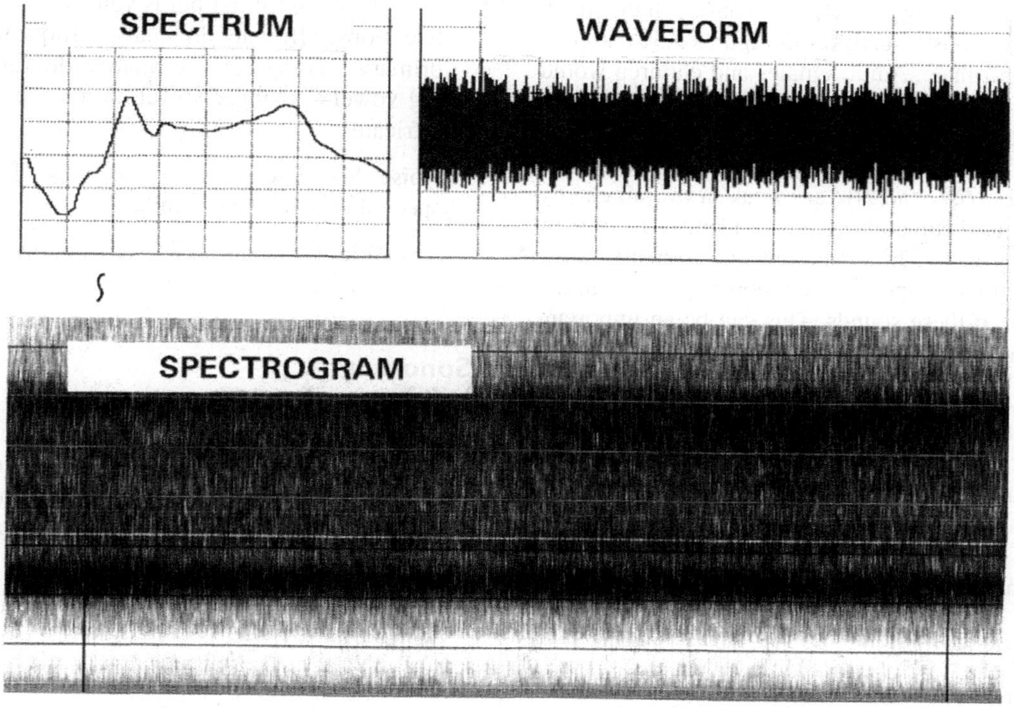

FIGURE 5.52
Spectrum, waveform, and spectrogram for the fricative /ʃ/. The spectrum at the top left is averaged over an interval represented by the vertical lines on the spectrogram.

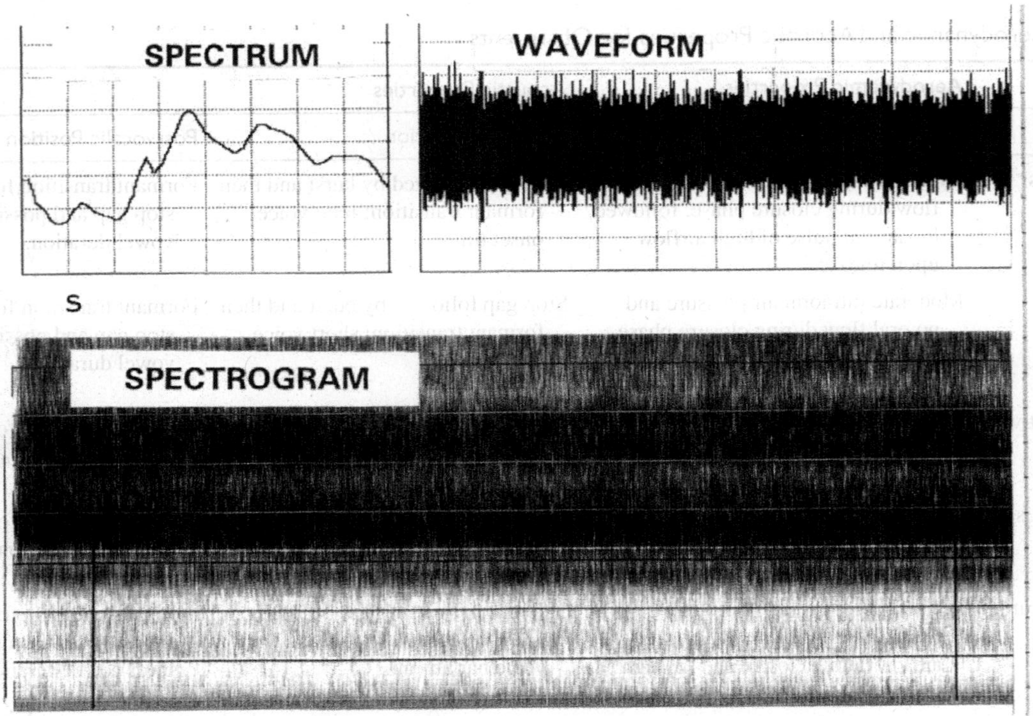

FIGURE 5.53
Spectrum, waveform, and spectrogram for the fricative /s/. The spectrogram at the top left is averaged over an interval represented by the vertical lines on the spectrogram.

difference explains why /s/ seems to have a higher pitch than /ʃ/. The acoustic analyses in Figures 5.52 and 5.53 are for an adult male. Adult females and children would have higher frequency values for the two fricatives, but the relative differences between /s/ and /ʃ/ would be similar to those for the adult male speaker. The fricatives /f/, /v/, /θ/, /ð/, and /h/ are weak in overall energy and are therefore sometimes hard to identify from their noise segment alone. In some contexts, formant transitions may be more important than noise spectrum in the identification of these sounds. This can be an important point in clinical assessment.

4. **Transitions**. The formant transitions are similar to those for stops with corresponding places of articulation. See Table 5.3 for a summary. As previously noted, the perceptual significance of the noise segment versus the formant transitions depends to a large extent on the energy of the noise. If the noise is weak, the listener may rely more on the transitional information to identify the fricative.

Affricates (/tʃ/ **and** /ʤ/).

1. **Silence**. Affricates have a silent interval that is similar to the stop gap of stops.
2. **Voicing**. The vocal folds vibrate for the production of /ʤ/, but not for /tʃ/. Therefore, the noise segment is voiced for the former but is voiceless for the latter. But, like stops, affricates in final position may have as the primary voicing cue the relative duration of a preceding vowel—a longer vowel duration before the voiced affricate.
3. **Noise**. See description of fricatives /ʃ/ and /ʒ/. The spectral properties are similar.
4. **Transitions**. See discussion of stops and fricatives, especially /ʃ/ and /ʒ/.

Sonorants

Nasals (/m/, /n/, **and** /ŋ/).

1. **Silence**. No silent gap occurs. But the nasals have less energy than surrounding vowels and therefore may be associated with a dip in overall energy compared to vowel sounds.
2. **Voicing**. Nasals are completely voiced except for whispered speech.
3. **Noise**. None, except in unusual circumstances.
4. **Transitions**. The nasals are similar to stops in their articulatory dynamics and therefore have similar transitions. See Table 5.3 for details on formant patterns.

Glides or Semivowels (/w/, /ʍ/, /j/). See Table 5.3 for a summary of articulatory–acoustic correlates.

1. **Silence**. None. Glides are typically weaker than neighboring vowels.
2. **Voicing**. Voicing continues throughout the glide articulation, except for whispered speech or the voiceless /ʍ/ (which may be disappearing from American English).
3. **Noise**. Rarely produced except for /ʍ/.
4. **Transitions**. As the vocal tract changes shape from glide to vowel (or vice versa), the acoustic resonances also change. Consequently, the formant frequencies undergo a gradual shift. These formant transitions for glides are longer in duration than those for stops, with continuous formant movements occurring for 100 ms or so. Glides can be distinguished from stops on the basis of transition durations, even when the extent of formant frequency change is similar. For example, when followed by the same vowel, the stop /b/ and the glide /w/ have similar changes in formant frequency values, but the change takes longer for the glide.

Liquids (/r/ and /l/).

1. **Silence**. None, but liquids have lower energy than adjacent vowels.
2. **Voicing**. Except in whispered speech, /r/ and /l/ are voiced.
3. **Noise**. None, except in unusual circumstances.
4. **Transitions**. The liquids are generally similar to stops in their articulatory dynamics and therefore have relatively short durations of formant transitions. One major difference between /r/ and /l/ is that /r/ is associated with a very low third-formant frequency (the lowest of any sound in American English). Therefore, the F_3 transition is a reliable cue for identifying the /r/ sound.

Acoustic Correlates of Suprasegmental Properties

To this point, the discussion pertains almost entirely to the acoustics of vowel and consonant segments. But acoustic methods are applicable to a host of issues in speech, including suprasegmental properties. We consider here acoustic studies relevant to loudness, vocal effort, and boundary effects.

Loudness and Vocal Effort

Loudness may seem to be a relatively straightforward aspect of speech, but an important complication should be noted. Current literature distinguishes loudness from vocal effort. Traunmuller and Eriksson (2000) defined vocal effort as "the quantity that ordinary speakers vary when they adapt their speech to the demands of increased or decreased communication distance" (p. 3438). In other words, vocal effort is the adjustment that we make when the distance between us and our listener(s) increases or decreases. Although vocal effort may be used for other purposes, it is the matter of distance between speaker and listener *(interlocutor distance)* that is of special concern. Now it may appear strange that we should speak of vocal effort rather than loudness when we try to account for adjustments in speech when there are changes in the distance between a speaker and listener. After all, intuition tells us that when people get farther away from us, we need to speak louder to be heard. This issue deserves some explanation.

Loudness is defined as the perception of the magnitude or strength of a sound and is usually scaled from soft to loud. To a first approximation, loudness is directly related to the physical measures of sound pressure level or intensity of a sound. So what happens when speakers adjust the loudness of their speech to be heard over varying distances from a listener? A very simple hypothesis is that speakers would follow the inverse square law, meaning that speakers would increase or decrease their vocal intensity by 6 dB for every doubling or halving of distance from the listener. If Listener A doubles his distance from Speaker B, then Speaker B should increase her vocal intensity by 6 dB. Interestingly, perceptual studies have shown that sound pressure level (or intensity) does not play a major role in judgments of vocal effort (Traunmuller & Eriksson, 2000). Although sound pressure level changes somewhat as speakers adjust their vocal effort, the relationship is variant, and the changes are often much smaller than would be predicted from the inverse square law. So what does change as the distance between speaker and listener increases? The most consistent changes that occur are those associated with increased vocal effort, specifically, increases in voice fundamental frequency (Rostolland, 1982; Traunmuller & Eriksson, 2000), increases in formant frequencies, especially for F_1 (Rostolland, 1982; Schulman, 1989; Junqua, 1993; Huber, Stathopoulos, Curione, Ash, & Johnson, 1999; Lienard & Di Benedetto, 1999; Traunmuller & Eriksson, 2000), increases in vowel duration (Fonagy & Fonagy, 1966; Bonnot & Chevrie-Muller, 1991), and changes in spectral emphasis or the tilt of the spectrum (Traunmuller & Eriksson, 2000). Vocal effort is a complex phenomenon that is not synonymous with loudness and is not directly related to physical measures of sound pressure level or intensity. The distinction between loudness and vocal effort is important when we try to understand what speakers actually do to make themselves understood to listeners who are positioned at various distances.

Boundary Cues

Boundary cues (or edge effects) are asymmetries in phonetic form that occur between internal positions and the edges of prosodic domains. In other words, a segment takes on different characteristics depending on whether it has an internal position as opposed to an edge or boundary position. The general pattern is that acoustic cues are enhanced for segments at the edges of prosodic domains. The enhancements take the form of lengthening of segments or pauses (Klatt, 1975, 1976; Beckman & Edwards, 1990; Wightman, Shattuck-Hufnagel, Ostendorf, & Price, 1992; de Pijper & Sanderman, 1994), strengthening (Fourgeron & Keating, 1997), changing the overlap between adjacent segments (Byrd, 1996; Byrd & Saltzman, 1998), and increasing the likelihood of glottalization of word-initial vowels (Dilley, Shattuck-Hufnagel, & Ostendorf, 1996). These effects distinguish a segment as occurring at a prosodic boundary and can help a listener to identify the boundary in question. De Pijper and Sanderman (1994) referred to the collective effects of these various cues as perceptual boundary strength. They showed that untrained listeners could reliably judge prosodic boundaries using these cues even when the lexical contents of the utterances were made unrecognizable.

A Look Toward the Future

The human ear is a marvelous sensory organ that has been the fundamental instrument in the history of phonetics research. Phoneticians have learned a great deal about speech by careful attention to the ear's auditory patterns. Similarly, auditory evaluation has contributed a great deal of information about speech disorders. But techniques for the physiologic and acoustic study of speech have expanded the potential of phonetic research and phonetic application, including the study of speech and language disorders. It is likely that many of the readers of this book will learn about phonetics and apply phonetic knowledge using acoustic analysis of some kind. Until fairly recently, acoustic analysis was found only in specialized laboratories. Today, the general user with a personal computer can perform some types of acoustic analysis with relatively low-cost software.

The essential step in using a personal computer to analyze speech is to digitize the speech waveform. Digitizing is a process of taking a continuously varying signal (the original speech waveform as recorded by a microphone) and converting it to a series of discrete samples. For a discussion of this process, see Kent and Read (2002). The digital signal processing that lies at the heart of modern systems for speech analysis offers a number of advantages, including the following:

- Visualization of speech patterns that are often too brief for confident perceptual analysis by the ear alone.
- Storage of speech samples as a digital file, which can be retrieved as desired.
- Editing of the digitized **waveforms** to extract an interval of special interest (such as isolating one fricative segment from a phonetic sequence).
- Measurement of speech features, including durations, fundamental frequency, formant frequencies, and various spectral features.
- Visual display of a client's speech pattern compared with a target pattern (for example, showing the /s/ sound produced by a child with an articulation disorder together with another /s/ sound that was correctly produced).

Acoustic analysis is a useful complement to phonetic transcription by ear. This book has barely touched on the acoustic aspects of speech, and we encourage interested readers to go beyond the introduction given here. Fortunately, acoustic analysis can be done effectively on many desktop and laptop computers. Some of the software is available as free downloads or at modest cost.

Exercises

1. Shown in Figure 5.54 are drawings of a side view of the vocal tract and the roof of the mouth. The ellipses (flattened circles) represent points of articulation. For both parts, identify by proper term the place of articulation represented by each ellipse.

2. For each consonant in the following word list, circle each letter for a consonant made with the tongue and underline each letter for a consonant made with the lips. Remember that two alphabet characters sometimes represent a single consonant phoneme, in which case you should circle or underline both letters.

(a) c o u g h	(i) p h o n e m e
(b) s c i s s o r s	(j) f i f t e e n
(c) p u f f	(k) b o o k m a r k
(d) m a n n i n g	(l) b a s e b a l l
(e) r a b b i t	(m) s h u f f l e
(f) v a l e n t i n e	(n) f e r v o r
(g) t h i c k e s t	(o) s n o w m a n
(h) w r i t h i n g	(p) o c e a n

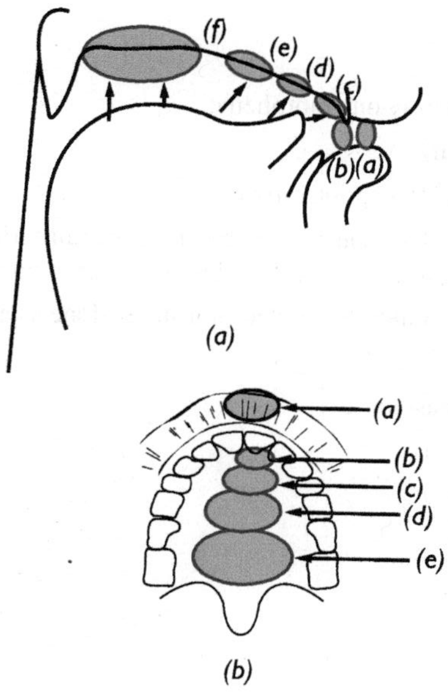

FIGURE 5.54
Ellipses showing places of consonant articulation: *(a)* lateral view of vocal tract; *(b)* view from below roof of mouth.

3. Verify the phonetic transcriptions provided for the standard pronunciation of the following words. Some of the transcriptions are in error because of incorrect consonant symbols. Circle each incorrect consonant and write the correct symbol above it.

Word	Transcription
(a) finger	[f ɪ n g ɚ]
(b) toothpaste	[t u ð p eɪ s t]
(c) hammer	[h æ m ɚ]
(d) wristwatch	[r ɪ s t w ɔ ʃ]
(e) curtains	[ʃ ɝ t n s]
(f) gasoline	[g æ s ə l i n]
(g) teenager	[t i n e] ʤ ɚ]
(h) telephone	[t ɛ l ə p h o n]

Word	Transcription
(i) bookshelf	[b ʊ k ʃ ɛ l f]
(j) thanksgiving	[ð æ ŋ k s g ɪ v ɪ n g]

4. Classify and group each of the following words according to the manner of articulation of the *first* consonant. List the words in six columns having the headings Stop, Nasal, Fricative, Affricate, Liquid, and Glide.

can	this	red	job	nose	pot	wine
keep	saw	choose	man	wail	show	lamb
wheel	name	bed	ring	phone	thigh	yes
gin	chorus	zipper	happy	knew	fate	

5. Write next to each word the phonetic symbol or symbols corresponding to the italicized letter(s). *Example:* tha*nks* [ŋ k s]

(a) fi*fths* [ ]
(b) mea*s*ure [ ]
(c) win*d*ow [ ]
(d) la*mpsh*ade [ ]
(e) tra*ct*or [ ]
(f) *squ*eal [ ]
(g) be*nch* [ ]
(h) nu*dged* [ ]
(i) swi*ms*uit [ ]
(j) *th*us [ ]
(k) boo*ked* [ ]
(l) fini*sh* [ ]
(m) (m) thi*stle* [ ]
(n) *sw*eet [ ]
(o) cru*nched* [ ]
(p) we*st* [ ]
(q) *c*ute [ ]
(r) *str*eak [ ]
(s) wi*thdr*aw [ ]
(t) wai*stl*ine [ ]

6. Write a phonetic transcription for each of the following words and then review the number of morphemes in the word.

Word	Transcription	Morphemes	Comment
(a) girl	[ ]	1	
(b) mission	[ ]	1	2 syllables but only one morpheme
(c) boys	[ ]	2	boys + s (plural)
(d) women's	[ ]	3	woman + (plural) + (possessive)
(e) svelte	[ ]	1	note violation of a phonetic sequencing constraint: English does not permit [sv] as a word-initial cluster except in borrowed words
(f) conceive	[ ]	2	note that second morpheme does not stand alone as a word
(g) reptilian	[ ]	2	reptile + ian
(h) demoted	[ ]	3	de + mote + (past tense)
(i) encryption	[ ]	3	en + crypt + ion
(j) transmission	[ ]	3	trans + mit + ion

Transcription Training

The items for transcription training are recorded on CD 1. They are the same lists that were used previously for vowel transcription. Transcribe the entire word and check your transcription against the key. Notice that each word list gives practice with a different group of consonants as follows:

Transcription List A— stops /b d g p t k/
nasals /m n ŋ/
liquids /r l/

(Most of these phonetic symbols use the alphabet letter ordinarily associated with the sound; only /ŋ/ does not have a corresponding alphabet character.)

Transcription List B— fricatives
/v f ð θ z s ʒ ʃ h/
affricates /ʤ ʧ/
glides /w ʍ j/

Transcription List C— all consonants introduced in lists A and B

Transcription List D— consonant review and introduction of syllabic consonants (see Chapter 6) and the alveolar flap

PROCEED TO: Clinical Phonetics CD 1, Tracks 1, 2, 3, 4: Transcription Lists A, B, C, D

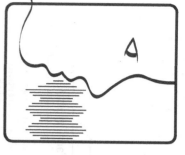

CHAPTER 6

SUPRASEGMENTALS AND NARROW TRANSCRIPTION

To this point, we have considered phonetics almost entirely in terms of its segmental structure, as a concatenation of vowels and consonants to represent an utterance of some kind. If this is as far as phonetic transcription goes, then the result is rather like a typescript, a string of phonemes. But speech is not like a series of keypresses. We talk with emphasis, emotion, loudness and rate changes, and a variety of touches that add color, meaning, and even melody to our utterances. The segmental structure of speech is accompanied by various vocal effects that extend over more than one sound segment in an utterance. These effects are called **suprasegmentals**.

It is easy to be confused by the various definitions that have been proposed for terms related to suprasegmentals. We need to proceed carefully to keep our terminology and concepts in order. Suprasegmentals is a general term for the various properties of speech that go beyond segmental representation. A similar term is **prosody** (from the Greek *prosōidía*, "song sung to music"). Suprasegmentals and prosody are used almost interchangeably in the phonetic literature, although some phoneticians strive to distinguish them. For the purposes of this text, the term *suprasegmentals* is regarded as the overarching category, with prosody being a major component. This approach is compatible with the general literature on clinical phonetics, but the reader is forewarned that terminological differences abound. A hint of the difficulties we face is expressed in the comment, "Although it is impossible to speak without using prosody, it is generally allotted comparatively little time or consideration in clinical training" (Peppe, 2009, p. 258). This quotation comes from a journal article with the title: *Why is prosody in speech-language pathology so difficult?* It appears that our work is cut out for us.

Most discussions of suprasegmentals (or prosody) list a number of component features, such as variations of tone, intonation, stress, timing, rhythm, loudness, and tempo. Therefore, suprasegmentals and prosody are a collection of variations and not a single feature. Each of the individual types of variation needs to be defined, which we do next. In the following discussion, the term prosody is used as one of two major aspects that fall under the larger category of suprasegmentals. The other aspect, **paralinguistics**, is discussed in a later section. Reference to Figure 6.1 should be helpful as you read this chapter. As you do so, remember that the information under consideration is a complement to the segmental information that has occupied our attention to this point. Segmental and suprasegmental aspects are tightly bound together in what we say.

PROSODY

The word **melody** sometimes is used as a synonym of prosody. Melody conveys the basic idea that prosody pertains to the intonation and rhythm of spoken language. But prosody unfolds into other categories as well, as we see below.

Intonation

Intonation may be defined as the pattern or melody of pitch changes in an utterance. Some definitions of intonation refer to the patterns of rises and falls, but even flat or unchanging intervals are part of the picture. Intonation should be distinguished from **pitch level**, which is the relative level of pitch that characterizes an utterance as a whole. That is, a speaker can produce an utterance with a pitch that is high, medium, or low. But for each of these average levels, it is still possible to produce dynamic changes in melody so that intonation is overlaid on a general pitch setting. An utterance can be described in terms of an overall **intonation contour**, sometimes called a **pitch contour**. This contour is shaped by several factors, as described in the following.

An important aspect of intonation is called **pitch declination** (sometimes called **sentence declination**), which is an overall fall in pitch over an utterance such as a sentence. When we speak, we usually begin at a relatively high pitch and then gradually reduce the pitch over an utterance (Figure 6.2a). This pitch change is one way of signaling the sentence structure of conversation—start high and end low. Because the main physical correlate of pitch is vocal f_0, phenomena such as pitch declination can be studied acoustically by determining the f_0 pattern. There are two major theories about how f_0 is regulated to achieve pitch declination.

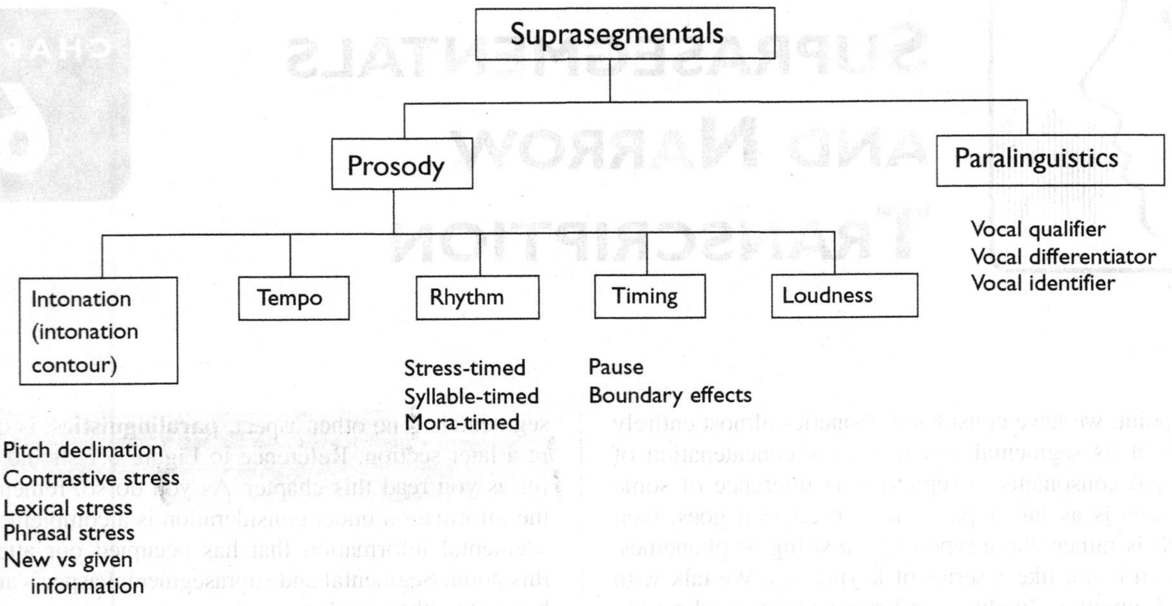

FIGURE 6.1
Components of suprasegmentals

One view, which we will call the **linear declination theory**, states that f_0 falls gradually and linearly throughout a sentence or clause (Maeda, 1976; Sorenson & Cooper, 1980; Thorsen, 1985). Lieberman (1967) proposed a contrasting theory, called the **breath-group theory**, which holds that a declarative sentence can be divided into nonterminal and terminal parts, and variation in f_0 is permitted only in the terminal part of the f_0 contour. Studies have shown that an important acoustic cue for syntactic structure is the fall of f_0 and intensity at the end of the breath group (Landahl, 1980; Lieberman & Tseng, 1981; Lieberman, Katz, Jongman, Zimmerman, & Miller, 1985). Pitch declination may be a universal property of languages, so that by listening for this pattern we can make some good guesses about the location of sentence boundaries even in languages that we do not understand. The sentence is not the only unit that determines pitch declination, because this phenomenon also can be used to delimit clauses or phrases within a sentences. The basic idea is that pitch can be reset to start at a higher level (**pitch resetting**) for each of these syntactic groupings. Resetting of pitch is a signal to the listener that a new syntactic unit is being produced.

Even the proponents of linear declination theory would readily admit that the f_0 contour of most utterances is not just a straight line that slants from high to low across the utterance. Rather, the contour is marked by a series of rises and falls superimposed on either a more gradual f_0 descent (linear declination theory) or a contour with a well-defined terminal fall in f_0 (breath-group theory). Figure 6.2b shows the way in which f_0 rises and falls are superimposed on a general f_0 decline. The moment-to-moment changes in f_0 are related to several other factors, as discussed next.

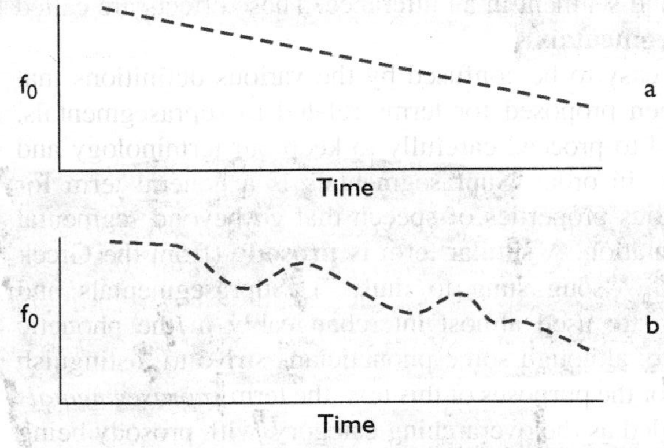

FIGURE 6.2
Illustration of pitch declination as an abstract pattern (a) and with local f_0 falls and rises superimposed (b).

Stress

Stress is the degree of prominence or emphasis associated with a particular syllable in a word or a word in a phrase, clause, or sentence. When we produce and perceive speech, we usually are aware that some syllables or words seem to stand out. They have prominence. One way of demonstrating this feature is to tap your finger as you speak, trying to tap once for each word. Most people will tap on the stressed syllable of the words. Acoustically, stress is conveyed by some combination of f_0, intensity, and duration. The actual variations in these three factors depend on the speaker and the utterance. Although all three can be used to signal a stress contrast, sometimes only one will be adjusted with the desired effect. But it is typical that f_0 will be regulated to mark stress, sometimes accompanied by changes in intensity and duration. For maximum effect, stress is conveyed by elevated pitch (or greater changes in pitch), increased intensity and lengthened duration.

Contrastive Stress. **Contrastive stress** is used when we wish to deviate from the usual or expected pattern of stress in an utterance. It is used to draw attention to a word. For example, consider the stress given to the word *of* in the phrase, *government of the people, by the people, for the people.* As one way of showing the parallel structure of the phrase, speakers often will stress the word *of,* even though this word is typically unstressed in general usage. Contrastive stress is flexibly applied depending on a speaker's intention. As another example, consider this dialog:

1. Britney: The term paper is due Friday.
2. Ashley: No, I am sure that it is due on Monday.
3. Britney: I think the paper is due on Friday and the quiz will be on Monday.

Read this dialog as though you are reading a script for a play. Do you notice that you have assigned an extra level of stress to the word *Monday* in (2) and the words *Friday* and *Monday* in (3)? Contrastive stress is used to emphasize the pivotal words in the dialog.

Lexical Stress. **Lexical stress** is a stress pattern intrinsic to a word. A frequently used example is the noun vs verb forms of words such as *protest, object, project, imprint,* and *research.* Each of these words has a noun or verb form that is distinguished by the stress pattern of the word. When the stress is placed on the first syllable, the word is understood as a noun. When the stress is on the second syllable, then the word is regarded as a verb. Notice that this kind of stress is based on our shared knowledge of the lexicon of a language. There are indications that the noun versus verb contrast just described is gradually disappearing. For example, for many speakers only one stress pattern suffices for the noun and verb forms of the word *research.*

Phrasal Stress. **Phrasal stress** is stress that is assigned beyond the level of lexical stress to apply in syntactic groupings of words, such as phrases, clauses, or sentences. When we produce a combination of words that form a particular grammatical grouping, we tend to produce differential levels of stress over the different word constituents. In other words, stress is not uniform across the words in a phrase.

New versus Given Information. **New versus given information** is a contrast related to the kind of information in a message, specifically, whether the information is expected to be new to the listener or already known by the listener. Speakers can use prosody to highlight words that present new information in a conversation or a message. When radio or television announcers introduce a new topic, they typically use prosody to cue listeners to the key word or words. We do the same in conversations when we want to mention a word that may be new to our listeners, or to mark a word that may not be expected or predicted. Given information is information that we expect can be assumed or inferred by a listener. This kind of information does not need to be highlighted or distinguished from the general flow of the conversation. New information is that which cannot necessarily be assumed or inferred. This kind of information often is marked by prosodic devices. An example comes from a study by Behne (1989), who described prosodic effects in a mini-discourse such as the following:

1. "Someone painted the fence."
2. "Who painted the fence?"
3. "PETE painted the fence."

In this exchange, the new information in sentence 3 is "Pete," who is identified as the individual who painted the fence. Try rehearsing this little exchange and try to describe how you might say "Pete" in sentence 3. Did you lengthen the word and produce with it a higher vocal pitch? That is what the subjects in Behne's study did. New information often is spoken with a lengthening of the critical word and with a higher pitch. Behne also showed that the same cues are used in French, but they are deployed somewhat differently.

Tempo

In music, **tempo** is the speed at which a piece is or should be played. More generally, tempo is rate of some activity. The tempo of spoken language is its rate, commonly expressed in units such as syllables/min or words/min. Tempo is generally regarded as a global property of speech, insofar as a given speech sample can be relatively slow, moderate, or fast. But in fact, tempo can change within a sample of speech derived from a given speaker. We often change the tempo of our speech depending on emotion, communicative setting, and other factors.

As tempo changes, the durations of phonetic segments change accordingly. At slow tempo, the durations are relatively long; at fast tempo, the durations are relatively short. The shortening and lengthening of phonetic segments are not necessarily uniform across different kinds of segments. For example, studies have shown that as speaking rate increases, the durations of pauses and steady-state segments for vowels and consonants are reduced proportionately more than the durations of transitional or dynamic segments. Generally, stressed vowels are preserved better than unstressed vowels. At very fast rates, segments and even syllables may be deleted. Another feature of rapid speaking rate is undershoot, which is a reduction of the extent of articulatory movement for a sound. Listeners expect these kinds of changes as speaking rate increases and usually can adapt to them without difficulty, even when entire syllables are deleted. Try saying the following words at your fastest rate and determine which syllable is likely to be deleted: *camera, definite, support, surprise.* Did you find that the syllable that has the least degree of stress is sacrificed at a fast speaking rate? For most speakers, the syllables that are deleted at a rapid speaking rate are the second syllables in *camera* and *definite,* and the first syllables in *support* and *surprise.*

Rhythm

Rhythm refers to the distribution of events in time. Most of us agree that speech seems to have a rhythm. This idea has led to formal proposals that speech can be described in terms of rhythmic units that tend to have about the same duration or length. This equivalence of units is called **isochrony** (which essentially means "same time").

It has also been proposed that different languages have different rhythmic units. A popular notion in the study of language is that English speech has a rhythm based on intervals called *feet,* which begin with a stressed syllable. The interval between stressed syllables is thought to be invariant. This idea gave rise to an important hypothesis that languages like English, German, and Dutch have a **stress-timed rhythm**. Some other languages have a different rhythm in which syllables have pretty much the same length regardless of whether they are stressed. These languages, which include Spanish and French, are said to have a **syllable-timed rhythm.** But it is probably inaccurate to say that most Indo-European languages must either be stress-timed or syllable-timed. Languages seem to fall on a continuum rather than a strict dichotomy. English (including UK and USA dialects) falls close to the stress-timed extreme and Spanish falls close to the syllable-timed extreme. French and Italian occupy intermediate positions on the continuum. If you are a native speaker of English learning a language such as French, Italian, or Spanish, you may have noticed that these other languages have a different rhythmic pattern.

Japanese, Estonian, and some other languages have been reported to have still another rhythm, this one based on a **mora**, to produce a **mora-timed rhythm.** Traditionally, it was claimed that moras are constant and serve as the basic unit of rhythm or timing. A common definition of a mora is that it is a unit of sound that determines syllable weight, which, in turn, determines stress or timing. Admittedly, this is a rather vague definition, so it may help to say further that the mora functions as a unit of duration in Japanese, serving as a measure of the length of words and syllables. In fact, the word *mora* means "to linger."

In summary, it has been proposed that languages can be described as stress-timed, syllable-timed, or mora-timed, depending on the presumed unit of rhythm. But it is best to think of these concepts as defining relative contrasts, and not necessarily strict categories, across languages. The impression that languages *have* a rhythm is perhaps the most important point to note. Whatever the rhythm of a given language might be, the timing of elements can be controlled to achieve various effects, such as those discussed next.

Timing

Pause (juncture). We might say that a **pause** is the sound of silence. It may seem strange that silence carries communicative value, but, in fact, pauses are part of the informational structure of speech, and listeners can use pauses to help them understand an utterance. Pauses appear for several reasons, such as when a speaker (1) marks boundaries between units such as phrases or clauses, (2) hesitates while retrieving a word or planning an utterances, or (3) desires to increase the sense of anticipation as a listener waits for information to follow (as in "and the winner of the contest is [pause] Joe Smith!"). The expression, "pause for effect," reflects the power of pause in spoken discourse.

Boundary or Edge Effects. **Boundary or edge effects** are phonological or phonetic characteristics that appear at the margins of a linguistic unit, especially a phrase. They can occur at either the right (leading) edge or left (terminating) edge of a unit. For the latter, these effects include a fall in f_0, a lengthening of the unit-final word or syllable, articulatory strengthening (more forceful articulation) for the final segments, and a pause at the end of the unit. Boundary effects are cues to the syntactic structure of a speaker's utterances and attending to them helps a listener to parse speech into grammatical constituents.

Loudness and Vocal Effort

Loudness is the perceived magnitude or strength of a sound. It varies along a perceptual dimension of weak (or soft) to strong (or loud). In general, the loudness of a sound (a perceptual judgment) varies with the intensity of the acoustic signal (a physical measure). A concept closely related to loudness is **vocal effort**, which is a quantity that a speaker regulates according to the distance between the speaker and the listener. As the communication distance increases, speakers typically increase their subglottal air pressure, the tension of the vocal folds, and the amount of jaw opening. These changes cause variations in the acoustic signal beyond an increase in vocal intensity. When researchers try to estimate vocal effort, they ask speakers or listeners to judge the physiological effort that goes into speaking. There is no generally accepted transcriptional device for loudness or vocal effort, but some symbols for discourse transcription are mentioned later in this chapter.

The Prosodic Unit or Intonational Unit

By this point, you probably have reached the conclusion that several different kinds of units and phenomena are nested within the overall suprasegmental structure or prosody of an utterance. The largest unit is known by several names in linguistics and phonetics: breath group, intonation unit, intonational phrase, tone unit, and prosodic unit, to mention a few. But whatever name we give it, the unit in question is distinguished by having a single pitch and rhythm contour, sometimes called a **prosodic contour**, schematically illustrated in Figure 6.3, which shows how four syllables of varying length are associated with a f_0 contour. This graph is one way of representing two major aspects of prosody, with f_0 being the vertical dimension and rhythm the horizontal dimension. Phonetic transcriptions of conversational or reading samples often identify this larger structure and then work out segmental and suprasegmental details as they relate to it. Although nomenclature is by no means standardized, there appears to be a preference for **intonational unit**, abbreviated IU. From the discussion in this chapter, you may be thinking that a better term would be prosodic unit, given that prosody is a larger construct that includes intonation as a component. And your thinking would be correct. So why not use the term prosodic unit? Mainly because the abbreviation PU can be used as an expression of disgust or displeasure, phonetically [piju]. Better to say IU than PU.

Examples of Prosodic Variations

Speakers rely on prosody to accomplish communicative goals in different situations. Furthermore, all speakers tend to make essentially the same kinds of prosodic adjustments, and this lends predictability to communication, making it easier for the listener to grasp the message.

Motherese. When adults speak to infants, they often use a style of speech called "**motherese**" (also known as **infant-directed speech** or **parentese**). Speech that is directed toward infants and young children is characterized by several features, including a higher pitch, exaggerated intonation, and increased repetition of words or other units. Many of these features are adjustments of the prosody of an utterance. It has been shown that infants prefer infant-directed speech to adult-directed speech, and some authorities believe that infant-directed speech helps infants to learn features of the language. Like much of language, motherese is not deliberately taught, although perhaps it is modeled from one generation to the next.

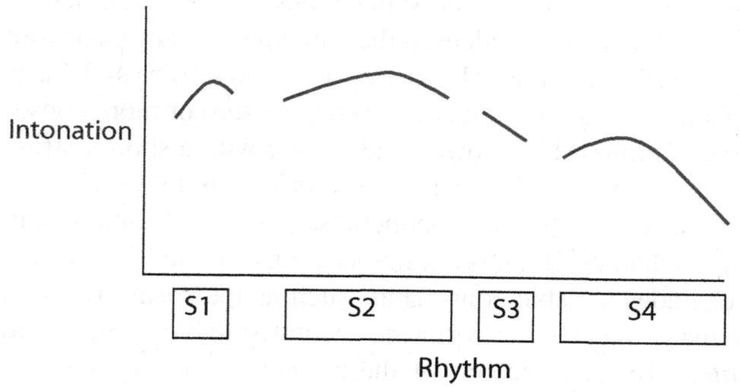

FIGURE 6.3
One graphical form of prosodic contour, with intonation as the vertical dimension and rhythm as the horizontal dimension. S1, S2, S3 and S4 are syllables.

Clear Speech. When we strive to be understood in a difficult listening situation, such as one with background noise, we adopt a style of speech called **clear speech**. This kind of speech typically is associated with prosodic changes including greater pitch variation and slowed rate. These adjustments are in addition to changes in articulatory properties such as producing stronger releases for stop consonants and increasing the articulatory movements for vowels. Clear speech can be contrasted with ordinary **conversational speech**, with the latter typically having a faster rate, smaller range for articulatory movements and deletion of some unstressed syllables. You can test your own production of clear versus conversational speech by talking under two different imaginary situations: first, talking to a young child over a noisy telephone signal and, second, talking to your best friend in a quiet, relaxed setting. What changes do you detect as you speak in the two conditions?

Other Prosodic Variations. We have considered just two examples of prosodic variations that speakers use in pretty much the same way in specific situations. But there are others. For example, it has been shown that speech-language pathologists use a different pattern of prosody when they provide therapy for language disorders compared to nontherapeutic situations (Reuvers & Hargrove, 1994). We can adopt a variety of prosodic variations in different communicative settings. Can you think of ways you change your prosodic patterns when speaking with your closest friend, a family member, an authority figure, or a stranger? Modifications of prosody are part of the adaptive nature of speech communication.

Paralinguistics

Beyond its segmental representation and prosody, speech is accompanied by a set of characteristics called **paralanguage**. The most typical definition of paralanguage is that is the nonverbal properties of speech that convey information about a speaker's emotion, attitude, and demeanor. A particular challenge is to draw a clear distinction between prosody and paralanguage, especially because some sources include intonation under paralanguage. One reason why it is difficult to separate prosody and paralanguage is that they sometimes employ similar vocal characteristics, such as pitch rises and falls, variations in loudness, and alterations in speaking rate. For the purposes of clinical phonetics, we define paralanguage (adjective *paralinguistic*) to be nonverbal characteristics related to emotion, speaking style, voice quality and voice qualifications. Note that *nonverbal* does not necessarily mean *nonvocal.* These characteristics influence the auditory pattern of speech, so they can be discerned from a telephone conversation or a radio broadcast, but they also can include nonauditory features, such as facial expressions and body language. We can accomplish a great deal with paralanguage, which enriches our communication in ways that are difficult to accomplish with texting or writing.

As an example of paralinguistic aspects of speech, consider a situation in which a group of college students on spring break in Florida are looking out the window at a drenching rain. One of them says, "It is a beautiful day on the beach!" Of course, this statement would be produced with irony. The ironic tone of voice is part of paralanguage and its use in this statement completely alters the received meaning. Suppose that another student in our spring break example says with a laugh, "Who brought a video game?" This disappointed student is not really expecting a reply, and the laugh is a paralinguistic component that signals its own meaning to the question.

Various elements of paralanguage have been described in the literature and we mention only a few here. **Vocal qualifier** is a technical term for tone of voice used to convey emotion or attitude. A **vocal differentiator** is a vocal expression of emotion including laughing and crying. A **vocal identifier** is a sound that is not necessarily a word but can express meaning. These include utterances such as "uh-huh," "oh," and "hmmm." Depending on the prosody of these utterances, they can convey quite different meanings or attitudes. Facial expressions, gestures, and body language are additional aspects of paralanguage.

THE BASES OF PROSODY

Speech Production Correlates

The lay listener, when asked to describe what stressed units in speech "sound like," usually says that a stressed syllable or word is "louder." Given that loudness is most directly related to sound intensity, we might expect that sound intensity is the physical correlate of our perception of stress. However, experimental studies show that stress perception is related to three acoustic parameters—duration, intensity, and fundamental frequency. It is questionable which of these is the most important, and it is possible that different speakers weight the acoustic cues differently. Generally, increased stress is associated with longer syllable durations, greater intensity of sound, and an elevation of the fundamental frequency. There are also acoustic changes in individual sound segments; for example, stressed vowels may assume a more distinctive acoustic structure. The literature on the acoustic correlates of prosody is too vast to be considered here, but it should be noted that the correlates are not simply specified and may vary across speakers and types of utterances. For further discussion, see the works of Fry (1955, 1958) and De Jong (1991).

It is important for clinical purposes that stress can alter vowel and consonantal articulation (Kent & Netsell, 1971; De Jong, 1991). When a syllable is stressed, its articulatory movements tend to become larger, so that the movements in stressed syllables are more contrastive. Both vowels and consonants are produced with more extreme articulatory positions. For instance, a strongly stressed production of the high-front vowel /i/ can be more fronted than a weakly stressed version of this vowel. The stressed production also has a longer duration. These are important considerations in speech training programs, many of which recommend the use of stressed forms for early training of a speech sound.

As noted earlier, tempo or speaking rate also affects articulation. As tempo increases, movements tend to be smaller in magnitude, and, in some speakers, the velocity of individual movements may increase.

Syllables and Prosody

The syllable plays a major role in most discussions of prosody. In fact, it is difficult to discuss prosody without referring to syllables. Edwards and Beckman (1988) concluded that the syllable is a necessary unit to describe stress patterns and the phonetic characteristics of larger units, such as phrases or clauses. The syllable would then appear to be central to the description of prosodic phenomena. But what is the syllable? Chapter 2 discussed the difficulties of defining it but left the real chore to this chapter. Most people have an intuitive sense of what a syllable is. Most of us can agree on the number of syllables contained in words like *bookshelf* (2), *territory* (4), and *computer* (3). Unhappily, intuition is not matched by an ease of formal definition. The syllable is not easy to define, and lengthy treatises have been written on this troublesome subject (Fudge, 1969; Hooper, 1972; Venneman, 1972; Kahn, 1980; Goldsmith, 1990). The following discussion is a selective review of a complicated literature.

Two general approaches have been taken to define the syllable. First, the syllable is recognized by many writers as a phonological constituent that is made up of phonetic segments. In other words, the syllable has an internal structure. Goldsmith (1990) condensed the outcome of traditional work on the syllable's internal structure as follows: "The syllable is a phonological constituent composed of zero or more consonants, followed by a vowel, and ending with a shorter string of zero or more consonants" (p. 108). This rather abstract statement describes how phonetic segments are combined to make syllables. But it is not fail-safe. One shortcoming is that it excludes syllabic consonants, such as the nasal /n/ used by many speakers to form the second syllable of the word *button.* To take account of these sounds, we might revise Goldsmith's statement as follows: "The syllable is a phonological constituent composed of (a) zero or more consonants, followed by a vowel, and ending with a shorter string of zero or more consonants, or (b) a sonorant consonant serving as a syllabic nucleus." This definition, however, would not win a prize in lexicography. Can we do better?

In the second general approach, the syllable has been described in relation to the overall sound pattern of the speech stream in which it occurs. Bloomfield ([1933] 1984) wrote of syllabicity in terms of the "force" that sounds have upon the ear. He used the term **sonority** in reference to this auditory force: "Evidently some of the phonemes are more sonorous than the phonemes (or the silence) which immediately precede or follow. . . ." (p. 120). Phonemes having a crest of sonority were said to be syllabic; other phonemes were considered nonsyllabic. Sonority is not without problems of its own. This concept has been criticized because of the difficulty of providing a suitable definition. The suggested correlates of sonority include degree of perceptual prominence, total acoustic energy, vocal tract openness, or the physiological effort given by the speaker to sound production. Highly sonorant sounds tend to be prominent perceptually, are associated with strong acoustic energy, have an open vocal tract, and involve a certain combination of respiratory and phonatory activity. These are relative terms, so that determination of degree of sonority depends on a sound's phonetic environment. For additional discussion, see the works of Christman (1992), Clements (1990), Keating (1983), Ladefoged (1993), and Price (1980).

If these two general approaches are combined, we could conclude that the syllable has a loosely specified internal structure and an auditory impact in the flow of speech. Any definition of the syllable must reconcile these internal and external criteria. The following comments work toward this goal.

As a further step toward a definition, Figure 6.4 shows the internal structure of the syllable commonly recognized in modern phonological theory. Hierarchically beneath the syllable are the components of **onset** and **rhyme**. The onset is either null (zero) or is realized as one or more consonants. The rhyme has two components, the **nucleus** (vowel element) and an optional **coda** (consonant or consonant cluster). This diagram roughly accords with the definition given earlier of a syllable's internal structure. But it goes further by proposing not only that the syllable is composed of phonetic segments, but that the syllable has the subdivisions of onset and rhyme, with the rhyme being composed of a nucleus and coda. This syllable structure helps to account for a variety of phonological and psychological phenomena, ranging from syllabic influences on phonological patterns to slips of the tongue in everyday speech.

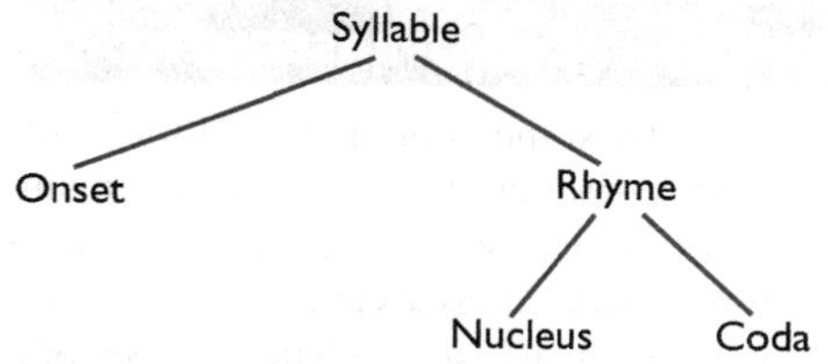

FIGURE 6.4
Basic structure of the syllable, as recognized by many linguists.

Understanding the internal structure of syllables is important because syllables are linked to their constituent segments through language-specific rules. Within a particular language, phonetic segments are regulated by principles that are based on syllable type and position of the segment within the syllable. A speaker of American English knows that *gvise* and *tleen* are not likely to be English words, because the initial consonant clusters violate the phoneme sequencing constraints of the language. Many important phonological principles are based on how segments relate to their parent syllables.

Now for the second part of the definition. Recall that syllables are identified within the prosodic flow of an utterance. Many linguists categorize syllables as heavy or light, depending on their prominence in this flow. A popular way of scaling this prominence is in terms of sonority. As Bloomfield ([1933] 1984) observed, some sounds are associated with a crest of sonority; these are syllabic sounds. This formulation suggests that there are two classes of sounds: sonorants and nonsonorants. However, sonority is perhaps better regarded as a scalar rather than a binary feature, meaning that sounds are not simply sonorant or nonsonorant, but that they have **degrees** of sonority. Sounds can be scaled according to the degree of sonority they typically have, as shown in Table 6.1.

Sonority values are important not only for understanding the relative prominence of a sound in the flow of speech but also for understanding the way in which phonetic constituents are arranged within the syllable. According to a principle called the Sonority Principle, consonant clusters are usually formed so that different manners of articulation are sequenced to allow one sonority peak for each syllable. For example, if the sounds [i], [t], [r], and [z] are to be arranged within a syllable, then [t r i z] is a good arrangement, providing for a sequence of sonority that builds up from [t] to [r] to [i] and then declines again to [z]. Think of the ideal pattern of

TABLE 6.1
Sonority Values Assigned to Selected Phonemes

Phoneme(s)	Value
/ɑ/	10
/e/, /o/	9
/i/, /u/	8
/r/, /w/	7
/l/	6
/m/, /n/	5
/s/	4
/v/, /z/, /ð/	3
/f/, /θ/	2
/b/, /d/, /g/	1
/p/, /t/	0.5

speech as a series of triangular peaks. Each peak is a sonorant crest and, thus, the nucleus of a syllable. Vowels are usually the sonorant crests because they are the most sonorant of all sounds. But sonorant consonants can also occur as crests. In a word such as *button,* the nasal /n/ can be a sonorant crest following the sonorant dip for [t]. There are certainly exceptions to the Sonority Principle in syllable structure; for example, words like *axe* and *lapse* do not conform to this principle. But it has general application to the syllables of English and most languages.

As noted in Chapter 2, the concept of sonority as the basis of syllabification encounters difficulties with some phonetic sequences. Consider vowel + vowel sequences in words like *trio, piano,* and *chaos.* The abutting vowels are not necessarily associated with two distinct crests of sonority but instead may be produced as one prolonged interval of sonority. The solution may take two different forms. One is to acknowledge that the prolonged sonority interval is related to two distinct sound patterns. That is, the interval contains two segments of high sonority that can potentially be separated by a short pause or a glottal stop without destroying the form of the word. The other solution is to allow segments of high sonority to occur in a single syllable only if they form a diphthong.

We take sonority as the *sine qua non* of syllabicity. Syllabic phonemes are relatively sonorous in the flow of speech, and segments within syllables are generally arranged to form a single sonorant peak within the syllable. The concept of sonority helps to explain the two major facets of a syllable, its internal organization and its identification in the flow of speech. Therefore, a syllable is a sonorant crest in the auditory pattern of speech. There are several advantages to this definition, but one in particular is that it affords a way to match up prosodic and segmental features of speech. Silverman and Pierrehumbert (1990) observe that associating prosodic specifications with sonority peaks is an effective way of coordinating prosodic and segmental features. Prosodic structure may be important to infants in their early learning about speech. Prosody, and its rhythmic base, is a possible foundation on which the infant can learn about the phonetic structure of a language (Kent, Mitchell, & Sancier, 1991).

Role of Prosody in Typical and Atypical Development of Speech and Language

The role of prosody in the development of speech and language has been studied in both typically and atypically developing children. Although many questions remain, some general ideas about prosodic development are coming into relief. One of the most conspicuous aspects in the development of prosody is that young children often omit unstressed or weak syllables. With maturation of speech and language skills, children are less likely to make these omissions and therefore can match more accurately the stress patterns of adult speech. This is one well-attested example of the importance of prosody in understanding the development of spoken language.

A good illustration of efforts to address the role of prosody in language development comes from Gerken and McGregor (1998). They described the development of prosody in both normal and disordered (or delayed) language, focusing on three aspects of prosody along with their developmental emergence:

1. Phrasal stress is a prosodic pattern for a phrase in which one word is more prominent or salient than other words by having a longer duration, greater loudness, or higher pitch. From their review of the research, Gerken and McGregor concluded that phrasal stress in compound nouns is established by the age of at least 3 years.
2. Prosodic boundary cues are cues that mark the ends of linguistic units, including pausing, pitch resetting, and syllable lengthening. Some boundary cues, such as sentence declination (which was termed pitch declination earlier in this chapter) and phrase final lengthening, are produced by the age of 2 years.
3. Meter is the pattern of stressed and unstressed syllables in an utterance, such as the tendency in English to alternate strong and weak syllables (e.g., the stress patterns in the words *Arizona* and *Americana*). One facet of meter, lexical stress assignment, appears to be fairly accurate and adult-like by the age of 3 years.

From the foregoing paragraph, it may seem reasonable to think that prosody is largely developed by the age of 3 years. However, studies indicate that both the perception and production of prosody are refined until at least the ages of 8 to 10 years (Doherty, Fitzsimmons, Asenbauer, & Staunton, 2007; Wells, Peppé, & Goulandris, 2004). We may conclude that although some features of prosody emerge in the vocalizations of infants, adult-like sophistication takes much longer and probably parallels the continuing development of language in childhood.

Not surprisingly, then, delayed or disordered prosody has been noted in a number of speech or language disorders including autism (Peppé, McCann, Gibbon, & Rutherford, 2007; Shriberg, Paul, McSweeny, Klin, Volkmar, & Cohen, 2001), Down syndrome (Stojanovik, 2011), dysarthria (Bunton, Kent, Kent, & Rosenbek, 2000), and language impairment in children (Gerken & McGregor, 1998). The general clinical need to characterize prosody has motivated the development of transcription systems and tests, as discussed in the following section.

Clinical Assessment of Suprasegmentals

This section mentions briefly some approaches for the clinical assessment of suprasegmental features. In the main, assessment of prosody traditionally has been accomplished within the general framework of assessment for specific disorders, such as aphasia, deafness, autism, and second language learning. Few general-purpose methods of prosodic assessment have been introduced.

Exclusion Codes

Content/Context	Environment	Register	States
C1 Automatic Sequential ___	E1 Interfering Noise ___	R1 Character Register ___	S1 Belch ___
C2 Back Channel/Aside ___	E2 Recorder Wow/Flutter ___	R2 Narrative Register ___	S2 Cough/Throat Clear ___
C3 I Don't Know ___	E3 Too Close to Microphone ___	R3 Negative Register ___	S3 Food in Mouth ___
C4 Imitation ___	E4 Too Far from Microphone ___	R4 Sound Effects ___	S4 Hiccup ___
C5 Interruption/Overtalk ___		R5 Whisper ___	S5 Laugh ___
C6 Not 4 (+) Words ___			S6 Lip Smack ___
C7 Only One Word ___			S7 Body Movement ___
C8 Only Person's Name ___			S8 Sneeze ___
C9 Reading ___			S9 Telegraphic ___
C10 Singing ___			S10 Yawn ___
C11 Second Repetition ___			
C12 Too Many Unintelligibles ___			

Prosody-Voice Codes

Prosody

Phrasing	Rate	Stress
1 Appropriate ___	1 Appropriate ___	1 Appropriate ___
2 Sound/Syllable Repetition ___	9 Slow Articulation/Pause Time ___	13 Multisyllabic Word Stress ___
3 Word Repetition ___	10 Slow/Pause Time ___	14 Reduced/Equal Stress ___
4 Sound/Syllable and Word Repetition ___	11 Fast ___	15 Excessive/Equal/Misplaced Stress ___
5 More than One Word Repetition ___	12 Fast/Acceleration ___	16 Multiple Stress Features ___
6 One Word Revision ___		
7 More than One Word Revision ___		
8 Repetition and Revision ___		

Voice

Loudness	Pitch	Quality: Laryngeal Features	Quality: Resonance Features
1 Appropriate ___	1 Appropriate ___	1 Appropriate ___	1 Appropriate ___
17 Soft ___	19 Low Pitch/Glottal Fry ___	23 Breathy ___	30 Nasal ___
18 Loud ___	20 Low Pitch ___	24 Rough ___	31 Denasal ___
	21 High Pitch/Falsetto ___	25 Strained ___	32 Nasopharyngeal ___
	22 High Pitch ___	26 Break/Shift/Tremulous ___	
		27 Register Break ___	
		28 Diplophonia ___	
		29 Multiple Laryngeal Features ___	

FIGURE 6.6
Exclusion codes and prosody-voice codes from *Prosody-Voice Screening Profile (PVSP)*. Shriberg, Kwiatkowski, and Rasmussen (1990). Tucson, AZ: Communication Skill Builders Inc. Reproduced with permission of the publisher.

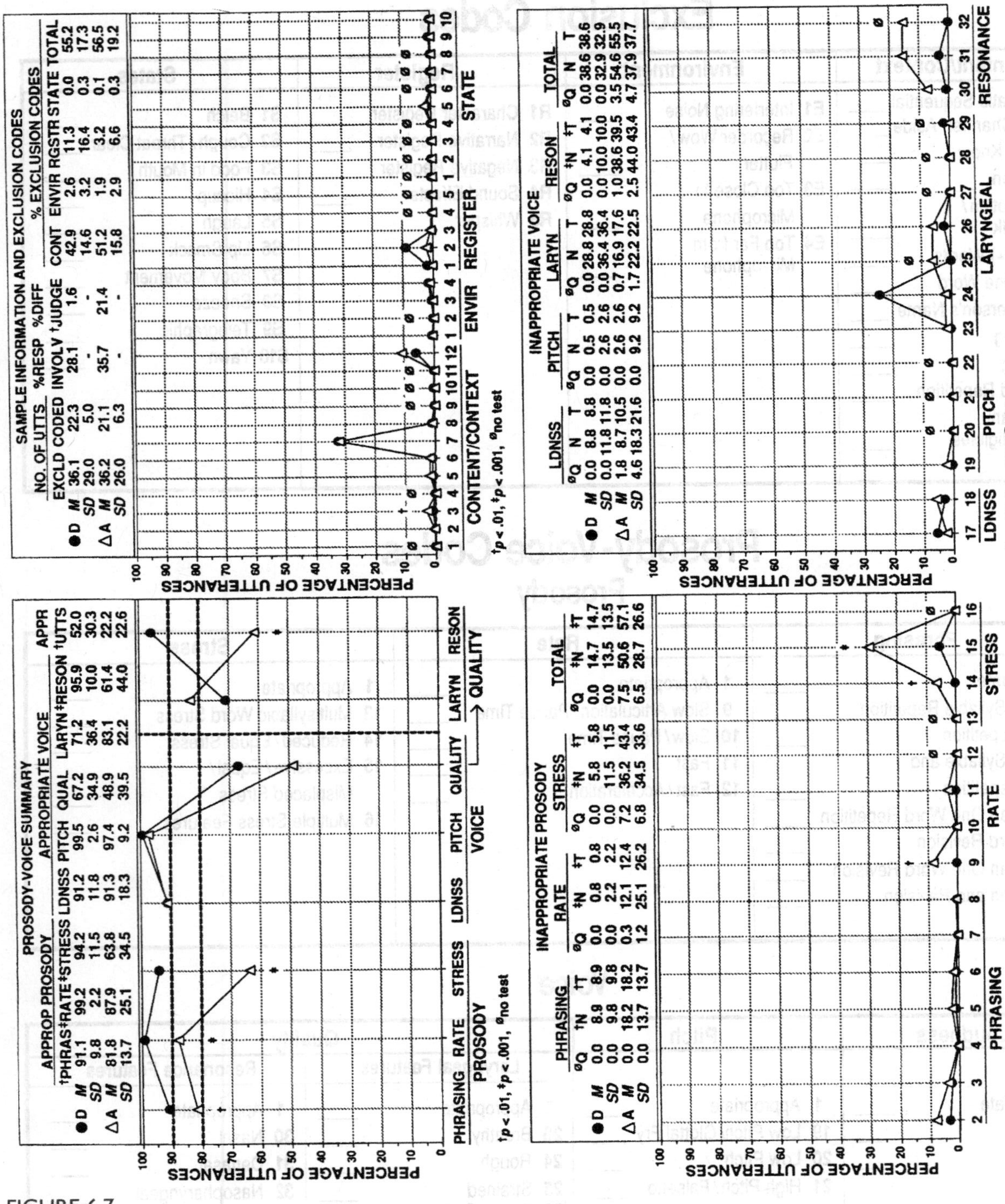

FIGURE 6.7
Illustration of clinical research use of *Prosody-Voice Screening Profile (PVSP)*. See Figure 6.6 for the key to each of the 31 exclusion codes and 31 prosody-voice codes. Shriberg (1993). Reproduced with permission of the publisher.

Selected Extensions to the International Phonetic Alphabet

As noted earlier, a special working party established by the International Phonetics Association adopted Laver's system for the transcription of voice quality. Laver's system affords a detailed description but requires some effort to learn and apply. Some of the IPA extensions for atypical speech (Duckworth et al., 1990) may suffice for some transcription purposes. Some examples of the extensions follow. In each example, the symbol **x** represents a phonetic symbol in a transcription.

Pausing is indicated by periods placed within parentheses, with the number of periods indicating the relative length of a pause:

[**x**(.)**x**]—short pause
[**x**(..)**x**]—medium-length pause
[**x**(...)**x**]—long pause

Loudness is indicated with the symbols **f** *(forte)* and **p** *(piano)* placed as subscripts around the affected portion of the transcription:

[xxx{$_{f}$xxx$_{f}$} xxx]—loud speech
[xxx{$_{ff}$xxx$_{ff}$} xxx]—louder speech
[xxx{$_{p}$xxx$_{p}$} xxx]—soft speech

Rate of speech is shown by use of the terms *allegro* and *lento:*

[xxx{$_{allegro}$xxx$_{allegro}$} xxx]—fast speech
[xxx{$_{lento}$xxx$_{lento}$} xxx]—slow speech

Voice quality is noted similarly with labeled braces. For example, use of falsetto voice is represented by the symbol **F:**

[xxx{$_{F}$xxx$_{F}$} xxx]

Symbols for Conversational Analysis

Transcription of conversational samples may require the use of symbols for situations that do not arise, or do not arise frequently, in other kinds of speech samples. Some conventions for conversational analysis are described as follows (drawn from French and Local, 1986):

=	Shows that one utterance follows immediately (no delay) from another.
(.)	marks a pause of less than a tenth of a second, which is a rather short pause in speech. Longer pauses can be noted quantitatively by entering the estimated duration of the pause within parentheses; e.g., (2.5) indicates a pause of 2.5 seconds.
:	indicates lengthening of the sound it follows.
.h (or h.)	represents outbreath. The symbol can be repeated to indicate longer outbreaths.
[	shows the point at which overlapping talking begins. A slash (/) is used to indicate where the overlapping talking ends.
<f>	is placed below an interval of talk to show that it is produced more loudly *(forte)* than is normal for the speaker.
<p>	is placed below an interval of talk to show that it is produced more quietly *(piano)* than is normal for the speaker.
<cr>	is placed below an interval of talk to show that it is produced with increasing loudness *(crescendo).*
<l>	is placed below an interval of talk to show that it is produced more slowly *(lento)* than is normal for the speaker.
...	marks an omission of a stretch of talk.
***	indicates an obscure or unintelligible utterance. Each asterisk represents one syllable.

Referring to these symbols, interpret the following conversational sample:

Well **<1.0>** I think that the problem is clear **h.h.h.**
|——————f——————|
They didn't read the directions = They just went on with it. **h.**
|——————f——————|
|————cr————|
No: wonder:, then, that it didn't work as expected. **h.**
This is the last time I will let them be unsupervised. **h.**
|——————p——————|

COARTICULATION

Consider the sentence, "Could you keep her stew steaming hot?" As produced by a speaker of General American English, this sentence would have a phonetic transcription like the following:

[kud ju kip hɝ stu stimɪŋ hɔt]

If we studied this utterance in detail with acoustic analysis or with an X-ray motion picture, we would discover these facts:

1. The [k] in *could* is produced with a back tongue articulation, but the [k] in *keep* is articulated with a relatively front tongue position.
2. The [h] in *her* is produced with an [ɝ]-like vocal tract configuration, but the [h] in *hot* has an [ɔ]-like vocal tract configuration.
3. The [s] in *stew* is produced with lip rounding, but the [s] in *steaming* is not.
4. The vowels in *steaming* are nasalized, but the vowel in *stew* is not.

These observations indicate that what we consider to be the same phonetic segment is not necessarily produced in the same way in different utterances. Actually, speech is replete with these modifications. Sounds are adapted to their phonetic contexts to make speech easier and faster. Many of these modifications are grouped together under the term **coarticulation**, which means that the production of a sound is influenced by other sounds around it, that is, by its phonetic context.

What are the contextual factors that cause coarticulation in items 1–4 of the list just identified?

In item 1, the [k] in *keep* is followed by the front vowel [i], whereas the [k] in *could* is followed by the back vowel [ʊ]. The exact place of articulation for the stop [k] is accommodated to the following vowel. If the vowel is front, then the [k] is made near the front of the oral cavity. But if the vowel is back, then the [k] also is made more as a back sound.

In item 2, the vocal tract configuration during the production of [h] anticipates the configuration of the following vowel. This is possible because the [h] sound does not have a highly specified position for the tongue, jaw, or lips. Therefore, the [h] in *her* can be produced with lip rounding and rhotic articulation suitable for vowel [ɝ]. Similarly, the [h] in *hot* can be produced with an open jaw and a low-back tongue position suitable for vowel [ɔ]. We can say that the [h] is *coproduced* with the following vowel.

In item 3, the [s] in *stew* is produced with lip rounding because this labial articulation is needed for the following vowel and does not interfere with production of the [s]. Lip rounding is not observed for the [s] in *steaming* because the following vowel [i] is not a rounded vowel. The fricative [s] can be rounded or not, depending on the following vowel.

In item 4, the vowels [i] and [ɪ] in *steaming* are both nasalized because they either precede a nasal consonant (in the case of [i]) or occur between two nasals (in the case of [ɪ]). Vowels can assume the nasalization of a neighboring consonant.

In each instance, the articulatory modification of a sound can be explained by a consideration of the phonetic context. These modifications give speech articulation a complex, highly overlapping character. The segments of speech interact, so that some of their features or properties are coarticulated (articulated together). Coarticulation refers to the various events in speech in which the vocal tract has simultaneous adjustments that are appropriate for two or more sounds. The direction of a coarticulatory effect can be described as forward (anticipatory) or backward (retentive). In forward coarticulation, an articulatory feature for a phonetic segment is evident in the production of an earlier segment. Nearly all the examples discussed above are forward coarticulation.

Backward coarticulation is illustrated with the utterance, "Please give me a cup of tea." An X-ray motion picture of most speakers would reveal that the velopharynx is open during the [i] of *me* but not during the [i] of *tea.* How do we explain this difference? Notice that the coarticulated property of velopharyngeal opening (nasalization) is attributable to the [m] that precedes the [i] in *me.* In this case, the direction of the coarticulatory effect is backward in the speech stream—hence, backward coarticulation.

Coarticulation usually is explained in terms of the concepts of spreading, shingling, or blending of articulatory properties across neighboring speech sounds. Although these three terms have a general similarity in their meaning, they are not identical in their implications for understanding the mechanisms of coarticulation.

Spreading (also called feature spreading) denotes an expansion or stretching of an articulatory feature. This concept seems especially appropriate if we think of features as being extendable to reach from one segment to another. This idea was often implemented as a spreading of binary feature values (e.g., spreading of nasalization as a [+nasal] and spreading of lip rounding as a [+round]) (Moll & Daniloff, 1971; Benguerel & Cowan, 1974). As applied to item 3 discussed earlier, the lip rounding feature for the vowel [u] would be spread or stretched to the preceding consonants [s] and [t]. As Boyce and Espy-Wilson (1997) explain, this account implies that "the underlying articulatory plan (including trajectory of movement, placement of movement in the vocal tract, etc.) for producing the target segment has been altered from the form it would take if it were bordered by different neighboring segments; in other words, *articulatory plan varies by segmental context*" (p. 3742; emphasis added). Shingling is a similar idea but denotes an overlapping such that a feature from one sound overlies an adjacent sound segment, rather like one roof tile covering another. Shingling allows a sound segment to be penetrated by a particular feature from another segment. For example, some accounts of nasalization propose that a nasality feature is shingled from a nasal phone to its preceding or succeeding phone.

Blending (also called coproduction) does not alter the segmental articulatory plan but rather supposes that coarticulation results from the overlap and blending of unaltered articulatory plans for adjacent segments. That is, the articulation is reshaped to accommodate the segment's phonetic neighbors, but the segment itself is not altered. The result is an articulation that takes into account the overall nature of one segment vis-à-vis the nature of the segments that surround it. Therefore, a modified movement is produced that can be intermediate to the movements for the two sounds in question.

These different accounts of coarticulation hold implications for the development of speech in children. The spreading and shingling accounts suggest that children must construct different articulatory plans for different segmental contexts. Blending, however, implies that children can rely on stable articulatory plans for individual segments but learn to overlap and blend these unchanged plans for adjacent segments. It is relevant to note that coarticulation may differ across individual speakers (Van den Heuvel, Cranen, & Rietveld, 1996), which may also favor the blending account, on the assumption that individual speakers develop unique strategies for blending segments. Coarticulation is one consideration in explaining why children may produce a given sound correctly in one phonetic context but not in another. By drawing on principles of coarticulation, it is possible to design contexts that facilitate correct sound production (Kent, 1982).

Coarticulation is limited primarily by the compatibility of two sounds. A common way of determining compatibility is to compare the phonetic features of the two sounds in question. Consider a consonant sound C and a vowel sound V that form a syllable CV. First, let us assume that C is the bilabial consonant /b/ and V is any vowel. Because the bilabial consonant can be produced with virtually any tongue position (so long as the vocal tract is not obstructed by the lingual articulation), the tongue is free to anticipate the lingual articulation for the vowel. Therefore, [b] in the word *bee* will be produced with an [i]-like tongue position, and the [b] in the word *boo* will be produced with an [u]-like tongue position. That is, /b/ offers very little coarticulation resistance to the vowel's lingual articulation. Both the bilabial stops and the labiodental fricatives have minimal coarticulation resistance (Recasens, 1985; Fowler & Brancazio, 2000). Coarticulation resistance depends especially on articulatory constraints that limit the physiological adjustments for a particular phone (Recasens, Pallares, & Fontdevila, 1997; Tabain, 2001). But now consider that consonant C is the lingua-palatal consonant /ʃ/. Because this consonant has a highly specified tongue position, it is not free to accommodate the lingual articulation of the following vowel. In other words, it has a high coarticulation resistance.

Keating (1990) proposed a window model of coarticulation that defines a permissible variation for an individual articulator, depending on the phonetic context. The "window" is the range of values that can be assumed by a particular articulatory dimension for a given feature. The window defines the allowable contextual variability for a phonetic feature; it specifies a range of possible positions. For example, the jaw has a certain range of positions that can be assumed for a given feature such as closed or open. Similarly, the velum has a certain range of positions that it can take for a feature such as closed (nonnasal). For some segments, the window is narrow, so that little contextual variation can occur. For other segments, the window is wide, so that contextual variation is considerable. According to this model, a speaker discovers the allowable tolerance for an articulatory dimension that is associated with a particular feature.

Diacritic Marks: An [æ̃] Is Not an [æ̤] Is Not an [æː]

As pointed by linguist J. C. Wells (2000), English is one of many languages that use the Latin alphabet, but only some of them rely on the basic set of 26 letters. English is one of those few. Most other languages supplement the basic set of letters by adding **diacritics** (accent marks). Reliance on the Latin alphabet causes a few problems for English, which has some sounds that were not used in Latin, such as the initial consonants in *sheep* and *cheap*. Both of these sounds are represented in English spelling by digraphs or combinations of letters (*sh* and *ch*).

A diacritic is a mark that is placed above, through, or below a letter to indicate a modification of the sound represented by the letter. You may have encountered diacritics if you studied other languages such as German (e.g., the diaeresis or umlaut as in *Götterdämmerung*) and Spanish (e.g., the tilde in *el Niño*). These languages extended their basic alphabet through the use of diacritics.

Diacritics in phonetics accomplish the same objective in that they indicate some kind of modification of the phoneme in question. The basic set of IPA symbols is extended by diacritics.

To this point in the book, we have been concerned with **broad transcription**, which makes use of phonemic symbols only. But when we transcribe the diverse allophonic variations (and misarticulations) that occur in speech, we have to use a finer, more detailed system than the set of phonemic symbols. For this kind of transcription, **narrow transcription**, it is necessary to use special modifiers called **diacritic marks**.

As a simple example, consider the speaker who tends to nasalize his speech. This speaker may produce the word *bad* with a nasalized vowel /æ̃/. This nasalization does not alter the selection of a phoneme symbol for the vowel, because in the English language, a nasalized /æ̃/ is still recognized as an [æ]. To indicate in the phonetic transcription that such a change in production has occurred, the diacritic mark [˜] is placed directly over the /æ/ symbol: [b æ̃ d]. Suppose that another speaker tends to produce vowels with a breathy voice, so that her production of the word *bad* has a conspicuous breathy quality. We can indicate this aspect of production by using the diacritic mark [̤], which is placed directly under the vowel symbol: [b æ̤ d].

The conventions for diacritic marks used in this book are not exactly the same as those of the International Phonetic Alphabet (IPA). We have departed slightly from the IPA system in favor of a system that we believe to be easier to learn and easier to use, especially as applied to communicative disorders. For the most part, our departures from the IPA system do not change the marks themselves but rather have to do with where the marks are placed. In the system used here, we have tried to be uniform by putting all the marks of a given category in a given position. For example, all the diacritic marks that refer to tongue position are placed directly under the phonemic symbol being modified, and all the diacritic marks that refer to lip position are placed directly over the phonemic symbol being modified.

The entire set of diacritic marks, or diacritics, is presented in Figure 6.8. Note that most of the diacritics are marked in one of six positions, represented by the numbers in Figure 6.8. A few miscellaneous marks are noted at the bottom right corner of the figure. Each numbered position is specified relative to the main symbol (IPA phonemic or phonetic symbol that is modified by the diacritic). The diacritic positions are as follows:

1. Onglide symbols, placed to the *upper left* of the main symbol.
2. Stress symbols, placed *over* the main symbol.
2. Nasal symbols, placed *over* the main symbol (and directly under the stress symbol if both are used).

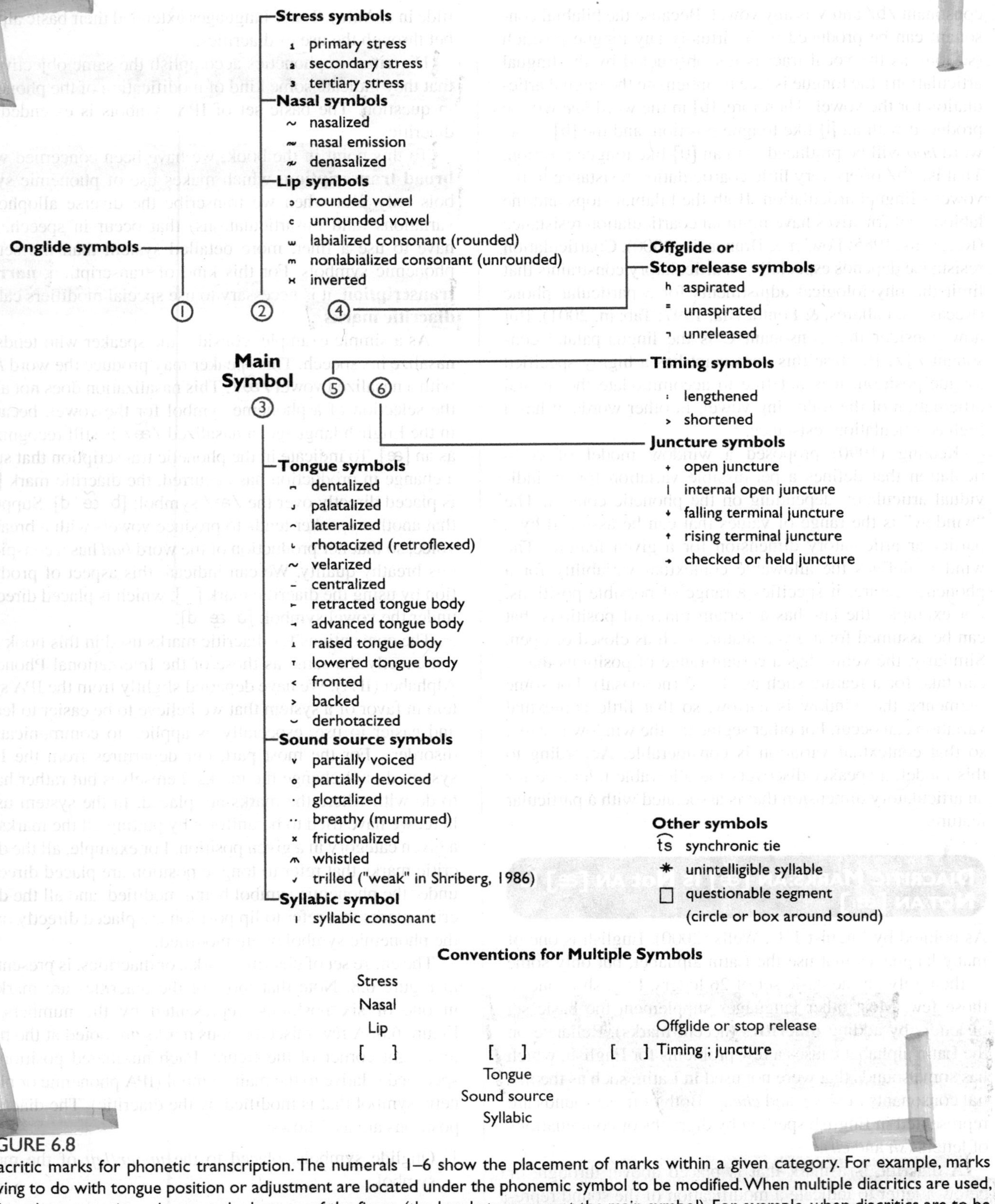

FIGURE 6.8
Diacritic marks for phonetic transcription. The numerals 1–6 show the placement of marks within a given category. For example, marks having to do with tongue position or adjustment are located under the phonemic symbol to be modified. When multiple diacritics are used, follow the conventions shown at the bottom of the figure (the brackets represent the main symbol). For example, when diacritics are to be used for both tongue and sound source, the tongue diacritic is written above that for sound source. Thus, a partially voiced, dentalized /s/ would be transcribed [s̪̬]. When diacritics from the same category are used together, they are written side by side; for example, a partially devoiced, trilled /r/ is transcribed [r̥̬].

2. Lip symbols, placed *over* the main symbol (and directly under any stress or nasal symbols).
3. Tongue symbols, placed *under* the main symbol.
3. Sound source or larynx symbols, placed *under* the main symbol (and directly under any tongue symbols that are used).
3. Syllabic symbol, placed *under* the main symbol (and directly under any tongue or source symbols).
4. Offglide symbols, placed to the *upper right* of the main symbol.
4. Stop release symbols, placed to the *upper right* of the main symbol.
5. Timing symbols, placed directly *to the right* of the main symbol.
6. Juncture symbols, placed directly *to the right* of the main symbol (and following any timing symbols).

The diacritic marks, together with the definitions of their associated terms, are discussed within each major category as follows. Later, we will suggest that you return to these descriptions as you listen to examples on the audio sample.

Onglide Symbols

Onglide symbols represent a brief or fragmentary sound that precedes the main symbol in a transcription. For example, if a very brief [ə] is heard at the onset of a fricative [s], then the transcription would be [ᵊ s].

Stress Symbols

Stress marking is discussed in some detail elsewhere in this chapter. For the present, note that three degrees of stress are marked with the numerals 1, 2, or 3 placed above the main symbol, which must be a vowel. When stress is marked with this number system, the top line of the transcription is reserved for stress marks.

Primary Stress [t u b ə]

The numeral 1 is placed over a vowel that is judged to carry **primary**, or first-level, **stress**. This is the highest degree of stress in an utterance, although it is possible for more than one syllable in an utterance to carry primary stress. It is assumed that every utterance has at least one primary stress.

Secondary Stress [ɛ m b ɑ r k]

The numeral 2 is placed over a vowel that is judged to carry **secondary**, or second-level, **stress**. It is possible for a multisyllable utterance to have two or more syllables with secondary stress.

Tertiary Stress [ə b aʊ t]

The numeral 3 is placed over a vowel that is judged to carry **tertiary**, or third-level, **stress**. This is the lowest degree of stress in an utterance, but it is possible for more than one syllable in an utterance to carry tertiary stress.

Nasal Symbols

The nasal symbols describe aspects of velopharyngeal function, that is, the valving between the oral cavity and the nasal cavity.

Nasalized [b æ̃ d]

A **nasalized** sound is produced with nasal resonance, which is created by an open velopharyngeal port allowing voicing energy to radiate through the nasal cavity. Velopharyngeal opening is illustrated for a vowel in Figure 4.30. In English, we normally nasalize vowels produced before or after nasal consonants. Compare the [æ] sounds in *man* and *bad,* the former of which is nasalized and the latter of which is not. Nasalization is essentially "talking through the nose."

Nasal Emission [s m aɪ l]

The sound of **nasal emission** is characterized by the release of noise energy through the nose. Nasal emission does not commonly occur in normal speech but is frequently noted in the speech of people with a cleft palate or other velopharyngeal incompetence. These speakers, who cannot close the velopharyngeal port tightly, may allow the noise energy of a fricative like /s/ to escape through the nose.

Denasalized [r æ n]

A **denasalized** segment is produced without nasalization or without an appropriate degree of nasalization. In normal English speech, this symbol rarely would be used, but it might be used for a speaker who failed to open the velopharyngeal port when it normally would open. If, for example, a child with cerebral palsy did not open the velopharynx for a vowel that is normally nasalized in English, one could mark the vowel as denasalized. In this case, the diacritic mark would indicate a deviation from the normal speech pattern of nasalization. A denasalized quality also may be heard for speakers with nasal congestion, as from a cold.

Lip Symbols

Rounded (or Protruded) Vowel [sw i t]

A **rounded** vowel is produced with a rounding, or protrusion, of the lips. In English, many of the back vowels are normally rounded, as in the case of /u/ and /o/. If you produce an /i/

while keeping the lips in a rounded state like that used for /u/, you should hear a marked difference in vowel quality. If a person uttered the word *sweet* but held the lip rounding needed for the /w/ throughout the word, then the vowel /i/ would be produced as a rounded vowel. The diacritic symbol for rounding may be easier to remember if you recall that ɔ is the symbol for a rounded vowel, phoneme /ɔ/.

Unrounded (or Unprotruded) Vowel [h u̹]

An unrounded vowel is produced without a rounding of the lips. Thus, if a speaker fails to round his or her lips for a vowel that is normally rounded, like /u/, this symbol would describe this deviation from the expected articulation.

Labialized Consonant [kʷ w i n]

A **labialized** consonant is produced with a constriction, or narrowing, of the lips (very much like rounding in the case of a vowel). In English, we tend to labialize many consonants when they are followed by a rounded vowel or by the /w/ sound. Thus, in the word *queen,* it is natural for a speaker to say a labialized /k/ in anticipation of the lip narrowing and protrusion for the /w/. This symbol is easy to remember if you recall that the /w/ is labialized and the diacritic mark is like a small *w* placed over the phonemic segment. Many English consonants tolerate labialization. For example, in the word *stew* /s t u/, lip rounding needed for the /u/ usually begins during the preceding /s/, so that both /s/ and /t/ are produced with lip rounding. Figure 6.9 illustrates the difference in lip configuration for a labialized and nonlabialized /s/.

Nonlabialized Consonant [w̼ i d]

The consonant is not articulated with a constriction, or narrowing, of the lips. If a speaker failed to narrow and protrude the lips for the /w/ in *weed,* the nonlabialization symbol would be appropriate. Try to say *weed* without labialization.

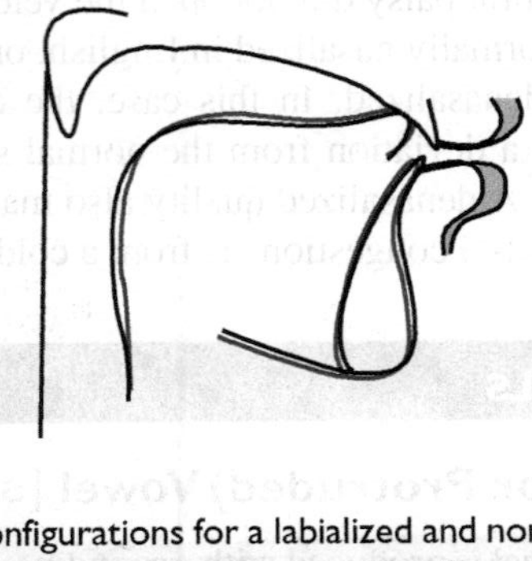

FIGURE 6.9
Articulatory configurations for a labialized and nonlabialized consonant /s/. The colored region shows the difference in lip position. For the labialized production, the vocal tract is lengthened in the forward direction.

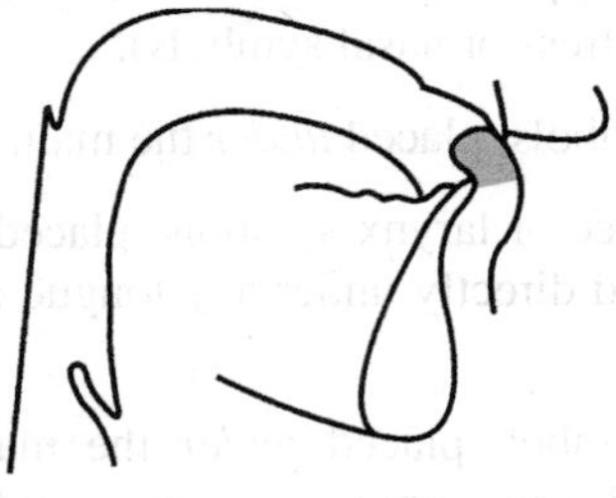

FIGURE 6.10
X-ray tracing of a child with cerebral palsy showing inversion of lower lip. Note that the lower lip is curled back behind the incisors.

Inverted Lip [b̆ i n]

Inversion, as illustrated in Figure 6.10, involves a curling back of the lip. In extreme inversion, the lip may be pulled back over the teeth. Inversion is not a common articulatory modification and is observed more often in neurologically or structurally impaired speakers than in normal speakers. Figure 6.10 is derived from an X-ray film of a child with cerebral palsy.

Tongue Symbols

The tongue symbols describe modifications of lingual articulation. Most of these symbols describe a modification in the place of articulation, but a few of them describe modifications in the manner of articulation.

Dentalized [w ɪ d̪ θ]

A **dentalized** consonant is articulated with the tip of the tongue against the back of the upper teeth (more precisely, the upper central incisors). Dentalization is illustrated in Figure 6.11. We normally dentalize the stop /d/ in words like *width,* where a dental fricative follows the stop. You should be able to feel a difference in the position of your tongue for the /d/ in *width* and the /d/ in *lid.* Of course, normally the /d/ is articulated as a lingua-alveolar stop. The dental allophone [d̪] is in complementary distribution

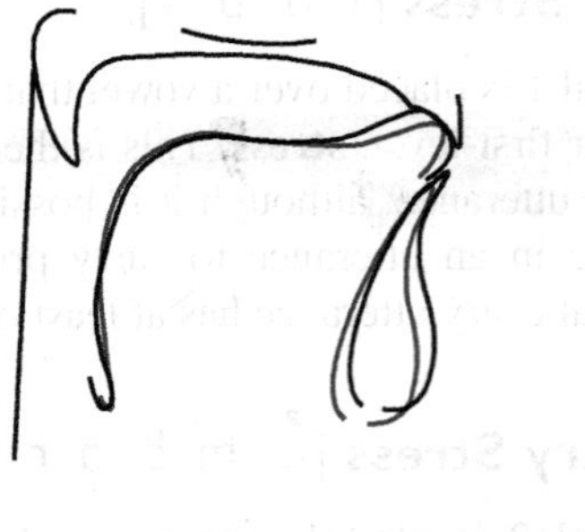

FIGURE 6.11
Articulatory configurations of an alveolar (black line) and dentalized (blue line) consonant made with tongue tip contact. In the dentalized production, the tongue tip is farther forward, making contact with the area behind the upper frontal incisors.

with the more usual alveolar [d]. Some children dentalize many or all of the sounds that are alveolar in adult speech. Note that dentalization of a normally alveolar sound is an example of fronting, or forward movement of place of articulation.

Palatalized [s̡ i l]

In **palatalized** consonant articulation, the blade, or front part of the tongue minus the tip, is close to the palatal area just behind the alveolar ridge. Perhaps the simplest way of viewing this modification is in its similarity to the normal articulation for the palatal fricative /ʃ/. A sketch of a palatalized and a normal (nonpalatalized) /s/ articulation is given in Figure 6.12. In Russian, which has both palatalized and nonpalatalized consonants, the former are called *soft* and the latter *hard* consonants, to signify the difference in auditory quality.

Lateralized [s̯ l i p]

The distinguishing property of a **lateralized** sound is the release of air through the sides (or at least one side) of the mouth. Thus, a lateralized /s/ is characterized by emission of the fricative air around the sides of the tongue, rather than through a narrow groove or slit in the midline of the articulator. One way of simulating lateral [s] is to place your tongue in position for an [l] and try to produce an [s]. You have succeeded if you produce a sound best described as "slurpy" or "lisping."

Rhotacized (or Retroflexed) [h ɑ r ʃ˞ ɚ]

As mentioned earlier, *r* coloring is a complicated articulation that takes at least two forms. One form is literally **retroflexion**, that is, involving a backward (*retro-*) turning (*flexion*) of the tongue tip. The other form takes the appearance of a bunching of the tongue in the front of the mouth, essentially in the palatal area. Ladefoged (1993) uses the term **rhotacized** to describe *r* coloring, whichever articulation may be involved, and we think this term is a good one because

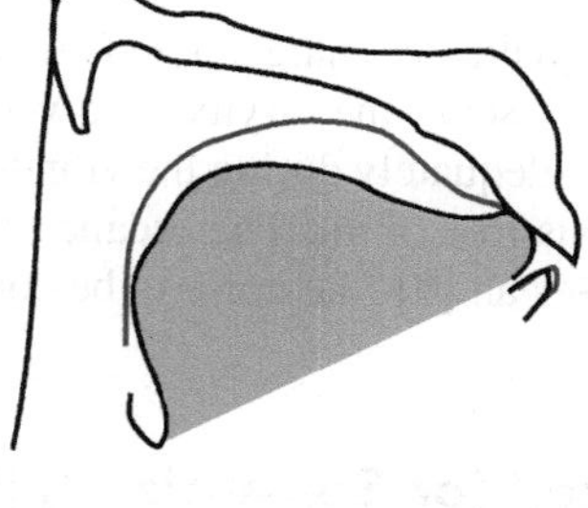

FIGURE 6.12
Articulatory configurations of a normal alveolar /s/ (black line) and a palatalized allophone (blue line). In the palatalized production, the blade of the tongue is raised toward the palatal area.

it does not have the inflexible and sometimes misleading articulatory interpretation of a word like retroflexion. At this point, it is sufficient to say that a sound with a retroflex modification has an *r* coloring or *r* similarity. This modification normally occurs in the word *harsher,* for which the /ʃ/ is rhotacized owing to the influence of the preceding and following *r* sounds. Although the difference is subtle to untrained ears, you might be able to perceive the effect of rhotacization by comparing the /ʃ/ sounds in the words *harsher* and *wishy.* It may help to prolong the fricative portions in the two words as you say them.

Velarized [f i l̴]

Velarization is a constriction of the vocal tract between the dorsum of the tongue and the posterior palate, or velum. Most speakers of English use a velarized [l̴], the so-called dark *l,* whenever /l/ is in postvocalic position at the end of a word. This /l/ usually is made with an elevated and back tongue body position and frequently without an anterior contact by the tongue tip. See the discussion of /l/ in Chapter 5 and note the drawings of /l/ articulation in that chapter.

Centralized [w ɪ n d o̱]

When a vowel is **centralized**, the tongue body is displaced toward the central region of the oral cavity. In its extreme form, centralization leads to a substitution of the schwa [ə] for the target sound. For example, with progressive centralization of the final vowel in *window,* the word would change from [w ɪ n d o] to [w ɪ n d o̱] to [w ɪ n d ə]. Notice that the particular direction of tongue displacement during centralization depends upon the articulation of the target sound. (See the diagram in Figure 4.14.) A centralized /i/ would move backward and downward (toward the center of the mouth), whereas a centralized /ɑ/ would involve a forward and upward movement. To some degree, centralization is a natural consequence of increased speaking rate or reduced stress. As a shorter period of time is allowed for a vowel articulation, the tongue undershoots, or falls short of its target position for the vowel, and thus exhibits a centralized articulation. Say the word *amputate* first very slowly and deliberately and then gradually faster and faster. You should be able to hear a change from [æm p j u t e͞ɪ t] to [æm p j ʊ t e͞ɪ t] to [æm p j ə t e͞ɪ t].

Retracted [b æ̠ t]

A **retracted** tongue position is one in which the tongue body is drawn back from the vowel target position. For example, a retracted /æ/ has a tongue position drawn back *toward* that for /ɑ/, without of course actually moving as far back as /ɑ/. The sound [æ̠] is intermediate in tongue position between a normal [æ] and a normal [ɑ]. The diacritic mark is easily remembered if you think of it as an arrow pointing toward the back (or right, by convention in this book, meaning back of the mouth).

Advanced [p ɑ̟ t]

An **advanced** tongue body position is forward, or anterior, to the target position. Thus, advanced /ɑ/ is more forward than a normal [ɑ] but not as far forward as a normal [æ]. Notice that the diacritic for advancement is an arrow pointing to the front of the mouth (left means front by the convention adopted in this book).

Raised [b ɛ̝ d]

A **raised** tongue body position is elevated above the usual, or target, position. A raised [ɛ̝] is higher than the usual [ɛ] but not so high as to sound like [ɪ].

Lowered [h ɛ̞ d]

A **lowered** tongue body position is lower than the usual, or target, position for a sound. Lowered [ɛ̞] is lower than the usual [ɛ] but not so low as to sound like [æ].

Fronted [s͔ n o͡ʊ]

A **fronted** consonant is one in which the place of articulation is unusually forward, but the exact modification is difficult to determine. Fronting applies to place of *consonant* articulation, whereas advancement refers to general tongue body position (usually for vowels but also for some consonants, like /k g/, involving the tongue body). In the example [s͔ n o͡ʊ], the transcriber might have been certain that the articulation was more anterior than it should have been but was uncertain as to exactly where the constriction was made. Whenever possible, the most explicit description should be given in the transcription, but a more general description like fronting is preferable to a highly questionable place specification.

Backed [z͕ u]

A **backed** consonant is one in which the place of articulation is unusually back, or posterior, but the exact modification is difficult to determine. See the comments immediately preceding for fronting. A back sound has a constriction that is in some sense farther back than the expected constriction for the phoneme symbol that is being modified.

Derhotacized [r̮ ɛ d]

A **derhotacized** sound is an /r/ consonant or an *r*-colored vowel that is significantly lacking in *r*-ness (rhotic or retroflex quality) but does not fall into another phonemic category of English. For example, a child who misarticulates /r/ may produce a sound that seems to be somewhere in between /r/ and /w/. Rather than assign this error production to the /w/ category, it is better to show by the transcription that the error sound is not a genuine substitution of /w/ for /r/. Hence, a derhotacized sound is one that lacks the expected /r/ quality that is accomplished by bunching or retroflexion of the tongue but is not so far removed from the target sound that a judgment of phonemic substitution is warranted.

Sound Source Symbols

The symbols in this category pertain to alterations of the source of sound energy; for example, sound generation at the larynx or noise generation at a site of fricative constriction.

Partially Voiced [æ b s̬ ə n t]

This diacritic is most frequently used to mark an unusual degree of voicing for a sound that is normally voiceless. It is not necessary that the segment be totally voiced; indeed, it often is of interest to describe partial voicing. Many normal speakers will voice the [s] in a word like *absurd* or *absent*, owing to the influence of the surrounding voiced sounds.

Partially Devoiced [d ɔ g̊]

In devoicing, a normally or typically voiced segment is partially or totally devoiced. In the example [d ɔ g̊], the [g] symbol might be retained in preference to the voiceless cognate [k] if some degree of voicing is maintained. Children have a tendency to devoice final obstruents; for example, [ʃ u z̥] for *shoes*, [d ɔ g̊] for *dog*, and [k ɑ r d̥] for *card*. Liquids and glides tend to be devoiced in normal adult speech when they follow voiceless sounds; for example, [p l̥ e͡ɪ] for *play*, [t r̥ i] for *tree*, and [t w̥ a͡ɪ s] for *twice*.

Glottalized (or Creaky Voice) [b ɑ̰ k s]

A **glottalized** sound has a creaky or irregular voice quality, often because of an aperiodicity in the laryngeal vibratory pattern. This feature and other phonatory deviations occur frequently in the speech of young children.

Breathy (or Murmured) [p l e͡ɪ̤ ɪ ŋ]

Breathy voice quality is characterized by air wastage, and therefore often noise, at the larynx. The vocal folds vibrate but do not close adequately during the vibratory cycle to prevent a continuous loss of air. The escape of air through the vocal folds causes an [h]-like noise to be combined with the voicing signal.

Frictionalized (or Spirantized) [s t͓ ɑ p]

A **frictionalized** or spirantized stop has noise energy caused by fricative-like airflow through a narrow oral constriction. This feature occurs through a failure of stop formation.

In normal speech, the dorsovelars /k g/ often are frictionalized because the tongue makes a sliding contact with the roof of the mouth and does not release the constriction as rapidly as the lips and tongue tip do for /p b/ and /t d/.

Whistled (or Hissed) [s̼ i]

Whistling, almost entirely restricted to fricatives, involves a sharply tuned noise source like that of normal whistling with the lips. This feature is most commonly heard with /s/and /ʃ/.

Trilled [t r̝ a͡ɪ]

A **trilled** sound is made with rapid, repetitive movements of alternating opening and closing, essentially vibratory in nature. Although trilled sounds do not commonly occur in English, they may be heard in other languages, such as German.

SYLLABIC SYMBOL

A small number of consonants can serve a syllabic function, meaning that they can serve as the nucleus of a syllable. The consonants most likely to do so are the nasals [m], [n], and [ŋ], the lateral [l], and the rhotic [r]. A syllabic consonant is indicated with a small vertical tic placed under the main symbol. For example, if the second syllable of the word *button* is produced with a syllabic nasal, the word would be transcribed as [b ʌ t n̩].

OFFGLIDE SYMBOLS

An offglide symbol is used to indicate the presence of a brief or fragmentary sound that immediately follows a more dominant, fully articulated sound. For example, if the word *her* is produced with a brief schwa vowel immediately following the vowel [ɝ], then the word would be transcribed as [h ɝ ə].

STOP RELEASE SYMBOLS

These symbols denote laryngeal and supralaryngeal characteristics associated with stop articulation, having to do primarily with (1) the relative timing of articulatory release and laryngeal valving, and (2) whether the stop closure is released with an audible burst.

Aspirated [tʰ ɑ p]

An **aspirated** stop has two intervals of noise, both of which typically are audible. The first noise segment is the release burst, the brief (5 to 20 ms) noise produced as the impounded air escapes in a plosive burst. This segment is followed by a generally longer interval of noise generated as air passes through the gradually closing vocal folds and the upper airway (an /h/-like sound). For voiceless stops in English, the vocal folds initially are open during the stop closure, so that the air pressure in the lungs can be fully transmitted to the oral cavity. The vocal folds then must close to allow voicing for a following voiced sound. But as the folds come together, the air passing between them generates a flat noise of rather weak intensity. Table 6.2 helps explain this sequence of events. During phase 1 of the stop articulation, the folds are open so that air from the lungs fills the closed oral cavity. Upon phase 2, the impounded air escapes with an audible explosion or burst. During phase 3, the folds are being brought together while the oral airway is open, so that air escapes through the mouth. This escaping air causes frication, or the aspiration noise. Finally, with phase 4, the folds are approximated so that voicing occurs, and the aspiration noise normally comes to an end.

TABLE 6.2
Vocal Fold Movements in the Production of Aspirated Stops

Phase 1	Phase 2	Phase 3	Phase 4
Folds are open.	Folds are open.	Folds begin to close.	Folds are brought together for voicing.
Stop closure is made.	Stop closure is released.	Oral airway is open.	Oral airway is open.

Unaspirated [s t̚ɑ p]

An unaspirated stop may have an audible release burst, but it does not have an aspiration interval. In English, unaspirated stops occur normally only when stops immediately follow fricatives, usually the /s/. Other released stops are aspirated. One possible explanation for the occurrence of unaspirated stops following fricatives is that the vocal folds begin their closing movement early during the consonant cluster, so that the folds are nearly approximated shortly after the stop is released. Interestingly, some children with /s/ omission produce the allophonically appropriate unaspirated stop even when the /s/ is judged to be omitted. That is, the child will say [t̚ɑ p] for the word *stop*.

Unreleased [l æ p˺]

An unreleased stop is one in which the articulatory closure is not broken with an audible burst of air (stop burst). For example, the final [p] in the word *lap* is not necessarily released. In fact, the lips can remain closed for a considerable period of time, virtually indefinitely, because the release burst is not a critical perceptual cue for the perception of an utterance-final stop. This fact can be demonstrated easily by saying the following words as you prolong the articulatory closure for the final stop: *rob, stop, road, seat, dog, trick.*

TIMING AND JUNCTURE SYMBOLS

These symbols are used to note variations in temporal pattern and intonation. For example, they may indicate that a sound is lengthened or prolonged, a pause occurs during an utterance, or a response is spoken as a question. Timing is concerned with durations, that is, whether sounds are long or short in their articulation. Juncture might be called "oral punctuation." Speech is produced with a number of cues that function somewhat like the commas, periods, and other punctuation marks used in writing. Juncture marks are used to indicate separation, pausing, and termination within speech. For example, a speaker can say *yes* in several ways: with finality, indicating an end to a conversation; with thoughtful prolongation and pause, as though he or she is still thinking about something; or with an interrogative intonation (questioning), to ask for repetition or clarification. The entertainer Victor Borge had a popular comical sketch in which he introduced special punctuation sounds (pops, splurts, raspberries, and the like) in conversational speech. For example, he used a special sound to show where an exclamation point might appear in a written transcript. Actually, a speaker normally uses a variety of sound pattern modifications to convey "punctuation" as well as attitudes, feelings, and other paralinguistic properties of speech.

Lengthened [s iː]

Lengthening means that a sound is prolonged; the duration of its articulation is conspicuously great or at least greater than what might ordinarily be expected. The transcription example indicates that vowel [i] is lengthened, that is, that the speaker held or maintained the vowel sound. In Southern speech, words like *lark* [l ɑ r k] may be produced without *r*-coloring but with a lengthened vowel so that the speaker still makes a phonetic distinction between *lock* [l ɑ k] and *lark* [l ɑː k]. Lengthening also occurs for some productions of geminate (double) consonants; for example, *that time* [ð æ tː a͡ɪm], *sad day* [s æ dː e͡ɪ], *some more* [s ʌ mː ɔ r]. Some phoneticians distinguish a single point [ˑ] from a double point [ː]. The single point is used to indicate a smaller degree of lengthening. However, we have found that such a distinction is difficult to teach and to use reliably; therefore, we recommend that the double-point symbol be used for most purposes. However, if you hear an extremely lengthened sound, such as a prolongation in stuttered speech, you can represent it with iterated double-point symbols; for example [sːːː iːː], for prolonged /s/ and prolonged /i/.

Shortened [w e ˃]

Shortening is indicated whenever a sound is conspicuously brief in duration. In the transcription example, the vowel [e] is marked as shortened. Shortening is appropriately marked for sounds that are abbreviated, truncated, or rushed in some respect. As another example, we sometimes hear children produce [s] segments that are almost so short as to sound like exploded [t]. But because the segment is perceptually identifiable as [s], the shortening mark is used rather than to transcribe the modification as a substitution of [t] for [s]: [s˃].

Close Juncture [a͡ɪ d ɪ d ɪ t] (*I Did It*)

Close juncture is not marked in a phonetic transcription because it implies that no special time separation occurs between elements; the transition between phones is made in a way that is physiologically convenient and should not interfere with the communication of meaning. Hence, close juncture is a kind of default juncture and occurs when no other junctural conditions apply. It does not alter a phonetic transcription.

Open Juncture [ə n a͡ɪ s + mæn] versus [ə n + a͡ɪ s mæn]

Open juncture is a short pause or gap that separates phone boundaries of syllables in ambiguous or confusable utterances. For example, the transcription examples distinguish *a nice man* from *an ice man.* Note that the segmental or phonemic content of these two phrases is identical but that they differ in timing or phrasing. Open juncture, which is represented phonetically by + or by a graphic space, is used in these transcriptions to show where a pause occurs. Open juncture also distinguishes confusable pairs like *nitrate* and *night rate. Nitrate* [n a͡ɪ + t r e͡ɪ t] differs from *night rate* [n a͡ɪ t + r e͡ɪ t] in pause or gap location.

Internal Open Juncture [l ɛ t s h ɛ l p | ʤ e͡ɪ n]

Internal open juncture generally is used to represent phrasing and is similar to commas, semicolons, and interjections in writing. The pause or gap indicated by internal open juncture usually is longer than that for the syllabic open junctures just discussed. In the transcription example of *Let's help, Jane,* the pause associated with the comma is represented in the phonetic transcription by the vertical line symbolic of internal open juncture. Notice that this juncture distinguishes the helper from the helpee.

Falling Terminal Juncture [t ʊ d e͡ɪ ↓]

Terminal juncture marks the end of an utterance (sentence, sentence fragment, or single-word response). Falling terminal juncture is associated with declarative statements in general and is conveyed acoustically by a falling fundamental frequency (voice pitch) on the last syllable. For example, the transcription example of *today* might be a reply to the question "When are you leaving for vacation?" The vertical arrow points downward to signify the falling fundamental frequency.

Rising Terminal Juncture [t ʊ d e͞ɪ ↑]

Rising terminal juncture generally represents interrogatives or questions. Questions are often signaled acoustically by a rise of fundamental frequency (voice pitch) on the final syllable. Thus, the transcription example of *today* indicates a question, "(Are you leaving) today?" The direction of the arrow indicates the rising fundamental frequency.

Checked or Held Juncture [t ʊ d e͞ɪ →]

Checked or held juncture may indicate either a speaker's intention to continue talking after a pause or an expression of continued interest in another speaker's utterance. For example, if a speaker is describing a list of activities for a week of vacation, *today* might be uttered with checked juncture to introduce the activities for the first day of the week. This type of juncture is frequently used by teachers when calling upon students to answer a question; [ʤ ɑ n →] (John. . .) identifies the student by name, and the checked juncture indicates that the teacher is waiting for the student's response. Checked juncture is expressed acoustically by a relatively flat or fixed fundamental frequency on the final syllable, often in association with a lengthening of that syllable.

OTHER SYMBOLS

Synchronic Tie [d͡z u]

A synchronic tie is used when two distinct articulations are linked or tied together in one segment. For example, the transcription [d͡z u] indicates that the [d] and [z] are produced synchronically, like an affricate. The tie symbol is used to represent this quality of linking or combination. The word *synchronic* literally means "together in time" or "at the same time" and is used here to denote that two sounds appear to occur together as one segment.

Unintelligible Syllable [✱]

Clinical transcription often presents situations in which a person's speech is not intelligible. For example, a child with a speech disorder might say a word or several words that the clinician fails to understand. An asterisk [✱] is used to represent each syllable in such words, for example, [✱ ✱ ✱ ✱ ✱ ✱]

Questionable Segment ⓐ or ⓘ

A circle is used around each segment in a transcription about which the transcriber is unsure. Either the questionable sound or sounds are circled (for example, (k) ɑ t, (k ɑ) t, (k ɑ t)) or a question mark representing questionable segments is circled (for example, k (?) t, (? ?) t, (? ? ?)). In computer fonts, circles may be replaced by rectangles.

STRESS AND OTHER SUPRASEGMENTAL FEATURES

Stress Marking in the IPA

The importance of stress can be shown by asking someone who can read phonetic transcription to say aloud the following utterances:

[ɛ s k ɔ r t] [p r o t ɛ s t] [ɪ n k l a͞ɪn]

Note that each of these words can be either a noun (having a greater level of stress on the first syllable) or a verb (having a greater level of stress on the second syllable). However, the segmental transcription alone does not indicate which form, noun or verb, is to be used. To make this distinction, some kind of stress marking is needed. The IPA convention is to mark the primary (highest level) stress with a small vertical mark above the line and before the affected syllable. Secondary (the next highest level) stress is marked with a similar vertical mark located below the line and before the affected syllable. The noun and verb forms of the words *escort, protest,* and *incline* are stress-marked as follows in the IPA:

Nouns	*Verbs*
[ˈɛ sˌ k ɔ r t]	[ˌɛ sˈ k ɔ r t]
[ˈp r oˌ t ɛ s t]	[ˌp r oˈ t ɛ s t]
[ˈɪ nˌ k l a͞ɪ n]	[ˌɪ nˈ k l a͞ɪ n]

A third (tertiary) level of stress is indicated in the IPA by the absence of a stress mark. For example, the weak second syllable of the words *father, city,* and *sofa* carries no special mark in the transcriptions [ˈf ɑ ð ɚ], [ˈs ɪ ɾ ɪ], and [ˈs o͞ʊ f ə]. The three levels of stress (primary, secondary, and tertiary) are represented in the words *ratify* [ˈr æ ɾ ɪ ˌf a͞ɪ] and *allophone* [ˈæ l əˌ f o͞ʊ n].

One disadvantage of the IPA stress marks is that they often are difficult to distinguish from the various diacritic marks used in a narrow transcription. Another disadvantage is that the marks are supposed to precede the affected syllable, which means that the transcriber must make decisions about syllabification (where one syllable ends and another begins). Syllabification decisions are not always obvious, so the requirement of syllable segregation for stress marking can stand in the way of transcription.

Stress Marking by Number

Because of these disadvantages in the IPA system of stress marking, we favor the method described previously in which stress level is represented simply as a number above the nucleus of the syllable (the nucleus being the vowel, diphthong, or syllabic consonant core of the syllable). Thus, the noun and verb forms of the word *incline* are represented as [ɪ n k l a͞ɪ n] (1 over ɪ, 2 over a͞ɪ) and [ɪ n k l a͞ɪ n] (2 over ɪ, 1 over a͞ɪ), respectively.

The numerals for stress marking are placed above any diacritics used in narrow transcription, such placement reflecting the suprasegmental nature of stress. The words *ratify* and *allophone* are stress marked as follows: [r $\overset{1}{\text{æ}}$ ɾ $\overset{3}{\text{ɪ}}$ f $\overset{2}{\text{aɪ}}$] and [$\overset{1}{\text{æ}}$ l $\overset{3}{\text{ə}}$ f $\overset{2}{\text{oʊ}}$ n].

The determination of stress level sometimes is a difficult judgment, as it requires that each syllable in an utterance be compared against others. Hence, stress is a relational feature, involving comparisons across syllables. We recommend that the beginning student first identify the syllable with primary stress and then make decisions about secondary and tertiary levels. Say each of the following words and place a "1" over the orthographic spelling of the syllable with primary stress. The correct answer is shown at the right.

t e l e p h o n e	tel
o c e a n	o
b u i l d i n g	build
W i s c o n s i n	con
N e b r a s k a	bras
s a l a d	sal
a g a i n	gain
w i n d o w	win
d i n o s a u r	di
W y o m i n g	o
g r e y h o u n d	both syllables have primary stress

Usually, only one syllable in a word has primary stress, but some words, like *greyhound,* typically have primary stress on both syllables. Two-syllable words having equal (primary) stress on both syllables are called **spondees**; other examples are the words *hothouse, horseshoe,* and *pathway.*

Polysyllabic words or phrases may contain more than one syllable of secondary or tertiary stress. For example, the word *relativity* has primary stress on the third syllable, secondary stress on the first syllable, and tertiary stress on the second, fourth, and fifth syllables.

[r $\overset{2}{\text{ɛ}}$ l $\overset{3}{\text{ə}}$ t $\overset{1}{\text{ɪ}}$ v $\overset{3}{\text{ɪ}}$ ɾ $\overset{3}{\text{i}}$]

Syllabification [b ʌ t n̩] [b æ t l̩] [r ʌ b m̩]

A special kind of reduced syllable is produced when the nucleic function ordinarily served by a vowel or diphthong is accomplished by a consonant, usually /m/, /n/, or /l/, but infrequently /r/. These consonants can, under certain conditions, become syllabic, meaning that they constitute in themselves a syllable. The syllabic function is indicated by a short vertical line directly under the consonant symbol. In the transcription examples, /n/, /l/, and /m/ are syllabic in *button, battle,* and *rub (the)m* ("rub'm"), respectively. **Syllabification** does not necessarily or always occur in these utterances, as they could be produced with the schwa vowel in the reduced syllable: [b ʌ t ə n], [b æ t ə l], and [r ʌ b ə m]. Syllabic consonants are most likely to occur when the consonant is homorganic (similar in place of articulation) with the boundary consonant in the preceding syllable. In the examples here, the homorganic pairings are /tn/, /tl/, and /bm/. When the homorganic condition is not satisfied, as in *tackle, trouble, siphon,* and *knock (the)m* ("knock'm"), a schwa vowel is more likely to be heard because the point of articulation necessarily changes between the consonants. In homorganic pairings, the articulatory contact can be maintained across the two sounds, and thus an open vocal tract (that is, a potential vowel) does not intervene. Some phoneticians use a syllable /r/ in words like *taper, tighter,* and *roller,* but we prefer the schwar /ɚ/ in these sequences.

Abbreviatory Devices in Phonetic Description

On occasion, the clinician may not want to take the time to record a detailed phonetic description of a client's speech. For example, it may be sufficient simply to listen to the client's conversational speech or a sample of reading and to record some general impressions about the phonetic behavior. For such an application, the clinician may proceed as follows.

First, to obtain phonetic information on at least broad categories of speech behavior, the clinician might consider the phonetic classes of stop, fricative, nasal, glide, liquid, and vowel-diphthongs, abbreviated S, F, N, G, L, and V, respectively. Then, upon hearing sounds in each category, the clinician notes errors, especially frequent or pervasive errors, for the major diacritic categories presented in this chapter, namely, lip articulation features, nasalization, tongue articulation features, source features, stop release features, and prosodic features. Because each of these categories of diacritics has a specified location in the diacritic marking system, a tally of errors can be kept by the diacritic location of the errors detected. Examples of an abbreviated phonetic description follow.

S̥ F̥	Devoicing of stops and fricatives.
Ṽ G̃	Nasalization of vowels and glides.
S˂ F˂ (< below)	Fronting of stops and fricatives.
V̥ V̤ Ṿ	Abnormal phonation of vowels: devoicing, breathiness, glottalization.
S͓	Spirantization of stops.
S̡ F̡	Palatalization of stops and fricatives.
S̪ F̪	Dentalization of stops and fricatives.
V̠	Retraction of tongue body for vowels.

Consider the following abbreviated phonetic description of a child's speech:

S F V

This description indicates that the child makes errors of tongue placement (fronting) for stops and fricatives, and errors of tongue body position (retraction) for vowels. In addition, the child frequently devoices segments and tends to use a breathy voice quality.

One reason for the modified system of diacritics in this book is that the system simplifies the tally of phonetic errors and allows a fairly easy and quick interpretation of the results with respect to major categories of error. In contrast, the diacritics used in the IPA to denote modifications of tongue articulation are variously placed with respect to phoneme symbols, so it is rather difficult to keep a record of these errors separate from errors of lip articulation, phonation, or nasalization. With the modified system used in this book, all errors of tongue articulation are marked in the same place, directly under the phoneme symbol. Therefore, a large number of errors affecting tongue position would be signified by the frequent appearance of diacritics in the slot directly under the phoneme symbol; for example, S F would indicate multiple errors of fronting, dentalization, and palatalization detected in a speech sample.

A system of abbreviation (we might call it phonetic shorthand) is especially important when the clinician is listening to conversational speech or reading. Phonetic decisions have to be made quickly, and there may not be time to write descriptive remarks such as "dentalized stops and fricatives." To use the shorthand system, the clinician might bear in mind the following configuration for diacritic marking. The blackened space is the position for a phonetic element or class symbol (such as V, S, F), and the bracketed words indicate positions for diacritics:

[Stress]
[Nasal]
[Lip]
■ [Release]
[Timing or juncture]
[Tongue]
[Source]

Whether a phonemic element or a class abbreviation is used in the black space depends on the degree of abstraction or generalization required. For example, if a phonetic modification applies to a class of sounds, like stops, then the abbreviation S (for stop) should be used. On the other hand, if the modification applies only to one stop, like [t], then the phonemic symbol [t] should be used.

In using the diacritic system for the first time, it may be helpful to circle the suitable diacritics from a list such as that shown in Figure 6.13. In this configuration, all diacritics

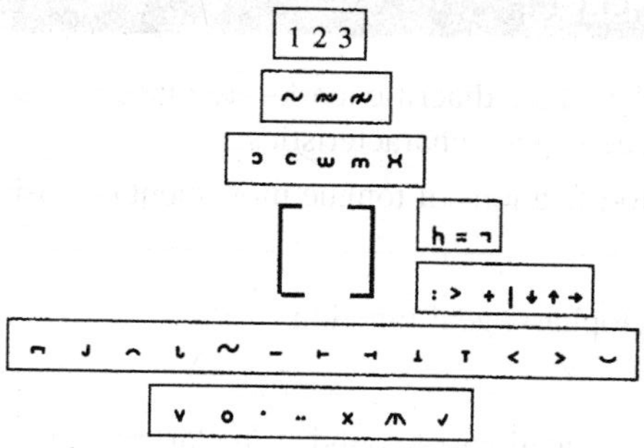

FIGURE 6.13

Complete set of diacritic marks arranged by placement relative to phonemic symbol (brackets). This composite diagram might be useful in early transcription practice using the diacritic system.

of a particular kind (for example, tongue modifications) are bracketed and placed in the appropriate location with respect to the symbol (phonetic element or class abbreviation) being modified. After some practice with the listed diacritic configuration, the clinician should acquire sufficient familiarity to rely on memory for the diacritics.

Some Guidelines for Using Diacritic Marks

The following questions might be useful to ask when using diacritic marks.

1. Which phonetic symbol best represents the sound in question? (Write the symbol in brackets: [æ], [s], [t].)
2. Is the sound produced with any modification of source? If so, write the appropriate diacritic *under* the phonetic symbol: [æ̤], [s̬], [t̽].
3. Is the sound a stop consonant? If so, is it unreleased [t˺]? If it is released, is it aspirated [tʰ] or unaspirated [t⁼]?
4. Is the sound produced with any modification of place of articulation? That is, is there any modification of lingual or labial articulation? If so, place the lingual [z̠] or labial [̑] diacritic in the appropriate place.
5. Is there any modification of velopharyngeal function, such as nasalization, nasal emission, or denasalization? If so, mark accordingly.
6. Is there any aspect of juncture or duration that should be indicated? Is there a pause or inflection (both are manifestations of juncture)? Is the sound abruptly terminated or prolonged? If so, mark appropriately.
7. Finally, are any of the miscellaneous special marks for stress of syllabification needed?

Chapters 7, 8, and 9 will give detailed consideration to the question of *when* diacritics should be used in clinical phonetics.

EXERCISES

1. Describe where diacritic marks are placed for the following speech sound characteristics:
   (a) Modifications of tongue movement or position ____________________
   (b) Velopharyngeal function ____________________
   (c) Modifications of sound at the larynx ____________________
   (d) Features of stop release ____________________
   (e) Juncture ____________________
   (f) Lip configuration ____________________

2. For each phonetic description, provide the phonetic symbol and appropriate diacritic mark. *Example:* Voiceless lingua-alveolar fricative with nasal emission—[s͌]
   (a) Nasalized high-front, tense vowel [ ]
   (b) Unaspirated voiceless bilabial stop [ ]
   (c) Labialized voiced lingua-dental fricative [ ]
   (d) Lengthened low-back, tense vowel [ ]
   (e) Lowered mid-front, lax vowel [ ]
   (f) Glottalized high-mid-back, lax vowel [ ]
   (g) Trilled voiceless lingua-alveolar stop [ ]
   (h) Devoiced bilabial nasal [ ]
   (i) Retroflex voiceless palatal fricative [ ]
   (j) Dentalized voiced lingua-alveolar fricative [ ]

3. For each phonetic symbol and multiple modifications given here, provide the appropriate diacritic marks.
   Example: [k̬ʷ], partially voiced and labialized
   (a) [æ], nasalized and lengthened
   (b) [d], devoiced and unreleased
   (c) [s], dentalized and lengthened
   (d) [ɪ], breathy and raised
   (e) [u], unrounded and nasalized
   (f) [l], velarized and devoiced
   (g) [tʃ], retroflexed and partially voiced
   (h) [t], aspirated and frictionalized

4. Using the number system for stress marking, transcribe the following words (General American pronunciation) and indicate the stress pattern.
   (a) transcribe ____________________
   (b) satisfy ____________________
   (c) legislature ____________________
   (d) furniture ____________________
   (e) Arizona ____________________
   (f) Chicago ____________________
   (g) overload ____________________
   (h) skyscraper ____________________
   (i) typewriter ____________________
   (j) Lithuania ____________________
   (k) masterpiece ____________________
   (l) Mississippi ____________________

5. Briefly describe the meaning of each diacritic in the following transcription.
   (a) [j e ᵊ →]
   (b) [w ɑ͞ɪ̃ ↑]
   (c) [h ɛ̈ l õ]
   (d) [p l̥̈ iː z →]
   (e) [k ʌ p $\overset{3}{\text{ə}}$ k $\overset{1}{\text{ɔ}}$ f $\overset{3}{\text{ɪ}}$]
   (f) [g ʊ̞ d m ɔ̃ r n ɪ̃ ŋ]
   (g) [ɑ͞ɪ d ɪ ʔ n o͞ʊː ð æᴵ t˺]

6. The following is an exercise in reading transcription—a linguistic potpourri. Try reading each transcription, referring to the International Phonetic Alphabet chart (inside cover) to guide your pronunciation of unfamiliar symbols. Stress is marked using the IPA system.

Spanish

jota	[ˈx o t a]
pegar	[p e ˈɣ a r]
la boca	[l ɑ ˈβ o k a]

French

peu	[p ø]
faim	[f ɛ̃]
Chopin	[ʃ ɔ ˈ p ɛ̃]
monsieur	[m ə ˈs j ø]

German

Tag	[t ɑ ː x]
Zug	[t s uː x]
spielen	[ˈʃ p iː l ə n]

Italian

Signori	[s iˈɲ ɔ r ɪ]
grazie	[ˈg r ɑ t s j e]

Russian
(trick) [ˈ ʃ t u k ə]
(good welfare) [ˈ b l a ɣ̊ ə]

Norwegian
dryppe [ˈ d r y pː ə]
dod [d oː]

Finnish
kiitos [ˈ k i t o s]
yksi [ˈy k s i̯]

TRANSCRIPTION TRAINING

Transcription List E

CD 1, Track 5, List E, provides practice in marking stress. Use the stress marking by number system above the phonetic transcription.

PROCEED TO: Clinical Phonetics CD 1, Track 5: Transcription List E

Transcription List F

Audio sample 1, Track 6 provides practice in transcribing casual speech, including terminal juncture symbols.

PROCEED TO: Clinical Phonetics CD 1, Track 6: Transcription List F

Vowels and Diphthongs Quiz

The next two audio sample training modules test phonetic transcription skills with children's speech. Each word was said by a child with normally developing speech. For this first quiz, transcribe only the vowels and diphthongs. Although you may hear some sound modifications that could be transcribed with diacritics, enter only the phoneme symbols in the brackets provided.

PROCEED TO: Clinical Phonetics CD 1, Track 7: Vowels and Diphthongs Quiz

Transcription Quiz

For this second introduction to children's speech, transcribe the entire word. Again, for clarity, possible diacritic modifications are not included in the key.

PROCEED TO: Clinical Phonetics CD 1, Track 8: Transcription Quiz

Diacritics Examples

The last training module on audio sample CD 1, Track 9 provides examples of sound modifications marked by diacritics. Their exercise provides a list of the 24 diacritic modifications, which are simulated here by two adult speakers. For each example, a speaker will say two sounds or words twice. Each sound or word will be said first with normal articulation, then with a sound modification. For example, the first set, which demonstrates nasalized vowels, is:

Normal [æ]	Nasalized [æ̃]
[i]	[ĩ]

As you listen to each example, follow the text descriptions beginning on page 109. These simulations also generally follow the ordering of symbols in Figure 6.8. Beginning in Chapter 8, you will have the opportunity to transcribe children's sound modifications as they occur in a clinical environment.

PROCEED TO: Clinical Phonetics CD I, Track 9: Diacritics Examples

CHAPTER 7

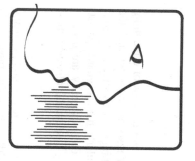

Clinical Scoring and Transcription

We are nearing the clinical training sections of this book. But some concepts and procedural issues require discussion before you tackle the text and audio materials in the next chapter. This chapter and associated appendixes should serve as a source for answers to questions that undoubtedly will arise as you attempt clinical phonetics.

Figure 7.1 illustrates the sequence of activities associated with scoring or phonetic transcription. These activities may be divided into three phases: (1) sampling and recording a child's speech, (2) playback and scoring or transcription, and (3) phonological analyses. This chapter is concerned primarily with events in the second phase, although we will discuss briefly issues in obtaining speech samples. Detailed procedures for digital audio recording and speech sampling are provided on the clinical phonetics website, formerly Appendix E.

Let us look first at some factors that influence scoring and transcription.

Factors that Influence Scoring and Transcription

Client Factors

Do characteristics of the person whose speech is being sampled affect the ease and accuracy of scoring and transcription? Unquestionably, they do. Some of the major individual differences are the person's age, dialect, and physical and personality characteristics.

Age. Children present many problems in transcription. For one thing, younger children have trouble understanding directions. The younger the child, the more difficult it is to have the child respond to formal testing. As an examiner, you need to devise effective and efficient ways to obtain speech samples for particular purposes. Procedures and findings for five types of speech samples—ranging from "non-directed" to "directed"—are described in Shriberg and Kwiatkowski (1985).

Children also behave in ways that interfere with transcription. For example, they frequently vary such voice characteristics as loudness and pitch, and they often fail to keep a fixed distance from the microphone of the recorder. They relish kicking tables and playing with microphone cords—all of which create noise on a recording. Occasionally, audio samples in this program will contain such child-generated noises.

The major reason that even the most well-mannered youngster is hard to score or transcribe is, of course, incomplete speech development. In fact, during the speech development period, children often produce sounds that are perceptually ambiguous. For example, Costely and Broen (1976) present acoustic data for a child whose voicing of alveolar stops /t/ and /d/ was indeterminate. Transcribers were baffled as to which stop consonant symbol was appropriate to use. Many studies since this one have shown that children produce sounds that do not clearly fall into adult categories. In the training samples to follow, we will be concerned with just these sorts of problems.

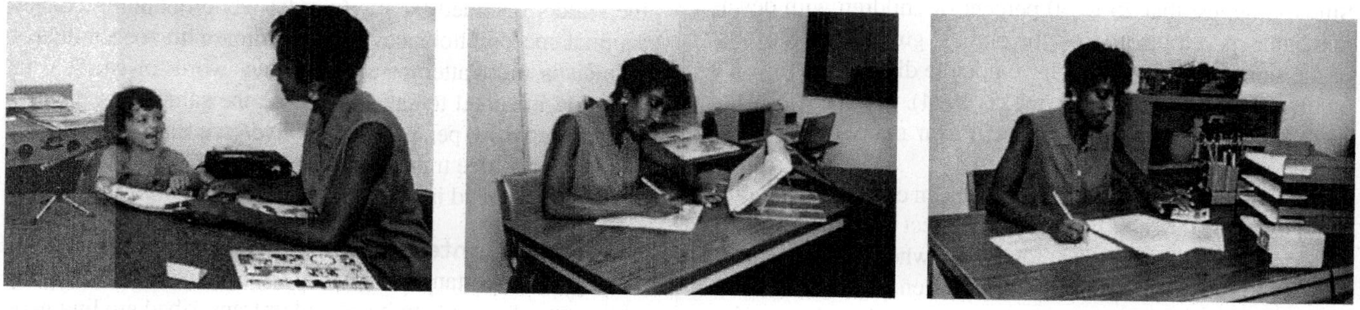

FIGURE 7.1
Obtaining, transcribing, and analyzing a speech sample.

Dialect. Another speech characteristic to consider is the client's dialect. In this text, as in most other American phonetics texts, General American speech is used as the reference dialect. Throughout the United States there are many regional dialects, as well as varieties of English spoken by those for whom English is a second language. For clinical work in communicative disorders, clinicians must learn to transcribe appropriately the dialect of the person with whom they will be working. Clinicians must learn both the phonological rules of the dialect and the boundaries for acceptable production of each allophone. The point to underscore is that dialect differences between speaker and transcriber must be placed in proper perspective. Chapter 10 provides a detailed review of dialectal issues as they impact phonetic transcription in the clinical environment.

Physical and Personality Characteristics. Included in this last category of individual differences among speakers are the many physical and personal factors that make one person's speech easier to score or transcribe than another's. A person who uses larger lip movements, for example, may be easier to transcribe than one who speaks with tight lips or clenched teeth. The term "easier" includes concepts of reliability and efficiency. It may be much more tedious and time-consuming to transcribe the speech of certain talkers, even though it is accomplished successfully in the end. Rate of speech is another critical variable. Some talkers speak or read so fast that transcription is extremely difficult, if not impossible.

Transcription may also be biased by more subtle speaker characteristics. For example, Stephens and Daniloff (1974) reported that one of their speakers who had normal *articulation* was perceived by a transcriber working from audiotape as making some /s/ distortions. Stephens and Daniloff suggested that perhaps this subject's atypical *voice quality* had influenced articulation judgments. One of our student clinicians noted a similar problem when transcribing tapes of some children. This student commented: "Sometimes it was hard to separate [the client's] articulation from laryngeal or resonant voice quality. This was especially true [on recordings] where there was a hypernasal resonant quality overriding the articulation." Such observations suggest that a person's voice quality can influence transcription of articulation (Ball, 1988). Studies suggest that 25 to 50 percent of children with developmental speech disorders—the clinical group used for most of the samples in this text—have notable differences in voice quality (Shriberg & Kwiatkowski, 1994). Therefore, in the training samples to follow, you will hear many examples of children with deviant voice quality.

The interpersonal relationship between client and clinician is yet another source of bias that may affect transcription data. Diedrich and Bangert (1981) found that when the examiner is also the child's clinician, the child will often be judged as more competent. Experienced clinicians will readily acknowledge this tendency to give their client "the benefit of the doubt," especially after a child has misarticulated several items in a row in a therapy session. Faced with the task of continuing to tell the child that a particular response was "wrong," the clinician will tend to credit an ambiguous response as "right." Interpersonal influence is particularly hard to guard against; perceptual decisions that affect others directly are hard to make reliably. In the clinic, the empathetic clinician must remain impartial.

Summary. Clients who are hard to test, who have many speech errors, or whose speech differs from the transcriber's are generally more difficult to score or transcribe reliably. The clinician must be aware of possible speaker characteristics, as well as interpersonal factors, that can bias perception and transcription reliability.

Task Factors

In addition to the client factors just reviewed, several characteristics of the speech task itself should be considered for possible influence on scoring or transcription.

Intelligibility. One important speech task factor is intelligibility. Do we transcribe differently when meaning can be ascribed to the string of sounds in an utterance, as opposed to when the sounds are "uninterpretable"? Oller and Eilers (1975), in a study of this question, found that knowledge of the intended lexical content of an utterance did alter transcription. Such findings, which have been replicated in several studies (clinical phonetics website, formerly Appendix D), present a disconcerting problem for clinical transcription. If the expectation of hearing a particular word yields a different transcription from that obtained when there is no such expectation, which transcription is more valid?

A phonetics "purist" might argue that the transcriber who is unaware of the intended sounds is more likely to produce valid transcription. In principle, it is hard to disagree with this view. In practice, however, such a view causes problems. Anyone who has had clinical experience with unintelligible children knows that transcription of speech, even when meaning is *known,* is difficult. When intended targets are unknown, transcription is almost impossible. As described in detail elsewhere (Shriberg, 1993; Shriberg & Kwiatkowski, 1980), we suggest that it is necessary for clinicians to gloss the child's intended targets (words) while obtaining conversational speech utterances from children with speech delays. Clinicians must attempt to determine, word-for-word, what the child intended to say at the time the sample is obtained. For an alternative perspective, however, see Ball (2008). In the following practice transcriptions, a gloss of the child's speech is always provided in the text.

Linguistic Context and Response Requirements. Two other important variables associated with the difficulty of the speech sample to be scored or transcribed are linguistic context and response complexity. These characteristics were introduced briefly in Chapter 1.

Linguistic context refers to the number and type of linguistic units (phonemes, syllables, words, and so forth) in which the target linguistic unit(s) is (are) embedded. Because of certain masking phenomena and memory constraints, it is easier to score or transcribe a sound when it occurs in a relatively simple context. For example, it is generally easier to transcribe a phoneme when it occurs in the context of a syllable, rather than a complete sentence. In the training program that follows, we begin with speech samples of relatively simple linguistic complexity.

Response complexity refers to the number of transcription responses per linguistic unit required of the clinician. Generally, it is easier to transcribe one target sound (or cluster) per unit (word, phrase, sentence, and so forth) than to transcribe two or more targets per unit. A case in point: Some clinical situations require that articulation errors for /r/ sounds only be transcribed; other situations require the clinician to keep track of both the /ɝ/ sounds and the /r/ phonemes. Experience in teaching transcription confirms that response requirements must be approached in steps—gradually increasing the number of responses the transcriber must make per linguistic unit.

These generalizations about hierarchies of linguistic context and response complexity can be overridden. For example, a child with a subtle /s/ distortion may be difficult to transcribe reliably when /s/ sounds are sampled in isolation. In contrast, it may be easy to transcribe reliably *both* /r/ and /s/ sounds in a continuous speech sample, provided the child has obvious substitutions for these sounds and speaks reasonably slowly. This is a case where client factors, as discussed earlier, affect the transcription task. The type of error a client makes may be more crucial than the linguistic context and response requirements of the task. Or, further, given two persons with comparable error types, each person's rate of speech or other speech/voice characteristics may substantially affect overall task difficulty.

Successive Judgments. In addition to intelligibility, linguistic context, and response requirements, a fourth speech task factor concerns the problem of maintaining independent judgment in a succession of perceptual decisions. If a sample contains ten successive target /s/ words and the first nine words are judged correct, the tenth word may have to be markedly "wrong" to be perceived as such. This situation is extremely common in clinical situations that emphasize high rates of target responses from clients. The clinician must make a series of rapid judgments. At some point in the series of judgments, the perceptual standard may become biased. Clinicians and speech aides who work daily with many children in such training programs should monitor their reliability. Routine intrajudge reliability checks, as defined and described on the clinical phonetics website, formerly Appendix D, will provide the needed data.

Summary. We have described four factors that influence task variables in transcription: (1) the need for transcribers to be aware of the intended target behaviors—that is, to have an accurate gloss of the child's utterance; the effects of (2) linguistic context and (3) response complexity on the ease and accuracy of transcription; and (4) the difficulty in keeping rapid successive judgments in a sample independent of one another. To determine if these factors are biasing scoring or transcription, clinicians should routinely obtain an estimate of their reliability, intrajudge and interjudge, as described in the clinical phonetics website, formerly Appendix D. Considering the central role of scoring or transcription in both assessment and management, periodic calibration of one's perceptual skills is necessary for "sound" clinical practice (pun intended).

Speech Sampling and Audio-Video Recording

In most clinical settings, a portable recorder is the constant companion of the speech-language clinician. Advancements in technology have made excellent recording equipment available and affordable. Portable videotape recorders are available to clinicians as well, but audio recorders are by far more prevalent.

In view of the widespread use of audio recorders, it is surprising that so few applied studies of recording variables have been undertaken. Two questions in the minds of many clinicians are: Is transcription from a recorded source as valid and reliable as transcription of live speech? And, is transcription from an audio source as valid and reliable as transcription from a video recording? Former Appendix D on the clinical phonetics website pursues the first question, including information from several studies and a comprehensive bibliography. Let us address the second question here. Video recording systems have two major advantages.

First, if certain basic prerequisites are met (adequate lighting, sharp focus, good close-ups) video recording allows us to preserve certain gestures associated with speech production. The necessity for observing such behavior, however, and the status of articulatory gestures for phonological analyses are perennial issues in the literature and depend on the purpose for scoring or transcription. Video recording allows you to see more articulatory behavior, but not all articulatory behavior is linguistically significant. A general argument can be made that phonetic transcription should be based on what you *hear,* not on what you *see.* Later we will offer specific suggestions for how to best use visual information obtained live or from a video recording for certain transcription needs.

A second advantage to video recording is the visibility of the context in which the utterances occur. Utterances that otherwise might not be intelligible on audio media may become so when accompanied by information on eye gaze, gestures, or manipulation of objects. For certain research purposes, such information is vital (e.g., when studying children with affective disorders such as autism). As discussed previously, however, we feel that interpretations should be validated immediately following each client utterance and recorded as the gloss spoken by the clinician. Accomplished in this way, audio recordings can be equally valid and certainly more efficient sources for clinical scoring or transcription than video, for certain research needs. Of course, for other clinical research purposes (e.g., observing lip movements in persons with motor speech disorders), video recordings may be the method of choice.

To summarize our observations on recording factors, advances in electronics have brought us from the era of disc recorders to wire recorders to the present-day technology of digital recorders (Shriberg et al., 2005). The small amount of data on the accuracy of transcribing live versus from audio or video sources has been equivocal. In the absence of data on audio–video recording effects on the validity of transcription, we can only point out some advantages and disadvantages of each type of recording system. In the following section, we suggest procedures that can minimize the main sources of unreliability introduced by the use of audio recordings. A good recorder is a clinician's trusted companion. Speech-language pathologists are well advised to become completely familiar with procedures that will yield high-quality recordings of the speech of their clients. Former Appendix E on the clinical phonetics website provides technical information and specific procedural guidelines.

Preparation for Clinical Transcription

We have just discussed factors that influence the scoring and transcription process. In this section, the step-by-step preparation for scoring or transcription will be inspected in detail. Preparation involves attention to five needs: (1) selecting a system, (2) selecting a set of symbols, (3) selecting a recording form, (4) determining response definitions, and (5) determining conventions (procedural rules).

Selecting a System

As described in Chapter 1, contemporary speech-language pathologists use three systems of clinical phonetics. We have labeled these systems *two-way scoring, five-way scoring,* and *phonetic transcription* (see Chapter 1, Figure 1.1). Two-way scoring organizes perceptual input into just two output categories—"right" and "wrong." Five-way scoring provides four categories of "wrong," including *deletion* (or *omission*), *distortion* (or *approximation*), *substitution,* and *addition* of another sound. Finally, phonetic transcription uses a large set of symbols to describe both normal and disordered speech.

Unfortunately, there have not been any published studies comparing the three systems of clinical phonetics. It would be interesting to know whether a decision is affected by the procedural system used to make it. For example, are listeners more likely to score a target sound as "wrong" when using a two-way system than when using a five-way system? Our experience in teaching the three systems has given us some insight into this question. A brief historical digression is needed to explain.

Over four decades ago (!), when we first attempted to program the learning of clinical phonetics (Shriberg & Swisher, 1972), we assumed that two-way scoring was the easiest of the three systems to learn. Thus, two-way scoring became the first step in our early teaching programs, using common error sounds in increasingly complex linguistic contexts, from sounds in isolation to sounds in words, phrases, and so forth. The results were less than successful. Frankly, our students complained a lot. They told us they liked the idea of programmed teaching, but they disagreed with many of the "right–wrong" decisions on the answer keys. Importantly, they also found it hard to tell us *why* they disagreed with an item. As we began to determine which items in the key the disagreements occurred on, we found ourselves using terms and concepts from phonetic transcription, such as allophone, diacritic marking, and so forth. It finally dawned on us that perhaps we should teach phonetic transcription *first.* Although phonetic transcription of speech errors was more difficult to learn, it provided a firm basis for the other two scoring systems. Using this arrangement in subsequent revisions of our program produced improved results. Although mutterings about the validity of our answer keys will never be entirely extinguished, at least disagreements can now be discussed in a more focused and productive manner.

In the training samples to follow, therefore, you will be taught phonetic transcription of children's speech errors from the start. This will seem difficult to begin with, particularly because we begin with vowels. Ultimately, however, it will prove efficient for the reasons just mentioned. Once you are able to identify feature errors such as lateralization, velarization, and so forth, you easily can sort these perceptions into two-way and five-way scoring decisions, which are used later in the program.

In summary, working clinicians should always be able to *choose* among systems to meet their clinical needs. Unfortunately, clinicians who do not use skills learned early in their training will not have this choice. We hope the audio samples and textual materials in this series will provide clinicians with some alternatives. Retrieving one's clinical skills in phonetic transcription may not be as easy as pedaling away on a bicycle after a long absence from biking. But we have seen many experienced clinicians "reacquire" transcription competence with a little effort. In the many years since the first edition of this text, narrow transcription skills have become a requirement for the contemporary clinician working with a variety of child and adult speech sound disorders.

Selecting a Set of Symbols

Once a system has been selected, the next order of business is to select a set of symbols to be used within that system. Table 7.1 is a list of the types of symbols that have been used in two-way and five-way scoring. Symbols for phonetic transcription were presented earlier in this text. Symbols for use of phonetic transcription are fixed; the symbols should be written exactly in the form presented by the International Phonetic Association and in diacritic systems such as the one used in this book. For two-way or five-way scoring, however, the clinician must select a set of symbols and use them consistently. Choosing a set of symbols should involve considerations of clarity, speed, and visibility to the client.

Clarity. Clarity refers to the amount of degradation a symbol can undergo and still retain its identity. For example, use of "+" for correct and "x" for incorrect could be troublesome for clinicians whose penmanship is not always clear, particularly under the press of rapid scoring. The two symbols might easily be confused later. A better decision would be to use "+" versus "0," or any two symbols sufficiently distinct to withstand a certain amount of degradation in the clinical setting.

Speed. Speed is another major consideration, one which requires the use of a symbol drawn with a brief, continuous stroke. For example, "c" is faster than writing out "correct" or "cor." or "OK" and so forth. People who habitually print find certain symbols easier to make than others. You should experiment with making 20 small "x's" rapidly versus 20 of some other symbol for "wrong." Which symbol permits the fastest scoring? You may wish to use the same symbol in all your work, provided it meets other criteria discussed in this section.

Visibility to Client. Visibility to the client refers to the ease with which a client can discern the symbols used for "correct" and "incorrect" responses. Children and motivated adults (who often view therapy as "back to school") will learn to watch the clinician's pencil to monitor the judgments being made about their responses. Such feedback during a therapy session can be counterproductive and, in a test situation, can invalidate test results. Therefore, the test administrator should avoid letting the client make inferences about the "correctness" of his or her responses by using a set of symbols involving similar hand movements, such as check (✔) and check-tail (✔̶) Here, the short tail added to the check to make the "incorrect" symbol is visually less obvious than the difference between a "+" and a "O," for example. If it is important to conceal your scoring of responses from the client, be sure to choose symbols that are made with ambiguous movements. Sometimes, however, the choice of symbols is dictated by the type of recording form used, which is discussed next.

Selecting a Recording Form

The purpose for which a sample is being transcribed will often suggest the type of recording form required. Published forms for scoring formal articulation tests are familiar to practicing clinicians. Figures 7.2, 7.3, and 7.4 are response forms from published articulation tests dating back several decades. Some of the test manuals for these and other recent articulation tests suggest how to use scoring symbols. Articulation test forms warrant two comments.

TABLE 7.1
Some Symbols Commonly Used in Two-Way and Five-Way Scoring of Speech Sound Changes

Correct	Incorrect	Substitution	Deletion	Distortion	Addition
Cor.	Incor.	Subst.	Del.	Dist.	Add.
C	I	X/Y[a]	Om. (omission)	D	^{X}Y[a]
✔	✔̶	X/	—	Lat. (lateralization)	Y^{X}
+	X		Ø	Dent. (dentalization)	
OK	—			Etc.	
G (good)	NG (not good)				
R (right)	W (wrong)				
A (acceptable)	NA (not acceptable)				

[a]These letters represent the target sound (Y) and the replacement or new sound (X).

9–62392

THE FISHER-LOGEMANN TEST OF ARTICULATION COMPETENCE

Screening ☐ Complete ☐

Record Form for the Picture Test

Name________ Date________ Examiner________

Age____ Grade (or Occupation)____ School (or Employer)________

Birthdate____ Home Address________

Native Dialect____ Foreign Language in home________

CONSONANT PHONEMES

						Manner of Formation																	
Card #	IPA Phoneme	Common Spelling	Dev. Age	Place of Articulation	Voicing	Stop			Fricative			Affricate			Glide			Lateral			Nasal		
						Pre.	Inter.	Post.	Pre.	Inter.	Post.	Pre.	Inter.	Post.	Pre.	Inter.	Post.	Pre.	Inter.	Post.	Pre.	Inter.	Post.
1 2 3 4 5	p b ʍ w m	p b wh w m	3 5 3 3	Bilabial	V̶	/p	/p	/p	/ʍ[1]														
					V	/b	/b	/b							/w	/w					/m	/m	/m
6 7	f v	f v	4 7	Labio-dental	V̶				/f	/f	/f												
					V				/v	/v	/v												
8 9	θ ð	th th	7 8	Tip-dental	V̶				/θ	/θ	/θ												
					V				/ð	/ð	/ð												
10 11 12 13	t d l n	t d l n	6 5 6 3	Tip-alveolar	V̶	/t	/t[2]	/t															
					V	/d	/d	/d										/l	/l	/l	/n	/n	/n
14 15	s z	s z	7 7	Blade-alveolar	V̶				/s	/s̲	/s												
					V				/z	/z	/z												
16 17 18 19	ʃ ʒ tʃ dʒ	sh zh ch j	6 7 6 7	Blade-prepalatal	V̶				/ʃ	/ʃ	/ʃ	/tʃ	/tʃ	/tʃ									
					V					/ʒ	/ʒ[3]	/dʒ	/dʒ	/dʒ									
20	j	y	5	Front-palatal	V̶																		
					V										/j	/j							
21	r	r	6	Central-palatal	V̶																		
					V										/r	/r	/r[4]						
22 23 24	k g ŋ	k g ng	4 4 5	Back-velar	V̶	/k	/k	/k															
					V	/g	/g	/g														/ŋ	/ŋ
25	h	h	3	Glottal	V̶				/h	/h													

Place of Articulation

SUMMARY OF MISARTICULATION PATTERNS:

MANNER OF FORMATION ERRORS:

PLACE OF ARTICULATION ERRORS:

VOICING ERRORS:

Notes: (These and additional notes are discussed in the Manual under "Dialectal Variations")
1. Either /ʍ/ or /w/
2. Either /t/ or /d/
3. Either /ʒ/ or /dʒ/.
4. Either /r/ or /ə/ or lengthening of the preceding vowel.

FIGURE 7.2
The Fisher-Logemann Test of Articulation Competence: Record Form for the Picture Test. H. Fisher and J. Logemann, The Fisher-Logemann Test of Articulation Competence. Record Form. Iowa City, IA: The Riverside Publishing Company, 1971. Reproduced with permission of The Riverside Publishing Company.

CONSONANT BLENDS

CARD & ITEM #	/s/ + CONSONANT	CARD & ITEM #	CONSONANT + /r/	CARD & ITEM #	CONSONANT + /l/
26–1	______/s spoon	28–1	______/r present	30–1	______/l sled
26–2	______/s star	28–2	______/r bread	30–2	______/l blue
26–3	______/s slide	28–3	______/r fruit	30–3	______/l plane
		28–4	______/r frying pan		
26–4	______/s snake	28–5	______/r three	30–4	______/l flag
27–1	______/s skate	29–1	______/r tree	31–1	______/l clown
27–2	______/s swing	29–2	______/r dress	31–2	______/l glass.
27–3	______/s smoke	29–3	______/r cry	31–3	______/l bottle
		29–4	______/r green		
Best Context: ______		Best Context: ______		Best Context: ______	
Worst Context: ______		Worst Context: ______		Worst Context: ______	

VOWEL PHONEMES

	FRONT	CENTRAL	BACK
HIGH	32–1. ______/i key 32–2. ______/ɪ mitten		34–4. ______/u two 34–3. ______/ʊ foot
MID	32–3. ______/e table 32–4. ______/ɛ bell	33–4. ______/ɝ shirt 33–3. ______/ə cup	34–2. ______/o phone
LOW	33–1. ______/æ hat		34–1. ______/ɔ ball 33–2. ______/ɑ sock

PHONEMIC DIPHTHONGS: 35–1. ______/aɪ eye 35–3. ______/ɔɪ boy

35–2. ______/aʊ house 35–4. ______/ju U

ANALYSIS OF VOWEL MISARTICULATIONS:

FIGURE 7.2
(continued)

PAT RECORDING SHEET

Name______________________ Date (Year ___ Month ___ Day ___)

School______________________ Birth ___ ___ ___

Grade__________ Age ___ ___ ___

Key: Omission (–); substitution (write phonetic symbol of sound substituted); severity of distortion (D1), (D2), (D3); ability to imitate (circle symbol or error).

Sound	Photograph	1	2	3	Vowels, Diph.		Comments
	I				III		
s	saw, pencil, house				aʊ house		
s bl	spoon, skates, stars						
z	zipper, scissors, keys						
ʃ	shoe, station, fish				u shoe		
tʃ	chair, matches, sandwich						
dʒ	jars, angels, orange						
t	table, potatoes, hat				æ hat		
d	dog, ladder, bed				ɔ dog		
n	nails, bananas, can				ə bananas		
l	lamp, balloons, bell				ɛ bell		
l bl	blocks, clock, flag				ɑ blocks		
θ	thumb, toothbrush, teeth				i teeth		
r	radio, carrots, car						
r bl	brush, crayons, train				e train		
k	cat, crackers, cake				ɚ-ə crackers		
g	gun, wagon, egg				ʌ gun		
	II						
f	fork, elephant, knife						
v	vacuum, TV, stove				ju vacuum		
p	pipe, apples, cup				aɪ pipe		
b	book, baby, bathtub				ʊ book		
m	monkey, hammer, comb				o comb		
w-hw	witch, flowers, whistle				ɪ witch		
	I						
ð	this, that, feathers, bathe						
h-ŋ	hanger, hanger, swing						
j	yes, thank you						
ʒ	measure, beige				ɔɪ boy		
	(story)				ɜ-ɜ bird		

SCORE

Sounds

I Tongue__________

II Lip __________

III Vowels__________

Total __________

FIGURE 7.3
PAT (Photo Articulation Test) Recording Sheet. Kathleen Pendergast et al., Photo Articulation Test. PAT Recording Sheet. Danville, IL: The Interstate Printers & Publishers, Inc., 1969. Reproduced with permission of the publisher.

CONNECTED SPEECH AND LANGUAGE

(Elicit story and conversation by using items 70 through 72. Note language, intelligibility, voice, fluency.)

ADDITIONAL DIAGNOSTIC INFORMATION

(Hearing loss, motor coordination, perceptual deficiencies, emotional factors, attitude toward disorder and treatment.)

THERAPY GOALS AND PROGRESS

Additional copies of this sheet available in pads of 96 each from
The Interstate Printers & Publishers, Inc., Danville, Illinois 61832
Reorder No. 1065

FIGURE 7.3
(*continued*)

INDIVIDUAL RECORD SHEET for A SCREENING DEEP TEST OF ARTICULATION

by Eugene T. McDonald

Name______ Birthdate______ School______ Grade______ Tester______ Date______

			[s]	[l]	[r]	[tʃ]	[θ]	[ʃ]	[k]	[f]	[t]
1 bus	fish	bʌ[s][f]ɪ[ʃ]	[ ]					[ ]		[ ]	
2 ball	chain	bɔ[l][tʃ]en		[ ]		[ ]					
3 watch	lock	wɔ[tʃ][l]ɑ[k]		[ ]		[ ]			[ ]		
4 house	flag	haʊ[s][f][l]æg	[ ]	[ ]						[ ]	
5 ring	witch	[r]iŋwɪ[tʃ]			[ ]	[ ]					
6 chair	sun	[tʃ]ɛ[r][s]ʌn	[ ]		[ ]	[ ]					
7 book	shoe	bʊ[k][ʃ]u						[ ]	[ ]		
8 cat	leaf	[k]æ[t][l]i[f]		[ ]					[ ]	[ ]	[ ]
9 star	thumb	[s][t]ɑ[r][θ]ʌm	[ ]		[ ]		[ ]				[ ]
10 horse	key	hɔ[r][s][k]i	[ ]		[ ]				[ ]		
11 cat	sheep	[k]æ[t][ʃ]ip						[ ]	[ ]		[ ]
12 ear	bell	ɪ[r]bɛ[l]		[ ]	[ ]						
13 tree	thumb	[t][r]i[θ]ʌm			[ ]		[ ]				[ ]
14 teeth	lock	[t]i[θ][l]ɑ[k]		[ ]			[ ]		[ ]		[ ]
15 tooth	brush	[t]u[θ]b[r]ʌ[ʃ]			[ ]		[ ]	[ ]			[ ]
16 knife	spoon	naɪ[f][s]pun	[ ]							[ ]	
17 leaf	chair	[l]i[f][tʃ]ɛ[r]		[ ]	[ ]	[ ]				[ ]	
18 glove	thumb	g[l]ʌv[θ]ʌm		[ ]			[ ]				
19 brush	five	b[r]ʌ[ʃ][f]aɪv			[ ]			[ ]		[ ]	
20 lock	fish	[l]ɑ[k][f]ɪ[ʃ]		[ ]				[ ]	[ ]	[ ]	
21 mouth	tie	maʊ[θ][t]aɪ					[ ]				[ ]
22 watch	fork	wɔ[tʃ][f]ɔ[r][k]			[ ]	[ ]			[ ]	[ ]	
23 fish	tooth	[f]ɪ[ʃ][t]u[θ]					[ ]	[ ]		[ ]	[ ]
24 sled	sheep	[s][l]ɛd[ʃ]ip	[ ]	[ ]				[ ]			
25 match	kite	mæ[tʃ][k]aɪ[t]				[ ]			[ ]		[ ]
26 sheep	chain	[ʃ]ip[tʃ]en				[ ]		[ ]			
27 fish	house	[f]ɪ[ʃ]haʊ[s]	[ ]					[ ]		[ ]	
28 thumb	saw	[θ]ʌm[s]ɔ	[ ]				[ ]				
29 saw	teeth	[s]ɔ[t]i[θ]	[ ]				[ ]				[ ]
30 witch	key	wɪ[tʃ][k]i				[ ]			[ ]		
31 mouth	match	maʊ[θ]mæ[tʃ]				[ ]	[ ]				

Summary of pertinent findings:

Recommendations:

No. contexts correct	[s]	[l]	[r]	[tʃ]	[θ]	[ʃ]	[k]	[f]	[t]
10	•	•	•	•	•	•	•	•	•
9	•	•	•	•	•	•	•	•	•
8	•	•	•	•	•	•	•	•	•
7	•	•	•	•	•	•	•	•	•
6	•	•	•	•	•	•	•	•	•
5	•	•	•	•	•	•	•	•	•
4	•	•	•	•	•	•	•	•	•
3	•	•	•	•	•	•	•	•	•
2	•	•	•	•	•	•	•	•	•
1	•	•	•	•	•	•	•	•	•
0	•	•	•	•	•	•	•	•	•

PHONETIC PROFILE

FIGURE 7.4
Individual Record Sheet for A Screening Deep Test of Articulation. Eugene McDonald, A Screening Deep Test of Articulation. Individual Record Sheet. Pittsburgh, PA: Stanwix House, Inc., 1968. Reproduced with permission of the publisher.

First, the space allotted to record a response is quite small on some forms, such as on the form for the McDonald Screening Deep Test of Articulation (Figure 7.4). When one is forced to write rapidly in such a small space, it is particularly important to use an easily distinguishable symbol system and to write legibly.

A second observation about articulation test forms is that they generally require particular care in five-way scoring of clusters. If the transcriber writes "D" or "distortion" in the box provided for a target cluster, the reader cannot discern which consonants in the cluster were distorted. The distortion could have occurred on one or more members of the cluster. A better practice is to transcribe the entire cluster, using "D" for any distorted segments within the cluster; for example [Dpl], [Dtr], [ntD], and so forth. This may look confusing but it actually gives the reader a clearer picture of what was spoken—whether one or more segments in the cluster were distorted and which ones were distorted.

In addition to forms for commercially available articulation tests, a variety of forms can be helpful for particular scoring or transcription needs. Figure 7.5, for example, is a simple form we have used for two-way scoring of a target sound in continuous speech. Figure 7.6 is a form we use for phonetic transcription of continuous speech. This information is subsequently entered into a computer program for phonetic and phonological analysis (Shriberg, Allen, McSweeny, & Wilson, 2001 Shriberg, Fourakis, et al., 2010a, 2010b). The selection of the proper recording form, as with other decisions that the clinician must make, is an important determinant of the efficiency and effectiveness of any clinical phonetics task.

Determining Response Definitions

Explicit response definitions are needed when using two-way or five-way scoring systems. A good response definition describes the attributes of each response in relation to the target behavior that make it correct, a distortion, a socially acceptable /s/, and so forth. The response definition should allow a clinician to make judgments rapidly and reliably. Good response definitions orient the listener to the crucial aspects of the stimuli requiring attention. Here are some actual response definitions taken from two-way scoring in the clinical literature; note the variety of approaches:

> *To be scored correct the test phoneme had to look and sound correct.* (Paynter, Ermey, Green, & Draper, 1978)
>
> *A correct response was defined as a sound production that conformed to Standard General American Speech.* (DuBois & Bernthal, 1978)
>
> *Subjects were reinforced with tokens when responses were considered "socially" acceptable (that is, neither drawing attention to the speaker nor interfering with communication).* (Irwin, Weston, Griffith, & Rocconi, 1976)
>
> *The teeth must be closed. You must not be concerned with the sound of [s] at this point, just the visual features of the mouth, teeth, and tongue.* (Mowrer, Baker, & Schutz, 1970)

In these response definitions, listeners are told to attend to visual, acoustic, or articulatory behaviors or combinations of these. By using a common response definition, listeners should be processing the stimuli in similar ways. Also, each will judge the stimuli in the same way on two separate occasions. The choice of response definitions, as seen in these examples, is arbitrary. Variations in response definitions arise from differences in theoretical positions, differences in goals, differences in the stage of clinical management, and so forth (Bow, Blarney, Paatsch, & Sarant, 2002).

One component that is missing in the response definitions just listed is a decision logic for dealing with questionable responses, that is, for responses that fall "between the cracks." A good response definition provides a rule for categorizing such behaviors. For some purposes, we might decide to generate a rule that discards questionable stimuli. Alternatively, a rule could assign questionable responses to one or another of the available categories. For example, in a two-way scoring task, the following three response definitions are possible (Figure 7.7):

1. Solution *(a)* is the conservative approach. Responses that seem to be in the "gray area" (shown here in blue) are simply discarded from subsequent analyses. Such a response definition could be used to purify data—only unambiguously judged responses will be preserved for some analysis procedure.

2. Solution *(b)* says to score responses correct unless they are heard as incorrect, just as one is "innocent until proven guilty" in jurisprudence. This criterion assumes that the population sampled has a higher probability of being innocent ("correct") *and* that *negative* judgments should not be made unless one is fairly certain of the data on which they are based. When screening a group of college students for errors in speech, for example, we might assign all questionable /s/ responses to "correct" because this is a normally speaking sample.

3. Solution *(c)* assumes the opposite position. Such a response definition might be used for the ultimate benefit of those already enrolled in a speech management program. Here, the approach is to assume that if a person's actual probability of correct responses is lower than 50 percent, questionable responses should be assigned to "incorrect." This criterion, "guilty until proven innocent," might be used constructively in a final phase of management or maintenance when a client benefits from feedback about marginally acceptable production while trying to maintain top performance.

NAME: ______________________ DATE: ______________________

SCHOOL/GRADE: ______________________ TARGET SOUND: ______________________

______________________ EXAMINER/CLINICIAN: ______________________

DESCRIPTION OF SAMPLE: ______________________

	1	2	3	4	5	6	7	8	9	10	11	12	13	14	15	16	17	18	19	20
Correct																				
Incorrect																				
	21	22	23	24	25	26	27	28	29	30	31	32	33	34	35	36	37	38	39	40
Correct																				
Incorrect																				
	41	42	43	44	45	46	47	48	49	50	51	52	53	54	55	56	57	58	59	60
Correct																				
Incorrect																				
	61	62	63	64	65	66	67	68	69	70	71	72	73	74	75	76	77	78	79	80
Correct																				
Incorrect																				
	81	82	83	84	85	86	87	88	89	90	91	92	93	94	95	96	97	98	99	100
Correct																				
Incorrect																				

No. Correct ______________________

No. Incorrect ______________________

Percentage Correct ______________________

FIGURE 7.5
A simple form for two-way scoring of a target sound in continuous speech.

PEPFORM: Cover Page | **Study** ______ **Peplog No.** ______ **Page** ______

Pepfile Name ______ Sampling Dates ______

Subject ______ Sampling Examiner ______

Age ______ Transcription Date ______

D.O.B. ______ Transcriber ______

Notes ______

Utterance No.	Counter No.	Line	Transcription and Comments
		X	
		Y	
		Z	
		X	
		Y	
		Z	
		X	
		Y	
		Z	
		X	
		Y	
		Z	
		X	
		Y	
		Z	
		X	
		Y	
		Z	

FIGURE 7.6

PEPPER (Programs to Examine Phonetic and Phonological Evaluation Records) Transcription Form—a form for phonetic transcription of continuous conversational speech. The orthographic form of a speaker's intended utterance is entered in the X line, the corresponding intended phonetic forms are entered in the Y line, and the realized phonetic forms are entered in the Z line. (Shriberg et al., 2001)

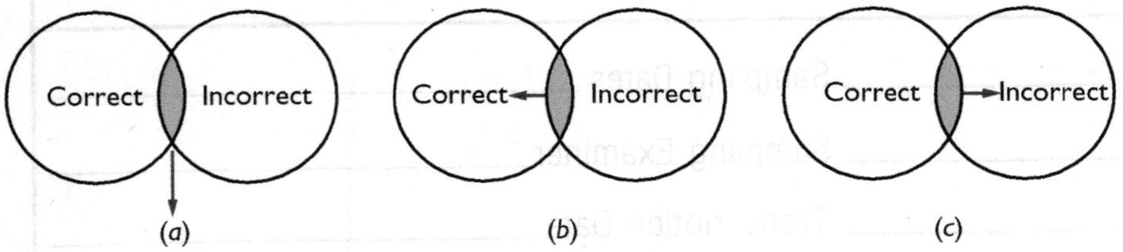

FIGURE 7.7
Three response definitions in a two-way scoring task.

The clinician must clearly formulate response definitions; in turn, response definitions will help the clinician accomplish the job. They should be explicit. They should tell the clinician precisely how to go about making judgments, including a decision rule for handling difficult judgments.

Determining Transcription Conventions

The final need in preparation for clinical transcription—after having selected a system, a set of symbols, a recording form, and response definitions—is to determine some conventions for transcription. Conventions are procedures that participants agree to abide by. Several types of conventions or "rules" are important to establish at the outset of any transcription endeavor.

Which Phonetic Behaviors Are to Be Transcribed and Which Can Be Ignored? A basic decision that will require a convention is whether the clinician must attend to every bit of the speaker's phonetic behavior. Should every normally occurring allophone, such as the aspiration of initial voiceless stops or assimilative nasality on vowels, be transcribed? Do we want to take the time to transcribe behaviors that are predictable in normal speech? The answer to this question hinges on the purposes of transcription. For the linguist, whose task might be to determine the sound system of an unknown language, it may be necessary to capture such detail. For a particular clinical task, however, such detail may not be of interest. The point is that whether a particular phonetic behavior is to be transcribed or ignored is an arbitrary or situationally determined matter. Confusion will result unless a convention for such decisions is explicit and made available to all parties involved. For example, here is a partial list of the conventions used with clinicians who transcribed continuous speech samples for one clinical research project:

1. Transcribe aspiration/nonaspiration only when it differs from the anticipated allophone.
2. Transcribe hypernasality only when it differs from the anticipated allophone.
3. Transcribe vowel duration only when it differs from the anticipated allophone.
4. Be most precise in your transcription for words that have primary stress; words having secondary stress or that are unstressed will be treated separately in the phonological analysis.
5. If you are undecided between two or more transcriptions of a consonant or consonant cluster, write your best estimate on the line and the alternative(s) above.

How Much of the Data Is to Be Transcribed Live Versus Transcribed Later from Audio or Video Recordings? It is very important to establish a convention for what will be scored or transcribed live as opposed to later from a recording. Stephens and Daniloff's (1974) position on this issue is that scoring of /s/ errors should be made live. As noted earlier in this chapter, these researchers found that live scoring of sibilants compared to audiotape scoring yielded different scores. Shriberg (1972) found that two-way judgments of /s/ errors were only 65 percent reliable from audiotape. Do these unhappy data on audio judgments indicate that we should throw away our recorders? Obviously not. The subject still requires a considerable amount of study. To date, the data are much too limited in scope and methodology to conclude that we should abandon use of the recorder. Furthermore, comparative linguistics has produced much valuable work based on recordings of languages made in the field. A more useful response is to ask what sorts of information are better to transcribe live when it is possible to do so.

One type of information the transcriber should attend to during the live recording session is the visual components of speech. Specifically, the transcriber should pay attention to *lip postures* and *lip closures.* Consider the word *cup* on an audio recording. If the final /p/ of *cup* is unreleased, there will not be an audible burst. If the examiner is audio recording, attention could be paid to transcribing lip closure live, which will resolve later questions about whether the child actually produced a final consonant /p/. Similarly, if /r/ is accompanied by lip rounding, such gestures are easier to observe live than to infer from listening to an audio recording.

If video recordings are made, live transcription might focus more on the acoustic characteristics of fricatives and affricates. The assumption is that the video signal will provide a faithful copy of visual information, while the audio signal on a videotape (but not on video disk) is less faithful in reproducing fricative sounds than the audio signal from a good audio recorder (Bunta, Ingram, & Ingram, 2003; Shriberg et al., 2005).

Summary

Much of the mystique about clinical phonetics is related simply to a lack of understanding about its basic clerical nature. We should not assume that every clinician recalls the symbols learned in the obligatory phonetics course taken in undergraduate programs. Clinicians may be baffled by reports from colleagues simply because they have forgotten how to interpret phonetic symbols rather than due to any other factor. Attention to each of the five preparation tasks described here—selecting a system, a set of symbols, and a response form and determining response definitions and transcription conventions—will provide the necessary base for the efficient use of clinical phonetics.

The Process of Scoring or Transcription

If you have "done your homework"—attended to all the preparatory needs just discussed—the process of scoring or transcription should go smoothly. It is the process itself that we now finally consider.

What takes place in the clinician's mind while doing clinical phonetics? It is tempting to try to model the process of scoring or transcription. Research in speech discrimination, decision theory, information processing, and related areas would provide relevant paradigms. As attractive as such model building would be, we will limit ourselves to a sketch of processes we have observed or readily can infer. Much of what we have learned about transcription comes from simply asking students what went on as they attempted to transcribe and from diaries students have kept while doing transcription tasks.

For ease of communication, we now slip into a "how to" manual style of discourse. Suggestions are made to you, the reader, now as a transcriber. We will assume that scoring or transcription is being accomplished from an audio recording except where otherwise indicated. Moreover, based on findings reported in Shriberg et al. (2005), transcriptions from CDs may differ in some ways from transcriptions that were done from audiotapes. Therefore, all our guidelines to follow (and elsewhere in this text) assume that you are transcribing from portable digital audio recorders. Specifically, you may experience some important validity, reliability, and/or efficiency differences transcribing CDs from your computer or portable device, compared to transcription from older audiotape devices.

Setting Up

Get Comfortable. Try to find an accommodating place for transcription. The lighting should be good, and the amount of distracting noise and potential visual distractions should be minimized. Be sure that you are comfortable and well oriented toward the playback device. Remote stop-start attachments are especially convenient, but most audiotape recorders require a mechanical, push-button arrangement on the machine itself. Unfortunately, when a recorder is lying flat on a table, you will be poorly oriented toward the loudspeaker. Try to set the recorder on an angle that allows you to manipulate the stop–rewind–start buttons while placing you squarely in front of the speaker. Surprisingly, it is little things like the angle of your wrist and fingers to the equipment that, over the course of a transcription session, begin to take their toll on the efficiency and general satisfaction with clinical transcription. Again, these same guidelines are relevant for playback functions using computer software, a keyboard, and a mouse.

Should I Use Headphones? The choice between using a set of headphones or listening to a recorder or speakers free-field involves several issues. Students we know who have used both generally prefer free-field listening to the use of headphones—especially if a lengthy session of listening is expected. For limited periods of scoring or transcription, headphones do have several advantages. A high-quality set of headphones will deliver excellent sound. By their very feel, headphones create a listening "set" for the student. Moreover, headphones block out competing noise. Especially when your listening place is shared with other students, roommates, and so forth, the headphones have the psychological effect of acting as a barrier to small talk and interruptions. On the negative side, however, headphone use becomes tedious after a certain amount of time, which varies from person to person. If you do use headphones, be sure that they are placed on your head comfortably and that they are in good repair. You will need to take more frequent breaks, but you may find that headphones enhance your overall efficiency.

Previewing the Recording

Undoubtedly, there are some situations where your very first impression of behavior is the most valid. Usually, however, preliminary play of the recording to be transcribed is desirable. Here are some comments from two student clinicians who transcribed speech samples from their clients:

> *It helped to listen to the whole tape once to get set.*
>
> *My approach was to listen to most of the tape without writing to get an idea of what to listen to.*

Note that these students' comments reflect some of the preparation tasks considered earlier. The preplay allows the transcriber to determine some conventions to be followed for the transcription; that is, what types of behaviors are to be transcribed and in what way. A preplay of the recording accomplishes other things: (1) It allows you to set the most appropriate playback level on the audio control and to desensitize yourself to sudden, unexpected intensity changes that invariably occur on speech samples from young children;

(2) it allows you to adjust the audio for background noise, such as hiss, to avoid confusing noise with fricative distortions; (3) it allows you to desensitize yourself to any biasing variables, such as voice characteristics of the client; (4) it allows you to adjust to the speech tempo of the client, to determine how much behavior you will be able to score or transcribe at a stretch.

There is one situation in which a preview is absolutely necessary. For unintelligible children or adults, it may be necessary to gloss the sample before a transcription can be made. As described earlier, a gloss is a word-by-word transcription of each word intended by the speaker, including fast speech forms and ungrammatical words. As you may imagine, glossing takes a good deal of time, and clinicians take such trouble only when a phonological analysis of continuous speech is required.

In summary, a preview lets you prepare for the task at hand—to determine what sorts of symbols will be needed and to predict how frequently certain types of behaviors will be occurring on the tape. Too often, if you begin "cold"—without a preview—some or all of the transcription will have to be redone. Guidelines for transcribing persons with dialects (Chapter 10) provide especially relevant rationale for previewing the sample.

A preplay may take away some of the drama of simply turning on the playback device and beginning transcription; but, in the long run, the extra time spent in previewing a sample will pay off.

First Presentation of the Target Behavior

After making all the preliminary arrangements covered to this point, you now are ready to score or transcribe. As we have reconstructed it, after you hear the first stimulus to be scored or transcribed, one of two things can happen: Either you score or transcribe it, or you will need to replay it. Let us look at each of these possibilities.

Immediate Recognition. The first possibility is that you may hear the target stimulus, for example, a w/r, an aspirated /k/, a correct /s/, and you instantly "compute." That is, you recognize immediately the scoring or transcription category that you should use to capture this response. Although you may have to pause to be sure you are using the right symbolization, you have made up your mind: It *is* a w/r, it *is* an aspirated /k/, it *is* a correct /s/. No mediation is necessary—at least you are not aware of any mediating processes. With practice, it is this type of instant processing that you will do more and more as you develop competence and confidence in discriminating the types of behaviors trained in this series. It is very similar to sight-reading music. Such symbolic conversions become so rapid that at some point you are not aware of any conscious effort to discriminate the correct symbols. It has become automatic.

Incomplete Recognition. A second possibility is that you will only partially discriminate a response category. Was the behavior a phonemic substitution, or was it a distortion of some sort? The information that we have put together indicates that, invariably, the strategy at this point is to *attempt a simulation of the behavior.* Producing the sound yourself, if you can articulate silently or even out loud a sound that matches the one heard, seems to aid in scoring or transcribing the target sound. The importance to clinical phonetics of being able to imitate deviant speech cannot be overstated. Here are some comments from student diaries:

> *I don't hear symbols. It's still a struggle for me to match my perceptual impressions against graphic representation, especially when I can't imitate it.*
>
> *The stimulus seemed so fleeting that I could not seem to get an accurate auditory image of it. If I was able to produce the child's production myself (what I thought was an accurate production), I was much more able to transcribe it.*
>
> *The better I could imitate, the easier it was to discriminate.*

These comments, particularly the first one, are telling. Clinicians need to learn to make the different types of speech sound errors made by their clients. Distortion-type errors, of course, are the most difficult. This strategy is not foolproof. But as long as a memory for the recorded sound (or live sound) lasts, you should attempt to match your production to that memory. The ability to imitate a child's speech error precisely is also an important skill in management programs when the clinician needs to demonstrate to the child exactly what the child is producing in place of the correct sound.

Second and Subsequent Presentations (Replays)

Replays may be necessary either to confirm the judgment made on the first trial or because a decision was not made as just described. Listeners seem compelled to use replays more often in phonetic transcription than when scoring by two-way or five-way systems. There seems to be an interaction between the level of intelligibility of the speaker, the complexity of the system, and the consequences of making hasty decisions. Ideally, of course, a listener should be equally careful about the discrimination task in all clinical phonetics situations.

One thing we have learned is that the tendency to call for a replay has to be guarded against. One student put it succinctly: "I allowed myself up to *10* repetitions for certain words—this was frustrating!!!" Our experience suggests that the following strategy for replays is best:

1. Play the word or larger sample two or three times without scoring or transcribing.

2. Score or transcribe.
3. Replay only if necessary.

What we are suggesting is that the target response may have to be repeated once or twice to encode it solidly in memory. However, unless it is lengthy, it should be repeated *only* once or twice.

We also suggest that a limitation be placed on the latency of your response, that is, the amount of time between listening and scoring or transcription. If a scoring or transcription response is not made within a given number of seconds, replay the item. If the target behaviors are such that auditory memory does decay with some regularity, such as in a 20-word listening task for /s/, setting an outside limit is useful. It is useful to say, for example, that you will allow no longer than three seconds for a decision or else replay the item. As one student wrote: "After two or three seconds, I just couldn't remember what I had heard." Knight (2010), however, recently demonstrated that accuracy may improve with repeated trials.

Strategies for Difficult Words

Another thing that we have observed is that clinicians devise interesting strategies when faced with behavior that is difficult to transcribe. Our diary studies indicate that students approach the transcription of difficult words in one of four ways:

1. Transcribe all the vowels first, then the singleton consonants, then the consonant clusters.
2. Transcribe syllable-by-syllable.
3. Transcribe all phoneme segments first, then add diacritics.
4. Transcribe the easiest behavior first, then go back as often as necessary to transcribe harder sounds.

The first two strategies have the value of forcing the transcriber to look at the syllable peaks, that is, the canonical structures of words (CV, CVC, CVCC, and so forth). The third strategy does most to capture the whole form of the word. Although we have tried all four methods to see which might force more rigor in transcription, the fourth strategy is easily the most used in our poll of students. From one of our student's diaries: "The first time I transcribed what was 'easiest'—what I was sure I heard. Next time, I transcribed what was next easiest. I used the same process until done with the utterance. The longer the utterance was, the more replays." And from another student: "I got the most 'remarkable' features written first."

Overall, then, there are many ways to deal with words that are not immediately transcribed. Try to observe the process you go through as you deal with difficult words. You may find that one or another of these four strategies works best for you.

Four Parameters of Phonetic Transcription

Former Appendix D now on the clinical phonetics website provides a review of research findings in phonetic transcription that your instructor may elect to pursue in class. As we conclude this chapter, it is useful to include findings from just one study that will be of interest in the present context.

The information in Table 7.2 was taken from the logbooks of a team of examiners who tested a series of job applicants for positions as research transcriptionists (Shriberg, Hinke, & Trost-Steffen, 1987). The application process used a job sample technique in which applicants were taught some skills in phonetic transcription, followed by criterion testing on those skills. The goal was to select from among all applicants the two persons who could best be trained to work closely with each other as a consensus transcription team for a research project in developmental phonological disorders.

The statements in Table 7.2 are observations about each of the applicants as he or she proceeded through the training tasks. The observations noted applicants' strengths and weaknesses in four parameters: *perceptual ability, efficiency and productivity, problem-solving ability,* and *interpersonal attitude.* The observations in Table 7.2 vividly convey the perceptual, cognitive, affective, and interpersonal processes that underlie phonetic transcription. Especially when you near the end of your coursework in phonetics, you may find it useful to compare some of your experiences and attitudes about transcription with these observations. Bottom line—would *you* get the job?!

Some Final Suggestions

Here is a roundup of some "dos and don'ts" that may make scoring or transcription successful and satisfying rather than frustrating.

1. Always use a pencil for transcription. Find the lead number that you like best. If you use a hard lead, be sure that it will photocopy (photocopying of clinical materials occurs regularly). Have several pencils available and a good eraser. If ever erasers were needed in adult writing, clinical phonetics is the place.
2. If you are transcribing in a group setting, develop a feeling of self-confidence (see Ramsdell, Oller, & Ethington, 2007). Try not to be unduly influenced by others, no matter what your stage of transcription skill (see entries in Table 7.2).
3. Try to keep successive items in a transcription task independent from one another. As discussed earlier, it is difficult to score or transcribe 50 items in a row without being influenced by a cumulative effect of your judgments or transcriptions. It may help to keep in mind that the original purpose for obtaining a series of such length must have included the belief that there would be some variability or

TABLE 7.2
Sample of Examiners' Comments about the Strengths and Weaknesses of Eight Job Applicants for a Consensus Transcription Team[a]

Type	Perceptual Ability	Efficiency and Productivity	Problem-Solving Ability	Interpersonal Attitude
Strengths:	• Seemed to have perceptual skills above what we have seen in other applicants. • Was able to make many of the error sounds, a strategy she used often. • Seemed able to concentrate on hearing what we described. • Seemed able to cross-check her perceptions. • Perception of small differences very good. • Seemed to form perceptual sets very well.	• Very much on task. • Asked questions to clarify what percept we heard. • No doubt she would be a hard worker and stay on task, deal with pertinent issues, etc. • Alert and conscientious. • Well-paced progress throughout the tasks. • Worked diligently to complete the individual sections. • Made lots of good comments focusing on the issues. • Concentrated on segments and seemed "hungry" to keep going. • Comments were consistently focused on primary issues. • Attitude reflected "get down to business" approach. • Comments reflected the pairing of prior learning with new information.	• Strong conceptual framework. • Used strategies to refresh memory and separate out how we were using diacritics. • Conceptually she seemed right on. • Even when her transcription was different from ours, it was very reasonable. • The way she described the process of coming to a decision was very logical.	• Seemed to care very much about the results. • Did not seem bothered by transcription that differed from hers. • Enthusiasm in the consensus process as well as in the transcription task. • She is the type of person it would be great to work with. • She said she loved transcription. • Although she could not hear differences, she said she felt very good about the session as a learning experience. • Eager to learn. • Felt that she would stick with her percept but was not defensive about someone else doing the same. • Enthusiastic and good dynamics in conversation. • Nice give-and-take in the consensus process. • Evidenced a flexible attitude about disagreements. • Took seriously all the components of the session. • Showed confidence but reasonable discussion when her percept didn't match the key.
Weaknesses:	• May experience fatigue more quickly. • Never seemed to use the training information to establish perceptual sets. • Never produced sounds herself for comparison. • Did not seem to be able to cross-check her perceptions. • Did not seem to be able to maintain a perceptual set for later use. • Did not seem to be able to tune in to small perceptual differences. • Changed percepts radically. • Weakness in ability to concentrate. • Evidence of not working at listening. • Could hear some differences but did not seem to work hard at hearing the difficult sounds.	• Her comments were not exactly tangential, but they did not reflect a lot of depth. • Did not ask questions that would probe our rationale for decisions. • Wasn't off task, but she didn't seem as though she would be productive at this type of task.	• Often remarked that she could not come up with any way to describe what she was hearing. • Used no apparent strategies to solve novel problems. • Seemed as if she was guessing instead of drawing logical conclusions. • When her transcriptions differed from ours, it did not always have a "reasonableness" to it. • The fricative distortions that she used did not follow any logical pattern. • It seemed that conceptually it was difficult for her to pull things together as we gave feedback. • Conceptual framework was there, but I'm not sure how often she used it. • Verbalizing strategies were there, but she didn't seem to have strategies to help in difficult situations.	• Give-and-take during consensus practice was skimpy. • Commented that the "test" was "no big deal." • In general, did not seem to exhibit much enthusiasm for the process. • Did not seem to be interested in why there were disagreements. • Perceived some defensiveness in some of her responses. • Didn't seem motivated or interested.

[a]The comments are lightly edited for clarity. Shriberg, Hinke, & Trost-Steffen, 1987. Reproduced with permission of the publisher.

inconsistency in production of target responses. Be alert for those new behaviors that may occur within a speech sample.

4. Students tell us that one hour is about as long as they can attend to scoring or transcription. Fatigue undoubtedly sets in even earlier in difficult tasks. The physical activity of stopping and starting a recording alone can be fatiguing. Therefore, breaks should be taken frequently. Learn to recognize your own personal signs of fatigue, be they physical signs or signs in your scoring or transcription that indicate increasingly less precise discriminations.

5. If you are transcribing from an audio recording only, do not become frustrated by the lack of visual information. Being able to watch a person as he or she is talking does help for certain transcription needs; but, for the reasons discussed earlier, the bulk of scoring or transcription across phonetic classes can be accomplished without visual cues. Of course, certain decisions will be just too difficult from an audio recording—particularly if it was not of good quality, if the speaker was not well oriented to the microphone, and so forth. In clinical practice, you will have to decide whether to try to score or transcribe the sample or whether to declare it invalid for such purposes.

6. Do not be worried if you miss some behaviors in a speech sample. Unless you have to account for every bit of speech, it usually is better to leave out questionable scoring or transcription decisions—at least to set them aside by circling them or using some other convention. Certain analysis procedures may be confounded because of some puzzling data that are unsupported anywhere else in the corpus. The advice is—try not to be "compulsive" about every bit of speech behavior. Avoid lingering on task decisions. Do what you can, then move on.

7. Finally, to score or transcribe efficiently, you must have absorbed the information discussed in this chapter and in the preceding chapters. To the extent that you do not really know the symbols or have not really established response definitions for yourself, scoring or phonetic transcription will be frustrating. If you cannot readily re-create in your mind where each vowel is made or where to place diacritic symbols, you will have persistent problems in clinical phonetics. Such deficits will increase your latency of transcription, and, in the extra time needed to recall a particular symbol, your memory of the stimulus itself will decay. For a period of time, you may need to work with a sheet listing all of the symbols needed for a particular task directly in front of you. Eventually, however, you must memorize all the symbols and their placements. Such preparation will pay off as you begin the discrimination training in the next chapter.

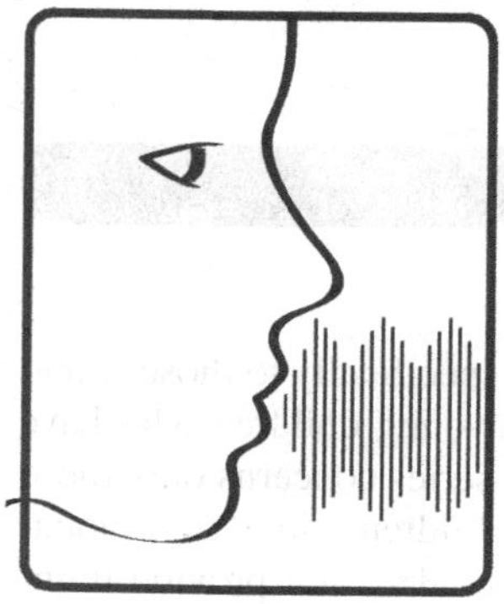

Transcription Training

CHAPTER 8

What follows is the first of five parts that provide training in discriminating speech sound changes. The parts are: (a) vowels/diphthongs, (b) stops, (c) fricatives/affricatives, (d) liquids/glides, and (e) nasals. Each part is divided into two sections. A background information section provides some relevant facts and observations about the sound class. A training modules section teaches the transcription skills for the sounds in the class that are most frequently needed in clinical practice. Training modules practice requires access to Clinical Phonetics Audio CDs 2, 3, and 4. Transcription keys, which include comments for each training module, are provided in a later section of this book on the left-hand pages. You should cover this page while writing answers in the spaces provided on the right-hand page transcription sheets. Discrimination skills may be practiced in many ways by creative use of these CDs and keys. You should experiment with various possibilities as you proceed through the CDs, adjusting your practice to the inherent difficulty of each module.[1]

PART A: TRANSCRIPTION OF VOWEL AND DIPHTHONG SOUND CHANGES

Background Information

As described in detail in Chapter 4, vowels (and diphthongs) are distinguished from one another by (1) position of tongue body within the oral cavity, (2) tenseness of tongue musculature or vowel duration, and (3) lip posture. Ready knowledge of how vowels and diphthongs differ on each of these features, as described in Chapter 4, is basic to transcription competence. One particular feature, lip rounding, warrants attention before proceeding to some distributional and frequency of occurrence facts.

The Problem of Transcribing Lip Rounding–Unrounding

Of the 13 vowels in English, only seven are normally rounded. Only vowels that have a relatively elevated jaw and mid or back tongue body are rounded. Such facts reflect universals of speech production as well as historical facts about the English vowel system. Certain clinical situations require accurate phonetic description of lip postures. For example, a young child who deletes final consonants may, by his or her lip postures on the preceding vowel, reveal his or her developing acquisition of the final consonant. This is discussed in more detail later. Lip posture information may also be useful when working with individuals who have neuromotor problems, for example, to describe the lip inversions seen in some types of cerebral palsy. Also, information on lip postures during vowels by children with severe hearing impairment may be useful in determining progress in speech development. For needs like these, symbols in addition to the five introduced in the diacritics chapter ([͗], [͑], [ᷱ], [ͫ], [ͯ]) may be required.

A problem with transcribing lip postures, as discussed in Chapter 7, is the availability of visual information, either live or from video sample. In our studies, diacritics indicating lip position on vowels and consonants were not transcribed reliably from audio samples alone. Therefore, the transcription of lip rounding has not been selected for training in this text. You may "hear" lip rounding or unrounding on the audio samples, and you will see lip posture symbols used here and there in the transcription keys. But we do not believe that transcription skills in lip posture diacritics can be learned solely from audio samples. Try to observe lip rounding–unrounding during live transcription sessions or transcription from video sample. When working with clients whose lip postures require modification, the clinician may need to adapt a system of lip gesture symbols that can be discriminated reliably by both the clinician and the client.

[1]Former Appendix D in the Clinical Phonetics website is a discussion of reliability, including procedures to assess your agreement with the answer keys. Before proceeding through the training modules, you should read this thoroughly. If these materials are used in connection with class assignments, you will need to check with your instructor to see how agreement will be assessed.

A clinical example of the use of special lip diacritics is described in Woodard (1991); see Appendix A for annotated references.

Distribution and Frequency of Occurrence Data for Vowels and Diphthongs: Implications for Clinical Transcription

Tables B.1 to B.15 in Appendix B contain many interesting facts about English vowels and diphthongs. For example:

1. Tense vowels occur in stressed syllables and in open syllables (syllables that are not closed by a consonant or a consonant cluster); lax vowels (excepting [ʌ, ə]) do not. Our language has words like *me* [mi] but not *mi* [mɪ], *two* [tu] but not *tuh* [tʊ]. Also, vowels occur in medial word position more frequently than initial or final word position (Table B.6).
2. Children use different vowels in the same proportion as adults do (Tables B.4, B.5). Schwa /ə/ is the most frequent of vowel sounds, about three times as frequent as the next most frequent vowel sound, /ɪ/. The vowel /ɪ/ is also used much more often than other vowels (Table B.8).

How are such data important for clinical transcription? For one thing, it is practical to become competent in transcribing sounds that occur frequently in English. According to these data in Table B.8, we should expect to hear a lot of front vowels, schwas, and centralized sounds. Therefore, the transcription training that follows will use these vowels more than the less frequently occurring vowels.

Another aspect of the statistics in Appendix B is their implications for management. Interestingly, vowels and diphthongs have received little attention by clinical speech-language pathologists. In the past, children who turned up in the clinics seldom had vowel or diphthong errors. As younger children are being served in public schools, however, statistical facts about vowels and diphthongs have become increasingly more useful (Otomo & Stoel-Gammon, 1992; Pollock, 1991; Pollock & Keiser, 1990; Stoel-Gammon & Harrington, 1990). To increase a child's intelligibility, it is prudent to select for management sounds that are distributed widely and occur frequently.

In sum, facts about vowels and diphthongs deserve close study, as is the case with all the data available in the tables in Appendix B. These tables contain the technical information needed for a variety of clinic decisions and for construction of management tasks. As introduced in Chapter 1, a primary goal of this book is to impress on student-clinicians the importance of such knowledge for the day-to-day practice of clinical speech-language pathology.

Training Modules

Overview

Transcription training is directed specifically to those sound changes that occur frequently in young children who have delayed speech. Importantly, this series concerns only those changes ("errors") that occur in children with developmental phonological delays. The series does not provide training on errors made by individuals with neuromotor, hearing, or orofacial involvement, although passing reference is made to sound changes that are relevant to involvements in these areas.

Before beginning practice on the audio samples, you should have immediate recall of each of the vowel and diphthong symbols introduced in the earlier chapters, as well as firm knowledge of the location and perceptual correlates of the following diacritics: [˔], [˕], [˖], [˗], [̠], [ː], and [˜]. Each diacritic describes a change in place or manner. As described in Chapter 6, each diacritic is always positioned above, below, or after the symbol it modifies. You should know these symbols and their conventional position well enough that you do not have to take time to look them up while you are working on the discrimination modules.

Training on the audio samples is divided into six vowel/diphthong sound changes: (1) substitutions, (2) modifications, (3) central vowels, (4) multiple element changes, (5) lengthening, and (6) nasalization. A total of eight transcription training modules, six covering the different changes plus two summary modules, are provided for you to learn to transcribe vowel and diphthong sound changes in children's speech. Here is how to proceed for each training module:

1. Read the text and be sure you understand what to listen for.
2. Proceed to the appropriate portion of the audio sample and transcribe items using the space provided on the transcription sheet (right-hand page). Be sure to write an alternative choice whenever you are undecided. Space is also provided for writing notes to yourself for later reference. The left-hand page, the transcription key, should be masked from view, using a sheet of paper or some other device.
3. When you have finished a training module, check your answers with those given in the transcription key. Note the "Alternatives," "Comments," and "Notes" sections provided in each module.
4. What you choose to do after the first time through each module is entirely up to you. Using transcription key

materials, you may wish to repeat the module with or without the transcription key in front of you, discuss your answers with a friend or the instructor, or complete remaining modules and return to particular modules later. These matters may be decided in conjunction with your instructor. Or, if you are proceeding through this series on your own, you may want to experiment until you find what works best for you.

Vowel and Diphthongs Module 1: Vowel and Diphthong Substitutions

Children's substitutions of one vowel for another usually follow closely the vowel quadrilateral (inside front cover). Substitutions generally involve a sound near the target sound, that is, in an adjacent cell (front, back, high, low, mid, etc.) on the quadrilateral. For example, [o] (mid-back) is a likely substitute for [ʊ] (mid-high-back).

PROCEED TO: Clinical Phonetics CD 2, Track 1: Vowels and Diphthongs Module 1: Vowel and Diphthong Substitutions

Vowels and Diphthongs Module 2: Vowel and Diphthong Modifications

Clinicians typically are more concerned with the consonant systems of children with delayed speech than with children's articulation of vowels. For certain clinical applications, however, close transcription of vowels and diphthongs may be required: for example, for analysis of phonological development, for an analysis of essentially "vowel speech," or for intelligibility programming for individuals with severe structural or functional deficits.

For example, clinicians may want to transcribe whether a child's /i/ is articulated appropriately as a high, tense sound [i] or as a somewhat lowered sound [i̞]. The diacritic symbols [̝], [̞], [̟], [̠], and [̈] are used to locate sounds relative to their customary positions within the vowel quadrilateral. Tongue raised [̝] and tongue lowered [̞] symbols may be used more often than tongue fronted [̟], tongue backed [̠], or tongue centralized [̈]. One reason for this difference is that changes in the front–back direction often are toward the *center* of the mouth, where the central vowels /ʌ/ and /ə/ are available to describe such perceptions.

One point of information before you begin this module—the task is going to be difficult! Transcribing vowel modifications is one of the most trying, least reliable tasks in all of phonetic transcription. Do the best you can. As you will see in the transcription key, even the "experts" have great difficulty agreeing on one best transcription for vowel modifications.

PROCEED TO: Clinical Phonetics CD 2, Track 2: Vowels and Diphthongs Module 2: Vowel and Diphthong Modifications

Vowels and Diphthongs Module 3: Central Vowels

As developed in Chapter 4, unstressed vowels in English are symbolized with /ə/, termed **schwa**. The schwa symbol occurs often in transcription to describe the unstressed vowels of polysyllabic words and of words in unstressed positions of phrases, sentences, and so forth. Only in very precise or unnaturally stressed speech are *all* vowels given full articulation. For example, the underlined vowels in the sentence "Alw<u>ay</u>s <u>e</u>nunciate pr<u>e</u>cisely" would be given full value ([eɪ], [i], [i]) only in overarticulated, careful speech. In normal speech they often are centralized to schwas.

Individuals with speech disorders may use /ə/ as a centralized vowel even more often than normal speakers. In listening to adults with motor speech disorders or children with delayed speech, for example, the effect of frequent /ə/ substitution is, in a cumulative way, quite pronounced.

If vowels are centralized extensively, as they might be if we talked with teeth clenched, speech will lose much of its clarity. Ogilvie and Rees (1969) describe the nature of schwa: "neutral, indeterminate, unstressed, *indefinite, weak*" (emphasis added). Many speakers we transcribe do, indeed, produce "indefinite" central vowels rather than the appropriate high-low-front-back vowels.

Transcription of /ə/ generally is not difficult; one problem does exist, however, which forms the basis of this module. It often is difficult to discriminate /ə/ and /ɪ/. Consider the word *mystic*. Do you hear a /ə/ or an /ɪ/ in the second syllable? The sound is very brief and indeterminate, and it could be transcribed either way. Most phoneticians prefer /ɪ/ in this position because the tongue is high and front as it travels between /t/ and /k/. Therefore the higher /ɪ/ is more likely to be produced in this context than the low /ə/.[2]

[2]The symbol [ɨ] is used by some phoneticians for a centralized /ɪ/. In this text, it is transcribed [ɪ̠].

When you are unsure of which unstressed vowel you hear, /ə/ versus /ɪ/, two guidelines may be followed:

1. /ɪ/ is somewhat more likely to occur when the original vowel is /i/; for example, "*be*fore" [b ɪ f ɔ r], "*be*cause" [b ɪ k ɔ z], "*re*hearse" [r ɪ h ɝ s], "beaut*i*ful" [b j u t ɪ f ə l], "Bill*y*" [b ɪ l ɪ].
2. Use /ɪ/ as the unstressed vowel before velars; for example, "majest*ic*" [m ʌ ʤ ɛ s t ɪ k], "cosm*ic*" [k ɔ z m ɪ k], "*be*gin" [b ɪ g ɪ n].

If neither of these contexts applies, and you are still unsure of which symbol to use, use /ə/.

PROCEED TO: Clinical Phonetics CD 2, Track 3: Vowels and Diphthongs Module 3: Central Vowels

Vowels and Diphthongs Module 4: Vowel–Diphthong Substitutions, Modifications, and Central Vowels

To this point, you have practiced three types of speech sound changes individually—substitutions, modifications, and central vowels. This module provides an opportunity to discriminate among these three changes in children's intended vowels and diphthongs. Before trying this module, be sure that you understand the bases for the transcription choices in each of the three previous keys.

PROCEED TO: Clinical Phonetics CD 2, Track 4: Vowels and Diphthongs Module 4: Vowel–Diphthong Substitutions, Modifications, and Central Vowels

Vowels and Diphthongs Module 5: Multiple Element Changes

Multiple element changes are changes of vowels and diphthongs that involve the *addition* of a sound element to the main vowel or diphthong. Such changes are of two types: on- or offglides and diphthongization.

Onglides and **offglides,** as described in Chapters 4 and 6, are intrusive sounds. A superscript notation is used to indicate that they sound like "intruders" on the primary pattern of the speech sounds, such as [ᵊɑ], [ɛ ᴵ]. Onglides and offglides are not fully realized, in terms of duration or loudness. Rather, they are short, transitional sounds that occur as the tongue travels to or from the target sound. As described in Module 3, the schwa [ə] is the most common realization of such indeterminate sounds. Listen to yourself produce the word *seal,* for example. You should hear a slight onglide just before the /l/, [s iᵊ l], yet Kenyon and Knott (1953), in their pronouncing dictionary of English, list the standard production of *seal* as [s i l] because the /ᵊ/ before the /l/ is predictable in this context. As the tongue travels from [i] to [l], [ᵊ] predictably occurs.

Diphthongization differs from on-/offglides only in degree. The difference between what could be described as an on- or offglide and what could be described as a diphthongized vowel is, in fact, quite slight. If the intrusive sound seems only transitional rather than intentional—if it is brief and unstressed—write it as a superscript as described above for on-/offglides. However, if the additional sound is longer in duration or more stressed, place the symbol on the line to indicate diphthongization. In this text, the class of multiple element sound changes includes both types of sound changes.

Before proceeding to training in discrimination of multiple element vowel/diphthong changes, practice in producing such sound changes should be helpful (recall a discussion of just this learning tactic in Chapter 7). Consider five possible *changes* of the vowel /i/ that have been introduced to this point; here is how each might be transcribed:

1. Vowel substitution /i/ → [ɪ], [ɛ], etc.
2. Vowel modification /i/ → [i̩], [i̠], etc.
3. Vowel centralization /i/ → [ə], [ʌ], etc.
4. Vowel onglide /i/ → [ᵊi]
   Vowel offglide /i/ → [iᵊ]
5. Vowel diphthongization /i/ → [iɑ], [iɛ], etc.

Now try to say each of the key words exactly as indicated in the phonetic transcription shown in Table 8.1.

TABLE 8.1
Vowel Changes Production Practice

Key Word	Substituted Vowel	Modified Vowel	Centralized Vowel	Onglide to Vowel	Offglide from Vowel	Vowel Diphthongization
help	[hɪlp]	[hɛ̝lp]	[hʌlp]	[hᴵɛlp]	[hɛᴵlp]	[heɛlp]
hat	[hɑt]	[hæ̞t]	[hʌt]	[hᵊæt]	[hæᵊt]	[hæɪt]

Practice the words in Table 8.1 with a friend or audio record them and play them back to yourself. Can you make these sound changes easily? Rapidly? As discussed earlier, phonetic transcription is more reliable if the transcriber is able to articulate faithfully each of the sound changes to be discriminated. Recall too that in the context of clinical management with a child who makes modification errors, the ability to demonstrate errors to the child is part of a clinician's clinical competence. Practice in making vowel modifications (and later in this series, fricative and liquid modifications) is especially beneficial.

PROCEED TO: Clinical Phonetics CD 2, Track 5: Vowels and Diphthongs Module 5: Multiple Element Changes

Vowels and Diphthongs Module 6: Vowel and Diphthong Lengthening

Vowel or diphthong **lengthening** is symbolized by [ː] immediately following the lengthened element. Use of this symbol often results from extremely subjective judgments. As discussed in Chapter 4, differences in vowel duration are measured in milliseconds. Yet, such differences *are* detectable, and we do have expectations of the relative duration of vowels in different phonetic environments. Such expectations are part of our phonological competence. Vowel length must be appropriate for a person to sound like a native speaker of a particular linguistic community. And for situations in which vowels may be the focus of management—such as with hearing-impaired individuals and individuals with severely impaired intelligibility due to structural or neuromotor deficits—vowel length is a feature that requires clinical attention.

One particular situation where vowel duration is important may occur when transcribing children with severely delayed speech. Some of these children delete the final consonants of words. This situation interacts with the fact that in English vowels are relatively longer before voiced obstruents than before voiceless obstruents. For example, the vowel /i/ is longer before voiced /d/ in *bead* than it is before voiceless /t/ in *beat*. The child with delayed speech who uses appropriate vowel duration preceding an omitted final consonant may be showing "knowledge" of this final sound, which he or she does not actually produce (Ingram, 1989; Renfrew, 1966; Shriberg & Kwiatkowski, 1980). If we listen closely to the child who deletes final /t/ and /d/ in the words *beat* and *bead*, for example, we may discover that the child actually makes the /i/ longer before /d/. We can thus give the child credit for observing this phonological regularity of English, which may also indicate knowledge of voicing distinctions in omitted final consonants (see Smit & Bernthal, 1983, for an extensive discussion).

One note before we begin transcription. Speech clinicians sometimes give exaggerated models of a sound within a stimulus word to make it more salient for the child. A problem with this technique is that children often will copy, faithfully, everything the clinician does, including exaggerated vowel duration. In addition, children may use a singsong pattern when reading or an overarticulated manner when "naming" objects, which may result in lengthened vowels.[3] These imitative behaviors are seldom of linguistic significance and should be differentiated in phonological analyses from behaviors that reflect a rule-governed aspect of the child's phonology.

[3]Many of the words on the training audio samples were edited from children's responses to articulation tests. Such responses sound different from candid samples of speech. Ladefoged (1993) refered to such speech as *citation forms,* nicely characterizing these isolated forms as "citing," in contrast to "talking," as in natural, continuous peech.

PROCEED TO: Clinical Phonetics CD 2, Track 6: Vowels and Diphthongs Module 6: Vowel and Diphthong Lengthening

Vowels and Diphthongs Module 7: Vowel and Diphthong Nasalization

A second change in vowel and diphthong manner occurs when nasal resonance is added to a vowel. **Nasalization** of vowels and diphthongs can be important for diagnostic purposes. The reasons are similar to those that we presented for transcribing on-/offglides, diphthongization, and duration. Nasalization may tell us something about the structural integrity of the speech mechanism and the regulation of articulatory timing. Nasality is an index of how well the velopharynx is functioning in speakers who have had a cleft palate or have a neuromotor problem. Some nasality on vowels will occur normally in conversational speech, especially when the vowels precede nasal consonants. In the word *man,* for example, the velum must be open for the two nasals but may be only partially closed for the vowel in between. This type of assimilation is termed **assimilative nasality**.

Transcription of nasalization can also yield information about the child with delayed speech development. The child who omits final /n/ and final /t/ will say [pæ] for both *pan* and *pat.* If we listen closely, however, we may hear a nasalized vowel [pæ̃] only in *pan.* What does this indicate? As with rule-governed vowel duration changes, it could indicate the child's awareness of the final nasal sound, even though he or she does not actually lift the tongue tip to say /n/ or /t/.

Problems in transcribing nasality are well known to speech clinicians. Researchers have attempted to develop objective ways of assessing relative nasality, although instrumental measures of nasality are validated ultimately by listeners' judgments. Clinicians must be alert to possible listener bias when transcribing nasality. For example, Ramig (1975) found that children were rated as more nasal when judges were aware of the children's cleft palate history. Such case-history information is not provided in the following module, although some of the samples are from people with repaired palatal clefts.

PROCEED TO: Clinical Phonetics CD 2, Track 7: Vowels and Diphthongs Module 7: Vowel and Diphthong Nasalization

Vowels and Diphthongs Module 8: Summary Quiz

Here's a chance to test your learning of all five types of sound changes that occur clinically on vowels and diphthongs. You may want to review each of the previous modules first—or perhaps spend more time on particular modules that were most difficult.

PROCEED TO: Clinical Phonetics CD 2, Track 8: Vowels and Diphthongs Module 8: Summary Quiz

PART B: TRANSCRIPTION OF STOP SOUND CHANGES

As in "Part A: Transcription of Vowel and Diphthong Sound Changes," stop training is divided into two sections—background information and training modules. Background information underscores facts about stop production and perception that should prove useful both for transcription and for clinical assessment and management. Modules for stop sound changes consist of six transcription training modules: (1) stop substitutions, (2) voicing of voiceless stops, (3) devoicing of voiced stops, (4) glottal stop substitutions, (5) stop deletions, and (6) frictionalized stops. Additionally, a seventh module provides a summary quiz of all stop sound changes. These transcription modules are recorded on Clinical Phonetics CD 2.

You may be happy to hear that transcription of stop changes generally is less taxing than vowel and diphthong transcription!

BACKGROUND INFORMATION

Description of Stops

As introduced in Chapter 5, page 58, stops are formed by ". . . a complete closure of the vocal tract, so that airflow ceases temporarily and air pressure builds up behind the point of closure." To review, the three cognate pairs, /pb/, /td/, and /kg/, are made along the vocal tract by the lips, tongue tip, and tongue dorsum, respectively. In addition to these six phonemes, American English speakers also have an allophone of /t/ and /d/, the flap [ɾ], and the glottal stop [ʔ]. The flap is used by most speakers of English in place of /t/ when it occurs between a preceding stressed vowel and a following unstressed vowel within a word (e.g., *letter* [l ɛ ɾ ɚ]) or between words (e.g., *quit it* [k w ɪ ɾ ɪ t]). The glottal stop sometimes occurs as an allophone of /t/ before syllabic nasals, such as *button* [b ʌ ʔ n̩] and in certain American dialectal forms, such as *bottle* [ˈb a ʔ l̩]. Glottal stops can also occur between two vowels and serve to separate them, such as *uh-oh* [ɔ ʔ o͡ʊ]. Although [ɾ] and [ʔ] are allophones that occur frequently in both normal and delayed speech, only the glottal stop [ʔ] will be considered in the training modules to follow.

Distribution and Frequency of Occurrence of Stops

Tables B.1 and B.2 in Appendix B present information on the distribution of stops in adult English in singletons and in clusters, respectively. Unlike vowels, which are distributed only in certain syllables, the six phonemic stop consonants occur in all word positions regardless of syllable stress. Stops also occur frequently in clusters, as indicated in Tables B.2 and B.11. Note that we can expect /t/ and /d/, the two alveolar stops, to occur most frequently in children's speech (Table B.10).

The broad distribution of stops in our language, together with the nature of stop production, yields a wide variety of stop allophones in spoken English. Thus, to sound like "native" speakers, children learning English, as well as adults learning English as a second language, must learn to produce these allophones under the appropriate conditions. For example, MacKay (1978) lists the allophones for /t/, as shown in Table 8.2.

Notice that from a management perspective, stimuli for a stop production program must account for these differing allophones. To promote *carryover* (generalization to free speech), the clinician should have the child practice making the target stop in diverse allophone contexts. Accordingly, clinicians must maintain consistent scoring or transcription skills across the wide variety of stop allophones.

TABLE 8.2
Allophones for /t/

Allophone Description		Symbol[a]	Word
Unaspirated	/t/	[t⁼]	s*t*op
Aspirated	/t/	[tʰ]	*t*op
Unreleased	/t/	[t ̚]	bough*t* two
Flapped	/t/	[ɾ]	bu*tt*er
Nasally released	/t/	[t̃]	bu*tt*on
Laterally released	/t/	[tᴸ]	li*tt*le
Dental	/t/	[t̪]	bo*th* *T*om and I
Back (alveopalatal)	/t/	[t̠]	mea*t* shop

[a]MacKay's diacritics.

Training Modules

Articulation errors on stops are rarely seen in school-aged children. Preschool children and people with structural and neuromotor problems, however, often have stop errors. Particularly for people with motor speech deficits, reduced intelligibility may be associated with imprecise stop articulation.

Our work with young children with moderate to severely delayed speech indicates that the majority of stop misarticulations can be divided into six clinical types: (1) stop substitutions, (2) voicing of voiceless stops, (3) devoicing of voiced stops, (4) glottal stop substitutions, (5) stop deletions, and (6) frictionalized stops.

Stops Module 1: Stop Substitutions

Stop substitutions made by a young child usually involve changes among the three primary stop positions of English. If stops are to be replaced by another phoneme (other than the voiced/voiceless cognate to be covered in the following module), they are almost invariably replaced by another stop. It is rare to see a stop replaced, for example, by a liquid, a glide, or a true fricative. Hence, we normally (abnormally!) get [t/k] or [d/g] (see Ingram's 1989 discussion of "fronting" phenomena), or sometimes sounds are "backed"—[k/t], [g/d]. Among the six stops, /p/ and /b/ are the most stable: They seldom are the "victims" in developmental substitutions. When they are replaced, it generally is due to assimilation influences (see Ingram, 1989, and Bankson, Bernthal, & Flipsen, 2008, for discussions of assimilation processes).

For this training module, we need concentrate only on stop substitutions *within* the voiceless series /ptk/ or within the voiced series /bdg/. We will hold voicing constant in the practice that follows next and reserve cognate substitution discrimination for separate practice.

Discriminating stop substitutions is usually a straightforward task, provided that the stop is loud enough. Be alert for one situation, however—the tendency to perceive /t/ for /k/ or /d/ for /g/ in clusters involving /l/ and /r/. For example, we tend to hear [t/k] in words like *clean* or [d/g] in words like *glee*. In these phonetic contexts, the /k/ and /g/ sounds may be made more forward in the mouth in anticipation of the more anterior /l/.

PROCEED TO: Clinical Phonetics CD 2, Track 9: Stops Module 1: Stop Substitutions

Stops Module 2: Voicing of Voiceless Stops

Discriminating voicing characteristics can be difficult. For example, deciding whether [p/b] or [b/p] substitutions have occurred are among the most troublesome of transcription tasks. You may have perceived voicing changes in some of the items in the previous module on stop substitutions. Given the complexity of the speech production and speech perception processes involved, it is not surprising that we have difficulty judging voicing changes. Before proceeding with the transcription training on voicing characteristics in this and the following module, review the discussion of stop production beginning on page 58. After you have reacquainted yourself with how voiced and voiceless consonants differ in word-initial and word-final position, continue with the following discussion.

In the word-initial position, the most common voicing error in young children is either to fully voice a voiceless stop (to substitute [d/t]; *two* [d u]) or to partially voice a voiceless stop ([t̬/t]; *two* [t̬u]). Strictly speaking, the "error" in each case may be related to voice onset time—voicing for the vowel starts too early for a "voiceless" stop to be made or heard. As developed earlier, differences in voice onset time of only 10 to 30 milliseconds can be very hard to discriminate. Normal children usually take many years before they can reliably coordinate voice onset time (Kent, 1976). Therefore, because voicing changes are the rule with many preschool children, they should not automatically be considered as "errors." Generally, we recognize cognate substitutions in the initial position—[b/p], [d/t], [g/k]. But how does the transcriber accurately perceive voice onset times that are just slightly advanced, that is, partially voiced?

Initial voiceless stops that sound partially voiced frequently should be transcribed as unaspirated. Thus, whenever initial /p/, /t/, or /k/ is perceived as partially voiced, it would be transcribed as [p˭], [t˭], and [k˭], respectively. Two considerations justify the use of this convention.

First, by using the aspiration symbol, we more accurately describe the factor that influences our perception of voicing in English. That is, the lack of aspiration of the initial voiceless sound makes it appear to be partially voiced. Therefore, [p˭], [t˭], and [k˭] are more appropriate than [p̬], [t̬], [k̬]. Second, by retaining the symbol of the target sound (such as [p˭]), rather than using a modified version of its cognate (such as [b̥]), a less severe claim is made about the child's phonological system. As discussed previously, it is more conservative to say that a child is modifying a certain phoneme than it is to say that he or she is *replacing* that phoneme with another phoneme or another modified phoneme. In general, we believe that substitution errors are more serious than some other error types; therefore, they should not be attributed to the child unless the evidence is clear-cut.

To sum up, the most common voicing "errors" in young children are to fully voice or partially voice an initial voiceless stop. On their way to adult speech, children require a lengthy period in which to acquire the motor control necessary for appropriate voice onset time values. Recall too that because voiceless sounds require more oral air pressure than voiced sounds, voiceless stops may be more difficult for the child or adult with a structural or neuromotor deficit. Initial voiceless sounds that are made weakly will also sound fully or partially voiced. We suggest that attention to the aspiration feature is the best approach for all such transcription situations. If initial voiceless stops /p/, /t/, or /k/ do not sound fully voiceless or fully aspirated, transcribe them as [p˭], [t˭], or [k˭].

PROCEED TO: Clinical Phonetics CD 2, Track 10:
Stops Module 2: Voicing of Voiceless Stops

Stops Module 3: Devoicing of Voiced Stops

The tendency toward partial devoicing of final voiced stops, particularly if they are unreleased, is common in casual or fast adult speech. In children, too, voicing of final voiced stops will often cease before articulation of the stop is completed. The symbol for partial devoicing is [̥].

Our strategy for discriminating *partially* devoiced final stops from those that are *fully* devoiced is to listen to the duration of the preceding vowel. If the length of the vowel seems appropriately long for a final voiced sound (relatively longer than before a final voiceless sound), the normally occurring partial devoicing is an appropriate allophone, such as [b̥], [d̥], and [g̊]. However, if you hear what appears to be a cognate substitution, such as [p/b], [t/d], or [k/g], and the length of the preceding vowel is too short for a final voiced stop, it is appropriate to use the symbol for the substituted cognate.

PROCEED TO: Clinical Phonetics CD 2, Track 11:
Stops Module 3: Devoicing of Voiced Stops

Stops Module 4: Glottal Stop Substitutions

As described in the first part of this text, a glottal stop is a stop made by a quick opening or closing, or both, of the vocal folds. It is heard as an abrupt onset of the vowel or an abrupt offset of the vowel. If you say the following two series of words rapidly, you should hear the similarity between the glottal stop and the other three voiceless stops: [pɑ], [tɑ], [kɑ], [ʔɑ]; [ɑp], [ɑt], [ɑk], [ɑʔ].

Part of the difficulty in perceiving glottal stops is due to the fact that the articulators involved in their production are the vocal folds. The "catch" glottal stop made by the vocal folds is not always easily distinguished from the normal onset or offset of phonation. Difficulty depends also, as with other discrimination tasks, on how forcefully the glottal stop is articulated. A forcefully produced glottal stop is much easier to identify than a lightly articulated glottal stop. In the latter case, it is very difficult to discriminate the glottal stop from normal voice onset or offset. For a prevocalic glottal stop, the basic cue is an abrupt onset often followed by an aspirated vowel (such as [ʔʰɑ]). For a postvocalic glottal stop, the cue is an abrupt offset (such as [ɑʔ]). Children with delayed speech generally use glottal stops as substitutions for final consonants. Children with repaired cleft palates may use glottal stops in all positions.

To summarize, listening for a glottal stop addition or substitution is difficult. In the initial position, the cue is an abrupt onset of the following vowel. In postvocalic or final position, the cue is an abrupt offset of the preceding vowel. In the final position, we also may hear a release of air comparable to released final /t/, /k/, or /p/ (such as *pet* [pɛʔʰ]).

PROCEED TO: Clinical Phonetics CD 2, Track 12: Stops Module 4: Glottal Stop Substitutions

Stops Module 5: Stop Deletions

Stop deletions occur frequently enough in children with both normal and delayed speech to warrant attention in this series.

Two types of situations arise. First, unreleased stop allophones occur in several phonetic contexts. In the following contexts, stops are likely to be perceived as having been deleted:

1. When followed by another stop (*cupcake* [kʌp˺kek]).
2. When between two consonants (*printshop* [prɪnt˺ʃɑp]).
3. When in a final homorganic cluster (*bank* [bæŋk˺]).

In each of these three phonetic contexts, stops generally are unreleased in adult speech as well as in children's speech. In such contexts, they may be perceived as deleted.

Second, there is one context in which stops actually are deleted that occurs uniquely in children with delayed speech—word-final stops. Final consonant deletion, including deletion of final stops, is a frequent error type in children with delayed speech. Knowing whether a child articulated a final stop can be important diagnostically, particularly because final /t/ and /d/ can mark past tense (*play* [pleɪ͡]; *played* [pleɪ͡d]).

Two strategies aid in discriminating stop deletions if the stop is only weakly articulated or unreleased. First, visual information is needed. Lip closure for /p/ and /b/ targets is most easily seen, whether live or from video recording. "Seeing" tongue activity for /t/, /d/, /k/, and /g/, however, depends on the size of the child's mouth, the angle of view, and so forth. If transcription of any of the six stops is important, as suggested in Chapter 7, try to make the necessary observations live while testing or later from a video recording.

The second strategy for transcribing stops in final position is to listen to the preceding vowel. As discussed earlier in the training for vowels, the child who deletes final stops may *mark* the preceding vowel in some way. Some possible situations, for example, are:

Stimulus Word	*Child's Production*
dog	[dɔː]
dot	[dɔ]
pin	[pɪ̃]
pick	[pɪ]
bike	[baɪ͡ᵊ]
bye	[baɪ͡]

The missing target phoneme in the stimulus words *dog, pin,* and *bike* is marked by the preceding vowel—by lengthening, by nasalization, and by an offglide, respectively. Compare these marked vowels to those said in response to the stimulus words *dot, pick,* and *bye.* Such subtle changes are important to transcribe when they affect our analysis of a child's speech development.

We use the "circle" convention and the question mark symbol quite often when we are unsure whether a final stop is present, such as *pat* [pæ(t)], [pæ(?)]. Rather than call a stop deleted or simply guess, we circle the questionable segment. Quite often, such difficult decisions involve possibly unreleased final stops, such as [dɔ(g˺)].

In summary, transcription of children with both normal and delayed speech will require careful attention to stop deletions, particularly final stop deletions. Visual verification of a stop gesture may be necessary to discriminate stops that are weakly articulated or not audibly released. Because articulation of vowels preceding final stops can be important for phonological analysis, the use of vowel diacritics to mark vowel characteristics is useful. Of course, the same types of agreement problems for vowel transcription are evident in such situations as those discussed in the vowel section. Specifically, you will need to use reliable symbols for duration, nasality, place modifications, and multiple element changes. Finally, use of the circle convention shown in Figure 6.6 ([t ɔ ⓟ]) or a question mark [p æ ?⃝]) should reflect the amount of confidence you place in your transcription.

PROCEED TO: Clinical Phonetics CD 2, Track 13:
Stops Module 5: Stop Deletions

Stops Module 6: Frictionalized Stops

One type of stop modification that occurs with some frequency in clinical populations is the **frictionalized stop** (also called a **spirantized stop**). Frictionalized stops, usually considered "distortions," do not have a crisp stop release; they have a gradual, rather than a sudden, movement away from the closure. Consequently, the resulting sound is less abrupt than the usual plosive burst of a stop release, sounding spirantized or more "drawn out." Frictionalized stops sound in between a stop and a fricative. You can simulate a frictionalized stop quite easily by making a /t/ and, while keeping oral pressure high, taking your tongue tip away from the alveolar ridge slowly rather than rapidly—[t͓].

We find occasion to use the frictionalized symbol [͓] often with young children and also with people who have neuromotor disorders. For young children with delayed speech, the frictionalized stop may indicate the beginning development of a new class of sounds, the fricatives—which initially appear at the same places of articulation (are homorganic to) as the previously acquired stops. A frictionalized /t/ ([t͓]) sound may be a transitional behavior before a child begins to make a good /s/. For children with neuromotor disorders, frictionalized stops may reflect difficulties in timing and other motor control domains, for stops require a rapid release.

It should be noted that we and others have also used "weakly released" to refer to stops that are not sharply released (the [̬] diacritic has been used to indicate "weak"). For example, Campbell and Dollaghan's (1995) description of the speech of a group of children and adolescents following traumatic brain injury includes the term "weak articulation of stop consonants" for four of the nine subjects.

PROCEED TO: Clinical Phonetics CD 2, Track 14:
Stops Module 6: Frictionalized Stops

Stops Module 7: Summary Quiz

Here is an opportunity to test your discrimination skills for all stop errors. Good luck!

PROCEED TO: Clinical Phonetics CD 2, Track 15:
Stops Module 7: Summary Quiz

PART C: TRANSCRIPTION OF FRICATIVES AND AFFRICATE SOUND CHANGES

The popular media tend to use the term *lisp* to refer to the use of any incorrect speech sound. Technically, however, a lisp refers only to substitution and distortion errors on fricatives and affricates, sounds we are concerned with in the modules to follow. Such errors are the most prevalent type of residual articulation error. Because of the high prevalence of fricative/affricate errors in school-aged children, some clinicians may find this training unit to be the most useful part of this chapter. We will need first to develop a clear understanding of the salient articulatory, acoustic, and linguistic differences among fricative and affricate sounds.

Background Information

Description of Fricatives

The terms **continuant, fricative,** and **sibilant** tend to be confused with one another. In the following list, note how these terms are superordinate to one another (see Appendix A, Table A.5 for a detailed review of relevant considerations).

Continuants: /θðfvszʃʒhlrwmnŋ/
Fricatives: /θðfvszʃʒh/
Sibilants: /szʃʒ/

Among the 15 continuant consonants, only nine are fricatives. And among these nine fricatives, only four are sibilants. Production of the English fricatives and affricates was described in Chapter 5. Here, four characteristics of fricative and affricate sounds are important to underscore for the purpose of clinical transcription.

Duration and Intensity Differences. The voiceless fricatives /θ/, /f/, /s/, /ʃ/ are often longer in duration and are more intense than their respective voiced cognates /ð/, /v/, /z/, /ʒ/. Increased duration and intensity of the noise segment were previously noted also for the voiceless stops /p/, /t/, /k/, as compared with their voiced cognates /b/, /d/, /g/. The clinical implication of this fact is that errors on voiceless sounds will be more noticeable than errors on voiced sounds. Because voiceless sounds normally are articulated longer and louder, errors on them are more obvious to a listener. For this reason, voiceless sounds are given priority in speech management programs.

Frequency (Pitch) Differences. As a general rule, as the place of articulation moves toward the back of the oral cavity, the pitch of the fricative noise gets lower. Try saying the following sounds in sequence, listening for the perception of a successively lowering noise pitch: /s/, /ʃ/, /h/. The noise pitch of fricatives is an important identifying characteristic, one that we will be using as a discrimination cue in an upcoming training module.

Tongue Configuration (Placement-Grooving) Differences. In production of /θ/, /ð/, /s/, /z/, /ʃ/, and /ʒ/, the sides of the tongue from front to back are in firm contact with the inner surface of the upper teeth or with the lateral portions of the alveolar ridge up to the canine teeth. The positioning for the tip of the tongue and the middle of the tongue changes most among these six sounds. For /θ/ and /ð/, there is no grooving of the tongue; it is flat. For /s/ and /z/, a narrow groove along the midline of the tongue is needed, with air funneled up to and out over the apex (not the very tip) of the tongue. The tongue tip, in fact, can be placed either somewhere just behind the upper teeth or somewhere behind the lower teeth. We tend to think that only the tip of the tongue is involved in /s/ production when, in fact, the whole apex usually is involved. Finally, for /ʃ/ and /ʒ/, grooving is not as narrow as for /s/ and /z/. The wider groove for /ʃ/ and /ʒ/ makes the friction noise much more diffuse than that for /s/ and /z/.

By sucking air inwards as you put your tongue in position for each sound, /θ/, /s/, /ʃ/, you should feel cool air passing over the point of the fricative source. Try it. Also, to feel the central emission of the airstream, for /s/ and /z/ in particular, make a sustained /s/ and run your finger from one side to the other directly along your teeth. The airstream will be partially interrupted as your finger passes by the central incisors.

Lip Position Differences. Lip position for all fricatives and affricates (excepting /f/ and /v/) is neutral or flat and spread. Some people round lips slightly for /ʃ/, /ʒ/, and /tʃ/, /ʤ/, however. The /h/ sound is entirely free of specifications for lip and tongue postures (as long as the vocal tract is open). Hence, lip and tongue positions for any given /h/ are determined by the shape of the vowel to follow. Consider the alternative lip and tongue positions for /h/ in the following words: *he, hot,* and *hoot.* Because it is free to assume the position of the following vowel (but, unlike the vowel, remains unvoiced), /h/ is sometimes called a "voiceless vowel" or "voiceless glide."

Distribution and Frequency of Occurrence of Fricatives

The distributional and frequency of occurrence data for fricatives and affricates are presented in Appendix B. With the exception of /ʒ/ and /h/, which do not occur in word-initial and word-final positions, respectively, these 11 sounds occur in all word positions. The cluster data are particularly relevant for such clinical tasks as the choice of management stimuli. In initial position, voiceless fricative clusters are more prevalent than voiced, with /s/ clusters by far the most widespread. Notice, too, that /s/ is the premier fricative, with /tʃ/ and especially /ʒ/ occurring much less frequently.

In summary, in consideration of all the characteristics reviewed here—intensity, duration, distribution, and frequency of occurrence—the sibilants /s/, /z/ (in word-final position as a grammatical morpheme), and /ʃ/ are the most important fricatives. Errors on these sounds are most "costly" to a child or adult, when we calculate their effects on intelligibility of speech or as a speech disability. Consequently, in the training modules to follow, a greater proportion of the training stimuli will be concerned with the transcription of /s/, /z/, and /ʃ/ errors.

TRAINING MODULES

Overview

Learning to transcribe errors on the nine fricatives and two affricates is going to be a large task. Before we subdivide them into modules on the basis of common discrimination problems, we will discuss errors that are common to all the fricatives and affricates, except /h/. Four errors are most frequent in the fricative and affricate production of young children with delayed speech, as follows.

Deletions. A major decision in transcribing fricatives of preschool children whose speech is delayed is whether any fricative noise is present. We can easily see why this is such a problem. Recall that fricatives, especially /θ/, /ð/, /f/, and /v/, are low-intensity sounds. These sounds may not be audible at all on audio recordings if a child makes them softly. And if the sibilants /s/, /z/, /ʃ/, and /ʒ/ are made weakly, they can be confused with audio hiss. We will need to practice hearing the presence or absence of any fricative-like sound for all of the fricatives.

Stopping. We find somewhat older (beyond preschool) children with delayed speech who very commonly replace fricatives with stops (**stopping**). Fricatives can be replaced by a stop that is made at the same place of articulation—for example, [b/v], [p/f], [d/z], [t/s]—or by a stop made at a different place.

Voicing Changes. As with stops, a number of factors related to stress may influence voicing changes in fricative production. Although our position has been to deemphasize the clinical importance of voicing "errors" in young children, some practice in discriminating voicing errors is provided.

Distortions. The last stage of fricative development begins when fricatives are distorted (approximated) in some manner. We will be using several diacritics for tongue changes involved in sibilant distortions in later training modules.

In summary, children with delayed speech may (1) delete, (2) stop, (3) voice/devoice, and/or (4) distort the 11 fricative and affricate sounds. The likelihood of each of these error types varies with the specific target sound involved. Accordingly, the training modules to follow are organized by target sound groups, with proportionately more practice on errors that occur more frequently in children with delayed speech.

Fricatives and Affricates Module 1: /f/ and /v/ Changes

Frequently occurring clinical problems with /f/ and /v/ fall into three types: (1) *deletions*—deciding whether the sound was present at all; (2) stop *substitutions*—deciding whether /f/ or /v/ was replaced by a stop (nearly always /p/ or /b/); or (3) *voicing* changes—deciding whether these sounds were correctly voiced. The practice module that follows provides examples of each of these sound changes.

PROCEED TO: Clinical Phonetics CD 2, Track 16: Fricatives and Affricates Module 1: /f/ and /v/ Changes

Fricatives and Affricates Module 2: /h/ Deletions

The only type of /h/ error that occurs with any frequency in delayed speech is /h/ deletion. Pronouns such as *him, her, his,* and *he* and auxiliary verbs such as *had* and *has* are likely to be said with /h/ deletions when they occur in an unstressed position in a sentence (*He put his hat on his head* [hipʊtɪzhætɔnɪzhɛd]). This is a casual speech phenomenon; we all "drop h's" when speaking casually or rapidly. Because /h/ deletions in such contexts are normal, only /h/ deletions in stressed positions (for example, the words *hat* and *head* in the previous sentence) might be of interest clinically. Nevertheless, clinicians should be able to transcribe /h/ deletions reliably whenever they occur.

PROCEED TO: Clinical Phonetics CD 2, Track 17: Fricatives and Affricates Module 2: /h/ Deletions

Fricatives and Affricates Module 3: Voiceless and Voiced *th* Changes

Studies of the prevalence of articulation errors have consistently found /θ/ and /ð/ to be among the last consonants articulated correctly in normal phonetic development. The usual "tongue between teeth" description of these sounds is not necessarily true of conversational speech. A wide range of placement of the tongue tip will produce /θ/ and /ð/, *as long as the tongue is in firm contact with the upper side teeth from front to back.* The tongue tip may be in light contact with the inner surface of the upper teeth or be placed between the upper and lower incisors. Because children evidently take longer to articulate these sounds correctly, we provide considerable practice on discrimination of errors in these sounds. This module will include the three types of errors found in children—deletions, substitutions, and distortions.

Deletions. In adult speech, /θ/ and /ð/ tend to be omitted in rapid speech (*Who's that* [huzæt]) and in clusters (*fifths* [fɪfs]). Because they are low in intensity, /θ/ and /ð/ are hard to identify auditorily.

Substitutions. The most likely substitution for /θ/ is /f/ or /t/; for /ð/, the most likely substitution is /v/ or /d/. Confirming /f/ or /v/ as the substituted sound, however, often requires visual evidence—seeing the teeth–lip closure. Again, the low intensity of these sounds makes them difficult to discriminate either live or from audio.

Distortions. The most common distortion for /θ/ and /ð/ are dentalized stops [t̪], [d̪]. By practicing making the following contrasts you can reacquaint yourself with dentalization of stops and fricatives. The tongue tip should be adjacent to or actually touching the inner margin of the teeth. Practice making the following contrasts.

1	2	3	4
Fricatives	Stops	Dentalized Stops	Dentalized Fricatives
those [ðoʊz]	[doʊz]	[d̪oʊz]	[z̪oʊz]
these [ðiz]	[diz]	[d̪iz]	[z̪iz]
thin [θɪn]	[tɪn]	[t̪ɪn]	[s̪ɪn]

Notice that the distortions in columns 3 and 4 are neither pure stops nor pure fricatives, respectively.

PROCEED TO: Clinical Phonetics CD 3, Track 1: Fricatives and Affricates Module 3: Voiceless and Voiced *th* Changes

Fricatives and Affricates Module 4: Fricative and Affricate Voicing Changes

Voicing changes of fricatives and affricates follow the same pattern as the voicing changes seen in the stops. Word-initial voiceless fricatives/affricates tend to be voiced; word-final fricative/affricates tend to be devoiced. Furthermore, the phonological rules for voicing assimilations in different phonetic contexts are essentially similar to those discussed for stops: fricatives and affricates tend to take on the voicing characteristics of adjacent consonants. The following module provides practice in discriminating voicing changes in certain fricatives and affricates.

PROCEED TO: Clinical Phonetics CD 3, Track 2: Fricatives and Affricates Module 4: Fricative and Affricate Voicing Changes

Fricatives and Affricates Module 5: Fricative and Affricate Substitutions

Substitution errors for fricatives and affricates generally involve either other fricatives or a stop. Seldom are fricatives replaced by sounds outside the class of obstruents; that is, not by nasal, liquid, or glide sounds. Our suggestions for transcribing fricative and affricate substitutions parallel those given for apparently phonemic substitutions for vowels and stops. We suggest a conservative approach. Do not label an error a fricative *substitution* unless the perceived sound is said essentially as it would be when used appropriately. Hence, for example, a perceived [t͡s/ʃ] is not the same as [tʃ/s]. Recall that in five-way scoring, tallying an error as a phonemic *substitution* rather than as a *distortion* could lead to incorrect analysis of the error pattern (see Chapter 7). The following module provides practice discriminating substitutions for fricatives and affricates; sounds for which substitutions are most common are: /s/, /z/, /ʃ/, /ʒ/, /tʃ/, and /ʤ/.

PROCEED TO: Clinical Phonetics CD 3, Track 3: Fricatives and Affricates Module 5: Fricative and Affricate Substitutions

Fricatives and Affricates Module 6: Dentalized Sibilants

This training module and the two following training modules focus on distortion errors on the sibilant sounds /s/, /z/, /ʃ/, and /ʒ/. The audio examples will focus primarily on the distortions of these sounds that most often occur. The task in these modules is to learn to discriminate among three possible distortion types. To aid in this difficult task, let us first review some information about the production and acoustics of sibilants (you may also wish to review the description of sibilant productions given on pages 59, 70, 88, and 150).

First, recall that tongue placement and tongue shape (grooving) play the principal role in our production of sibilants. The front sounds made at the alveolar ridge, /s/ and /z/, are less intense (perceptually, they are softer) than the palatals /ʃ/ and /ʒ/. Recall also that the frequency (perceptually, the noise pitch) of lingual fricatives generally goes down as the point of articulation progresses from the front to the back of the oral cavity. That is, /s/ sounds higher pitched than /ʃ/. Both intensity and frequency factors, which result from the positioning of the tongue, will figure in our discussion of differences among distortion errors.

Finally, recall that although the tongue is the primary agent for sibilant production, both the teeth and the lips play important secondary roles. If you grasp your bottom lip between your fingers and alternately pull it down and back up while making a sustained fricative /s/, you will hear /s/ change in pitch. And if you slowly protrude your lower teeth forward while making /s/, you will hear /s/ change in pitch. Further, if you say /s/ with neutral or slightly rounded lips, then say it with lips fully rounded, you will hear /s/ change in pitch. The point is that although tongue shape and placement play the primary role in sibilant production, the teeth and the lips (particularly the bottom lip) do play an important secondary role. As clinicians are well aware, slight-to-severe sibilant distortions may be caused by structural abnormalities in a client's oral mechanism.

With these overall descriptive facts in mind, let us now consider the most frequent of all articulation errors, the dentalized /s/ [s̪]. Any distortion of /s/ or /z/ wherein the tongue gets too close to or actually abuts the alveolar ridge or teeth may be transcribed as [s̪] or [z̪]. A host of symbols has been proposed to capture subtle differences among /s/ distortions in this area. Trim (1953), for example, proposed 18 symbols to represent /s/ distortions. Although highly trained phoneticians can become skilled in using many of these symbols reliably, such discriminations are difficult, if not impossible, to teach on audio sample. Moreover, the clinical need for and benefits to be derived from such close transcription have yet to be demonstrated. In any case, we encompass the many possible frontal variants of /s/ sounds with the single symbol [s̪].

The ability to discriminate the varieties of dentalized /s/ [s̪] sounds from "normal" /s/ is markedly facilitated when the student-clinician can produce these distortion errors. Try pushing your tongue tip just millimeters forward and reducing the narrow groove along the middle of the tongue while making /s/. You should be able to make a variety of sounds, each of which is neither a correct /s/ nor a correct /θ/. These sounds should be somewhere in between /s/ and /θ/. The key perceptual feature of dentalized /s/ [s̪] is that in some way the fricative sound is "flattened." The high-pitched "sharpness" of /s/ is lost; instead it sounds anywhere from almost completely stopped to "flat." Also, because it is more forward and less sibilant, dentalized /s/ should seem less loud than correct /s/.

Be sure you can make the many varieties of dentalized /s/ and /z/ readily before proceeding to the following training module. Practice making the many varieties of dentalized /s/ by yourself and with a colleague. See if your friend can discriminate your intended distortions from your intended correct /s/. Pulling down your bottom lip during [s] and [s̪] production will allow you to more clearly hear the difference.

PROCEED TO: Clinical Phonetics CD 3, Track 4: Fricatives and Affricates Module 6: Dentalized Sibilants

Fricatives and Affricates Module 7: Lateralized Sibilants

Lateral "lisps" ([s̺], [z̺], [ʃ̺] [ʒ̺]) have been referred to as sounding "wet" or "slurpy." These terms do, in fact, capture a perceptual aspect of the lateralized sibilant. Once this percept is learned, lateralization of /s/ and other sounds is readily recognized.

Here is how to teach yourself to make a lateral lisp. Place your tongue in the position that you would to say /l/ as in *look*. Now, keep your tongue tip *firmly* anchored on your alveolar ridge and try to say /s/. What you should generate is air turbulence over the *sides* of the tongue. Hence, the term *lateral* /s/. You can confirm the lateral air emission by tapping your cheek as you sustain the lateralized /s/ [s̺]. The sound will change in its quality as you divert the airstream by tapping your cheeks. In fact, you can shunt the air from one side to the other with your tongue, creating either a unilateral lisp or, if directed around both sides at once, a bilateral lisp. In our experience, most children with lateral lisps will have air coming out both sides.

Be sure you can make a "respectable" [s̺], [z̺], [ʃ̺], and [ʒ̺] before proceeding to the audio sample training on discrimination of lateralization. You should not hear or feel air coming across the central incisors. You can check for this by placing a single strip of tissue in front of your incisors, with or without your bottom lip pulled down. The tissue should not flutter; it should flutter only as you bring the tissue to the side(s) of the lips to which the airstream has been diverted. Again, practice with a colleague should be helpful.

PROCEED TO: Clinical Phonetics CD 3, Track 5: Fricatives and Affricates Module 7: Lateralized Sibilants

Fricatives and Affricates Module 8: Retroflexed Sibilants

The last type of sibilant distortion, retroflexed [s̢], [z̢], [ʃ̢], [ʒ̢], occurs only infrequently in children.[4] Retroflexed /s/, [s̢], with or without a whistling component, [ŝ̢], is a common /s/ variant in certain Southern and rural communities. Also, Rousey and Moriarity (1965) present some evidence that a form of a whistling, retroflexed /s/ may occur temporarily when a person is nervous.

To make [s̢], first put your tongue in the position you normally would for /r/ or /ɝ/ as in *run* or *earn*. Now, keep your tongue poised in this retroflex position and try making /s/—try to generate a friction sound while your tongue is in the retroflex position. As you tense your tongue and experiment with different approximations of your tongue tip to the roof of your mouth, you should be able to make a retroflexed /s/, including a whistle component [ŝ̢]. The trick is to make a very narrow groove in the center of the tongue and to tighten up the tongue as it curls backwards. Because the sound is made so far back in the oral cavity, its pitch should be lower than the dentalized /s/ [s̪] or the lateralized /s/ [s̺]. Try saying *bursar* [bɝs̢ɚ], *purse* [pɝs̢], *mercy* [mɝs̢ɪ]. Now try making retroflexed /s/ in words like *see, say,* and *Mississippi.* If your tongue is properly rolled back, your retroflexed /s/'s will sound like Humphrey Bogart's ("play it again, Sam").

[4]Another type of /s/ distortion, palatalized /s/ [sʲ], is perceptually quite similar to retroflexed /s/. Palatalized /s/ has a flattened tongue in the region of the turbulence. If you say the words "gas shortage" and freeze on the underlined continuant, you should be making [sʲ]. The [s] sounds like a sibilant midway between /s/ and /ʃ/. Palatalized /s/'s occur often in children. Unfortunately, however, we have not been able to teach reliable discrimination of this sound by audio recordings.

PROCEED TO: Clinical Phonetics CD 3, Track 6: Fricatives and Affricates Module 8: Retroflexed Sibilants

Fricatives and Affricates Module 9: Sibilants Quiz

Here is an opportunity to test your skill in discriminating sibilant distortions. The following module contains a variety of the sibilant distortions practiced up to this point—the emphasis will be on /s/ and /z/ distortions.

PROCEED TO: Clinical Phonetics CD 3, Track 7: Fricatives and Affricates Module 9: Sibilants Quiz

Fricatives and Affricates Module 10: Summary Quiz

Summary Quiz time once more! As in Part A for vowels and Part B for stops, this final quiz in Part C provides a good chance for you to review all the fricative and affricate errors taught to this point. You may want to review your work on the previous modules before beginning here. *Bonne chance!*

PROCEED TO: Clinical Phonetics CD 3, Track 8: Fricatives and Affricates Module 10: Summary Quiz

PART D: TRANSCRIPTION OF GLIDE AND LIQUID SOUND CHANGES

BACKGROUND INFORMATION

Description of Glides and Liquids

Glides and liquids are grouped together for this next series of training modules. The reason for this is that these two sound classes have much in common, as the following outline of their phonetic relationships clearly shows (see also Appendix A, Table A.5).

Sonorants (versus the **obstruents,** which are **stops, fricatives,** and **affricates**)

- **Nasals**
- **Vowels and diphthongs**
- **Glides**—/w/, /j/
- **Liquids**—/l/, /r/

Thus, the two glide sounds /w/, /j/ and the two liquid sounds /l/, /r/ all share a family tie to the class of sonorants. As noted for stop errors in Part B, children's errors on /w/, /j/, /l/, and /r/ are most likely to remain within class. That is, these four sonorant sounds are not likely to be replaced by obstruents when a substitution error occurs; they most likely will be replaced by another sonorant.

Distribution

The frequency of occurrence of each of the two glides and the two liquids differs markedly, as indicated in Appendix B. The consonant /r/, for example, ranks among the most frequent sounds, whereas /j/ is a very infrequent sound. The fact that many languages have only one liquid or none at all suggests that liquids are difficult to discriminate and to produce. English-speaking children must learn to differentiate among four glides and liquids. As we will discuss, they generally have little or no trouble with glides, but they have a great deal of difficulty with the two liquids.

Appendix B, Table B.1, includes a summary of the distributional rules for the occurrence of liquids and glides. Note that /w/ and /j/, which require a tense onset followed by a gliding movement, do not occur in word-final position. Because our orthography uses the letters "w" and "y" to end words (*tomorrow* and *buy*), we tend to forget this distributional characteristic of the glides /w/ and /j/. Note also (Table B.2) that glides and liquids are the only sounds permitted in the third position in an initial three-consonant cluster, such as [s k w] or [s p l], and that clusters containing glides and liquids occur frequently (Table B.11).

TRAINING MODULES

The glides /w/ and /j/ are among the first consonants that children articulate correctly. Therefore, children who have significant errors on /w/ and /j/ generally have extremely delayed speech. Substitutions for glides occur frequently enough to warrant the discrimination training presented in the following module.[5]

[5] The distinction between /w/ ([w]) and /hw/ ([ʍ]) (*witch–which; wail–whale*) is not preserved in many American English dialects. For convenience, we use [w] for all training stimuli.

Glides and Liquids Module 1: Glide Changes

The task in this brief training module is straightforward. Here is an opportunity to transcribe changes for the glides /w/ and /j/.

PROCEED TO: Clinical Phonetics CD 3, Track 9: Glides and Liquids Module 1: Glide Changes

Glides and Liquids Module 2: /l/ Substitutions

The liquids /l/ and /r/ generally are conceded to be among the most difficult sounds in a language to articulate. Among the 24 English consonants, only /l/ requires the airstream to be emitted laterally—over the sides of the tongue. In the first of two /l/ sound change training modules, we are concerned with substitutions of other phonemes for /l/. As noted earlier, substitutions for /l/ generally will be one of the other sonorants—either a glide, a liquid, or a vowel-like sound.

Clinicians typically have difficulty discriminating whether a child said final /l/ correctly or whether there was a vowel substitution (for example, *tail* [teɪ o]). Clinicians may be unaware that /l/ in this position is normally velarized, making it more similar acoustically to back vowels, and that tongue tip contact is not always made for postvocalic /l/. In the training module immediately following this one, a more detailed description of velarized /l/ will be provided. Here, it is sufficient to note that a velarized /l/ allophone occurs in the postvocalic position.

PROCEED TO: Clinical Phonetics CD 3, Track 10: Glides and Liquids Module 2: /l/ Substitutions

Glides and Liquids Module 3: Velarized /l/

As introduced in the previous module, velarized /l/ [l̴] is an allophone of /l/ that occurs primarily after a vowel at the ends of words. For the purposes of clinical phonetics, a velarized or "dark" /l/ can be differentiated from a "clear" /l/ by the activity of the back of the tongue during the articulation of this lateral sound (recall the discussion of the use of these terms beginning on page 64). For normal or "clear" /l/, the back of the tongue is positioned low in the oral cavity, and the high point of the tongue is at the alveolar ridge. Consider the position of the front and back of the tongue for [l] in the word *leap*.

For a "dark" or velarized /l/ [l̴], the back of the tongue is close to the velum. Our perception of a "darker" quality to the /l/ is associated with this secondary articulation within the oral cavity. The tongue tip may not even touch the alveolar ridge during velarized /l/ production. Consider the position of the front and back of the tongue for /l/ in the word *peal*. Now compare *leap* [l i p] and *peal* [pil̴] to appreciate the different qualities.

Whereas velarized /l/ [l̴] is a predictable allophone in postvocalic, word-final position, some individuals use a dark /l/ habitually in all phonetic positions. Such errors in adults generally go unnoticed by most people. Occasionally, however, the velarization is so pronounced that it draws attention to itself. The following module provides practice in hearing clear and dark /l/'s in an adult who could produce either at will after a program of speech management to correct velarized /l/.

PROCEED TO: Clinical Phonetics CD 3, Track 11: Glides and Liquids Module 3: Velarized /l/

Glides and Liquids Module 4: Derhotacized /r/, /ɝ/, /ɚ/

Whether due to their perceptual characteristics, their articulatory demands, or some combination of both, /r/ and /ɝ/ seem to be hard for children to acquire. Children who make errors on one of these sounds (including also the unstressed vowel [ɚ]) usually make errors on the other (Shriberg, 1975, 1980b). Notice that the onset position for the consonant /r/

is the vowel /ɝ/, just as the consonants /w/ and /j/ have onsets similar to /u/ and /i/, respectively. In addition to the derhotacized /r/ [r̮] that we will learn to discriminate in this module, two other types of errors on /r/, /ɝ/, and /ɚ/ will require discrimination training: w/r and velarized /r/ [r̃].

Derhotacized /r/ [r̮] is the most common error type for /r/ in school-aged children and in adults. In overall prevalence of articulation error types, it ranks second only to dentalized /s/ [s̪].

To make a derhotacized /r/, put your tongue in the position you would to say /ʃ/—as though you were going to say *shoe*. Now glide away from this position as you say... *rue*. Try beginning in the /ʃ/ position as you say *read, ride, road*. You should hear a slightly lengthened derhotacized /r/ [r̮] that may vary with the height of the following vowel. Derhotacized /r/ sounds cover a wide range of "*r*-ness," from just a trace of *r* coloring to almost [r]. As you attempt to make derhotacized /r/ sounds, [r̮], be sure to focus on tongue postures, not lip gestures such as rounding or protrusion. Lip rounding of /r/ is determined partly by the following vowel, not only by the "*r*-ness" of the consonant itself (contrast the amount of lip rounding in *read* versus that in *rude*).

Here are some examples that should reacquaint you with the proper use of the symbols for derhotacized /r/ introduced earlier in this text.

Item	*If Correct*	*If Derhotacized*
read	[rid]	[r̮id]
early	[ɝlɪ]	[ɝ̮lɪ]
crayon	[kreɪ͡ an]	[kr̮eɪ͡ an]
acre	[eɪ͡ kɚ]	[eɪ͡ kɚ̮]
brewers	[bruɚz]	[br̮uɚ̮z]

PROCEED TO: Clinical Phonetics CD 3, Track 12: Glides and Liquids Module 4: Derhotacized /r/, /ɝ/, /ɚ/

Glides and Liquids Module 5: /r/ Quiz

The previous training module provided practice in transcribing derhotacized /r/ sounds. The following module provides practice in contrasting correct /r/, derhotacized /r/ [r̮], and w/r substitutions. Our suggestion for transcribing what appears to be w/r is consistent with all previous cautions about use of substitutions—be sure you really hear [w] (Chaney, 1988). Derhotacized /r/ [r̮] is much more prevalent than w/r in school-aged children and adults, while w/r is heard in very young children. This /r/ quiz provides an excellent opportunity to practice an important discrimination, one that clinicians often report difficulty in making in the course of their work with school-aged children with /r/ problems.

PROCEED TO: Clinical Phonetics CD 3, Track 13: Glides and Liquids Module 5: /r/ Quiz

Glides and Liquids Module 6: Velarized /r/

Velarized /r/ [r̃] is an infrequent error in children. In one study of 50 children with /r/ errors, we found only one child with velarized /r/ (Shriberg, 1975). We include brief training on this error type.

A velarized /r/ [r̃] is essentially the same sound as a velarized /l/[l̃]. Both are made by a gliding movement of the back of the tongue; they both are substitutes for liquids; hence, velarized /l/ and velarized /r/ sound essentially the same. Follow the same procedure to make a velarized /r/ [r̃] that was suggested for making a velarized /l/ [l̃]. Put the back of your tongue up toward /g/ or /k/, but do not allow the tongue to actually touch the velum. Now, with a gliding movement of the back of the tongue, say the words *red, run, room*. In practicing [r̃], you may notice that you are saying a fricative-like sound or even a stoplike sound. Neither of these is what you are aiming at. Rather, it should be a gliding movement away from the soft palate. The sound should be "dark"—as though it is coming from the very back of the oral cavity.

PROCEED TO: Clinical Phonetics CD 4, Track 1: Glides and Liquids Module 6: Velarized /r/

Glides and Liquids Module 7: Summary Quiz

It's that time again.... The following 25-item module should afford a good opportunity to test your clinical transcription skill on glides and liquids. In keeping with their clinical prevalence, /l/ and /r/ errors will receive the most emphasis. *¡Buena suerte!*

PROCEED TO: Clinical Phonetics CD 4, Track 2: Glides and Liquids Module 7: Summary Quiz

PART E: TRANSCRIPTION OF NASAL SOUND CHANGES

BACKGROUND INFORMATION

Description and Distribution of Nasals

The three nasals, /m/, /n/, and /ŋ/, are among the easiest sounds to make. The lips [m], tongue apex or tip [n], and back of tongue [ŋ] only need to close off the oral cavity; the velum remains open. Notice also that it does not matter how tightly the lips are pressed for an acceptable /m/ or exactly where the tip of the tongue is for an acceptable /n/.

Appendix B contains a summary of the distributional and frequency of occurrence characteristics of /m/, /n/, and /ŋ/. /n/ is among the most frequent of the English consonants, with only /t/ occurring more frequently in some studies. /m/ and /n/ also occur frequently in clusters, particularly in word-final position. Only /ŋ/ is restricted in its position of occurrence—it cannot be used to begin a word.

TRAINING MODULES

Nasals are generally acquired early by normal-speaking children. Nasal errors and the problems associated with their transcription only occur, therefore, in very young, rather than older, children. And unless one considers n/ŋ in word-final position to be an error (which we generally do not when it occurs in an unstressed syllable), nasal errors are actually seen very seldom. The few errors that do occur may be divided into: (1) deletions and (2) an assortment of variations that we will present subsequently in the form of a summary quiz.

Nasals Module 1: Nasal Deletions

The most difficult problem you are likely to experience in transcribing /m/, /n/, and /ŋ/ is deciding whether a nasal was deleted. Consider a word such as *can.* The assimilative nasality that is normal on the preceding vowel [kæ̃n] may be sufficient to create the impression of the final /n/ without the final /n/ actually being articulated ([kæ̃]). Even in clusters, as in *bent,* assimilative vowel nasalization can suffice for a perception of /n/ ([bɛ̃]). Particularly in the speech of very young children, it can be difficult to decide whether /n/ and, to a lesser degree, /m/ and /ŋ/ were actually produced or whether we are responding only to assimilative nasality on the preceding vowel. In the training module that follows, keep in mind that you are lacking the visual information that will make this task somewhat easier in the live situation.

PROCEED TO: Clinical Phonetics CD 4, Track 3: Nasals Module 1: Nasal Deletions

Nasals Module 2: Summary Quiz

This summary quiz contains a collection of errors on nasals taken from our clinical tape collection. These sound changes can be categorized into three types.

Denasalized. Denasalization occurs when a nasal is articulated as the homorganic stop, that is, [b/m], [d/n], and [g/ŋ]. Children with a common cold, sinusitus (inflammation of a sinus), a deviated septum, enlarged adenoids, or other nasal obstructions may consistently denasalize nasal consonants. The result may be perceived either as a complete substitution by the voiced homorganic stop (*Pam* [pæ̃b]) or as a nasal followed by an intrusive homorganic voiced stop (*Pam* [pæ̃m^b]).

Devoiced Nasals. When children delete /s/ in an initial /sn/ or /sm/ cluster, the nasals may sound devoiced. For example, *Snoopy* [n̥͌upɪ], *smoke* [m̥͌oʊ̃k]. Here we have used the nasal emission diacritic [͌] as well as the devoicing symbol [̥]; children often mark the missing fricative /s/ by voiceless emission of the nasal. Nasal emission also occurs frequently in the speech of children with repaired cleft palates.

Nasal Substitutions. Substitution of one nasal for another is generally restricted to certain lexical items (*balentime* for *valentine*). Less frequently, nasal confusions may be a consistent pattern in the child's phonological system. In the latter case, substitutions are almost invariably [m/n] or [n/m]. In word-final position, /ŋ/ may appear to be replaced by /n/(n/ŋ); but, more likely, the /ŋ/ was said as a syllabic, such as *walking* [wɔkŋ̍]. As noted before, these latter differences generally are not of clinical significance.

PROCEED TO: Clinical Phonetics CD 4, Track 4: Nasals
Module 2: Summary Quiz

GRAND QUIZ

You knew this was coming! This final module of Chapter 8 gives you a chance to transcribe 45 words completely. You will hear many "old friends"... sound changes of every type practiced in the preceding 34 training modules. Take time with each word. You may want to reread the discussion beginning on page 136 for suggestions on whole word transcription strategies. *Alles Gute!*

PROCEED TO: Clinical Phonetics CD 4, Track 5:
Grand Quiz

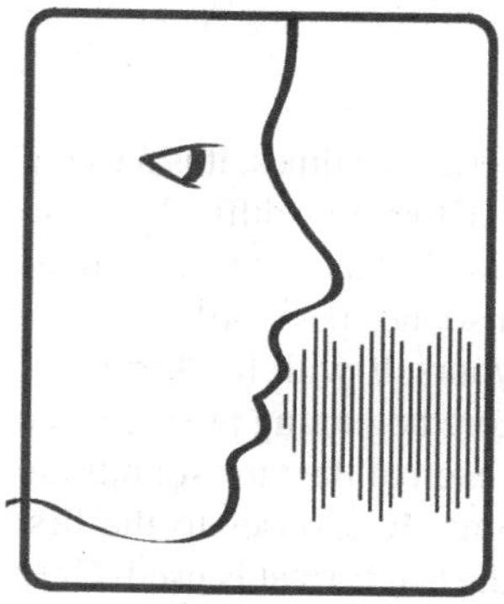

CHAPTER 9

Transcription and Scoring Practice

To this point in the training series, you have learned:

1. How the sounds of English are made and how they are distributed in the language.
2. The most frequently occurring sound changes made by children with delayed speech and how to discriminate among them.
3. A set of symbols to represent both the normal sounds and a variety of sound changes.

This chapter will build upon these skills. The goal is to provide you with transcription practice on a variety of clinical tasks. Materials are presented that provide:

- Practice using two-way scoring, five-way scoring, and phonetic transcription.
- Practice in building transcription speed. Materials reflect the pace of transcription that occurs in the clinic (repetitions of items are *not* provided in these transcription modules).
- Exposure to some of the primary sampling procedures clinicians use to assess a child's speech, including several articulation tests and free speech samples.
- Further exposure to the variety of errors seen clinically.

The transcription exercises referred to in this chapter, like the previous one, consist of blank forms on the right-hand page and a completed key on the left-hand page. To allow for training in all three systems used by clinicians—two-way scoring, five-way scoring, and phonetic transcription—additional blank forms and keys are provided for certain modules. Feedback comments follow some of the modules.

The Clinical Phonetics website includes additional transcription practice materials including, most recently, samples of children and adolescents with motor speech disorders.

Practice Modules

Practice Module 1: Single-Sound Articulation Test

Speech-language clinicians commonly use forms of speech sampling that, for convenience, are termed **single-sound** articulation tests. These tests assess a target sound in three positions within a word—initial, medial, and final. As described in Chapter 7 (see also Figure 1.1), the **response complexity** for the clinician involves only one target sound per word. The clinician may ask a child to name a picture (elicitation) or to say a word after him or her (imitation). References and comparative discussion of some of the more widely used measures may be found in several textbooks on developmental phonological disorders, including Bernthal and Bankson (1993).

The single-sound articulation test used in this module is the Developmental Articulation Test (Hejna, 1955), administered by imitation to a 7-year-old girl with moderately to severely delayed speech. In this test, the girl attempts 17 of the consonant sounds as they occur in word-initial, word-medial, and word-final position (except /ŋ/, /w/, and /j/, which are tested only in the two positions in which they occur). For each word spoken by the child, score/transcribe *only* the target sound. Three blank test forms are presented, one each for two-way scoring, five-way scoring, and phonetic transcription, respectively. You may wish to gain practice using any or all of the three systems. For two-way scoring, use "plus" (+) and "zero" (0). For five-way scoring, use "plus" (+) for correct, "minus" (–) for deletion, "D" for distortion, and write in the symbol perceived for an addition and for a substitution; for example, [w] (for [w/r]), [t] (for [t/k]), and so forth. For phonetic transcription, use the symbols and diacritics that you have learned in previous chapters. Score or transcribe only the target sound in the space under each column. The first three columns for /m/ are completed to illustrate the procedure. Only the first 17 items have been dubbed for training.

PROCEED TO: Clinical Phonetics CD 4, Track 6: Practice Module 1: Single-Sound Articulation Test

Practice Module 2: Multiple-Sound Articulation Test

Multiple-sound articulation tests require the clinician to score or transcribe more than one target sound per item (see Figure 1.1). A wealth of technical issues has emerged from the comparison of the results of such tests to those obtained with single-sound measures. Such controversies are beyond the scope of this program, but discussions are available in many sources, including Bankson, Bernthal, and Flipsen (2008) and Morrison and Shriberg (1992).

The multiple-sound articulation test selected for this module is the McDonald Screening Test, which follows from a view of speech production developed by McDonald (1964, 1968) that emphasizes the role of phonetic context on the articulation of target sounds. Because the McDonald Screening Test yields information on nine sounds, each tested 10 times, it is a useful clinical measure; *however,* it is one of the more difficult tests to administer and to score or transcribe because clinicians must make decisions on as many as four sounds per word.

You will need to familiarize yourself with the format of the McDonald Screening Test before beginning practice (see page 278). Note that responses to each of the nine sounds are recorded in spaces within a column. Responses to the first item are completed to show how the test format is used. Only the first 21 items will be presented. Once again, your goal is to play each recorded stimulus only once. Try to minimize playbacks. Blanks are provided for two-way scoring, five-way scoring, and phonetic transcription. The child whose speech is being tested is 5 years old; his speech may be considered moderately delayed.

PROCEED TO: Clinical Phonetics CD 4, Track 7: Practice Module 2: Multiple-Sound Articulation Test

Practice Module 3: /s/ in Continuous Speech; Sample I

This transcription practice module and the two immediately following contain samples of continuous speech by children who have errors on /s/. As we discussed earlier, /s/ errors are the most prevalent type of residual articulation error. Clinicians commonly obtain continuous speech samples from children with /s/ errors to probe how well a child is generalizing and maintaining articulatory skills in a continuous speech situation. For such monitoring tasks, two-way scoring usually is sufficient. What the clinician generally needs is a statement of the percentage of items for which the child is correctly articulating the target sound. These data, in such forms as "percentage correct per minute" or "percentage correct per sample" are used in different phases of management programs.

We have found that a two-step approach for acquisition of this skill works well. First, students need to learn to *identify* a target sound each time it occurs in free speech. When accuracy in identifying target sounds as they occur in free speech is high enough, the next task is to *discriminate* correct production of target sounds from incorrect ones. The practice modules in this section follow this two-step approach.

Preliminary Practice—Identifying /s/ in Continuous Speech. Frequency of occurrence data (Appendix B) and research by Diedrich and Bangert (1981) indicate that /s/ occurs often in normal speech, approximately seven times per minute. When clinicians first try to *identify* each occurrence of /s/ in continuous speech, two types of errors are often made:

1. The most frequent error students make when counting /s/ in a speech sample is to include /z/. Try to disregard how words are spelled—think of how words sound (*pays* [pe͞ɪz], *pads* [pædz], and so forth).
2. Another error is to miss /s/ sounds in words that have two or more /s/ sounds per word. Usually one or more of the /s/'s occur in a cluster (*stamps*).

Before listening to the continuous speech samples, see how often you can correctly identify the occurrence of /s/ in words. For each word in the following list—as rapidly as you can—say the word out loud and decide how many /s/ *sounds* it contains:

Item	*Number of /s/ Sounds*
1. stores	________
2. simplex	________
3. substantial	________
4. scissors	________
5. Mississippi	________
6. Missouri	________
7. transcribers	________
8. stencils	________
9. scratches	________
10. taxes	________

You can gain further practice by counting sounds in a number of ways. You can listen to the radio or television and count the number of /s/'s produced by a particular speaker. You can do the same while listening to a friend. Another excellent way to develop this skill is to record yourself reading or talking. The advantage here is that after listening and counting the /s/'s that occurred, you can replay the recording as often as needed to determine the actual count. Accuracy within 85 to 90 percent of the actual tally should be your objective before proceeding to the next stage.

Transcription Practice—Discriminating /s/ Errors in Continuous Speech. The following pages contain the transcripts (right-hand page) and the keys (left-hand page) for each of three speech samples. You can practice in either of two ways. First, you may wish to tally the correct and incorrect /s/'s without reference to the transcription. To do this, simply use a piece of scrap paper and tally each correct versus incorrect /s/ as you hear it on the recording. Alternately, you may wish to use the transcript to follow along and mark your decision over each /s/ that occurs as a phoneme on the transcript (watch those /z/'s). Keeping a tally without a transcript is what clinicians ordinarily do in the clinical situation. However, use of a transcript allows you to compare your answers item by item with the key. What you should be aiming for is a total percent correct figure that agrees with the key about 85 percent or more of the time.

Because the perceptual events in this task are fleeting, do not expect to agree exactly item by item with the key—our panel of listeners certainly did not agree with each other all the time.

The three children in these samples were either in kindergarten or first grade. They all are interviewed by the same clinician; the tapes have been edited only slightly. As you will hear, "kids say the darndest things."

PROCEED TO: Clinical Phonetics CD 4, Track 8: Practice Module 3: /s/ in Continuous Speech; Sample 1

Practice Module 4: /s/ in Continuous Speech; Sample 2

PROCEED TO: Clinical Phonetics CD 4, Track 9: Practice Module 4: /s/ in Continuous Speech; Sample 2

Practice Module 5: /s/ in Continuous Speech; Sample 3

PROCEED TO: Clinical Phonetics CD 4, Track 10: Practice Module 5: /s/ in Continuous Speech; Sample 3

Practice Module 6: /r/ in Continuous Speech; Sample 1

A second group of target sounds that speech-language pathologists must learn to identify and discriminate in continuous speech is the /r/, /ɝ/, and /ɚ/ sounds. Errors on *r* sounds are second only to /s/ in terms of their prevalence as a residual speech sound error.

The two-step approach for learning to transcribe /s/ in continuous speech also is suggested for *r* errors. Clinicians may or may not wish to include the three *r* types in the same tally. For some clinical purposes, a combined tally may be sufficient; however, for more discriminating purposes, separate counts of errors on /r/, /ɝ/, and /ɚ/ may be useful. Because every orthographic *r* is said as either /r/, /ɝ/, or /ɚ/, the *s–z* confusion experienced on /s/ does not occur. Rather, the opposite problem of *underestimating* the occurrence of /r/, /ɝ/, and /ɚ/ crops up. When a word contains two or more *r* sounds (*brother* [b r ʌ ð ɚ]; *Barbara* [b ɑ r b ə r ə]), it becomes especially difficult to identify and transcribe each *r* sound. The task also is more difficult for speakers with inconsistent *r* errors.

Once again, before proceeding to the speech sample modules, first develop your skill in counting *r* sounds in continuous speech. Use the procedures suggested for /s/—by listening to the radio or television or by recording yourself, and so forth. Try to keep separate tallies for the occurrence of /r/, /ɝ/, and /ɚ/; /r/ will occur most frequently among the three sounds, by about a 3:1 ratio over the long term. Your counts should be reliable within 85 to 90 percent (see former Appendix D on website) before proceeding to the speech samples for error discrimination training.

PROCEED TO: Clinical Phonetics CD 4, Track 11: Practice Module 6: /ɾ/ in Continuous Speech; Sample 1

Practice Module 7: /ɾ/ in Continuous Speech; Sample 2

PROCEED TO: Clinical Phonetics CD 4, Track 12: Practice Module 7: /ɾ/ in Continuous Speech; Sample 2

Practice Module 8: /ɾ/ in Continuous Speech; Sample 3

PROCEED TO: Clinical Phonetics CD 4, Track 13: Practice Module 8: /ɾ/ in Continuous Speech; Sample 3

Practice Module 9: All Sounds in Continuous Speech; Sample 1

Transcribing all sounds in continuous speech can be considered the "grand quiz" of this chapter. Your task in these two modules is to transcribe each word in a series of continuous speech samples using all the appropriate symbols and diacritics for phonetic transcription. If it has been some time since you have used all the phonetic and diacritic symbols, review Chapter 6 and the material in Chapter 8. Obviously, this task ranks as the most difficult in the realm of clinical transcription (Figure 1.1, cell 24). The gloss provided on the left-hand page is the *consensus* from our panel—you may not agree with each and every transcription. You may wish to transcribe each of the two samples once without reference to the gloss. As discussed in Chapter 7, having available a gloss of what the child intended to say can influence markedly our perception of speech.

PROCEED TO: Clinical Phonetics CD 4, Track 14: Practice Module 9: All Sounds in Continuous Speech; Sample 1

Practice Module 10: All Sounds in Continuous Speech; Sample 2

PROCEED TO: Clinical Phonetics CD 4, Track 15: Practice Module 10: All Sounds in Continuous Speech; Sample 2

CHAPTER 10

PHONETIC VARIATION

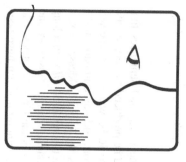

This chapter describes phonetic variation in American English. *Clinical Phonetics* has focused on teaching you how to phonetically transcribe speech in typically developing children and the speech of children and adults with speech sound disorders. In this final chapter we continue to use the term **articulation** to refer to articulatory placement and the term **pronunciation** to indicate the choices that speakers make in production. For example, the vowel /æ/ has different *pronunciations* across dialects; each dialect *articulates* the /æ/ vowel differently. We look at both *how* and *why* people differ in their pronunciation of speech sounds.

Examples of variation in pronunciation across different talkers are not hard to find. For example, it is almost a rite of passage for students going away to college to compare their pronunciation to that of their new classmates who grew up in different regions of the country or other countries. The author of this chapter, who grew up in Buffalo, was surprised in his freshman year of college to find his dorm mates from the northeastern United States commenting on his pronunciation of the words *Mary*, *merry*, and *marry*. The author articulated all three words as [merɪ] and his dorm mates produced them as [merɪ], [mɛrɪ], and [mærɪ], respectively. Each of these three pronunciations sounded identical to his ears!

The author now observes the ritual of phonetic variation comparisons among his own students at the University of Minnesota. The students, most of whom come from many regions of Minnesota and Eastern Wisconsin, often have markedly different pronunciations of certain classes of words. For example, many of the Northern Minnesotans produce the word *bag* as /beːg/, whereas their peers from Southern Minnesota pronounce it /bæg/. Some students from Eastern Wisconsin pronounce *bag* with a complex diphthong, as in /bi͡əg/. Students from Waterloo, Iowa, for example, produce the vowel in *pen* like the vowel in *head*, and the vowel in *pin* like the vowel in *hid*. A student who grew up in rural southwestern Georgia, however, would be more likely to produce *pen* with a vowel that sounds like the one in *pin*.

This chapter was authored by Benjamin Munson.

Phonetic variation is not just confined to vowels, as in each of the preceding examples. Consider the articulation of the words *straw* and *sock*. In addition to differences in vowel productions in each word, some people produce the initial sound in the word *straw* with a voiceless fricative that is more similar to the initial sound in the word *shock*. Someone who learned to speak in South Boston, Massachusetts, is not likely to produce /r/ in *par*, resulting in productions of *par* and *pa* (i.e., "dad") that sound alike.

The goal of this chapter is to introduce the topic of these types of phonetic variation. There are four chapter objectives. The first is to familiarize you with different sources of variation in pronunciation. Because the focus of this book is on phonetics, our discussion is limited to speech variation, rather than to variation in other linguistic domains, such as variation in word choice or sentence structure. We will not be discussing examples likely to be familiar to many readers, such as whether carbonated soft drinks are called *pop*, *soda*, or *tonic*, or whether a speaker uses sentences like *these clothes need washed* or *she doesn't have anything,* instead of *these clothes need to be washed* or *she ain't got nothing*.

The second objective is to describe some of the features that differ across various types of English. This will be illustrated by phonetic descriptions of different varieties of English. The emphasis in this chapter is on the varieties of English spoken in North America, although there will be some discussion of varieties of English spoken outside of the United States.

The third objective is to discuss speech in the context of clinical practice in speech-language pathology. Consider, for example, two reasons why a child might produce *part* without an audible /r/ sound. The first is that the child was exposed to adults producing the word without an /r/, and these /r/-less pronunciations are the norm for that speech community's dialect. In that case, the child is successfully copying the adults she was exposed to during language acquisition. A second explanation is that the child was exposed to productions of *part* with the /r/ present, but failed to learn to produce that sound. The second possibility may call for speech therapy. Speech and language professionals must know the variations in English spoken around them so they can differentiate between cases where an individual's pronunciation reflects normal variation and cases in which there may be a mild to severe speech sound disorder. Moreover, awareness of variation is important during the assessment of others' speech production. Regardless of whether we realize it, we have quite a bit of knowledge of the ways pronunciation varies. This knowledge leads us to have expectations about how others should talk, which in turn affects how we perceive the sounds that other people produce. Being aware of this tendency might help suppress this ***perceptual bias***.

The fourth objective of this chapter is to understand why languages vary, how they vary, and the consequences of this variation for individual speakers and the societies in which they live.

LEARNING GOALS

By the end of this chapter, you should be able to:

1. Define linguistic variation, especially as it relates to variation in pronunciation.
2. Describe differences in vowel and consonant production among different regional dialects of American English, African American Vernacular English, and foreign-accented English.
3. Differentiate production patterns due to normal linguistic variation from those that meet criteria for a speech sound disorder.
4. Describe why dialectal variation occurs and make predictions about how differences across dialects might affect the ease of communication between speakers of different dialects.

SOURCES OF PHONETIC VARIATION

Dialects

Imagine an ambitious research project that obtained a high-quality recording of the same set of words and sentences from every English-speaking person in the world without a speech, language, or hearing disorder, or any other disorder that might have a secondary effect on speech. Because samples of the same words and sentences would be obtained, there would be no speaker variations due to word choice or sentence structure. The only variation would be in how the words and sentences were spoken. Detailed demographic information similar to what might be included in the long form of the U.S. census would also be obtained from each speaker. Imagine transcribing these speech samples using the narrow phonetic transcription methods that have been taught in this book. Further, imagine that all transcriptions were made by the most skilled transcriber possible, such that all differences across the transcriptions could be attributed to differences in the speech of each speaker rather than differences among transcribers or to poor transcription ability.

In this hypothetical study, the words and sentences that were transcribed similarly would be produced by people who shared some traits. One trait would be where each speaker was born and raised. Speakers born and raised in parts of the southern United States, such as the city of Odessa, Texas, would be more likely to produce the vowel in *oil* with a long [ɔː] component and no [ɪ] component, whereas those born and raised and/or living in other parts of the United States would be more likely to produce the diphthong that you have been taught to transcribe in this word up to this point, [ɔ]. Speakers from parts of the southern United States would also be more likely to produce the voiced fricative /z/ in the word *greasy*.

A project almost equal in ambition to the project above (although obviously narrower in scope) was undertaken by the linguists Sharon Ash, Charles Boberg, and William Labov. The results of their project are published in the ***Atlas of North American English*** (ANAE, Labov, Ash, & Boberg, 2006, formerly called the *Phonological Atlas of North America*). The ANAE project conducted linguistic interviews with a large number of individuals in a variety of locations in the United States. The ANAE focused on speakers from urban areas who were natives of the regions in which they lived. Urban areas were selected because the ANAE investigators were particularly interested in how sounds change over generations, and people from urban areas tend to change their pronunciation patterns more rapidly than those in rural areas. Because the definition of *urban area* was based on U.S. census criteria and not by popular-culture notions of urban, the sample did include a number of relatively small cities, like Brainerd, Minnesota; Linden, Alabama; and Minot, North Dakota. The result is a fascinating illustration of the geographic distribution of pronunciation variants in North America.

A specific example of regional aspects of phonetic variation concerns whether speakers produce merged (i.e., the same) pronunciations of the low back vowels in words like *Don* and *dawn*. Data from the ANAE, shown at www.ling.upenn.edu/phono_atlas/maps/Map1.html, show that speakers from two areas produce these vowels differently: ones from cities around the Great Lakes—such as Buffalo, Cleveland, Detroit, Chicago, and Milwaukee—as well as ones from locations on and near the East Coast—such as Boston, New York, Philadelphia, Charlotte, North Carolina, and Atlanta, among others. Speakers in other parts of the country produce the same vowels in these words.

Systematic variation in speech in different geographic regions is evidence of the existence of **regional dialects** of American English. Later in this chapter, regional dialects of English, especially American English, are discussed in detail. For now, let us consider what it means for something to be a dialect. The word **dialect** is used widely both in technical studies of human communication and in our popular culture. In this textbook we use dialect in the more technical sense to mean a variety of a language (in this case, English) that is **mutually intelligible** with all other dialects of that language. That is, it can be understood by other speakers of that language. Transient miscommunications can occur between speakers of two dialects when there is a mismatch between the ways that two speakers pronounce a word. For example, a person from the northern United States might not know whether a speaker from the southern United States is referring to a *pen* or a *pin* when the Southern speaker says [pɪn], because Southern speakers often produce the /ɪ/ and /ɛ/ vowels as /ɪ/ before nasals, a process called the **pin-pen *merger***. However, such cases do not prevent messages from being transmittable by supplementing them with other information. After the northern U.S. speaker indicates that he doesn't understand the southern U.S. speaker, the southern speaker can disambiguate a production by saying, for example, *an ink* [pɪn] or *a safety* [pɪn]. Moreover, for two varieties to be considered dialects, they should have evolved from a single ancestral language. From this perspective, the distinctive regional variants of American English are labeled dialects. Moreover, southern and northern U.S. dialects are distinct modern versions of the variety of English spoken by the English colonists in North America. Their evolution as distinct dialects can be traced from written archives and, in the twentieth century and beyond, recordings of speech.

Another use of the term dialect, one often used in the popular culture, will likely be more familiar to most readers of this chapter. This definition labels varieties as dialects if they are subordinate to a **standard language** spoken in the same area. A good illustration of this is the categorization of languages in mainland China. China has a standard language, Putonghua (普通话, literally translated as *common speech*). This is based on (but not identical to) the variety of Mandarin Chinese spoken in China's capital city, Beijing. This variety is used in national broadcast and print media and is taught in schools. There are many other languages spoken in China. These include Beijing Mandarin (the variety on which Putonghua is based), Ji-Lu Mandarin (spoken in the northern port city of Tianjin and adjacent areas), Cantonese (spoken in southern China and in Hong Kong), and Hakka (spoken in a small portion of Southeastern China and in small groups elsewhere in China), among many other cities and areas. Of these four languages, only Beijing Mandarin and Ji-Lu Mandarin are intelligible with one another, and with Putonghua. Cantonese and Hakka are neither mutually intelligible nor are they intelligible to speakers of Putonghua, Beijing Mandarin, or Ji-Lu Mandarin.

In this second sense of the word dialect, Beijing Mandarin, Ji-Lu Mandarin, Cantonese, and Hakka are all dialects: They differ from the official standard language, Putonghua, and the fact that they are not used in official government communication or in education reduces their prestige. However, under the definition of dialects presented earlier and used to describe southern and northern U.S. English, only Beijing Mandarin, Ji-Lu Mandarin, and Putonghua are dialects, as they are the only languages that are mutually intelligible. Moreover, although all of these languages arise from a common ancestral language, the divergence of Ji-Lu and Beijing Mandarin occurred much more recently than the divergence of Hakka and Cantonese from the other two.

How would southern U.S. and northern U.S. speech be classified under this sense of the word dialect? This question is difficult to answer because the U.S. has no **official language** or **standard dialect.** Contrast this with the state of affairs in France. In France, there is a body called the **Académie Française** that acts as a *de facto* national authority and advisory board on the variety of the French language used in France (as opposed to the varieties used in other French-speaking areas, like Quebec or Senegal). The *Académie Française* publishes a dictionary and guidelines on grammar and usage. One of its stated goals is to monitor changes in usage that become necessary when new words are coined. It has in times during its history taken very strong stances on ongoing changes in French vocabulary and usage. For example, *the Académie Française* has developed French translations of technological terms to use in place of English borrowings (i.e., *le courriel* instead of *l'email* as a translation of the newly coined English word *e-mail*).

The United States has no organization equivalent to the *Académie Française*. However, there is an implicit standard in the United States that is reflected in the variety of English that is taught in schools and that is used in broadcast and print media. Readers of this chapter will agree that it is unlikely that sentences like *the car needs washed*, *borrow me a dollar*, and *he ain't got nothin' to give* are less likely to be taught in schools and used in national media than are the sentences *the car needs to be washed*, *lend me a dollar*, and *he doesn't have anything to give*. Indeed, the author of this chapter was tested in a Buffalo, New York, citywide middle-school English examination on his knowledge that *borrow me a dollar* was an ungrammatical sentence. Yet at least some readers (including the author of this chapter) are likely to have used or heard someone else use one of the former set of sentences, or ones like them, in conversation. We will call utterances that deviate from the predominant form of a language **vernacular forms,** following the usage developed by the linguist William Labov cited previously. Other textbooks might refer to these as **nonstandard forms.** We avoid the term *nonstandard* to circumvent the problem that the standard for North American English is based on a common set of language practices in schools and the media, whereas the standard of Putongua or Continental French is more rigidly and officially codified and enforced.

The focus of this book is phonetics, and readers may be wondering—are there *any* standards for pronunciation of American English words? Given that American English is not codified in the same way that European French is, we have only two sources within which to look to for an answer: instructional materials used in schools and pronunciation by people in the media. For children without speech, language, or hearing disorders, pronunciation *per se* is not typically a part of elementary schools' curricula, but there are two subjects in which pronunciation is critical: word-learning and reading. In early elementary school, children are taught words both as a string of letters and as a sequence of sounds. In very early instruction, this curriculum is often supplemented by explicit instruction of the correspondences between the letters and sounds that comprise the word. The curriculum enforces some standard pronunciations. For example, the standard pronunciation of *coyote* as [kʰaɪoʊ̍tɪ] and not [kʰaɪ̍oʊt] or [kʰaɪoʊ̍t] is enforced through instruction, even though the latter pronunciation would be predicted based on the pronunciation of word-final *ote* sequences in words like *tote* and *remote*. Further examples of standards from instruction can be found in dictionary pronunciation guides. These show that the word *banal* should be pronounced [bənɑ̍l] or [bənæ̍l] rather than [be̍ɪnəl], and that *dour* should pronounced [dur] rather than [daʊ̍ɚ] even though the latter pronunciations are predicted by the pronunciations of words with similar spelling, like *anal* and *sour*. But dictionary pronunciation guides often include multiple acceptable variants for a word. The Merriam-Webster online dictionary lists [bənɑ̍l] (i.e., using Clinical Phonetics symbols) as the first pronunciation of the word *banal*, but lists [be̍ɪnəl] as one acceptable variant. In this sense, dictionary definitions are one standard for pronunciation. A cursory look at pronunciations of words described previously (*pin*, *pen*, *don*, *dawn*, *cat*, and *cart*) shows a bias in dictionaries to pronunciations that are distinct from one another. That is, the pronunciations reflect the Midwestern post-vocalic /r/ in *cart*, as well as distinct vowels in *pin* and *pen* and in *don* and *dawn*.

What about the standards of pronunciation in the national media of radio and television? Crucially, one hears very few pronunciations on national radio and television news that are markedly vernacular. Three national television network news anchors at the time of the writing of this chapter—Katie Couric, Diane Sawyer, and Brian Williams—were raised in three distinct dialect regions, according to the ANAE. Couric was raised in Virginia, Sawyer in Kentucky, and Williams in northern New Jersey and western New York State. Yet their pronunciations are remarkably similar to one another. Just as with dictionary pronunciations, these pronunciations favor distinctive pronunciations (i.e., phonetically distinct *pen* and *pin*, *caught* and *cot*), rather than a particular regional variety. The situation is different in the United Kingdom, where a variant termed **Received Pronunciation** (RP) serves as a quasi-standard variety and is used in a great deal of the broadcast media, including the British Broadcasting Corporation.

Consistent with the discussion to this point, the phonetic domains of a dialect can be defined as patterns of pronunciation that are specific to a particular region. The origin of regional dialects is a subject of much debate. One widely accepted hypothesis is that regional dialects arise from the interaction of two factors: language contact and ongoing language change. The influence of language contact on the formation of U.S. dialects can be seen in the variety of English spoken in the Mississippi Delta region of the United States. This area was settled initially by French colonists before it became a territory of the United States and later part of the country, and hence, the distinctive variety of English spoken there likely reflects the early influence of French. A notable influence is expressed in French syllable stress, which, unlike English, includes syllable stress later in many words. For example, consider the differences in syllable stress placement in the English word *automobile*, in which stress is on the first syllable, and the French word *garage*, where it is on the last syllable.

Ongoing change is a pervasive feature of human language. The pronunciation of the word *knight* in 2010, /na̍ɪt/, is different from its pronunciation 1000 years ago, which was something like /kniʒt/, with an initial /kn/ consonant cluster (a combination that we don't have in any current English words), the vowel /i/ instead of /aɪ/, and the voiceless velar fricative /ʒ/ (a sound that we don't have in any current English words, but which exists in the Scottish pronunciation of the word *Lo<u>ch</u>* or the German pronunciation of the name *Ba<u>ch</u>*). The factors that cause language change depend, in part, on the structure of the language undergoing change. Language change resulting from contacts with speakers with different first languages influences dialect formation. For example, Southern English reflects, in part, the nature of the languages originally spoken by other persons in the region. Although the origin of dialects is a matter of debate, one fact about them is not disputed: Dialects do not reflect the perceptual, motoric, or cognitive skills of the speakers of different languages. They are indicative of normal variation.

Other Sources of Phonetic Variation

Recall our hypothetical study of variations in phonetically transcribed speech of typical speakers. Much of that variation would not be random, and not all of it would relate to where a speaker learned to talk. Our hypothetical project would also have a rich set of **demographic** data on the speakers—information like their age, sex, and level of education. What other demographic factors might predict speakers who produce sounds similarly from those who produce sounds differently?

Not surprisingly, you may have been challenged by the question just raised and find yourself at a loss to come up with explanatory factors for phonetic variation other than geographic regions of the country. There are far more stereotypes about how people from different dialect regions speak than there are stereotypes about different groups within dialects. A closer look, however, indicates that there are significant variations in pronunciation among speakers of the same regional dialect. As discussed in the following section, for example, consider the dialect of English spoken in New York City. One clear characteristic of this dialect is that post-vocalic /r/ is often absent in words that speakers of other dialects typically produce with post-vocalic /r/.

Words like *core* and *heart* sound similar to—although not identical to—*caw* and *hot*. The distribution of word-final /r/ has in New York has been studied extensively. It has been shown to be associated with three demographic variables. The first of these is age: the /r/-less productions (like *hot* for *heart*) are more likely to be used by older New York English speakers than by younger ones. The second is sex: Men are more likely to use /r/-less productions than women. The third is **socioeconomic status**: Studies indicate that salespeople at department stores serving people from lower socioeconomic strata use /r/-less variants more than salespeople in stores serving customers from higher socioeconomic status. Thus, it is clearly an oversimplification to describe New York English as having no post-vocalic /r/.

Why is phonetic variation this complex? Why don't all speakers of New York English produce words the same way? Just as there is no uniform answer to the question "Why are there dialects?", there is also no clear-cut answer to this question. But many of the principles that help us understand why different dialects exist also help us understand why there is variation within dialects. Languages change over time and these changes are one reason why dialects exist. Phonetic changes do not occur instantaneously. Sometimes they begin in very small, very localized contexts. For example, deletion of post-vocalic /r/ in New York City may have emerged in a small core of people in a particular socioeconomic class, then gradually, over generations, spread to members of other speech communities. As Labov (2001) reviews, the origin and spread of sound changes appears to happen in systematic ways, associated with characteristics of the speakers of who are engaging in the sound change and the structure of their social networks. This can give rise to fine-grained social stratification in sound production within communities.

The sources of phonetic variation can be even more local than might be inferred from the preceding discussion. Think back to the scenario of a person entering college and encountering significantly different pronunciation variants from those to which he or she is accustomed. It is likely that each of these variants will be associated with a particular meaning in the speech community. To return to the earlier discussion, Minnesotans' different pronunciations of *bag* are strongly associated with whether the speaker is from the North-Central dialect region, where [be͡ɪg] is more common than [bæg]. However, if individuals are able to develop conscious awareness of that relationship, they can use their control of the production of the word *bag* to convey different attributes—real or imagined—about themselves. For example, if the author of this chapter, whose native pronunciation of *bag* is [bæg], is in a social situation where he wants to show solidarity with other Minnesotans, he might pronounce the word [be͡ɪg] to convey familiarity and hope this his pronunciation leads them to think of him as a member of their group.

The literature on sociolinguistics includes many examples of the above example, termed **stylistic variation**. Detailed studies of adolescents' speech have found that members of social groups within schools sometimes mark their membership in their groups with distinctive pronunciation. A study by Drager (2008), for example, showed that two groups of girls in a high school in Christchurch, New Zealand (ones who were very engaged in school activities, versus ones who were relatively disengaged), marked their membership with distinctive pronunciations of the word *like*. Mendoza-Denton (2008) showed that high school-aged members of different Latina gangs marked their membership in the gang with distinctive pronunciations of the word *nothing*, a frequently occurring discourse marker in that speech community.

We can also find examples of pronunciation variation that convey different speaker attitudes in studies of pronunciation in the media. One such example comes from studies of the word *Iraq*. The pronunciation of this word is highly variable: the vowel in the first syllable can be either [ɑ͡ɪ] or [ə], and the vowel in the second syllable can be either [æ] or [ɑ]. A study by Hall-Lew, Coppock, and Starr (2010) examined different pronunciations of this word during debates in the U.S. House of Representatives in early 2007 regarding the proposal to send extra troops to that country (the so-called "surge" strategy). They found that during these debates Democrats were more likely than Republicans to use the [ɑ] vowel than the [æ] vowel in the second syllable, even when other factors related to the pronunciation of the word (i.e., regional dialect) were controlled.

Stereotypes about speakers of different parts of the United States abound. The linguist Dennis Preston conducted a series of studies in which he asked linguistically naïve people (i.e., people without any specialized training or coursework in speech, language, or hearing) from different parts of the United States to divide the U.S. map into different regions and to label them. One student's dialect labels reflect stereotyped perceptions of different regions ("boring Midwest" for a large area of the Midwest; "fully ivy league influence" for New England), different speakers ("surf-ubian, totally!" for California and Nevada), and different styles ("bird talk" for a region in the Northwest). Preston's (1989) book *Perceptual Dialectology* is a fascinating and detailed review of how people from different parts of the United States perceive the country to be divided into different dialect regions and how they perceive people in those regions.

STEREOTYPES

As you read the next section, think of what, if any, stereotypes you hold about different varieties of English. Ask yourself the following questions: Where do you suppose you learned those stereotypes? How are they represented, if at all, in media like radio, film, and television? Does the information in this chapter prompt you to reevaluate those stereotypes?

Regional U.S. Dialects

Vowels

Our discussion now turns to the phonetic characteristics of different regional dialects in the United States, which are differentiated primarily by differences in vowel pronunciations. The question of how to divide the United States into dialect regions has been considered many times. The linguistic atlases (maps of the United States that show dialect regions) that have resulted from various projects differ greatly, due in part to the linguistic focus in each project. Maps of variation in word-choice yield different dialect regions (i.e., locations where *pop* versus *soda* is used) than maps of phonetic variation (i.e., the locations in the same area in which the vowel in *light* is pronounced as either /a͡ɪ/ or /ʌɪ/). Moreover, given that the unique pronunciations of dialects are likely due, in part, to ongoing sound changes, the features of dialects are likely to change over generations. Hence, atlases capture variation at a moment in time, but do not show the change—sometimes quite rapid—that happens within and across generations of speakers.

With these several caveats in mind, we begin our discussion of phonetic dialect regions. In this first section we focus on vowel differences; a later section describes consonant differences associated with regional dialects. The division of dialects that we use is shown in Figure 10.1.

The ANAE's general tactic to defining dialect is to identify patterns of pronunciation and to find unique intersections of those patterns. For example, a dialect region might be defined as the intersection of two patterns, each of which spans multiple dialects.

Western United States.

West. The first U.S. dialect region to consider, the West, spans the largest geographic area in the country. This dialect region's eastern boundary is a few hundred miles east of the eastern edge of the Rocky Mountains. One particularly strong defining feature of the West dialect is fronting of /u/. This is enshrined in popular culture in stereotypic pronunciations of words like *dude* (and even in invented spelling of this word as *<dewd>*). This vowel fronting results in an /u/ whose acoustic quality is intermediate between /u/ and /i/ (i.e., [du̟d]).

A second feature of at least one sub-region of the Western dialects is a set of pronunciation variants known as the California Chain Shift. A *chain shift* is a set of sound changes in which the position of an entire group of vowels shifts around in the vowel space. Figure 10.2 is a schematic picture of the California Chain Shift adapted

The West A vast area that includes all or nearly all of the states of CA, CO, ID, NV, MT, NM, NV, OR, WA, WY, along with the westernmost parts of KS, NE, OK, SD

North Central A band that crosses the northernmost parts of MI, MN, MT, ND, WI

The North The northern Midwest and East, including parts of CT, IA, IL, IN, MA, MI, MN, NE, NY, OH, PA, SD, WI

Inland North Primarily the southern Great Lakes region, including parts of IA, IL, MI, NY, OH, PA, WI

The Midland a central region that includes parts of several states, including IA, IL, IN, KS, MO, OH, NE

St. Louis Corridor A narrow strip running northeasterly from St. Louis into Central IL

The South A broad region containing much of OK and TX and all or almost all of AL, AR, GA, KY, LA, MS, TN, SC, VA

Texas South A region of north-central TX

Inland South A small region that includes northern AL, Eastern TN, Western NC, and western SC.

Western Pennsylvania the western part of the state, along with bordering regions of OH, WV

Western New England Parts of CT, MA, NY, VT

Eastern New England Eastern portions of CT MA, NH, southern part of ME, all of RI

New York City

Mid Atlantic parts of DE, MD, NJ, PA

FIGURE 10.1
Dialect regions of the United States, as defined in the Atlas of North American English (Labov, Ash, & Boberg, 2006).

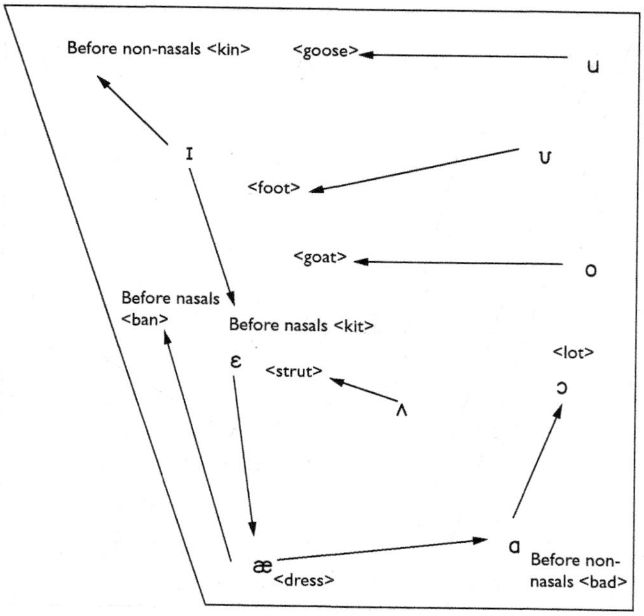

FIGURE 10.2
The California Chain Shift.

from research by Penelope Eckert. The arrows in this figure show the movement of vowels from their position in the American English vowel space (i.e., the vowel space shown in the inside front cover of this book) to their position in the California Chain Shift vowel space. At the end of the arrow, Figure 10.2 includes an example of a word that would contain the shifted vowel. The /u/ in American English is shown in the high-back portion of the vowel space, with an arrow pointing to the high-central portion of the vowel space and the word, *goose*. This means that *goose* would be pronounced [gu̟s] in this dialect.

As shown in Figure 10.2, the California Chain Shift includes the fronting of /u/ characteristic of the entire Western dialect region. It also has a lowering of mid-front vowels, and the retraction of low vowels. For example, the low vowel /ɑ/ is pronounced with a very back tongue position, resulting in similar pronunciations of the vowels in the words *lot* and *cloth*. Moreover, when it occurs before non-nasal consonants, the vowel /æ/ is produced with a markedly back tongue position, in a way that makes Californian pronunciations of the word *cat* sound like speakers of other dialects' pronunciations of the word *cot*. Before nasals, the vowel moves in the other direction and is produced with a relatively high tongue position. The vowel /ɛ/ is also produced with a markedly lower tongue position. Before non-nasal consonants, the vowel /ɪ/ is moving lower, although before nasals it is produced with a high tongue position, nearly merging with /i/ in pairs of words like *bin* and *bean*.

Seattle. Characterization of the western United States as a single dialect region has been disputed by some researchers. Ingle, Wright, and Wassink (2005) examined vowel production in one Seattle neighborhood, Ballard, which was historically home to Scandinavian immigrants who worked as fishermen. Ingle and colleagues showed that some Ballard residents produced a very back, rounded /u/. That is, these speakers resisted the /u/-fronting pattern that is characteristic of the broader Western dialect region.

Middle United States. The second and third U.S. dialect regions, respectively, are the termed the Midland and the St. Louis Corridor.

Midland. The Midland dialect spans Western Ohio, Southern Indiana, much of Central and Southern Illinois, Missouri, and Eastern Kansas. The Midland region, like the Western region, is characterized by very fronted pronunciations of /u/ and /o͡ʊ/ and, like the North region, by a merger between the *cloth* and *lot* vowels, such that words like *caught* and *cot* both sound like [kɑt].

St. Louis Corridor. The St. Louis Corridor includes the city of St. Louis, Missouri, and a relatively long but narrow area between St. Louis and Chicago, roughly along U.S. Interstate 55. This area is marked by speakers with the product of a Northern Cities Vowel Shift (to be described), as well as pronunciations of *barn* and *far* with the vowel /ɔ/.

Southern United States. The fifth through seventh dialect regions are the South, the Inland South, and the Texas South.

South. The South is bounded approximately by the Ohio River, the Missouri-Arkansas border, and the Texas-Oklahoma border on the north, the Texas-New Mexico border on the west, and the Florida-Alabama and Florida-Georgia borders on the south. The Texas South and Inland South are subsets of this larger region. One feature that cuts across the entire South is the production of the phonemic diphthongs /ɑ͡ɪ/ and /ɔ͡ɪ/ as monophthongs. Although most of the South shows this feature to some degree, it is particularly prevalent in the Inland South (comprising roughly the region along the Southern Appalachian mountains) and the Texas South (comprising North and Central Texas). Monophthongization is a very salient feature of Southern English. Indeed, Americans readily identify people who produce, for example, the diphthong /ɑ͡ɪ/ as the monophthong /ɑ/ as being from the South (Plichta & Preston, 2005).

Figure 10.3 shows another feature characteristic of the South, the Southern Chain Shift.

The /u/ and /o/ fronting in South dialect is a feature found in many U.S. dialects. South dialect reflects a complex pattern of front-vowel shifts. Whereas the vowel shift in Figure 10.3 suggests that the tense-lax pairs /i/-/ɪ/ and /e͡ɪ/-/ɛ/ are swapping positions in the vowel space, closer analyses of these vowels indicates that they are undergoing patterns of complex diphthongization, such

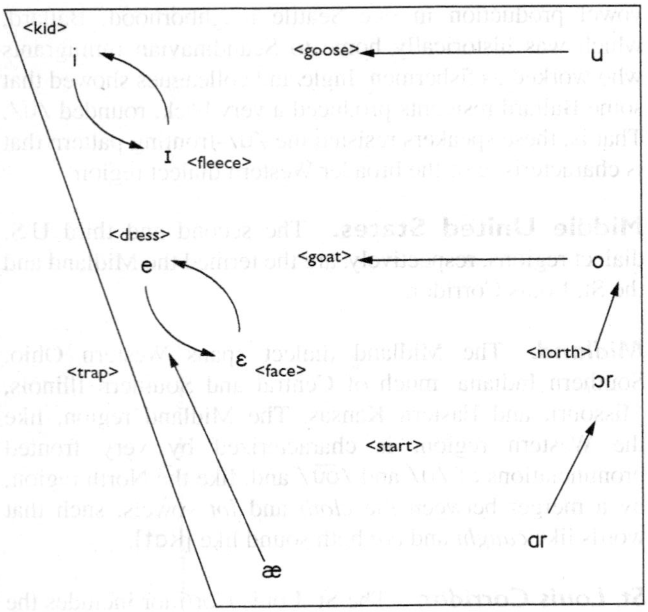

FIGURE 10.3
The Southern Chain Shift.

that *kid*, *dress*, and *trap* are produced [kiəd], [dreəs], and [treəp] respectively, whereas *keep* and *face* are produced as [kʌɪp] and [fʌəs]. In addition, the back vowel-plus /r/ sequences are moving up in the vowel space.

Northern United States. The eighth through eleventh dialect regions are the North-Central, North, Inland North, and Western Pennsylvania dialects.

North-Central. The North-Central dialect region spans Northern Minnesota, Eastern Montana, and North Dakota. A defining characteristic of this dialect region is a very back-round /u/ and /o/. The similarity of Ballard /u/ (recall the discussion of the Seattle region Western dialect) and North /u/ may not be coincidental: The North-Central dialect region was settled by Scandinavian immigrants, much as was the Ballard neighborhood of Seattle. A second characteristic of the North-Central dialect region is the distinctive pronunciation of the vowel /æ/ before syllable-final /g/ and /ŋ/, such that the words *bag* and *fang* are pronounced [beːg] and [feːŋ], respectively. There is also a tendency in these regions to produce /e͡ɪ/ and /o͡ʊ/ without a great deal of diphthongization (Watson & Munson, 2007). This is why the symbol [eː] was used in the above transcriptions of *bag* and *fang*. Words like *boat* would be transcribed as [boːt] in this dialect.

North. Just south of the North-Central dialect is the North dialect region, covering central and southern Minnesota, eastern South Dakota, and northern Iowa. One feature that differentiates the North dialect from North-Central dialect is that speakers in the North region engage in a pattern of

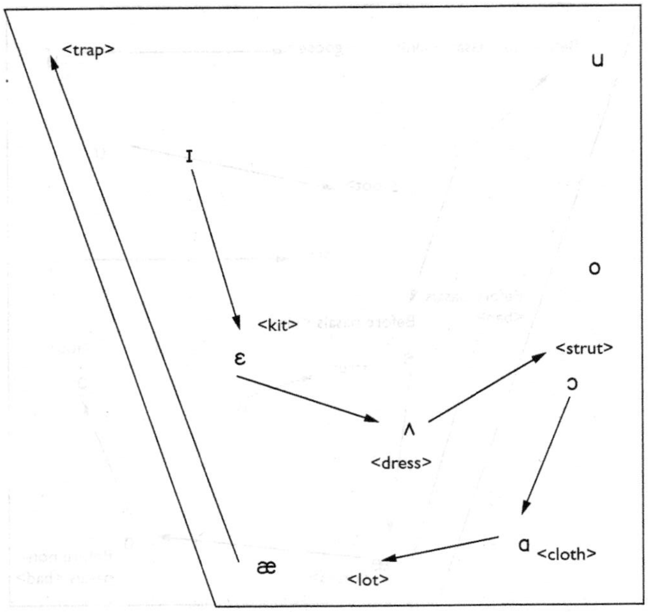

FIGURE 10.4
The Northern Cities Chain Shift.

pronunciations shown in Figure 10.4 termed the **Northern Cities Chain Shift**. One of the most perceptually salient features of the Northern Cities Chain Shift is the realization of /æ/, sometimes termed *tense* /æ/. This vowel is produced as a diphthong with a high-front on-glide, such that the word *cat* is pronounced as [kiət]. Another important feature of the Northern Cities Chain Shift is the status of the low-back vowels, as in the words *cloth* and *lot*. In general, speakers of the North dialect region merge these two vowels, such that the words *cot* and *caught* are pronounced very similarly, and close to the vowel [ɑ]. Indeed, as discussed next, it is this feature that differentiates the North-Central dialect from the Inland North.

Inland North. The Inland North dialect region includes the regions on the southern and eastern shores of the Great Lakes. Speakers in this dialect region undergo the Northern Cities Chain Shift, but generally maintain a distinction between the *lot* and *cloth* vowels. As in the North dialect region, the speakers in the Inland North undergo a process called *Canadian Raising*, where the diphthong [ɑ͡ɪ] becomes [ʌɪ] before voiceless obstruent consonants, as in the pronunciations of [mʌɪs] for *mice* and [fʌɪt] for *fight*.

Western Pennsylvania. The Western Pennsylvania dialect is characterized by a unique pronunciation of the diphthong /ɑ͡ʊ/ as monophthongal /ɑ/. This feature is so salient among residents of that region that individuals from the city of Pittsburgh joke about their pronunciation of downtown as [dɑntɑn], even spelling that word as *dahntahn* in folk descriptions of this dialect.

TALKING ABOUT DIALECTS

Stereotypes about Western Pennsylvania English can be found in souvenirs of the city of Pittsburgh, such as shirts that include the phrase "dahntahn Pittsburgh." How did people talk about the dialect that was spoken where you grew up? Did they have distinctive spellings for local pronunciations or stereotypes about the way that different groups in your area spoke?

Northeastern United States. The last four dialect regions (twelfth through fifteenth) are those spoken in the Northeastern United States: the Mid-Atlantic, New York City, Eastern New England, and Western New England.

Mid-Atlantic. The Mid-Atlantic dialect is spoken in the areas of Maryland (including Washington, DC, southern New Jersey, and eastern Pennsylvania). This dialect region is characterized by fronted /u/ and /o/, and the upward movement of back vowels—/r/ combinations, such that the word *part* is produced as [pɔrt] and *port* is produced as [pʊrt]. Pronunciation patterns in the city of Philadelphia include a fronted nucleus in the diphthong /a͡ʊ/, such that *house* is pronounced [hæʊs].

New York City. The English spoken in New York City has been studied extensively and has a special status among dialects of English, inasmuch as it is associated with the largest city in the United States and is extensively portrayed—both authentically and by actors—in film, television, and music. As discussed previously, a particularly salient feature of this dialect is the lack of post-vocalic /r/ in syllable codas in words like *car, horse, poor*, and *fair*, as well as the maintenance of a three-way distinction among the vowels /ɑ/, /ɛ/, and /æ/ before an /r/ in syllable onset, as in our earlier examples of the words *Mary, merry*, and *marry*, respectively. A second feature of this dialect that has been well studied is the different pronunciations of the vowel /æ/. A tense pronunciation—much like the tense /æ/ of the Northern Cities Chain Shift—occurs in most closed syllables, like *lamb* and *had*, whereas a lax pronunciation occurs in open syllables or before /n/, as in *manner, happy*, and *hand*. This pattern is noteworthy because it interacts with the morphological structure of words in interesting ways. For example, the tense /æ/ occurs in the word *planning* but not *planet*, even though the two words have identical CVCVC (consonant-vowel-consonant-vowel-consonant) syllable structures. The presence of tense /æ/ in *planning* is presumably because the root word *plan* would have a tense /æ/ in it. The word *planet* is not morphologically complex and hence would not have a tense /æ/ in it.

Eastern New England. The Eastern New England dialect region includes extreme Eastern Connecticut, Rhode Island, eastern Massachusetts, southern New Hampshire, and southern Maine. It shares with New York City the lack of a postvocalic /r/. The feature that arguably defines this region is that it merges the *lot* and *cloth* vowels to the vowel /ɔ/.

Western New England. Western New England includes the Hudson River Valley, Vermont, western Massachusetts, and western Connecticut. This dialect region is intermediate between the Eastern New England and New York City dialects and the dialects undergoing the Northern Cities Chain Shift. Hence, the signature of this dialect is a mild engagement in the Northern Cities Chain Shift, as documented by a difference between the /ɛ/ and /ɑ/ phonemes that is smaller than those seen in the Eastern New England and New York City dialects, but not as extreme as in Northern Cities Chain Shift speakers.

TEACHING YOURSELF DIALECTS BY PREDICTING CONFUSIONS

Given the vowel differences we see across dialects, we might predict that speakers of different dialects would have a difficult time understanding one another. Fortunately, confusions rarely occur. Listeners do a good job using context to understand what another speaker is saying and can adapt to a new accent relatively rapidly. However, when cross-dialect confusions exist, they are in the directions that you would predict from the descriptions in this section. When a speaker from the Midlands hears a speaker from the Inland North say [kɑt], he or she is sometimes unsure whether the intended target was *cot* or *caught*, while speakers from the Inland North interpret it only as *cot*. As we have seen, this is because speakers from the Midlands produce both *cot* and *caught* with the same vowel, [ɑ]. Consider any of the dialects we have described. Imagine a conversation between two speakers of any two of these dialects. Try to find pairs of words (like the *cot-caught* pair) that might be subject to confusion. How might the two people misperceive each other? For example, imagine a conversation between someone whose vowels undergo the California Chain Shift and someone whose vowels undergo the Southern Chain Shift.

A Note on Acoustic Methods. To this point we have not described the methods researchers have used in studies of regional dialects. It is important to note that in addition to perceptual phonetics, acoustic phonetic procedures such as those noted throughout this book have been used to validate both the vowel and consonant (described next) differences found in the fifteen U.S. regions. Acoustic studies have been especially helpful to validate dialectal variations in vowels. For example, Clopper, Pisoni, and de Jong (2005) obtained acoustic measures of duration and first and second formant frequencies from five repetitions of 11 different vowels produced by 48 talkers representing both genders and six regional varieties of American English. Analysis of the recordings indicated consistent variation associated with region of origin, especially in the production of low and high back vowels. In particular, the northern talkers produced shifted low vowels consistent with the Northern

Cities Chain Shift, the southern talkers produced fronted back vowels consistent with the Southern Vowel Shift, and the New England, Midland, and Western talkers produced the low back vowel merger. More recently, Jacewicz, Fox, and Salmons (2011) showed that the acoustic characteristics of school-aged children's productions were also dialect specific, when speakers from the Inland South, the Inland North, and the Midlands were compared.

Consonants

The ANAE described previously focused almost exclusively on vowel variation in the 15 dialects. The notable exception is information on dialectal differences in the pronunciation of postvocalic /ɾ/, which is absent in the New York City and Eastern New England dialect regions. As we have seen previously in this text and transcription practice modules, speech-language pathologists focus on consonant sounds because they are important to intelligibility and are frequently in error in children and adults with speech disorders.

Unfortunately, there is no single resource on dialectal variation in consonants that is as comprehensive a resource as the ANAE is for vowels. There is, however, some evidence of systematic variation in consonant production in North American English. One prominent consonantal feature that differs across U.S. dialects relates to the production of syllable-final /l/. This element is sometimes pronounced as a vowel similar to [ʊ], as in a Columbus, Ohio disc-jockey's pronunciation of [go͡ʊdən o͡ʊdiz] for *golden oldies* (Dodsworth, 2005). The geographic distribution of this pronunciation has not been as well studied as the variant vowel pronunciations. However, this vocalic pronunciation has been noted in New York, Philadelphia, rural Wisconsin, and Columbus, Ohio. It is particularly important for speech-language pathologists, as it mirrors /l/ vocalization as a common articulation error in young children (i.e., /l/ is replaced by a vowel). Thus, as with all potential dialectal differences, speech-language pathologists who observe /l/ vocalization in a child need to determine whether it is a common feature of the child's ambient dialect before classifying this phonetic variation as an articulation error.

A second consonantal feature that has been shown to differ across U.S. dialects is the production of the consonant /s/ in word-initial clusters. Baker, Mielke, and Archangeli (2006) found that some speakers produce the /s/ in /s/-plus-stop clusters similar to how they produce /ʃ/. The trend was to produce an increasingly less /s/-like and more /ʃ/-like sound in /st/, /spr/, /skr/, and /str/ clusters, in that order. No systematic studies of the distribution of this variant in American English have been conducted; it has also been noted in one non-U.S. dialect: New Zealand English (Lawrence, 2000). A clear illustration of this can be seen in an advertising campaign by the U.S. Army that highlights the slogan "Not just strong, Army strong." Commercials promoting the army with this slogan (including one that can be viewed on the video-sharing site YouTube.com, at www.youtube.com/watch?v=hosiAsy8dhA) illustrate this /ʃ/ pronunciation multiple times.

EXERCISE: LISTENING FOR DIALECTS ON THE NEWS

National network news is a rich source of samples of speech from different dialect regions. Whereas the anchors generally use "standard" pronunciations, the local people they interview often use vernacular forms. Since the advent of video-sharing websites, many clips are archived and can be viewed long after events have happened. Searching for specific news events can help you locate specific dialect regions. Some examples: Coverage of the September 11, 2001, terror attacks in New York included many examples of New York English; coverage of the 2010 Gulf of Mexico oil spill included examples of the distinctive variety of English spoken in rural southern Louisiana; coverage of the 2010 Upper Big Branch Coal Mine disaster in West Virginia provided many examples of speech from the Inland South; coverage of the assassination of Osama bin Laden in 2011 (which was announced at a Philadelphia Phillies baseball game) provided interesting samples of the mid-Atlantic dialect; and coverage of the tornado outbreak in Alabama in 2011 provided numerous samples of Southern English.

BEYOND REGIONAL DIALECTS

African American English

This section discusses dialects that are not defined by geographic regions, but instead characterize different social groups. In this chapter, we refer to these as **social dialects**, following a (1983) position paper by the American Speech-Language-Hearing Association. One social dialect that has been particularly well studied is African American Vernacular English [AAVE]. This variant goes by a variety of names, including Black English [BE] and African American English [AAE]. AAE is sometimes used to describe linguistic variants that are used across different social classes, whereas AAVE is reserved for variants that are used predominantly by working-class speakers. Any discussion of AAVE should begin with an important caveat: Not all African Americans use AAVE. Indeed, not all AAVE speakers use AAVE all the time. As with other dialects, some speakers show most or all features of the dialects, while others show few.

Unlike most other topics in this book, AAVE has more than once been at the center of heated and sometimes rancorous debates in the public sphere. It is unlikely that you and any of your phonetics classmates will get in a heated political debate over whether the medial /k/ in Wisconsin should be transcribed with a diacritic indicating aspiration, or whether the last syllable of *happy* should be transcribed with /ɪ/, as this book recommends, or /i/, as some other texts do. You may, however, argue about AAVE. Events that have put AAVE in the national spotlight—such as the

"Ebonics debate" following a 1996 policy decision by the city of Oakland, California, school board regarding AAVE—bring out a diversity of very strong opinions. Readers of this chapter are encouraged to read Lakoff's (2000) essay "Ebonics—It's Chronic," which provides valuable context to our discussion of AAVE.

One influential theory about the origin of AAVE is that it is a *creole* language. Creoles are languages that arise when speakers of different languages come in contact and must develop a way to communicate with one another. The language devised by the first generation of mixed-language speakers is called a *pidgin*, and when it is acquired by children and begins to be used widely among members of a community, it is termed a creole. AAVE is thought to be a creole that arose from the different West African languages spoken by African slaves brought to the American colonies and the English spoken by their captors. Just as with other varieties of English, AAVE has been the subject of language change in the many centuries since it first developed. The AAVE spoken today is not like the AAVE spoken 200 years ago.

AAVE has distinctive syntactic, morphological, lexical, and phonological features. A discussion of the first three of these linguistic domains is beyond the scope of this text. Interested readers are encouraged to consult Rickford (1999) for a discussion of the history and sociocultural implications of AAVE, Green (2002) for a linguistic analysis of AAVE, and Craig and Washington (2005) for a discussion of the impact of AAVE on educational outcomes in children in schools where other dialects are spoken. Although AAVE is often characterized as one dialect, recent studies have shown that it is not a monolithic dialect uninfluenced by regional dialects. Rather, for example, Hinton and Pollock (2000) showed that AAVE users from Davenport, Iowa, differed from those in Memphis, Tennessee, in their production of postvocalic /r/. Those in Davenport used it consistently, whereas those in Memphis were more variable in their usage.

The rest of this section is a brief summary of the comprehensive characteristics of the phonetic and phonological characteristics of AAVE presented by Thomas (2007). As in Thomas, we describe the features of AAVE relative to features of other North American dialects. Our use of terms like deletion or substitution does not mean to indicate, of course, that AAVE pronunciation is the consequence of widespread, chronic speech errors, like the deletion and substitution errors that children make. They are used merely for convenience and to make this discussion comparable to other descriptions of AAVE.

Metathesis. One feature of AAVE is occasional *metathesis*, i.e., switching of the order of sounds. An often-cited example is changing the order of word-final /s/-plus-stop consonant clusters, as in the pronunciation [æks] for *ask*.

Interdental Fricative Deletion. A second AAVE feature is the occasional absence of /θ/ or /ð/. Sometimes these are produced as a dentalized /t/ or /d/, as in [d̪ɪs] for *this*, or [wɪt̪] for *with*. Other times, they are produced as /f/ or /v/, respectively, as in [bæf] for *bath*, or [brʌvə] for *brother*.

Postvocalic /r/ Deletion. As indicated in the above transcription of *brother*, another characteristic of AAVE is the absence of postvocalic /r/. As mentioned earlier, this feature of AAVE is variable across different geographic regions. Even in the dialect, where /r/ production is variable, postvocalic /r/ was present in over 50 percent of utterances. One pattern related to /r/ that appears to be unique to AAVE is its deletion in word-medial position, as in the pronunciation [flɑːdə] for *Florida*, and after /θ/ in word-initial clusters, as in [θo͡ʊ] for *throw*.

/l/ Vocalization. AAVE also has a pattern of /l/ vocalization that parallels its postvocalic /r/ deletion. As described by Thomas (2007), there are three potential results of /l/ vocalization in AAVE. "One is vocalization to a mid- to high-back, rounded vowel or semivowel in the range of /o/ or /w/, as in *feel* produced as /fio/. This variant is common and widespread in European American speech as well as African American speech. A second variant is vocalization to schwa, as in [fiə] for *feel*. This variant is strongly associated with African American speech. The third variant is deletion of historical /l/, as in [pʰʊ] for *pull*." (p. 454). At least one study has compared African American and Caucasian speakers in a single dialect region, New York City, and found higher rates of /l/ vocalization in the AAVE speakers than in the non-AAVE speakers (Labov, Cohen, Robins, & Lewis, 1968).

Cluster Differences. AAVE has distinctive patterns of pronunciation of consonant clusters. In AAVE, the initial clusters /ʃr/ and /str/ are sometimes pronounced /sr/, as in [srɪmp] for *shrimp*; /str/ may be produced as /skr/ as in [skrit] for *street*. Word-final cluster differences include deletion of the stop in fricative-stop clusters, as in [tɛs] for *test*. Notice that such deletions are not uncommon in most dialects of American English at fast rates of speech and in certain phonological environments, such as when the next word begins with a consonant. However, cluster reduction is more consistent across different contexts in AAVE speakers than in speakers of other North American English dialects.

Researchers have documented a number of significant findings associated with phonetic variation in AAVE clusters. For example, the plural form of words like *desk* is produced by some AAVE speakers as [dɛsɪz], suggesting that these speakers' underlying representation of this word is /dɛs/ and not /dɛsk/. Wolfram and Thomas (2002) have reported that cluster reduction does not occur across the board in AAVE. As indicated previously, it is more common in word-final fricative-plus-stop and liquid-plus-stop sequences (i.e., *desk*, *hold*) than in stop-stop or nasal-stop sequences (i.e., *fact, lamp*). One particularly interesting aspect of cluster reduction in AAVE is that it interacts with a word's morphological structure: Consonants are less likely to be deleted when they code a regular past tense than when they do not. Hence, the same sequence, /pæst/, is more likely to be pronounced /pæs/ when it refers to the word *past* than the word *passed*.

Monopthongization. Many vowel-production patterns in AAVE mirror those in Southern regional dialects, such as the monophthongization of /a͡ɪ/ and /ɔ͡ɪ/, the fronting of /u/, and the merger of /ɪ/ and /ɛ/ before nasals.

Glide-Onset Differences. One vowel pronunciation pattern that appears to be unique to AAVE is the production of the sequence /ju/. In many British dialects of English, this sequence is produced after alveolar stops, as in the words *tune* and *noon*, as well as after bilabial and velar stops, as in *computer* and *cute*. Many North American dialects also produce /ju/ after bilabials and velars, but not after alveolars, where it is pronounced simply /u/ (i.e. [tun] and [nun]). In contrast, some AAVE speakers pronounce this sequence as /u/ in bilabial and velar contexts, as in [kəmputə] for *computer*.

Regional AAVE Differences. The label AAVE suggests a dialect common to African Americans regardless of geographic region. However, some studies have shown regional differences in AAVE, as discussed earlier in this section. For example, AAVE speakers in some regions appear to resist engaging in ongoing sound changes such as the several sound shifts we have described. Gordon (2000) examined AAVE speakers' engagement in the Northern Cities Chain Shift and found that AAVE speakers were less likely than Caucasian speakers to have that shift.

Dialectal Differences versus Speech-Sound Disorders. Finally, it is important to underscore that when features of AAVE discussed in this section are compared with features of children raised in Mainstream American English environments who have speech sound disorders, there are several superficial similarities. Some examples in both groups as discussed in this book are production of [f] or [v] in words with target /θ/ and /ð/, deletions of sounds in consonant clusters, or the vocalization of /r/ and /l/. Although the pronunciations are superficially similar, they arise from very different origins. The AAVE child speakers who produce these patterns do so because they have successfully emulated the language around them, whereas the pronunciations of children with a speech sound disorder reflect a delay or disorder in learning the target language. Clearly, speech-language pathologists who work with diverse populations—including children who speak AAVE—have to assess carefully the nature of the language input that children receive to determine the clinical significance of their speech patterns.

L1-Influenced English

The last type of phonetic variation we discuss in this chapter relates to people who speak English as a second language (L2), with their pronunciation of L2 being a consequence of the influence of the first language (L1). The pronunciation patterns of L2 English speakers result from a complicated interaction among many factors, including the similarity of the sound structures of English and those of the first language, the age at which English began, and the circumstances under which English was learned (i.e., whether through formal instruction in a non-English-speaking country, formal instruction in an English-speaking country, or naturalistically through exposure to English in an English-speaking country.) In general, the smallest phonetic differences between L2 speakers and native speakers of English will be in circumstances in which English was learned very early and where there is a strong similarity between English and the first language. In these circumstances, there is a good likelihood that the L2 speaker will sound like a native speaker.

To illustrate the role of the phonetic similarity of L1 and L2, consider some of the differences between English and Spanish. Spanish is the second most widely spoken language in the United States. According to the U.S. census, approximately 45 million Hispanic Americans speak Spanish as a first or second language. Many other Americans take courses in Spanish in school or university and have varying degrees of proficiency. Like many of the world's languages, Spanish has only five vowels, /i/, /e/, /ɑ/, /o/, /u/, whereas English has many more singleton (monophthong) vowels and diphthongs. Spanish speakers who do not know any English generally perceive the English vowels /i/ and /ɪ/ as instances of the Spanish vowel /i/. Not surprisingly, when these Spanish speakers learn English as a second language, they pronounce words like *Pete* and *pit* similarly, i.e., [pit]. Another example is the Spanish sounds /p/, /t/, and /k/, which are produced without aspiration (see Chapter 6). Consequently, L2 productions of these voiceless unaspirated stops in words like *Pete* and *pit* would be produced by a Spanish-influenced L2 English speaker with an unaspirated stop, i.e. [p˭it]. Again, this tendency would be strongest in people who learned English later in life. Finally, the Spanish vowels /e/ and /o/ are produced with little to no diphthongization; hence, words like *say* and *so* are pronounced [se] and [so] rather than [se͡ɪ] and [so͡ʊ]. In each of these examples, Spanish-speaking children who are exposed to English earlier have more native-sounding productions than children or adults who acquire English later in life.

One special case of L1-influenced English is Chicano English. Chicano English is a variety of English used by some members of Chicano communities (i.e., communities of people with Mexican heritage) in the southwestern United States. It is distinguished from Spanish-influenced English in that it is acquired from birth. That is, the distinctive pronunciation is not the result of the influence of Spanish on individuals' acquisition of English, but rather the influence of Spanish pronunciation on an entire speech community's pronunciations. A full description of the sound structure of Chicano English can be found in Santa Ana and Bayley (2004). The distinctive pronunciation patterns follow from Spanish-English differences. Spanish does not have the voiced alveolar fricative /z/; hence, words like *clothes* and *easy* are pronounced [klos] and [isi]. This pattern also occurs for /v/ in final position (as in [sef] for *save*). Elsewhere, words that are pronounced with /v/ in other North American dialects are pronounced with [b] (as in [bæli] for *valley*). Similarly, the interdental fricatives /θ/ and /ð/ are variably produced as [t̪], [f], or [s].

Spanish and English are very much global languages. As with English, there is substantial dialectal variation in Spanish. Speakers of Iberian Peninsula dialects pronounce the word *raza* ("race") as [raθa], whereas most speakers in Latin America pronounce it [rasa]. Speakers in Argentina pronounce the sequence *ll* in *caballo* as /ʃ/, as in the word [kaˈβaco], whereas those in Mexico say, [ʎ], as in [kaˈβaʎo]. The sound [ʎ] is a palatal lateral approximant, similar to the sequence of sounds /lj/ in the middle of words like million. The sound [β] is a voiced bilabial fricative, produced by moving the upper and lower lips close enough to one another to cause frication, but not close enough to cease airflow. It is an allophone of /b/ between vowels in many Latin American Spanish dialects. All of those differences would lead to slightly different Spanish-influenced English. In comparison to Mexican speakers, Argentine speakers are predicted to more closely produce English /ʃ/; compared to Latin American speakers, Peninsular speakers are predicted to more closely produce English /θ/.

The topic of why people produce particular patterns of variation has been debated extensively and is well outside of the scope of this introductory textbook. Given the complex influences that result in accented speech, it is impossible to determine with perfect accuracy how an L2 speaker "should" sound. As we have seen with regional and vernacular phonetic variation, this becomes challenging when a speech-language pathologist must determine whether a given child's pronunciation reflects the typical processes of acquiring a second language or a speech disorder that prevents successful first- or second-language acquisition. However, given a detailed understanding of the phonological structure of two languages, intelligent predictions and interpretations can be made.

An L2 Case Study

The Somali language is historically spoken in the horn of East Africa, in and around the country of Somalia. Long-standing political strife in that country has led to a substantial Somali population in Diaspora. A sizable population of Somali people has located in Minneapolis, as well as in Columbus, Ohio. Many Somali-speaking children attend the three largest school districts in Minnesota: Minneapolis, Saint Paul, and Anoka-Hennepin Public Schools. Therefore, there is a great need for Columbus, Ohio, and Central Minnesota speech-language pathologists to develop a knowledge base to determine which Somali children's pronunciations reflect typical L2 English pronunciation and which might reflect speech sound disorders. How might knowledge of the phonetic systems of Somali and English help us start to build this knowledge base?

Table 10.1 is a chart of a subset of Somali consonants, adapted from Orwin (1990). As shown, Somali and English have three fricatives in common, /f/, /s/, and /h/. Somali also has three fricatives that do not occur in English: the velar fricative /ʒ/, the palatal fricative /ç/ (a sound that is produced with a more-anterior tongue position than English /ʃ/, and both voiceless and voiced pharyngeal fricatives, [ħ] and [ʕ] (an additional Somali epiglottal fricative has been omitted and Somali does not have voiced fricatives). Unlike English, it has dental stops [t̪] and [d̪] and does not have alveolar stops /t/ and /d/. It has an additional stop place, the uvular /æ/. Based on the consonant information in Table 10.1, we might expect that Somali speakers learning English would produce words like *very* and *zoo* as [fɛrɪ] and [su], that is, substituting the most similar sounds that are shared by both languages, /f/ and /s/, for those that

TABLE 10.1
A Subset of the Somali Consonant System

	Bilabial	Dental	Alveolar	Retroflex	Palatal	Velar	Uvular	Pharyngeal	Glottal
Oral Stops	b	t̪ d̪		ɖ		k g	q		ʔ
Fricatives/ Affricate	f		s		ç t͡ʃ	x	χ	ħ ʕ	h
Nasal Stops	m		n						
Trill			r						
Lateral Approximant			l						
Glides	w				j				

(Adapted from Orwin, 1990).

are unique to English, /v/ and /z/. Somali has only one bilabial stop, /b/, whereas English has /b/ and /p/. Again, we might expect that Somali learners of English would produce words like *pen* as [bɛn], substituting the most similar sound shared by both languages, /b/, with the one unique to English, /p/. These are just a few of the differences in pronunciation that are predicted from Somali and English consonant systems. They illustrate how an understanding of the phonetic systems of two languages can help speech-language pathologists develop informed hypotheses about typical L2 differences based on the influence of L1.

DIFFERENCE OR DISORDER?

In several places we have tried to illustrate that the task of differentiating between difference and disorder is challenging for clinicians working with clients from diverse cultural and linguistic backgrounds. The challenge is great, in part, due to the complex and highly individual interactions within clients. Their cultures and the language(s) they speak make it challenging to develop lists of typical "differences" and differences that indicate "disorder." Yet in any large group of children, the probability is that some will have a speech disorder, and therefore speech-language pathologists must develop a set of skills to identify such children. Developing these skills is, of course, beyond the scope of this book. Interested readers are referred to Kohnert (2007). As an exercise in the clinical implication of differences versus disorder, find a standardized test of articulation for children. Transcribe the words in the test as they would be spoken in standard American English. Next, transcribe them as they would be spoken in any of the regional dialects, AAVE, or Spanish-Influenced American English. If, for example a typically developing AAVE-speaking child were to take this test and have all of her AAVE pronunciations counted as errors, how many of the test words would be scored as having errors? Finally, take the same test and make intelligent guesses of how a Somali L1 speaker would pronounce the words, based on the discussion above.

WORLD ENGLISHES

English is the official language or one of the official languages in many countries. Some obvious countries are Australia, New Zealand, and countries in the United Kingdom, whereas others might be more surprising, like Ghana, the Philippines, and Hong Kong. Importantly, English is an official language in four of the world's most populous countries, Bangladesh, India, Nigeria, and the United States. Not surprisingly, the variants spoken in India, Bangladesh, and Nigeria sound markedly different from one another and from the variety spoken in the United States and Canada. A discussion of the characteristics of each one of these variants is far outside of the scope of this chapter. However, it's important to keep in mind that many people who were born outside of North America speak a variety of English very different from North American dialects, even though they may have acquired it very early in life. A good example of this is the English spoken by people in the second most-populous country in the world, India, in which a great many people speak English. India is a multilingual country with a large number of official languages. Not surprisingly, many people in India speak two or more languages.

The considerable phonetic variation in the English spoken in India is due, in part, to the number and type of other languages a speaker knows and the frequency with which she or he listens to and speaks English on a daily basis. Nonetheless, some phonetic features of Indian-influenced English are relatively common. For example, Indian English speakers may have different patterns of stress placement than North American speakers, as in [sentɛ̍nsɪz] for *sentences* or [mɪ̍steɪk] for *mistake*. Indian English speakers may also produce unaspirated variants of /p/, /t/, and /k/, [d] and [t] in place of /ð/ and /θ/, and produce a labiodental approximant [ʋ] for /w/ and /v/. A full discussion of the sound structure of Indian English can be found in Gargesh (2008). These features potentially reduce the intelligibility of Indian English speakers for American English listeners. And as we saw previously with AAVE, certain errors also sound like the errors made by children with speech sound disorders, such as the lack of aspiration in word-initial /p/, /t/, and /k/, which mirrors the initial voicing errors made by some children with speech–sound disorder.

What about other Asian languages? Asia is the most populous continent on Earth. Over one billion people live in Mainland China. The majority speak a variety of Mandarin. In Japan, 130 million people speak Japanese. Seventy-two million people live on the Korean peninsula and speak Korean. Just as with other languages, people who speak Japanese, Mandarin, and Korean natively and who acquire English beyond adolescence have English that is phonetically distinctive.

Information about the Mandarin sound system should, once again, help you make predictions about the influence of Mandarin on English. For example, Mandarin has no non-nasal syllable-final consonants. Not surprisingly, heavily Mandarin-accented English is characterized by numerous errors in word-final consonants. Japanese and Korean have no phonemic distinction between /r/ and /l/, and Japanese- and Korean-accented English is characterized by a similar lack of contrast between these sounds. The lack of an /r/-/l/ contrast is arguably a widely held stereotype about all people from Asia. Interestingly, this is not a characteristic of Mandarin-accented English, because Mandarin, like English, has a contrast between /r/ and /l/.

PERSONAL CONSEQUENCES OF PHONETIC VARIATION

We have illustrated in this chapter that the pronunciation of sounds varies as a function of many considerations. In a more personal way, phonetic variation can encode various attributes of a speaker and hence can be used by listeners to make inferences about those attributes. Unfortunately, distinctive patterns of pronunciation have the potential to activate stereotypes of the attributes that different pronunciation patterns convey. One striking example is described in Purnell, Idsardi, and Baugh's (1999) study of the perception of phonetic variation in San Francisco. One of the three researchers made telephone calls to landlords in five different San Francisco-area communities, pretending to be interested in renting an apartment. In approximately equal numbers of calls, he used mainstream American English, Chicano English, or AAVE, all of which he self-reports speaking natively and having been exposed to during language development. This use of vocal disguise is called the "matched-guise" technique. In one of the five communities, a predominantly white community, fewer successful appointments to view the property were made when the Chicano English or AAVE guise were used than when the mainstream American English guise was used. In predominantly African American neighborhoods, more appointments were made when using the AAVE guise than the other two, although the size of the difference across guises was smaller than that for the white neighborhoods. Subsequent perception studies showed that the author's three speaking styles were readily identified by a different group of naïve listeners in a laboratory perception study simply from his pronunciations of the word *hello*. This study provides strong support to the perspective that subtle differences in pronunciation can underlie significant differences in social perceptions and interactions.

Knowledge of phonetic variation can also affect how people perceive phonemes. There is evidence that people identify the very same sound differently depending on what they believe about the person who produced it. One interesting example of this is presented by Drager (2011), who studied the perception of vowels spoken in New Zealand. In New Zealand English, the vowels in the words *dress* and *trap* have been changing over time. Older speakers of New Zealand English produce something close to [ɛ] in *dress*, and [æ] in *trap*, much as speakers of North American varieties of English. Younger speakers have begun to use different pronunciations. The vowel in *dress* is close to [ɪ], and their pronunciations and the vowel in *trap* is close to [ɛ]. These pronunciation differences reflect a normal sound change, as discussed earlier. That means that when New Zealanders hear the word [sɛt] they may be unclear whether it should be interpreted as the word *sat* or *set* because older speakers would use this pronunciation for the word *set* and younger speakers for the word *sat*. Drager used computer speech synthesis to make a continuum of sounds between [ɛ] and [æ]. The continuum was based on small changes in vowel formant frequencies. She then played these sounds to listeners accompanied by a picture of an older or a younger person and asked them to select the vowel they heard. When listeners were presented with a clear example of [æ], they labeled it as the vowel in the word *trap* regardless of whether it was paired with an older or a younger talker's face. But when a sound that wasn't quite [ɛ] or [æ] was presented, the apparent age of the talker affected the vowel they chose. Listeners were biased to label it as the vowel in *sat* when they thought it was a younger talker, and the vowel in *set* when they thought it was an older speaker. That is, when they thought it was a younger talker, they presumed that this talker would produce the vowel in *sat* similar to how an older talker would produce the vowel in *set*. They did so without being asked to pay attention to the age of the talker.

Drager's study is one of many showing that perception can be biased by expectations. Other work has shown that people's expectations about someone's age and sex affect how they perceive voiceless fricatives (Munson, 2009; Strand & Johnson, 1996), their beliefs about differences between Canadian and American English affecting vowel perception (Niedzielski, 1999), and their beliefs about how differences between black and white speakers of American English affect people's perception of final consonants (Staum Casasanto, 2008).

The studies noted above have examined social perceptions of adults' speech. Some studies have shown that these same biases affect the perception of children's speech. Munson, Edwards, Schellinger, Beckman, and Meyer (2010) showed that listeners are more likely to rate children's productions of frontally misarticulated /s/ as incorrect when they are led to believe that the child is younger (by presenting the child's fricative production preceded by the carrier phrase [a͡ɪ wɪwɪ ja͡ɪk], i.e., a misarticulated version of the sentence *I really like*) than when they are led to believe that the child is older (by presenting the same fricative after the same phrase produced correctly).

It is the position of the American Speech-Language-Hearing Association (ASHA, 1983) that "no dialectal variety of American English is a disorder or a pathological form of speech or language. Each dialect is adequate as a functional and effective variety of American English. Each serves a communicative function as well as a social-solidarity function. Each dialect maintains the communication network and the social construct of the community of speakers who use it. Furthermore, each is a symbolic representation of the geographic, historical, social, and cultural background of its speakers." Students are encouraged to read the entire text of this seminal position statement, available at from the ASHA website at www.asha.org/policy.

Conclusion

The phonetic transcription skills that you have gained by completing the practice modules and associated text in this book have given you the skills that you need to use narrow phonetic transcription in the clinic. This chapter has given you a guide for what you might expect in providing clinical services to people with speech disorders in different areas of the United States. We hope these same transcription skills and knowledge base about phonetics also enable you to be a good "dialect geographer"—that is, to learn and represent phonetically the local norms for pronunciation in the area in which you practice. More generally, we hope that this chapter has inspired you to be a linguistic ethnographer—someone who actively seeks to understand relevant social groupings and relevant social behaviors of members of different speech communities. This is not an ivory-tower venture: Understanding which pronunciations reflect typical variation and which indicate disorder is critical to assessing communication impairments in children. Doing this task accurately will rely on your careful, critical, and thoughtful observations about how language lives in the world around you. Recall that people's knowledge of variation affects how they hear speech sounds. Simply put, our ears can deceive us as well as inform us, and one of the sources of deception comes from our knowledge of how talkers vary from one another. Although there is no sure way to avoid biases, we can say with great certainty that acknowledging that they exist and knowing why they exist is a valuable first step to arriving at maximally objective phonetic transcription.

Further Reading

Students interested in a comprehensive and technical introduction to dialectal variation are referred to William Labov's three-volume work *Principles of Linguistic Change, Volume 1, Internal Factors* (1994), *Volume 2, Social Factors* (2001), and *Volume 3, Cognitive and Cultural Factors* (2010). This work reviews Labov's decades-long research on linguistic variation in the United States, particularly in New York City and in Philadelphia. Readers are also referred to Penelope Eckert's (2000) *Language Variation as Social Practice: The Linguistic Construction of Identity in Belten High*. This work complements that of Labov, in that it is an intensive observational study of linguistic variation in a suburban Detroit high school. It argues that different social groups construct and convey their identities through patterns of linguistic variation. Readers who are interested in a more general discussion of linguistic variation are referred to the books *The Story of English* and *Do You Speak American?*, both of which were produced for Public Television. The journals *American Speech*, published by the American Dialect Society, and *Language Variation and Change* regularly publish articles on speech-sound variation.

Other Resources

The World Wide Web is filled with resources on dialects, some of which are listed in this section. As is true with all information on the web, this information is maintained by different groups, and therefore reflects different standards of data collection and transcription. None of the sites is maintained by the authors of this book, and the transcription systems that are used by these sites sometimes differ from that used in this book. Nonetheless, they contain valuable pieces of information and interesting audio samples.

The International Dialects of English (IDEA) website (http://web.ku.edu/~idea) is maintained by the Department of Theater at the University of Kansas. The fact that this site is maintained by a theater program is not accidental: Being able to convincingly mimic a regional accent is a valuable skill for an actor to have. The IDEA website has numerous samples of varying quality, along with an orthographic transcription. It is a useful resource for students who want to simply listen to differences among different dialects.

The website http://csumc.wisc.edu/wep/index.html provides podcasts regarding the varieties of English used in the state of Wisconsin.

The Speech Accent Archive (http://accent.gmu.edu), has recordings of first- and second-language speakers of English from a wide variety of geographic regions in the United States and abroad. It is maintained by scholars in the George Mason University Department of English. The samples are phonetically transcribed. The level of transcription detail is different from that used in this book, although the website carefully details the different principles that were used in making the transcriptions.

The website www.soundcomparisons.com is maintained by researchers at the University of Edinburgh in Scotland. It has a large number of speakers producing a consistent set of words. Although there are relatively few samples from the United States, the website does have two productions by AAVE speakers, one from Chicago and one from North Carolina. Detailed phonetic transcriptions are provided.

The website http://aschmann.net/AmEng is maintained by a hobbyist with an interest in dialects. In addition to providing numerous original samples, it is a centralized archive of materials on dialects from other sources, such as the video-sharing site youtube.com. There are numerous links to videos of politicians and other public figures that illustrate different dialects. This Web page is extremely dense and contains a great deal of information.

Finally, the website www.pbs.org/speak is associated with the *Do You Speak American?* book and television series. This site has a quiz that tests your ability to categorize speakers' dialects (www.pbs.org/speak/seatosea/americanvarieties/map/map.html) and a quiz to measure how easily you can perceive the productions of someone who speaks an unfamiliar dialect (www.pbs.org/speak/ahead/change/vowelpower/vowel.html), along with many other interesting resources.

TRANSCRIPTION EXERCISES

MODULE TIME	
TOTAL	6:22
ELAPSED	00:00–06:22

Clinical Phonetics CD 1, Track 1
Transcription List A

TRANSCRIPTION KEY

1	me	[mi]	26	ramp	[ræmp]
2	on	[ɑn]	27	blue	[blu]
3	at	[æt]	28	treat	[trit]
4	two	[tu]	29	talc	[tælk]
5	top	[tɑp]	30	real	[ril]
6	keep	[kip]	31	ghoul	[gul] or [guəl]
7	moon	[mun]	32	nude	[nud]
8	knee	[ni]	33	calm	[kɑm]
9	back	[bæk]	34	barn	[bɑrn]
10	gap	[gæp]	35	rank	[ræŋk]
11	gang	[gæŋ]	36	creed	[krid]
12	dot	[dɑt]	37	tool	[tul] or [tuəl]
13	peaked	[pikt]	38	bomb	[bɑm]
14	ruined	[rund]	39	trapped	[træpt]
15	pond	[pɑnd]	40	clean	[klin]
16	poor	[pur]	41	long	[lɔŋ]
17	boot	[but]	42	rang	[ræŋ]
18	bat	[bæt]	43	tank	[tæŋk]
19	drop	[drɑp]	44	group	[grup]
20	teamed	[timd]	45	keel	[kil] or [kiəl]
21	league	[lig]	46	banged	[bæŋd]
22	loot	[lut]	47	lock	[lɑk]
23	wrong	[rɔŋ]	48	bleed	[blid]
24	lagged	[lægd]	49	clue	[klu]
25	bald	[bɔld]	50	grew	[gru]

MODULE TIME	
TOTAL	6:22
ELAPSED	00:00–06:22

Clinical Phonetics CD 1, Track 1
Transcription List A

TRANSCRIPTION SHEET

1	me	[ ]	26	ramp	[ ]
2	on	[ ]	27	blue	[ ]
3	at	[ ]	28	treat	[ ]
4	two	[ ]	29	talc	[ ]
5	top	[ ]	30	real	[ ]
6	keep	[ ]	31	ghoul	[ ]
7	moon	[ ]	32	nude	[ ]
8	knee	[ ]	33	calm	[ ]
9	back	[ ]	34	barn	[ ]
10	gap	[ ]	35	rank	[ ]
11	gang	[ ]	36	creed	[ ]
12	dot	[ ]	37	tool	[ ]
13	peaked	[ ]	38	bomb	[ ]
14	ruined	[ ]	39	trapped	[ ]
15	pond	[ ]	40	clean	[ ]
16	poor	[ ]	41	long	[ ]
17	boot	[ ]	42	rang	[ ]
18	bat	[ ]	43	tank	[ ]
19	drop	[ ]	44	group	[ ]
20	teamed	[ ]	45	keel	[ ]
21	league	[ ]	46	banged	[ ]
22	loot	[ ]	47	lock	[ ]
23	wrong	[ ]	48	bleed	[ ]
24	lagged	[ ]	49	clue	[ ]
25	bald	[ ]	50	grew	[ ]

MODULE TIME	
TOTAL	6:03
ELAPSED	06:22–12:25

Clinical Phonetics CD 1, Track 2
Transcription List B

TRANSCRIPTION KEY

1	yes	[j ɛ s]	26	rich	[r ɪ ʧ]
2	wish	[w ɪ ʃ]	27	veal	[v i l] or [v i ə l]
3	sheep	[ʃ i p]	28	Yale	[j e͡ɪ l]
4	faith	[f e͡ɪ θ]	29	jazz	[ʤ æ z]
5	thanks	[θ æ ŋ k s]	30	fence	[f e n s] or [f ɛ n t s]
6	rash	[r æ ʃ]	31	that	[ð æ t]
7	weaved	[w i v d]	32	whale	[w e͡ɪ l]
8	this	[ð ɪ s]	33	fish	[f ɪ ʃ]
9	waste	[w e͡ɪ s t]	34	yeast	[j i s t]
10	when	[ʍ ɛ n]	35	fizz	[f ɪ z]
11	fast	[f æ s t]	36	seethe	[s i ð]
12	vest	[v ɛ s t]	37	dwell	[d w ɛ l]
13	wage	[w e͡ɪ ʤ]	38	vast	[v æ s t]
14	cheese	[ʧ i z]	39	eighth	[e͡ɪ t θ]
15	thing	[θ ɪ ŋ]	40	hatch	[h æ ʧ]
16	thief	[θ i f]	41	sting	[s t ɪ ŋ]
17	stretch	[s t r ɛ ʧ]	42	hedge	[h ɛ ʤ]
18	badge	[b æ ʤ]	43	haze	[h e͡ɪ z]
19	share	[ʃ ɛ r]	44	his	[h ɪ z]
20	they	[ð e͡ɪ]	45	bear	[b ɛ r]
21	which	[ʍ ɪ ʧ]	46	heave	[h i v]
22	teach	[t i ʧ]	47	bath	[b æ θ]
23	yams	[j æ m z]	48	freeze	[f r i z]
24	gems	[ʤ ɛ m z]	49	shrill	[ʃ r ɪ l]
25	check	[ʧ ɛ k]	50	staged	[s t e͡ɪ ʤ d]

MODULE TIME	
TOTAL	6:03
ELAPSED	06:22–12:25

Clinical Phonetics CD 1, Track 2
Transcription List B

TRANSCRIPTION SHEET

1	yes	[ ]	26	rich	[ ]
2	wish	[ ]	27	veal	[ ]
3	sheep	[ ]	28	Yale	[ ]
4	faith	[ ]	29	jazz	[ ]
5	thanks	[ ]	30	fence	[ ]
6	rash	[ ]	31	that	[ ]
7	weaved	[ ]	32	whale	[ ]
8	this	[ ]	33	fish	[ ]
9	waste	[ ]	34	yeast	[ ]
10	when	[ ]	35	fizz	[ ]
11	fast	[ ]	36	seethe	[ ]
12	vest	[ ]	37	dwell	[ ]
13	wage	[ ]	38	vast	[ ]
14	cheese	[ ]	39	eighth	[ ]
15	thing	[ ]	40	hatch	[ ]
16	thief	[ ]	41	sting	[ ]
17	stretch	[ ]	42	hedge	[ ]
18	badge	[ ]	43	haze	[ ]
19	share	[ ]	44	his	[ ]
20	they	[ ]	45	bear	[ ]
21	which	[ ]	46	heave	[ ]
22	teach	[ ]	47	bath	[ ]
23	yams	[ ]	48	freeze	[ ]
24	gems	[ ]	49	shrill	[ ]
25	check	[ ]	50	staged	[ ]

MODULE TIME	
TOTAL	5:51
ELAPSED	12:25–18:16

Clinical Phonetics CD 1, Track 3
Transcription List C

TRANSCRIPTION KEY

1	jaw	[ʤ ɔ]	26	shoes	[ʃ u z]
2	joke	[ʤ o͡ʊ k]	27	alms	[ɑ m z]
3	psalm	[s ɑ m]	28	gold	[g o͡ʊ l d]
4	shoot	[ʃ u t]	29	crook	[k r ʊ k]
5	should	[ʃ ʊ d]	30	books	[b ʊ k s]
6	though	[ð o͡ʊ]	31	cough	[k ɔ f]
7	could	[k ʊ d]	32	whole	[h o͡ʊ l]
8	rouge	[r u ʒ]	33	thought	[θ ɔ t]
9	shawl	[ʃ ɔ l]	34	vault	[v ɔ l t]
10	Vaughn	[v ɔ n]	35	groom	[g r u m]
11	through	[θ r u]	36	looked	[l ʊ k t]
12	wash	[w ɔ ʃ] or [w ɑ ʃ]	37	yawn	[j ɔ n]
13	woods	[w ʊ d z]	38	slew	[s l u]
14	throw	[θ r o͡ʊ]	39	both	[b o͡ʊ θ]
15	stone	[s t o͡ʊ n]	40	gone	[g ɔ n]
16	halls	[h ɔ l z]	41	would	[w ʊ d]
17	strewn	[s t r u n]	42	nook	[n ʊ k]
18	palms	[p ɑ m z]	43	soul	[s o͡ʊ l]
19	stood	[s t ʊ d]	44	room	[r u m]
20	salt	[s ɔ l t]	45	whom	[h u m]
21	squaw	[s k w ɔ]	46	haunt	[h ɔ n t]
22	flowed	[f l o͡ʊ d]	47	those	[ð o͡ʊ z]
23	shook	[ʃ ʊ k]	48	swath	[s w ɑ θ]
24	food	[f u d]	49	draw	[d r ɔ]
25	spot	[s p ɑ t]	50	ought	[ɔ t]

MODULE TIME	
TOTAL	5:51
ELAPSED	12:25–18:16

Clinical Phonetics CD 1, Track 3
Transcription List C

TRANSCRIPTION SHEET

1	jaw	[ ]	26	shoes	[ ]
2	joke	[ ]	27	alms	[ ]
3	psalm	[ ]	28	gold	[ ]
4	shoot	[ ]	29	crook	[ ]
5	should	[ ]	30	books	[ ]
6	though	[ ]	31	cough	[ ]
7	could	[ ]	32	whole	[ ]
8	rouge	[ ]	33	thought	[ ]
9	shawl	[ ]	34	vault	[ ]
10	Vaughn	[ ]	35	groom	[ ]
11	through	[ ]	36	looked	[ ]
12	wash	[ ]	37	yawn	[ ]
13	woods	[ ]	38	slew	[ ]
14	throw	[ ]	39	both	[ ]
15	stone	[ ]	40	gone	[ ]
16	halls	[ ]	41	would	[ ]
17	strewn	[ ]	42	nook	[ ]
18	palms	[ ]	43	soul	[ ]
19	stood	[ ]	44	room	[ ]
20	salt	[ ]	45	whom	[ ]
21	squaw	[ ]	46	haunt	[ ]
22	flowed	[ ]	47	those	[ ]
23	shook	[ ]	48	swath	[ ]
24	food	[ ]	49	draw	[ ]
25	spot	[ ]	50	ought	[ ]

MODULE TIME	
TOTAL	9:29
ELAPSED	18:16–27:45

Clinical Phonetics CD 1, Track 4
Transcription List D

TRANSCRIPTION KEY

1	eyebrow	[a͡ɪ b r a͡ʊ]	32	ruckus	[r ʌ k ə s]
2	cowboy	[k a͡ʊ b ɔ͡ɪ]	33	foyer	[f ɔ͡ɪ ɚ]
3	rainbow	[r e͡ɪ n b o͡ʊ]	34	murder	[m ɝ d ɚ]
4	daylight	[d e͡ɪ l a͡ɪ t]	35	hurdle	[h ɝ d l̩][a]
5	highway	[h a͡ɪ w e͡ɪ]	36	cupboard	[k ʌ b ɚ d]
6	thyroid	[θ a͡ɪ r ɔ͡ɪ d]	37	turtle	[t ɝ t l̩][a]
7	lifeboat	[l a͡ɪ f b o͡ʊ t]	38	sister	[s ɪ s t ɚ]
8	railroad	[r e͡ɪ l r o͡ʊ d]	39	further	[f ɝ ð ɚ]
9	greyhound	[g r e͡ɪ h a͡ʊ n d]	40	sirloin	[s ɝ l ɔ͡ɪ n]
10	housewife	[h a͡ʊ s w a͡ɪ f]	41	surround	[s ɝ a͡ʊ n d]
11	boathouse	[b o͡ʊ t h a͡ʊ s]	42	station	[s t e͡ɪ ʃ ə n]
12	outside	[a͡ʊ t s a͡ɪ d]	43	acre	[e͡ɪ k ɚ]
13	lifeline	[l a͡ɪ f l a͡ɪ n]	44	survive	[s ɚ v a͡ɪ v]
14	downspout	[d a͡ʊ n s p a͡ʊ t]	45	alike	[ə l a͡ɪ k]
15	hyoid	[h a͡ɪ ɔ͡ɪ d]	46	buttons	[b ʌ t n̩ z][a]
16	roadhouse	[r o͡ʊ d h a͡ʊ s]	47	rusted	[r ʌ s t ɪ d]
17	skylight	[s k a͡ɪ l a͡ɪ t]	48	annoy	[ə n ɔ͡ɪ]
18	daytime	[d e͡ɪ t a͡ɪ m]	49	butter	[b ʌ ɾ ɚ]
19	townhouse	[t a͡ʊ n h a͡ʊ s]	50	certain	[s ɝ t n̩][a]
20	Friday	[f r a͡ɪ d e͡ɪ]	51	cradle	[k r e͡ɪ d l̩][a]
21	outline	[a͡ʊ t l a͡ɪ n]	52	surly	[s ɝ l ɪ]
22	rowboat	[r o͡ʊ b o͡ʊ t]	53	cousin	[k ʌ z n̩][a]
23	highlight	[h a͡ɪ l a͡ɪ t]	54	lighter	[l a͡ɪ t ɚ]
24	pie plate	[p a͡ɪ p l e͡ɪ t]	55	person	[p ɝ s ə n]
25	houseboy	[h a͡ʊ s b ɔ͡ɪ]	56	towers	[t a͡ʊ ɚ z]
26	slurred	[s l ɝ d]	57	subtle	[s ʌ t l̩][a]
27	suburb	[s ʌ b ɚ b]	58	putty	[p ʌ ɾ ɪ]
28	astound	[ə s t a͡ʊ n d]	59	pious	[p a͡ɪ ə s]
29	joyous	[ʤ ɔ͡ɪ ə s]	60	writer	[r a͡ɪ t ɚ]
30	rubber	[r ʌ b ɚ]	61	worthy	[w ɝ ð ɪ]
31	curtain	[k ɝ t n̩][a]	62	perturb	[p ɝ t ɝ b]

MODULE TIME	
TOTAL	9:29
ELAPSED	18:16–27:45

Clinical Phonetics CD 1, Track 4
Transcription List D

TRANSCRIPTION SHEET

1	eyebrow	[ ]	32	ruckus	[ ]
2	cowboy	[ ]	33	foyer	[ ]
3	rainbow	[ ]	34	murder	[ ]
4	daylight	[ ]	35	hurdle	[ ]
5	highway	[ ]	36	cupboard	[ ]
6	thyroid	[ ]	37	turtle	[ ]
7	lifeboat	[ ]	38	sister	[ ]
8	railroad	[ ]	39	further	[ ]
9	greyhound	[ ]	40	sirloin	[ ]
10	housewife	[ ]	41	surround	[ ]
11	boathouse	[ ]	42	station	[ ]
12	outside	[ ]	43	acre	[ ]
13	lifeline	[ ]	44	survive	[ ]
14	downspout	[ ]	45	alike	[ ]
15	hyoid	[ ]	46	buttons	[ ]
16	roadhouse	[ ]	47	rusted	[ ]
17	skylight	[ ]	48	annoy	[ ]
18	daytime	[ ]	49	butter	[ ]
19	townhouse	[ ]	50	certain	[ ]
20	Friday	[ ]	51	cradle	[ ]
21	outline	[ ]	52	surly	[ ]
22	rowboat	[ ]	53	cousin	[ ]
23	highlight	[ ]	54	lighter	[ ]
24	pie plate	[ ]	55	person	[ ]
25	houseboy	[ ]	56	towers	[ ]
26	slurred	[ ]	57	subtle	[ ]
27	suburb	[ ]	58	putty	[ ]
28	astound	[ ]	59	pious	[ ]
29	joyous	[ ]	60	writer	[ ]
30	rubber	[ ]	61	worthy	[ ]
31	curtain	[ ]	62	perturb	[ ]

MODULE TIME	
TOTAL	9:29
ELAPSED	18:16–27:45

Clinical Phonetics CD 1, Track 4
Transcription List D, Continued

TRANSCRIPTION KEY

63	dirty	[d ɝ ɾ ɪ]	67	mercy	[m ɝ s ɪ]
64	muscle	[m ʌ s l̩][a]	68	litter	[l ɪ t ɚ]
65	sucker	[s ʌ k ɚ]	69	mutton	[m ʌ t n̩][a]
66	lighter	[l a͡ɪ t ɚ]	70	tighten	[t a͡ɪ t n̩][a]

[a]Syllabic sounds [n̩] and [l̩] will be discussed in Chapter 6.

MODULE TIME	
TOTAL	9:29
ELAPSED	18:16–27:45

Clinical Phonetics CD 1, Track 4
Transcription List D, Continued

TRANSCRIPTION SHEET

63	dirty	[ ]	67	mercy	[ ]
64	muscle	[ ]	68	litter	[ ]
65	sucker	[ ]	69	mutton	[ ]
66	lighter	[ ]	70	tighten	[ ]

Clinical Phonetics CD 1, Track 5
Transcription List E

MODULE TIME	
TOTAL	5:00
ELAPSED	00:00–05:00

TRANSCRIPTION KEY

1	gasoline	[gæsəlin]	21	ratify	[ræɪfaɪ]
2	stationary	[steɪʃənɛrɪ]	22	tobacco	[tʊbæko]
3	bookshelf	[bʊkʃɛlf]	23	typewriter	[taɪpraɪɚ]
4	Arizona	[ɛrɪzoʊnə]	24	community	[kəmjunɪɾɪ]
5	vacation	[vekeɪʃən]	25	quarterback	[kwɔrtɚbæk]
6	sanctuary	[sæŋktʃuɛrɪ]	26	thesaurus	[θisɔrəs]
7	adjustment	[ədʒʌstmənt]	27	united	[junaɪɾəd]
8	Ohio	[ohaɪo]	28	dedication	[dɛdɪkeɪʃən]
9	Miami	[maɪæmɪ]	29	California	[kælɪfɔrnjə]
10	edition	[ɛdɪʃən]	30	atmosphere	[ætməsfɪr]
11	relinquish	[rɪlɪŋkwɪʃ]	31	substance	[sʌbstəns]
12	Chicago	[ʃɪkɑgo]	32	geography	[dʒiɑgrəfɪ]
13	university	[junɪvɝsɪɾɪ]	33	Wyoming	[waɪomɪŋ]
14	boisterous	[bɔɪstrəs]	34	dictionary	[dɪkʃənɛrɪ]
15	redeemer	[ridimɚ]	35	reduction	[rɪdʌkʃən]
16	rotation	[roteɪʃən]	36	multiply	[mʌltɪplaɪ]
17	decision	[disɪʒən]	37	television	[tɛləvɪʒən]
18	Seattle	[siætl̩]	38	Argentina	[ɑrdʒəntinə]
19	irritation	[ɪrɪteɪʃən]	39	profession	[profɛʃən]
20	Wisconsin	[wɪskɑnsɪn]	40	religion	[rɪlɪdʒɪn]

MODULE TIME	
TOTAL	5:00
ELAPSED	00:00–05:00

Clinical Phonetics CD 1, Track 5
Transcription List E

TRANSCRIPTION SHEET

1	gasoline	[ ]	21	ratify	[ ]
2	stationary	[ ]	22	tobacco	[ ]
3	bookshelf	[ ]	23	typewriter	[ ]
4	Arizona	[ ]	24	community	[ ]
5	vacation	[ ]	25	quarterback	[ ]
6	sanctuary	[ ]	26	thesaurus	[ ]
7	adjustment	[ ]	27	united	[ ]
8	Ohio	[ ]	28	dedication	[ ]
9	Miami	[ ]	29	California	[ ]
10	edition	[ ]	30	atmosphere	[ ]
11	relinquish	[ ]	31	substance	[ ]
12	Chicago	[ ]	32	geography	[ ]
13	university	[ ]	33	Wyoming	[ ]
14	boisterous	[ ]	34	dictionary	[ ]
15	redeemer	[ ]	35	reduction	[ ]
16	rotation	[ ]	36	multiply	[ ]
17	decision	[ ]	37	television	[ ]
18	Seattle	[ ]	38	Argentina	[ ]
19	irritation	[ ]	39	profession	[ ]
20	Wisconsin	[ ]	40	religion	[ ]

MODULE TIME	
TOTAL	2:34
ELAPSED	05:00–07:34

Clinical Phonetics CD 1, Track 6
Transcription List F

TRANSCRIPTION KEY

(Note: These samples represent casual, slurred speech.)

1	Where did you go?	[w ɛ r ʤ ə g o͡ʊ ↑]
2	He isn't here.	[h i ɪ z n h ɪ r ↓]
3	I don't know.	[a͡ɪ ɾ o n o͡ʊ ↓]
4	What are you going to do?	[w ʌ ʧ ə g ɔ n ə d u ↑]
5	It's something new.	[ɪ t s ʌ m ʔ m̩ n u ↓]
6	She's around the corner.	[ʃ i z ə r a͡ʊ n ə k ɔ r n ɚ ↓]
7	What's the time?	[w ʌ t s ə t a͡ɪ m ↑]
8	How do you spell it?	[h a͡ʊ j ə s p ɛ l ɪ t →]
9	It's in the red car.	[ɪ t s ɪ n ə r ɛ k ɑ r ↓]
10	Didn't you know that?	[d ɪ n ʧ ə n o͡ʊ æ t ↑]
11	I'm going now.	[a͡ɪ g o ɪ nː a͡ʊ ↓]
12	Want to stay here?	[w ɑ n ə s t e͡ɪ h ɪ r ↑]
13	Up and away.	[ʌ p m̩ ə w e͡ɪ ↓]
14	I've got to write it.	[a͡ɪ g ɑ ə r a͡ɪ ɾ ɪ t ↓]
15	Did you finish?	[d ɪ ʤ u f ɪ n ɪ ʃ ↑]

MODULE TIME	
TOTAL	2:34
ELAPSED	05:00–07:34

Clinical Phonetics CD 1, Track 6
Transcription List F

TRANSCRIPTION SHEET

(Note: These samples represent casual, slurred speech.)

1	Where did you go?	[ ]
2	He isn't here.	[ ]
3	I don't know.	[ ]
4	What are you going to do?	[ ]
5	It's something new.	[ ]
6	She's around the corner.	[ ]
7	What's the time?	[ ]
8	How do you spell it?	[ ]
9	It's in the red car.	[ ]
10	Didn't you know that?	[ ]
11	I'm going now.	[ ]
12	Want to stay here?	[ ]
13	Up and away.	[ ]
14	I've got to write it.	[ ]
15	Did you finish?	[ ]

MODULE TIME	
TOTAL	5:53
ELAPSED	07:34–13:27

Clinical Phonetics CD 1, Track 7
Vowels and Diphthongs Quiz

TRANSCRIPTION KEY

1	grass	[æ]	16	toes	[o͡ʊ]
2	house	[a͡ʊ]	17	twins	[ɪ]
3	man	[æ]	18	bird	[ɝ]
4	bed	[ɛ]	19	teeth	[i]
5	witch	[ɪ]	20	brush	[ʌ]
6	egg	[ɛ]	21	third	[ɝ]
7	book	[ʊ]	22	knife	[a͡ɪ]
8	five	[a͡ɪ]	23	saw	[ɔ] or [ɒ]
9	can	[æ]	24	play	[e͡ɪ]
10	keys	[i]	25	stove	[o͡ʊ]
11	flower	[a͡ʊ]	26	first	[ɝ]
12	box	[ɑ]	27	clown	[a͡ʊ]
13	cup	[ʌ]	28	boy	[ɔ͡ɪ]
14	hat	[æ]	29	fish	[ɪ]
15	tail	[e͡ɪ]	30	smoke	[o͡ʊ]

MODULE TIME	
TOTAL	5:53
ELAPSED	07:34–13:27

Clinical Phonetics CD 1, Track 7
Vowels and Diphthongs Quiz

TRANSCRIPTION SHEET

1	grass	[ ]	16	toes	[ ]
2	house	[ ]	17	twins	[ ]
3	man	[ ]	18	bird	[ ]
4	bed	[ ]	19	teeth	[ ]
5	witch	[ ]	20	brush	[ ]
6	egg	[ ]	21	third	[ ]
7	book	[ ]	22	knife	[ ]
8	five	[ ]	23	saw	[ ]
9	can	[ ]	24	play	[ ]
10	keys	[ ]	25	stove	[ ]
11	flower	[ ]	26	first	[ ]
12	box	[ ]	27	clown	[ ]
13	cup	[ ]	28	boy	[ ]
14	hat	[ ]	29	fish	[ ]
15	tail	[ ]	30	smoke	[ ]

MODULE TIME	
TOTAL	7:28
ELAPSED	13:27–20:55

Clinical Phonetics CD 1, Track 8
Transcription Quiz

TRANSCRIPTION KEY

1	rabbit	[r æ b ɪ t]	21	monkey	[m ʌ ŋ k ɪ]
2	glasses	[g l æ s ɪ z]	22	boat	[b o͡ʊ t]
3	chair	[t ʃ e͡ɪ r] or [t ʃ ɛ r]	23	wagon	[w e g ɪ n] or [w e͡ɪ g ɪ n]
4	teeth	[t i θ]	24	smooth	[s m u ð]
5	shoe	[ʃ u]	25	fish	[f ɪ ʃ]
6	this	[ð ɪ s]	26	measuring cup	[m ɛ ʒ ɚ ɪ ŋ k ʌ p]
7	ladder	[l æ d ɚ]	27	jumping	[ʤ ʌ m p ɪ ŋ]
8	station	[s t e͡ɪ ʃ ɪ n]	28	husky	[h ʌ s k ɪ]
9	seal	[s i l]	29	matches	[m æʧ ə z]
10	pages	[p e͡ɪ ʤ ɪ z]	30	hat	[h æ t]
11	hanger	[h e͡ɪ ŋ ɚ]	31	toast	[t o͡ʊ s t]
12	beige	[b e͡ɪ ʒ] or [p e͡ɪ ʒ]	32	cage	[k e͡ɪ ʤ]
13	toes	[t o͡ʊ z]	33	thumb	[θ ʌ m]
14	garage	[g ə r ɑ ʤ]	34	household	[h a͡ʊ s h o͡ʊ l d]
15	valentine	[v æ l ɛ n t a͡ɪ n]	35	carrots	[k ɛ r ɪ t s]
16	baby	[b e͡ɪ b ɪ]	36	pages	[p e͡ɪ ʤ ɪ z]
17	feather	[f ɛ ð ɚ]	37	boat	[b o͡ʊ t]
18	car	[k ɑ r]	38	bus	[b ʌ s]
19	toothache	[t u θ e͡ɪ k]	39	pipe	[p a͡ɪ p]
20	dishes	[d ɪ ʃ ɪ z]	40	toothache	[t u θ e͡ɪ k]

MODULE TIME	
TOTAL	7:28
ELAPSED	13:27–20:55

Clinical Phonetics CD 1, Track 8
Transcription Quiz

TRANSCRIPTION SHEET

1	rabbit	[ ]	21	monkey	[ ]
2	glasses	[ ]	22	boat	[ ]
3	chair	[ ]	23	wagon	[ ]
4	teeth	[ ]	24	smooth	[ ]
5	shoe	[ ]	25	fish	[ ]
6	this	[ ]	26	measuring cup	[ ]
7	ladder	[ ]	27	jumping	[ ]
8	station	[ ]	28	husky	[ ]
9	seal	[ ]	29	matches	[ ]
10	pages	[ ]	30	hat	[ ]
11	hanger	[ ]	31	toast	[ ]
12	beige	[ ]	32	cage	[ ]
13	toes	[ ]	33	thumb	[ ]
14	garage	[ ]	34	household	[ ]
15	valentine	[ ]	35	carrots	[ ]
16	baby	[ ]	36	pages	[ ]
17	feather	[ ]	37	boat	[ ]
18	car	[ ]	38	bus	[ ]
19	toothache	[ ]	39	pipe	[ ]
20	dishes	[ ]	40	toothache	[ ]

MODULE TIME	
TOTAL	7:05
ELAPSED	20:55–28:00

Clinical Phonetics CD 1, Track 9
Diacritics Examples

TRANSCRIPTION KEY

	NORMAL SOUND	MODIFIED SOUND	DISTORTION	COMMENTS[1]
1	[æ]	[æ̃]	Nasalized vowel	
	[i]	[ĩ]		
2	[s]	[s͋]	Fricative with nasal emission	
	[ʃ]	[ʃ͋]		This distortion is typically difficult to perceive.
3	ran [ræn]	ran [ræ͊n]	Denasalized vowel	The nasal consonant is also denasalized.
	mean [min]	mean [mi͊n]		The nasal consonants are also denasalized.
4	[e]	[eɪ̹]	Rounded vowel	(Diphthong)
	[i]	[iˀ]		
5	[u]	[uͨ]	Unrounded vowel	
	[oʊ]	[oʊͨ]		(Diphthong)
6	[s]	[sᷱ]	Labialized fricative	Somewhat whistled [͎] as well
	she [ʃi]	shoe [ʃᷱu]		
7	we [wi]	we [wͫi]	Nonlabialized consonant	
	way [we]	way [wͫeɪ]		
8	see [si]	see [s̪i]	Dentalized/s/	
	ice [aɪs]	ice [aɪs̪]		
9	see [si]	see [sʲi]	Palatalized /s/	
	ice [aɪs]	ice [aɪsʲ]		
10	see [si]	see [s̭i]	Lateralized /s/	
	ice [aɪs]	ice [aɪs̭]		
11	see [si]	see [s̢i]	Retroflexed /s/	
	ice [aɪs]	ice [aɪs̭]		Hear the whistle [͎].
12	law [lɔ]	law [l̰ɔ]	Velarized /l/	
	all [ɔl]	all [ɔl̰]		
13	[eɪ]	[e̠ɪ]	Centralized vowel	(Diphthong)
	sit [sɪt]	sit [sɪ̠t]		

[1]Some of these exemplars sound "unnatural" or forced, relative to the way they sound in the examples from speakers with disorders to follow. You may want to write in your own comments and questions at this point, in preparation for the training modules in Chapters 8 and 9.

MODULE TIME	
TOTAL	7:05
ELAPSED	20:55–28:00

Clinical Phonetics CD 1, Track 9
Diacritics Examples, Continued

TRANSCRIPTION KEY

14		[æ]		[æ̠]	Retracted vowel	
	her	[hɚ]	her	[hɚ̠]		
15		[o͡ʊ]		[o͡ʊ̟]	Advanced vowel	(Diphthong)
	paw	[pɔ]	paw	[pɔ̟]		
16		[æ]		[æ̝]	Raised vowel	
	men	[mɛn]	men	[mɛ̝n]		
17		[e͡ɪ]		[e͡ɪ̞]	Lowered vowel	(Diphthong)
	hid	[hɪd]	hid	[hɪ̞d]		
18	see	[si]	see	[s̬i]	Partially voiced consonant	
	ice	[a͡ɪs]	ice	[a͡ɪs̬]		
19	zoo	[zu]	zoo	[z̥u]	Partially devoiced consonant	
	is	[ɪz]	is	[ɪz̥]		
20		[ɑ]		[ɑ̣]	Glottalized vowel	
	man	[mæn]	man	[mæ̣n]		
21		[ɑ]		[ɑ̤]	Breathy vowel	
		[i]		[i̤]		
22	key	[ki]	key	[k͓i]	Frictionalized stop	
	stay	[ste͡ɪ]	stay	[st͓e͡ɪ]		
23		[pɑ]		[p˭ɑ]	Unaspirated stop	
	too	[tu]	too	[t˭u]		
24	up	[ʌp]	up	[ʌp̚]	Unreleased stop	
	sat	[sæt]	sat	[sæt̚]		

MODULE TIME	
TOTAL	3:14
ELAPSED	00:00–03:14

Clinical Phonetics CD 2, Track 1
Vowels and Diphthongs Module 1: Vowel and Diphthong Substitutions
TRANSCRIPTION KEY

	STIMULUS WORD	INTENDED	CONSENSUS	ALTERNATIVES	COMMENTS
1	sheep	[i]	[ɪ]		Make no mistake about the [p]!
2	penny	[ɛ]	[ʌ]		
3	bib	[ɪ]	[ʌ]	[æ], [æ̞], [æᵊ]	
4	wagon	[æ]	[æ]	[æ̞], [ɛᴵ]	
5	book	[ʊ]	[ʌ]		
6	light	[a͡ɪ]	[a͡ɪ]		
7	house	[a͡ʊ]	[ɔ]		
8	feather	[ɛ]	[ɑ]		
9	fish	[ɪ]	[ʌ]	[ɛ]	
10	rabbit	[æ]	[ʌ]	[a], [ɔ]	
11	toothache	[u]	[u]		
12	behind	[ə] or [ɪ]	[i]		Normally unstressed . . . as a preposition!
13	potatoes	[e͡ɪ]	[a͡ɪ]	[e͡ɪ]	
14	chair	[e]	[ɛ]	[e̝], [ɛ̞]	
15	baby	[e͡ɪ]	[i]	[i̝]	
16	crackers	[æ]	[ɑ]		

Notes: Students typically do well on this first module. If you did not, you may want to review the vowel and diphthong symbols. You will have difficulty with the vowel and diphthong modules that follow if you are not yet comfortable with all vowel and diphthong symbols. Try to arrange for a practice session with someone else to be sure you are symbolizing all the vowels and diphthongs correctly. Differences in dialectal background may be a factor. Before proceeding to the remaining modules, be sure you can discriminate and symbolize each of the vowels and diphthongs.

MODULE TIME	
TOTAL	3:14
ELAPSED	00:00–03:14

Clinical Phonetics CD 2, Track 1
Vowels and Diphthongs Module 1: Vowel and Diphthong Substitutions

TRANSCRIPTION SHEET

	STIMULUS WORD	INTENDED	PERCEIVED	ALTERNATIVES	COMMENTS
1	sh<u>ee</u>p	[i]	[ ]		
2	p<u>e</u>nny	[ɛ]	[ ]		
3	b<u>i</u>b	[ɪ]	[ ]		
4	w<u>a</u>gon	[æ]	[ ]		
5	b<u>oo</u>k	[ʊ]	[ ]		
6	l<u>igh</u>t	[a͡ɪ]	[ ]		
7	h<u>ou</u>se	[a͡ʊ]	[ ]		
8	f<u>ea</u>ther	[ɛ]	[ ]		
9	f<u>i</u>sh	[ɪ]	[ ]		
10	r<u>a</u>bbit	[æ]	[ ]		
11	t<u>oo</u>thache	[u]	[ ]		
12	b<u>e</u>hind	[ə] or [ɪ]	[ ]		
13	pot<u>a</u>toes	[e͡ɪ]	[ ]		
14	ch<u>ai</u>r	[e]	[ ]		
15	b<u>a</u>by	[e͡ɪ]	[ ]		
16	cr<u>a</u>ckers	[æ]	[ ]		

Clinical Phonetics CD 2, Track 2
Vowels and Diphthongs Module 2: Vowel and Diphthong Modifications

TRANSCRIPTION KEY

MODULE TIME	
TOTAL	5:07
ELAPSED	03:14–08:21

EXAMPLES

NORMAL	[æ]	RETRACTED	[æ̠]
	[hɝ]		[hɝ̠]
NORMAL	[o]	ADVANCED	[o̟]
	[pɑ]		[pɑ̟]
NORMAL	[æ]	RAISED	[æ̝a]
	[mɛn]		[mɛ̝n]
NORMAL	[e]	LOWERED	[e̞]
	[hɪd]		[hɪ̞d]
NORMAL	[e]	CENTRALIZED	[e̱]
	[sɪt]		[sɪ̱t]

	STIMULUS WORD	INTENDED	CONSENSUS	ALTERNATIVES	COMMENTS
1	pa<u>g</u>es	[e͡ɪ]	[e͡ɪ]	[i̞]	
2	be<u>d</u>	[ɛ]	[ɛ̞]	[æ̝], [æ]	
3	ma<u>t</u>ches	[æ]	[æ̠]	[a]	
4	ha<u>t</u>	[æ]	[æ̠]	[ʌ]	
5	ho<u>m</u>e	[o͡ʊ]	[o͡ʊ]		
6	ca<u>r</u>	[ɑ]	[ɑ]	[ɑ̟]	
7	ha<u>m</u>mer	[æ]	[æ̝]	[e͡ɪ̞]	
8	do<u>g</u>	[ɔ]	[ɔː]		Lengthened (see Module 6)
9	wi<u>t</u>ch	[ɪ]	[ɪ]	[ɪ̞], [ɛ̝]	Centralized: [_]
10	fo<u>r</u>k	[ɔ]	[ʊ]	[ʊ̝], [o]	
11	ca<u>t</u>	[æ]	[ɑ]	[ɑ̟], [ɔ̟], [a]	
12	ca<u>n</u>	[æ]	[æ̠]	[ɑ], [ɑ̟]	Slightly lengthened; breathy
13	to<u>p</u>	[ɔ]	[ɔ]	[ɑ]	Dialectal variants [ɔ] versus [ɑ]
14	wa<u>t</u>ch	[ɔ]	[ʌ]	[ʌ̠], [ɔ̟]	Notable
15	na<u>i</u>ls	[e͡ɪ]	[e͡ɪ]	[æ], [a͡ɪ̊]	Lower and retracted
16	pe<u>n</u>cil	[ɛ]	[ɪ̞]	[ɛ̝]	
17	ba<u>b</u>y	[e͡ɪ]	[e͡ɪ]		Almost [ɪ]
18	be<u>d</u>	[ɛ]	[æ̝]	[ɛ̞]	
19	blo<u>c</u>ks	[ɑ]	[ɑ]	[ɑ̟]	Normal for this dialect
20	la<u>m</u>p	[æ]	[æ̝]		

Notes: As you can see, agreement among transcribers for vowel–diphthong modification is seldom very high. A good way to review these materials is to replay the tape, repeating out loud after each item what you transcribed and the consensus judgment. Another helpful procedure is to say the target vowel and the vowel closest to the modification—then try to make the consensus intermediate vowel. Be sure to assess your agreement by a "liberal" criterion, using the concept of *functional equivalence* described in former Appendix D on the website.

Clinical Phonetics CD 2, Track 2
Vowels and Diphthongs Module 2:
Vowel and Diphthong Modifications

TRANSCRIPTION SHEET

MODULE TIME	
TOTAL	5:07
ELAPSED	03:14–08:21

EXAMPLES			
NORMAL	[æ]	RETRACTED	[æ̠]
	[hɝ]		[hɝ̠]
NORMAL	[o]	ADVANCED	[o̟]
	[pɑ]		[pɑ̟]
NORMAL	[æ]	RAISED	[æ̝]
	[mɛn]		[mɛ̝n]
NORMAL	[e]	LOWERED	[e̞]
	[hɪd]		[hɪ̞d]
NORMAL	[e]	CENTRALIZED	[e̱]
	[sɪt]		[sɪ̱t]

	STIMULUS WORD	INTENDED	PERCEIVED	ALTERNATIVES	COMMENTS
1	pages	[e͡ɪ]	[ ]		
2	bed	[ɛ]	[ ]		
3	matches	[æ]	[ ]		
4	hat	[æ]	[ ]		
5	home	[o͡ʊ]	[ ]		
6	car	[ɑ]	[ ]		
7	hammer	[æ]	[ ]		
8	dog	[ɔ]	[ ]		
9	witch	[ɪ]	[ ]		
10	fork	[ɔ]	[ ]		
11	cat	[æ]	[ ]		
12	can	[æ]	[ ]		
13	top	[ɔ]	[ ]		
14	watch	[ɔ]	[ ]		
15	nails	[e͡ɪ]	[ ]		
16	pencil	[ɛ]	[ ]		
17	baby	[e͡ɪ]	[ ]		
18	bed	[ɛ]	[ ]		
19	blocks	[ɑ]	[ ]		
20	lamp	[æ]	[ ]		

MODULE TIME	
TOTAL	1:46
ELAPSED	08:21–10:07

Clinical Phonetics CD 2, Track 3
Vowels and Diphthongs Module 3: Central Vowels

TRANSCRIPTION KEY

	STIMULUS WORD	INTENDED	CONSENSUS	ALTERNATIVES	COMMENTS
1	lion	[ə] or [ɪ]	[ɪ]		[l ɑ ɪ n]
2	scissors	[ɚ]	[ɪ]	[ɪ̞], [ɪ̠], [ɛ̠]	
3	flower	[ɚ]	[ʌ]	[ɑ̘]	Note final stress.
4	behind	[ə] or [ɪ]	[ɪ]	[ɪ̝], [ɪ̞]	
5	garage	[ə]	[ə]		
6	glasses	[ə] or [ɪ]	[ə]	[ɪ̠]	
7	carrots	[ə]	[ɪ]	[ɛ̠]	
8	dishes	[ə] or [ɪ]	[ə]		

Notes: As discussed in the text, discrimination of vowels in unstressed syllables is difficult. However, these discriminations do become of interest diagnostically in the case of people who have difficulty acquiring the stress patterns of English. Suggestions for "hearing" these modifications are the same as those for the preceding module.

MODULE TIME	
TOTAL	1:46
ELAPSED	08:21–10:07

Clinical Phonetics CD 2, Track 3
Vowels and Diphthongs Module 3: Central Vowels

TRANSCRIPTION SHEET

	STIMULUS WORD	INTENDED	PERCEIVED	ALTERNATIVES	COMMENTS
1	li<u>o</u>n	[ə] or [ɪ]	[ ]		
2	sciss<u>or</u>s	[ɚ]	[ ]		
3	flow<u>er</u>	[ɚ]	[ ]		
4	b<u>e</u>hind	[ə] or [ɪ]	[ ]		
5	g<u>a</u>rage	[ə]	[ ]		
6	glass<u>e</u>s	[ə] or [ɪ]	[ ]		
7	carr<u>o</u>ts	[ə]	[ ]		
8	dish<u>e</u>s	[ə] or [ɪ]	[ ]		

MODULE TIME	
TOTAL	3:44
ELAPSED	10:07–13:51

Clinical Phonetics CD 2, Track 4 Vowels and Diphthongs Module 4: Vowel–Diphthong Substitutions, Modifications, and Central Vowels

TRANSCRIPTION KEY

	STIMULUS WORD	INTENDED	CONSENSUS	ALTERNATIVES	COMMENTS
1	cake	[eɪ]	[eɪ]		
2	bed	[ɛ]	[ʌ]		
3	table	[eɪ]	[ɑɪ]	[ɛᶦ]	
4	blocks	[ɑ]	[ʌ]		
5	light	[ɑɪ]	[ɑɪ]		
6	book	[ʊ]	[ʌ]		
7	dishes	[ɪ], [ə]	[ɪ], [ɪ]	[ɛ], [ɪ̝]	Said with equal stress
8	gun	[ʌ]	[ʌ]		
9	angels	[eɪ]	[eɪ]		[ẽɪ n ʤ oʊ z̥]
10	ladder	[æ]	[ɑ]	[æ̟]	
11	hat	[æ]	[a]	[ʌ̠], [æ̟]	For discussion, see Chapter 4, Front Series
12	apple	[æ]	[ɑ]	[ɑ̠], [æ̟]	
13	bunny likes carrots	[ɛ], [ə]	[ɛ], [ʌ]		[b ʌ n ɪ lak k ɛ w ʌ]
14	elephant	[ɛ], [ə]	[ɛ̝], [ɛ]	[ɛ]	[ɛ̝ l̰ f ɛ n t]
15	scissors	[ɪ], [ɚ]	[ɪ], [ə]		
16	plane	[eɪ]	[ɑɪ]	[eɪ̝], [ɑ̞]	
17	baby	[eɪ], [ɪ]	[eɪ], [ɪ]	[eɪ̝]	
18	ring	[ɪ]	[ɪ̠]	[ɛ]	[r̫ ɪ̠̃ ŋ]

Notes: Here's a good place to calculate your agreement with the transcription key. Appendix D on the website presents the procedures. Try calculating your exact agreement with either the "consensus" entry or any of the alternative entries. How are you doing? Look at those items in which you *disagree*. Can you determine any pattern to your differences with the key? Which types of sound changes will require more practice?

MODULE TIME	
TOTAL	3:44
ELAPSED	10:07–13:51

Clinical Phonetics CD 2, Track 4 Vowels and Diphthongs Module 4: Vowel–Diphthong Substitutions, Modifications, and Central Vowels

TRANSCRIPTION SHEET

	STIMULUS WORD	INTENDED	PERCEIVED	ALTERNATIVES	COMMENTS
1	cake	[e͡ɪ]	[ ]		
2	bed	[ɛ]	[ ]		
3	table	[e͡ɪ]	[ ]		
4	blocks	[ɑ]	[ ]		
5	light	[a͡ɪ]	[ ]		
6	book	[ʊ]	[ ]		
7	dishes	[ɪ], [ə]	[ ], [ ]		
8	gun	[ʌ]	[ ]		
9	angels	[e͡ɪ]	[ ]		
10	ladder	[æ]	[ ]		
11	hat	[æ]	[ ]		
12	apple	[æ]	[ ]		
13	bunny likes carrots	[ɛ], [ə]	[ ], [ ]		
14	elephant	[ɛ], [ə]	[ ], [ ]		
15	scissors	[ɪ], [ɚ]	[ ], [ ]		
16	plane	[e͡ɪ]	[ ]		
17	baby	[e͡ɪ], [ɪ]	[ ], [ ]		
18	ring	[ɪ]	[ ]		

MODULE TIME	
TOTAL	4:09
ELAPSED	13:51–18:00

Clinical Phonetics CD 2, Track 5
Vowels and Diphthongs Module 5: Multiple Element Changes

TRANSCRIPTION KEY

	STIMULUS WORD	INTENDED	CONSENSUS	ALTERNATIVES	COMMENTS
1	dog	[ɔ]	[a͡ʊ]	[ʌʊ], [a͡ʊ]	
2	swing	[ɪ]	[ɪ]	[ɪ̞], [ɛ̝]	
3	hat	[æ]	[æ ^{ə}]		[h æ ^{ə} t]!
4	shoe	[u]	[u ^{ɪ}]	[u ^{ə}]	Breathy offglide
5	bell	[ɛ]	[ɛ]		
6	toothbrush	[u]	[u ^{ɪ}]		
7	smooth	[u]	[u ^{ə}]		Hoarse voice; breathy offglide
8	key	[i]	[iː ^{ə}]	[iː ^{ɪ}]	
9	hat	[æ]	[e ^{ɪ}]	[æ̝ ^{ɪ}], [ɛ̞ ^{ɪ}]	
10	saw	[ɔ]	[a͡ʊ]	[ɑ ^{o}], [ɔ ^{o}]	
11	keys	[i]	[i]		
12	box	[ɑ]	[ɑ ^{ʊ}]	[ɑ ^{ə}], [ɑ ^{ɔ}]	
13	man	[æ]	[ẽ ^{ə}]	[æ̃ə]	
14	shoe	[u]	[u ^{ə}]	[u ː^{ə}]	
15	house	[a͡ʊ]	[a͡ʊ ^{ə}]		
16	tree	[i]	[i]	[ə i]	Slight onglide?
17	gun	[ʌ]	[ʌ]		
18	saw	[ɔ]	[ɔ ^{ə}]		
19	on	[ɔ]	[ʊ ^{ə}]	[ɔ ^{ə}]	
20	tree	[i]	[i ^{ə}]		

Notes: For all but the most detailed phonological inquiry, the distinction between an on-/offglide and diphthongization is unimportant. However, most of the multiple elements here (the addition of a vowel) should be readily discriminable. Practice of the type suggested in the text, making diphthongs from monophthongs, should be helpful if you are having difficulty hearing the intrusive vowels.

MODULE TIME	
TOTAL	4:09
ELAPSED	13:51–18:00

Clinical Phonetics CD 2, Track 5 Vowels and Diphthongs Module 5: Multiple Element Changes

TRANSCRIPTION SHEET

	STIMULUS WORD	INTENDED	PERCEIVED	ALTERNATIVES	COMMENTS
1	dog	[ɔ]	[ ]		
2	swing	[ɪ]	[ ]		
3	hat	[æ]	[ ]		
4	shoe	[u]	[ ]		
5	bell	[ɛ]	[ ]		
6	toothbrush	[u]	[ ]		
7	smooth	[u]	[ ]		
8	key	[i]	[ ]		
9	hat	[æ]	[ ]		
10	saw	[ɔ]	[ ]		
11	keys	[i]	[ ]		
12	box	[ɑ]	[ ]		
13	man	[æ]	[ ]		
14	shoe	[u]	[ ]		
15	house	[a͡ʊ]	[ ]		
16	tree	[i]	[ ]		
17	gun	[ʌ]	[ ]		
18	saw	[ɔ]	[ ]		
19	on	[ɔ]	[ ]		
20	tree	[i]	[ ]		

MODULE TIME	
TOTAL	3:28
ELAPSED	18:00–21:28

Clinical Phonetics CD 2, Track 6
Vowels and Diphthongs Module 6: Vowel and Diphthong Lengthening

TRANSCRIPTION KEY

	STIMULUS WORD	INTENDED	CONSENSUS	ALTERNATIVES	COMMENTS
1	he's running in a pile of dirt	[i]	[iː]		
2	chicken	[ɪ]	[ɪ]		
3	zipper	[ɚ]	[ɝ]	[ɝ ᵊ]	Change in stress
4	ladder	[æ]	[aː]	[æː]	
5	car	[ɑ]	[ɑː]		
6	elephant	[ɛ]	[aː]	[ɛ̝ː], [æ̞]	Almost sounds like "Alan Funt"!
7	finger	[ɪ]	[ɪ]		
8	bathe	[e͡ɪ]	[e͡ɪː]		
9	shoe	[u]	[uː]		
10	bell	[ɛ]	[ɛː]	[ɛ̝ː]	
11	blocks	[ɑ]	[ɑː]		
12	balloons	[u]	[uː]		The /n/ is slightly lengthened also.
13	top	[ɔ]	[ɔ]		
14	saw	[ɔ]	[ɑːᵊ]	[ɑːᶷᵊ], [ɔːᶷᵊ]	The vowel changes.
15	potato	[e͡ɪ]	[e͡ɪː]		

Notes: Your response should be in fairly high agreement with the key for this module. Notice that use of the lengthening diacritic is a dichotomous matter: You either perceived the target sound as lengthened or you did not. Did you use this diacritic more or less often than the key? Keep in mind that the consensus entry represents a conservative use of this diacritic. That is, the diacritic is used only when the vowel is readily perceived as lengthened. This is a conservative response definition, as illustrated in Chapter 7—"innocent until proven guilty."

MODULE TIME	
TOTAL	3:28
ELAPSED	18:00–21:28

Clinical Phonetics CD 2, Track 6
Vowels and Diphthongs Module 6:
Vowel and Diphthong Lengthening

TRANSCRIPTION SHEET

	STIMULUS WORD	INTENDED	PERCEIVED	ALTERNATIVES	COMMENTS
1	he's running in a pile of dirt	[i]	[ ]		
2	chicken	[ɪ]	[ ]		
3	zipper	[ɚ]	[ ]		
4	ladder	[æ]	[ ]		
5	car	[ɑ]	[ ]		
6	elephant	[ɛ]	[ ]		
7	finger	[ɪ]	[ ]		
8	bathe	[e͡ɪ]	[ ]		
9	shoe	[u]	[ ]		
10	bell	[ɛ]	[ ]		
11	blocks	[ɑ]	[ ]		
12	balloons	[u]	[ ]		
13	top	[ɔ]	[ ]		
14	saw	[ɔ]	[ ]		
15	potato	[e͡ɪ]	[ ]		

MODULE TIME	
TOTAL	3:37
ELAPSED	21:28–25:05

Clinical Phonetics CD 2, Track 7
Vowels and Diphthongs Module 7: Vowel and Diphthong Nasalization

TRANSCRIPTION KEY

	STIMULUS WORD	INTENDED	CONSENSUS	ALTERNATIVES	COMMENTS
1	kiss	[ɪ]	[ɪ̃]		
2	a knife	[a͡ɪ]	[ã͡ɪ̃]		Slight
3	bicycle	[a͡ɪ]	[ã͡ɪ̃]		
4	a window	[ɪ],[o͡ʊ]	[ɪ̃], [õ͡ʊ̃]		
5	sky	[a͡ɪ]	[a͡ɪ]		
6	a bunny rabbit	[ʌ], [æ],[ɪ]	[ʌ̃], [æ̃], [ɪ̃]		
7	I like ice cream	[a͡ɪ], [a͡ɪ],[a͡ɪ], [i]	[ɑ̃], [ã͡ɪ̃], [ã͡ɪ̃], [ĩ]		All nasalized
8	baby	[e͡ɪ], [ɪ]	[e͡ɪ], [ɪ]	[ẽ͡ɪ̃]	
9	wagon	[æ]	[æ̃]		
10	soap	[o͡ʊ]	[õ͡ʊ̃]		
11	grass	[æ]	[æ̃]		
12	cracker	[æ], [ɚ]	[æ̃], [ɚ̃]		[æ̃] is only slight.
13	orange	[ɔ], [ɪ]	[ɔ̃], [ɪ̃]	[ɔ̃͡ɪ̃]	Sounds like a diphthong
14	banana	[æ]	[æ̃]	[æ̃˕ ː], [ɑ̃]	
15	lamp	[æ]	[ɑ̃]		[j ɑ̃ m̃ p]
16	balloon	[u]	[ũ]		[b ɪ j ũ ː]

Notes: Most of these items keyed for nasality were quite obviously nasalized. You should readily be able to produce nasalized vowels throughout the entire vowel quadrilateral. Practice in minimal pairs too, *man–pat*, should sharpen your discrimination skills for assimilative nasality.

MODULE TIME	
TOTAL	3:37
ELAPSED	21:28–25:05

Clinical Phonetics CD 2, Track 7 Vowels and Diphthongs Module 7: Vowel and Diphthong Nasalization

TRANSCRIPTION SHEET

	STIMULUS WORD	INTENDED	PERCEIVED	ALTERNATIVES	COMMENTS
1	kiss	[ɪ]	[ ]		
2	a knife	[a͡ɪ]	[ ]		
3	bicycle	[a͡ɪ]	[ ]		
4	a window	[ɪ], [o͡ʊ]	[ ], [ ]		
5	sky	[a͡ɪ]	[ ]		
6	a bunny rabbit	[ʌ], [æ], [ɪ]	[ ], [ ], [ ]		
7	I like ice cream	[a͡ɪ], [a͡ɪ], [a͡ɪ],[i]	[ ], [ ], [ ], [ ]		
8	baby	[e], [ɪ]	[ ], [ ]		
9	wagon	[æ]	[ ]		
10	soap	[o͡ʊ]	[ ]		
11	grass	[æ]	[ ]		
12	cracker	[æ], [ɚ]	[ ], [ ]		
13	orange	[ɔ],[ɪ]	[ ], [ ]		
14	banana	[æ]	[ ]		
15	lamp	[æ]	[ ]		
16	balloon	[u]	[ ]		

MODULE TIME	
TOTAL	4:18
ELAPSED	25:05–29:23

Clinical Phonetics CD 2, Track 8
Vowels and Diphthongs Module 8: Summary Quiz

TRANSCRIPTION KEY

	STIMULUS WORD	INTENDED	CONSENSUS	ALTERNATIVES	COMMENTS
1	spider web	[ɛ]	[ʌ]		[w ʌ b̥]
2	baby	[e͡ɪ]	[e̞]	[e̞ᴵ]	
3	cat	[æ]	[æᵊ]	[æ ː]	
4	skates	[e͡ɪ]	[e͡ɪ]		
5	saw	[ɔ]	[ɑᶷ]	[ɑ°], [ɔ°]	
6	jars	[ɑ]	[ɑː]		
7	yes	[ɛ]	[ɛ]		
8	bed	[ɛ]	[ʌ]		
9	scissors	[ɪ]	[i]		
10	feather	[ɛ]	[ɛ̞]	[ɛ]	
11	hat	[æ]	[æᴵ]		
12	dog	[ɔ]	[ɔː]		
13	blue	[u]	[u̝]	[ᵊu], [u͗], [ʊᶷ]	Really difficult!
14	balloons	[u]	[ũ]		[b l ũ n z̥]
15	boat	[o͡ʊ]	[o̞͡ʊ]	[ʊᶷ], [ᶷu]	
16	garage	[ɑ]	[ɑː]		
17	matches	[ə]	[ʌ]		
18	fork	[ɔ]	[ɔ]	[oᵊ]	
19	cracker	[æ]	[æ̃]		
20	tongue	[ʌ]	[ʌ]		
21	he's so funny	[i], [o͡ʊ], [ʌ], [ɪ]	[ɪ], [o͡ʊ], [ʌ], [ɪ]		

Notes: If you agree with the "consensus" or "alternative" key somewhere above 75 percent on these 24 vowels/diphthongs, you are doing very nicely. After this quiz, you should be able to analyze quite closely where you should concentrate your efforts for additional practice. Keep in mind that you would undoubtedly do better with a *live* child in front of you.

MODULE TIME	
TOTAL	4:18
ELAPSED	25:05–29:23

Clinical Phonetics CD 2, Track 8
Vowels and Diphthongs Module 8: Summary Quiz

TRANSCRIPTION SHEET

	STIMULUS WORD	INTENDED	PERCEIVED	ALTERNATIVES	COMMENTS
1	spider web	[ɛ]	[ ]		
2	baby	[e͡ɪ]	[ ]		
3	cat	[æ]	[ ]		
4	skates	[e͡ɪ]	[ ]		
5	saw	[ɔ]	[ ]		
6	jars	[ɑ]	[ ]		
7	yes	[ɛ]	[ ]		
8	bed	[ɛ]	[ ]		
9	scissors	[ɪ]	[ ]		
10	feather	[ɛ]	[ ]		
11	hat	[æ]	[ ]		
12	dog	[ɔ]	[ ]		
13	blue	[u]	[ ]		
14	balloons	[u]	[ ]		
15	boat	[o͡ʊ]	[ ]		
16	garage	[ɑ]	[ ]		
17	matches	[ə]	[ ]		
18	fork	[ɔ]	[ ]		
19	cracker	[æ]	[ ]		
20	tongue	[ʌ]	[ ]		
21	he's so funny	[i], [o͡ʊ], [ʌ], [ɪ]	[ ], [ ], [ ], [ ]		

MODULE TIME	
TOTAL	2:54
ELAPSED	00:00–02:54

Clinical Phonetics CD 2, Track 9
Stops Module 1:
Stop Substitutions

TRANSCRIPTION KEY

	STIMULUS WORD	INTENDED	CONSENSUS	ALTERNATIVES	COMMENTS
1	table	[b]	[d]		
2	crackers	[k]	[t]		
3	cake	[k]	[t]		
4	gun	[g]	[d]		
5	dog	[d]	[d]		
6	apple	[p]	[p]		
7	bus	[b]	[d]		
8	pin	[p]	[p]		
9	dog	[d]	[d]		
10	can	[k]	[p]	[t]	Judges were split evenly on this one.
11	carrot	[k]	[t]		
12	wagon	[g]	[d]		
13	clock	[k]	[t]		
14	boat	[b], [t]	[b], [t]		
15	book	[b], [k]	[p], [k]	[t]	
16	pocket	[p], [k], [t]	[p], [p], [t]		

Note: This array of stop substitutions should be fairly easy to discriminate.

MODULE TIME	
TOTAL	2:54
ELAPSED	00:00–02:54

Clinical Phonetics CD 2, Track 9
Stops Module 1:
Stop Substitutions

TRANSCRIPTION SHEET

	STIMULUS WORD	INTENDED	PERCEIVED	ALTERNATIVES	COMMENTS
1	table	[b]	[ ]		
2	crackers	[k]	[ ]		
3	cake	[k]	[ ]		
4	gun	[g]	[ ]		
5	dog	[d]	[ ]		
6	apple	[p]	[ ]		
7	bus	[b]	[ ]		
8	pin	[p]	[ ]		
9	dog	[d]	[ ]		
10	can	[k]	[ ]		
11	carrot	[k]	[ ]		
12	wagon	[g]	[ ]		
13	clock	[k]	[ ]		
14	boat	[b], [t]	[ ], [ ]		
15	book	[b], [k]	[ ], [ ]		
16	pocket	[p], [k], [t]	[ ], [ ], [ ]		

Clinical Phonetics CD 2, Track 10
Stops Module 2:
Voicing of Voiceless Stops

TRANSCRIPTION KEY

MODULE TIME	
TOTAL	1:57
ELAPSED	02:54–04:51

EXAMPLES			
ASPIRATED	[pʰɑ]	UNASPIRATED	[p˭ɑ]
	[tʰu]		[t˭u]

	STIMULUS WORD	INTENDED	CONSENSUS	ALTERNATIVES	COMMENTS
1	potato	[pʰ]	[pʰ]	[p˭], [b]	
2	potato	[pʰ]	[p˭]	[b]	
3	cat	[kʰ]	[kʰ]		
4	potatoes	[pʰ]	[p˭]		Change of stress [b ə ˈ t e͡ɪ t o z]?
5	spoon	[p˭]	[pʰ]		This is not an example of devoicing.
6	star	[t˭]	[t˭]		
7	skates	[k˭]	[k˭]		
8	spoon	[p˭]	[p˭]		

Notes: Another way to practice making this sound change is to contrast voiceless stop contrasts as they occur initially as singletons and as the second member of a cluster. In item 6, for example, practice saying /t/ in the word *star* [t˭] versus / t / in *tar* [tʰ].

Clinical Phonetics CD 2, Track 10
Stops Module 2:
Voicing of Voiceless Stops

TRANSCRIPTION SHEET

MODULE TIME	
TOTAL	1:57
ELAPSED	02:54–04:51

EXAMPLES			
ASPIRATED	[pʰa]	UNASPIRATED	[p˭a]
	[tʰu]		[t˭u]

	STIMULUS WORD	INTENDED	PERCEIVED	ALTERNATIVES	COMMENTS
1	potato	[pʰ]	[ ]		
2	potato	[pʰ]	[ ]		
3	cat	[kʰ]	[ ]		
4	potatoes	[pʰ]	[ ]		
5	spoon	[p˭]	[ ]		
6	star	[t˭]	[ ]		
7	skates	[k˭]	[ ]		
8	spoon	[p˭]	[ ]		

MODULE TIME	
TOTAL	3:19
ELAPSED	04:51–08:10

Clinical Phonetics CD 2, Track 11
Stops Module 3:
Devoicing of Voiced Stops

TRANSCRIPTION KEY

	STIMULUS WORD	INTENDED	CONSENSUS	ALTERNATIVES	COMMENTS
1	egg	[g]	[kʰ]		
2	bathtub	[b]	[pʰ]		
3	the bird	[d]	[d̥]		"Almost" [t]
4	dog	[g]	[g̊]		
5	egg	[g]	[g̊ʰ]		Compare to no. 1.
6	bathtub	[b]	[b]		Slight devoicing at end
7	bed	[d]	[d̥ʰ]		
8	spider web	[b]	[p]		
9	bib	[b]	[b̥ʰ]		Close to [p]
10	pig	[g]	[k]		Short vowel
11	bed	[d]	[tʰ]		Long vowel
12	bed	[d]	[d]		Compare to nos. 7, 11.
13	wagon	[g]	[g̊]		
14	window	[d]	[d]		
15	blue	[b]	[b̥]	[b]	
16	brush	[b]	[b̥]	[b]	
17	doggie, a big dog	[g], [b], [g]	[g], [p], [g̥ʰ]	[g]	

Note: Judges agreed quite well on almost all items.

MODULE TIME	
TOTAL	3:19
ELAPSED	04:51–08:10

Clinical Phonetics CD 2, Track 11
Stops Module 3:
Devoicing of Voiced Stops

TRANSCRIPTION SHEET

	STIMULUS WORD	INTENDED	PERCEIVED	ALTERNATIVES	COMMENTS
1	egg	[g]	[ ]		
2	bathtub	[b]	[ ]		
3	the bird	[d]	[ ]		
4	dog	[g]	[ ]		
5	egg	[g]	[ ]		
6	bathtub	[b]	[ ]		
7	bed	[d]	[ ]		
8	spider web	[b]	[ ]		
9	bib	[b]	[ ]		
10	pig	[g]	[ ]		
11	bed	[d]	[ ]		
12	bed	[d]	[ ]		
13	wagon	[g]	[ ]		
14	window	[d]	[ ]		
15	blue	[b]	[ ]		
16	brush	[b]	[ ]		
17	doggie, a big dog	[g], [b], [g]	[ ], [ ], [ ]		

MODULE TIME	
TOTAL	1:49
ELAPSED	08:10–09:59

Clinical Phonetics CD 2, Track 12
Stops Module 4:
Glottal Stop Substitutions

TRANSCRIPTION KEY

	STIMULUS WORD	INTENDED	CONSENSUS	ALTERNATIVES	COMMENTS
1	sheep	[p]	[ʔ]		Shortened vowel
2	monkey	[k]	[ʔ]		
3	table	[b]	[ʔ]		
4	apple	[p]	[ʔ]		
5	monkey	[k]	[k]		
6	matches	[tʃ]	[ʔ]		
7	dishes	[ʃ]	[ʔ]		The "click" after the word is from a counter used in management.
8	ladder	[d]	[ʔ]		

Notes: Items that clearly demonstrate glottal stop substitutions were difficult to isolate from our audiotapes of children with delayed speech. Particularly in postvocalic, word-final position, glottal stops are difficult to discriminate by perceptual phonetics, such as item 1 above.

MODULE TIME	
TOTAL	1:49
ELAPSED	08:10–09:59

Clinical Phonetics CD 2, Track 12
Stops Module 4:
Glottal Stop Substitutions

TRANSCRIPTION SHEET

	STIMULUS WORD	INTENDED	PERCEIVED	ALTERNATIVES	COMMENTS
1	shee<u>p</u>	[p]	[ ]		
2	mon<u>k</u>ey	[k]	[ ]		
3	ta<u>b</u>le	[b]	[ ]		
4	a<u>pp</u>le	[p]	[ ]		
5	mon<u>k</u>ey	[k]	[ ]		
6	ma<u>tch</u>es	[tʃ]	[ ]		
7	di<u>sh</u>es	[ʃ]	[ ]		
8	la<u>dd</u>er	[d]	[ ]		

MODULE TIME	
TOTAL	4:12
ELAPSED	09:59–14:11

Clinical Phonetics CD 2, Track 13
Stops Module 5:
Stop Deletions

TRANSCRIPTION KEY

	STIMULUS WORD	INTENDED	CONSENSUS	ALTERNATIVES	COMMENTS
1	some might not	[t]	[ø]		Because /t/ is homorganic with /n/, a deletion here is not unusual.
2	cup	[p]	[pʰ]		"Popping" release
3	glasses	[g]	[ø]		Something here?
4	black	[k]	[ø]	[k˺]	No voicing at release
5	hat	[t]	[tʰ]		Breathy voice
6	book	[k]	[k˺]	[t˺], [ʔ]	Note vowel [a].
7	lamp	[p]	[pʰ]		
8	cake	[k]	[kʰ]		
9	thank you	[k]	[ø]		
10	dog	[g]	[ø]		
11	soft	[t]	[ø]		
12	bird	[d]	[ø]		
13	top	[p]	[pʰ]		
14	ladder	[d]	[ø]		
15	radio	[d]	[ø]	[ʔ]	/d/ replaced by a voiceless segment
16	bed	[d]	[ø]		[b ɛ ᵊ ø]
17	jump	[p]	[pʰ]		
18	that	[t]	[ø]		
19	that bite	[t], [t]	[ø], [ø]		
20	kitty cat	[t], [t]	[ø], [ø]		

MODULE TIME	
TOTAL	4:12
ELAPSED	09:59–14:11

Clinical Phonetics CD 2, Track 13
Stops Module 5:
Stop Deletions

TRANSCRIPTION SHEET

	STIMULUS WORD	INTENDED	PERCEIVED	ALTERNATIVES	COMMENTS
1	some might not	[t]	[ ]		
2	cup	[p]	[ ]		
3	glasses	[g]	[ ]		
4	black	[k]	[ ]		
5	hat	[t]	[ ]		
6	book	[k]	[ ]		
7	lamp	[p]	[ ]		
8	cake	[k]	[ ]		
9	thank you	[k]	[ ]		
10	dog	[g]	[ ]		
11	soft	[t]	[ ]		
12	bird	[d]	[ ]		
13	top	[p]	[ ]		
14	ladder	[d]	[ ]		
15	radio	[d]	[ ]		
16	bed	[d]	[ ]		
17	jump	[p]	[ ]		
18	that	[t]	[ ]		
19	that bite	[t], [t]	[ ], [ ]		
20	kitty cat	[t], [t]	[ ], [ ]		

Clinical Phonetics CD 2, Track 14
Stops Module 6:
Frictionalized Stops

TRANSCRIPTION KEY

MODULE TIME	
TOTAL	1:36
ELAPSED	14:11–15:47

EXAMPLES			
NORMAL	[ki]	FRICTIONALIZED	[k͓i]
	[steɪ͡]		[st͓eɪ͡]

	STIMULUS WORD	INTENDED	CONSENSUS	ALTERNATIVES	COMMENTS
1	train	[t]	[t͓]		
2	soap	[p]	[pʰ]		
3	truck	[t]	[t͓]		
4	comb	[k]	[k͓]	[t͡s]	
5	car	[k]	[kʰ]		Note that even a normally released /k/ sounds "noisy."
6	with its path	[p]	[p͓]		Not stop closure

Notes: Clear examples of frictionalized stops are difficult to isolate. Keep in mind that this diacritic symbolizes a range of sound changes, from almost /s/-like to barely any closure for the stop. The speaker in item 6, for example, was a dysarthric individual whose articulation of stops was consistently imprecise.

Clinical Phonetics CD 2, Track 14
Stops Module 6:
Frictionalized Stops

TRANSCRIPTION SHEET

MODULE TIME	
TOTAL	1:36
ELAPSED	14:11–15:47

EXAMPLES			
NORMAL	[ki]	FRICTIONALIZED	[k̽i]
	[s t eɪ]		[s t̽ eɪ]

	STIMULUS WORD	INTENDED	PERCEIVED	ALTERNATIVES	COMMENTS
1	<u>t</u>rain	[t]	[ ]		
2	soa<u>p</u>	[p]	[ ]		
3	<u>t</u>ruck	[t]	[ ]		
4	<u>c</u>omb	[k]	[ ]		
5	<u>c</u>ar	[k]	[ ]		
6	with its <u>p</u>ath	[p]	[ ]		

MODULE TIME	
TOTAL	5:02
ELAPSED	15:47–20:49

Clinical Phonetics CD 2, Track 15
Stops Module 7: Summary Quiz

TRANSCRIPTION KEY

	STIMULUS WORD	INTENDED	CONSENSUS	ALTERNATIVES	COMMENTS
1	bed	[b], [d]	[b], [d]		
2	bib	[b], [b]	[b], [b^{h}]		
3	bread	[b], [d]	[ø], [d̥]		
4	gun	[g]	[d]		
5	kitty cat	[k], [t], [k], [t]	[k], [t], [t], [t]		
6	toothbrush	[t], [b]	[t͓^{h}]*, [b]		*Aspirated and frictionalized release
7	frog	[g]	[g̊]		
8	bird	[b], [d]	[b], [d̥]		
9	dishes	[d]	[d]		[d ɪ ʔ ɪ]
10	a ladder	[d]	[t^{h}]		
11	paper	[p], [p]	[p^{h}], [p]		
12	monkey	[k]	[b̥]	[p^{b}]	[m ʌ p^{b} i]; [m ʌ > b i]
13	bird	[b], [d]	[b], [d̥]		
14	radio	[d]	[ø]		
15	carrot	[k], [t]	[t$^{=}$], [t]		
16	bed	[b], [d]	[b], [t]		[b æ ː t]
17	cup	[k], [p]	[t], [p̚]		[t ʌ p̚]
18	book	[b], [k]	[p], [p]	[k], [ʔ]	Not enough to tell which
19	dog	[d], [g]	[d], [g̊]		
20	pig	[p], [g]	[p], [k]		
21	baby	[b], [b]	[b], [b]		
22	bed	[b], [d]	[b], [ø]		
23	tail	[t]	[t]		
24	TV	[t]	[p]		[p i f i] !
25	dog	[d], [g]	[d], [ø]		

Notes: There are 44 stops to discriminate; each agreement is worth approximately 2.3 points. Which error types do you consistently discriminate correctly? Which need more practice? Which diacritics do you tend to overuse? underuse?

MODULE TIME	
TOTAL	5:02
ELAPSED	15:47–20:49

Clinical Phonetics CD 2, Track 15
Stops Module 7:
Summary Quiz

TRANSCRIPTION SHEET

	STIMULUS WORD	INTENDED	PERCEIVED	ALTERNATIVES	COMMENTS
1	bed	[b], [d]	[ ], [ ]		
2	bib	[b], [b]	[ ], [ ]		
3	bread	[b], [d]	[ ], [ ]		
4	gun	[g]	[ ]		
5	kitty cat	[k], [t], [k], [t]	[ ], [ ], [ ], [ ]		
6	toothbrush	[t], [b]	[ ], [ ]		
7	frog	[g]	[ ]		
8	bird	[b], [d]	[ ], [ ]		
9	dishes	[d]	[ ]		
10	a ladder	[d]	[ ]		
11	paper	[p], [p]	[ ], [ ]		
12	monkey	[k]	[ ]		
13	bird	[b], [d]	[ ], [ ]		
14	radio	[d]	[ ]		
15	carrot	[k], [t]	[ ], [ ]		
16	bed	[b], [d]	[ ], [ ]		
17	cup	[k], [p]	[ ], [ ]		
18	book	[b], [k]	[ ], [ ]		
19	dog	[d], [g]	[ ], [ ]		
20	pig	[p], [g]	[ ], [ ]		
21	baby	[b], [b]	[ ], [ ]		
22	bed	[b], [d]	[ ], [ ]		
23	tail	[t]	[ ]		
24	TV	[t]	[ ]		
25	dog	[d], [g]	[ ], [ ]		

MODULE TIME	
TOTAL	5:35
ELAPSED	20:49–26:24

Clinical Phonetics CD 2, Track 16
Fricatives and Affricates Module 1: /f/ and /v/ Changes

TRANSCRIPTION KEY

	STIMULUS WORD	INTENDED	CONSENSUS	ALTERNATIVES	COMMENTS
1	leaf	[f]	[ø]		
2	knife	[f]	[f]		
3	telephone	[f]	[f]		
4	fork	[f]	[ø]		
5	vacuum	[v]	[v]		
6	vacuum	[v]	[ø]		
7	TV	[v]	[t]		Noisy
8	knife	[f]	[s]		
9	fork	[f]	[p˭]		
10	vacuum	[v]	[b]		
11	knife	[f]	[f]		
12	stove	[v]	[b̥]		
13	a leaf	[f]	[f]		
14	TV	[v]	[f]		
15	five	[v]	[v̥]		
16	vacuum	[v]	[v̥]		
17	stove	[v]	[v̥]		
18	leaf	[f]	[v]		
19	TV	[v]	[v̥]	[b v̥]	
20	stove	[v]	[v̥]		
21	elephant	[f]	[f]		
22	vacuum	[v]	[w]		
23	knife	[f]	[t]		
24	a feather	[f]	[f]		
25	TV	[v]	[v̥]		

MODULE TIME	
TOTAL	5:35
ELAPSED	20:49–26:24

Clinical Phonetics CD 2, Track 16
Fricatives and Affricates Module 1: /f/ and /v/ Changes

TRANSCRIPTION SHEET

	STIMULUS WORD	INTENDED	PERCEIVED	ALTERNATIVES	COMMENTS
1	leaf	[f]	[ ]		
2	knife	[f]	[ ]		
3	telephone	[f]	[ ]		
4	fork	[f]	[ ]		
5	vacuum	[v]	[ ]		
6	vacuum	[v]	[ ]		
7	TV	[v]	[ ]		
8	knife	[f]	[ ]		
9	fork	[f]	[ ]		
10	vacuum	[v]	[ ]		
11	knife	[f]	[ ]		
12	stove	[v]	[ ]		
13	a leaf	[f]	[ ]		
14	TV	[v]	[ ]		
15	five	[v]	[ ]		
16	vacuum	[v]	[ ]		
17	stove	[v]	[ ]		
18	leaf	[f]	[ ]		
19	TV	[v]	[ ]		
20	stove	[v]	[ ]		
21	elephant	[f]	[ ]		
22	vacuum	[v]	[ ]		
23	knife	[f]	[ ]		
24	a feather	[f]	[ ]		
25	TV	[v]	[ ]		

MODULE TIME	
TOTAL	1:48
ELAPSED	26:24–28:12

Clinical Phonetics CD 2, Track 17
Fricatives and Affricates Module 2:
/h/ Deletions

TRANSCRIPTION KEY

	STIMULUS WORD	INTENDED	CONSENSUS	ALTERNATIVES	COMMENTS
1	house	[h]	[ø]		ø/s also
2	dog house	[h]	[ø]		
3	he's this high	[h], [h]	[h], [h]		
4	and he's a poodle	[h]	[ø]		Normal in this context
5	house	[h]	[h]		
6	they were voting for him	[h]	[ø]		Same as no. 4
7	hanger	[h]	[h]		
8	hammer	[h]	[ø]		

MODULE TIME	
TOTAL	1:48
ELAPSED	26:24–28:12

Clinical Phonetics CD 2, Track 17
Fricatives and Affricates Module 2: /h/ Deletions

TRANSCRIPTION SHEET

	STIMULUS WORD	INTENDED	PERCEIVED	ALTERNATIVES	COMMENTS
1	house	[h]	[ ]		
2	dog house	[h]	[ ]		
3	he's this high	[h], [h]	[ ], [ ]		
4	and he's a poodle	[h]	[ ]		
5	house	[h]	[ ]		
6	they were voting for him	[h]	[ ]		
7	hanger	[h]	[ ]		
8	hammer	[h]	[ ]		

MODULE TIME	
TOTAL	6:32
ELAPSED	00:00–06:32

Clinical Phonetics CD 3, Track 1
Fricatives and Affricates Module 3: *th* Changes

TRANSCRIPTION KEY

	STIMULUS WORD	INTENDED	CONSENSUS	ALTERNATIVES	COMMENTS
	DELETIONS				
1	bathe	[ð]	[ø]		[θ]?
2	toothbrush	[θ]	[ø]		
3	brother	[ð]	[ð]		
4	that apple	[ð]	[ð]		
5	feather	[ð]	[ø]	[ʔ]	Abrupt onset of second syllable
6	bath	[θ]	[ø]		[θ]?
7	teeth	[θ]	[θ]		
	SUBSTITUTIONS				
8	feather	[ð]	[l]		
9	that	[ð]	[d]		
10	bathtub	[θ]	[s]		
11	feather	[ð]	[d]		
12	teeth	[θ]	[f]		
13	smooth	[ð]	[ð]	[ð̥]	
14	this	[ð]	[d]		
15	bathe	[ð]	[v]	[v̥]	
	DISTORTIONS				
16	that	[ð]	[z̪]	[z̪̥]	
17	three	[θ]	[s̪]		
18	feather	[ð]	[ð]		
19	this	[ð]	[t͓]		
20	bath	[θ]	[θ]	[tð̥], [t͓]	
21	teeth	[θ]	[θt]		
22	that	[ð]	[ð̯]		Lateralized?
	ANY ERROR				
23	toothache	[θ]	[θ]		
24	thumb	[θ]	[s]		
25	this	[ð]	[z̪]		One judge heard as a palatalized /z/, [zʲ].
26	this apple	[ð]	[d]		
27	thank you	[θ]	[s]		
28	bathtub	[θ]	[ø]		
29	thank you	[θ]	[θ̯]		
30	a thumb	[θ]	[f]		

MODULE TIME	
TOTAL	6:32
ELAPSED	00:00–06:32

Clinical Phonetics CD 3, Track 1
Fricatives and Affricates Module 3: *th* Changes

TRANSCRIPTION SHEET

	STIMULUS WORD	INTENDED	PERCEIVED	ALTERNATIVES	COMMENTS
	DELETIONS				
1	bathe	[ð]	[ ]		
2	toothbrush	[θ]	[ ]		
3	brother	[ð]	[ ]		
4	that apple	[ð]	[ ]		
5	feather	[ð]	[ ]		
6	bath	[θ]	[ ]		
7	teeth	[θ]	[ ]		
	SUBSTITUTIONS				
8	feather	[ð]	[ ]		
9	that	[ð]	[ ]		
10	bathtub	[θ]	[ ]		
11	feather	[ð]	[ ]		
12	teeth	[θ]	[ ]		
13	smooth	[ð]	[ ]		
14	this	[ð]	[ ]		
15	bathe	[ð]	[ ]		
	DISTORTIONS				
16	that	[ð]	[ ]		
17	three	[θ]	[ ]		
18	feather	[ð]	[ ]		
19	this	[ð]	[ ]		
20	bath	[θ]	[ ]		
21	teeth	[θ]	[ ]		
22	that	[ð]	[ ]		
	ANY ERROR				
23	toothache	[θ]	[ ]		
24	thumb	[θ]	[ ]		
25	this	[ð]	[ ]		
26	this apple	[ð]	[ ]		
27	thank you	[θ]	[ ]		
28	bathtub	[θ]	[ ]		
29	thank you	[θ]	[ ]		
30	a thumb	[θ]	[ ]		

Clinical Phonetics CD 3, Track 2
Fricatives and Affricates Module 4: Fricative and Affricate Voicing Changes

TRANSCRIPTION KEY

MODULE TIME	
TOTAL	5:53
ELAPSED	06:32–12:25

EXAMPLES			
NORMAL	[zu]	DEVOICED	[z̥u]
	[ɪz]		[ɪz̥]

	STIMULUS WORD	INTENDED	CONSENSUS	ALTERNATIVES	COMMENTS
	PREVOCALIC POSITION				
1	vacuum	[v]	[v]		
2	zebra	[z]	[z̥͎]		Whistled
3	zipper	[z]	[z̥]		
4	vacuum	[v]	[v̥]		Slightly devoiced
5	jumping	[ʤ]	[ʤ]		Slightly devoiced
6	jars	[ʤ]	[ʤ̥]		
	INTERVOCALIC POSITION				
7	TV	[v]	[v]		Noisy
8	feather	[ð]	[ð]		
9	pages	[ʤ]	[ʤ̥]		Second syllable is breathy.
10	scissors	[z]	[z]		
11	seven	[v]	[v]		
12	feather	[ð]	[ð̥]		
13	scissors	[z]	[z̥]		Almost [s]
	POSTVOCALIC POSITION				
14	five	[v]	[v̥]		
15	stove	[v]	[v̥]		
16	smooth	[ð]	[ð̥]	[θ]	
17	glasses	[z]	[z̥]	[z]	Devoiced only at the very end
18	feathers	[z]	[s͎]	[z̥͎]	
19	toes	[z]	[z̥]	[z̪̥]	
20	smooth	[ð]	[ð̥]		
21	dishes	[z]	[z̥]		
	ASSORTED POSITIONS				
22	telephone	[f]	[f]		
23	TV	[v]	[v̥]		Noise
24	cage	[ʤ]	[ʤ̥]		
25	matches	[z]	[z]		
26	toes	[z]	[z̥]		
27	garage	[ʤ]	[ʤ̥]		
28	zebra	[z]	[z̥]	[s]	

Note: One of the best comparisons is between the final /z/ in no. 25 *matches* versus no. 26 *toes*.

Clinical Phonetics CD 3, Track 2
Fricatives and Affricates Module 4: Fricative and Affricate Voicing Changes

TRANSCRIPTION SHEET

MODULE TIME	
TOTAL	5:53
ELAPSED	06:32–12:25

EXAMPLES			
NORMAL	[zu]	DEVOICED	[z̥u]
	[ɪz]		[ɪz̥]

	STIMULUS WORD	INTENDED	PERCEIVED	ALTERNATIVES	COMMENTS
	PREVOCALIC POSITION				
1	vacuum	[v]	[ ]		
2	zebra	[z]	[ ]		
3	zipper	[z]	[ ]		
4	vacuum	[v]	[ ]		
5	jumping	[ʤ]	[ ]		
6	jars	[ʤ]	[ ]		
	INTERVOCALIC POSITION				
7	TV	[v]	[ ]		
8	feather	[ð]	[ ]		
9	pages	[ʤ]	[ ]		
10	scissors	[z]	[ ]		
11	seven	[v]	[ ]		
12	feather	[ð]	[ ]		
13	scissors	[z]	[ ]		
	POSTVOCALIC POSITION				
14	five	[v]	[ ]		
15	stove	[v]	[ ]		
16	smooth	[ð]	[ ]		
17	glasses	[z]	[ ]		
18	feathers	[z]	[ ]		
19	toes	[z]	[ ]		
20	smooth	[ð]	[ ]		
21	dishes	[z]	[ ]		
	ASSORTED POSITIONS				
22	telephone	[f]	[ ]		
23	TV	[v]	[ ]		
24	cage	[ʤ]	[ ]		
25	matches	[z]	[ ]		
26	toes	[z]	[ ]		
27	garage	[ʤ]	[ ]		
28	zebra	[z]	[ ]		

MODULE TIME	
TOTAL	5:49
ELAPSED	12:25–18:14

Clinical Phonetics CD 3, Track 3
Fricatives and Affricates Module 5:
Fricative and Affricate Substitutions

TRANSCRIPTION KEY

	STIMULUS WORD	INTENDED	CONSENSUS	ALTERNATIVES	COMMENTS
	/s/				
1	saw	[s]	[θ]		
2	house	[s]	[t]		
3	saw	[s]	[t]		
4	whistle	[s]	[s]		
5	seal	[s]	[s]		
	/z/				
6	zipper	[z]	[d͡ʒ]	[ʤ]	
7	a zebra	[z]	[z]		
8	scissors	[z]	[d]		
9	toes	[z]	[z̥]		
10	zipper	[z]	[j]		
11	hose	[z]	[d]		
	/ʃ/				
12	brush	[ʃ]	[s]		
13	fish	[ʃ]	[t]		[tʰ]
14	shoe	[ʃ]	[ʃ]		
15	station	[ʃ]	[s]		
16	dishes	[ʃ]	[ʃ]		
17	shoe	[ʃ]	[s]		
	/ʒ/				
18	measuring cup	[ʒ]	[ʒ]		
19	television	[ʒ]	[z̥]	[z̥]	
20	beige	[ʒ]	[z]		
21	measure	[ʒ]	[n]		
	/ʧ/				
22	chair	[ʧ]	[ʃ]		
23	watch	[ʧ]	[ʧ]		
24	sandwich	[ʧ]	[k͡s]	[t͡s]	[s] distorted?
25	matches	[ʧ]	[ʧ]		Stress change
26	chicken	[ʧ]	[t]		
	/ʤ/				
27	jar	[ʤ]	[s]	[s̻]	
28	orange juice	[ʤ]	[d]		
29	GI Joe	[ʤ], [ʤ]	[ʤ], [ʤ]		!!

MODULE TIME	
TOTAL	5:49
ELAPSED	12:25–18:14

Clinical Phonetics CD 3, Track 3
Fricatives and Affricates Module 5: Fricative and Affricate Substitutions

TRANSCRIPTION SHEET

	STIMULUS WORD	INTENDED	PERCEIVED	ALTERNATIVES	COMMENTS
	/s/				
1	saw	[s]	[ ]		
2	house	[s]	[ ]		
3	saw	[s]	[ ]		
4	whistle	[s]	[ ]		
5	seal	[s]	[ ]		
	/z/				
6	zipper	[z]	[ ]		
7	a zebra	[z]	[ ]		
8	scissors	[z]	[ ]		
9	toes	[z]	[ ]		
10	zipper	[z]	[ ]		
11	hose	[z]	[ ]		
	/ʃ/				
12	brush	[ʃ]	[ ]		
13	fish	[ʃ]	[ ]		
14	shoe	[ʃ]	[ ]		
15	station	[ʃ]	[ ]		
16	dishes	[ʃ]	[ ]		
17	shoe	[ʃ]	[ ]		
	/ʒ/				
18	measuring cup	[ʒ]	[ ]		
19	television	[ʒ]	[ ]		
20	beige	[ʒ]	[ ]		
21	measure	[ʒ]	[ ]		
	/tʃ/				
22	chair	[tʃ]	[ ]		
23	watch	[tʃ]	[ ]		
24	sandwich	[tʃ]	[ ]		
25	matches	[tʃ]	[ ]		
26	chicken	[tʃ]	[ ]		
	/ʤ/				
27	jar	[ʤ]	[ ]		
28	orange juice	[ʤ]	[ ]		
29	GI Joe	[ʤ], [ʤ]	[ ], [ ]		

Clinical Phonetics CD 3, Track 4
Fricatives and Affricates Module 6: Dentalized Sibilants

TRANSCRIPTION KEY

MODULE TIME	
TOTAL	5:16
ELAPSED	18:14–23:30

EXAMPLES			
NORMAL	[si]	DENTALIZED	[s̪i]
	[a͡ɪs]		[a͡ɪs̪]

	STIMULUS WORD	INTENDED	CONSENSUS	ALTERNATIVES	COMMENTS
	FINAL POSITION				
1	crayons	[z]	[z̥]	[t͡s̪]	Intrusive [t̪]?
2	doghouse	[s]	[s]		
3	fingers	[z]	[z̪̥]		
4	potatoes	[z]	[z̪]		
5	stories	[z]	[z]	[z̥]	
6	glasses	[z]	[z]		The intervocalic /s/ may be dentalized.
7	nose	[z]	[z̪]		
8	bus	[s]	[s]		Slightly dentalized
9	matches	[z]	[z]		
10	house	[s]	[s̪]	[sʲ]	One judge heard as palatalized /s/.
	INITIAL POSITION				
11	saw	[s]	[s̪]		
12	a zebra	[z]	[z̪]		Slightly
13	smooth	[s]	[s̪]	[θ͡s̪]	Close to [θ/s]
14	spoon	[s]	[s]		
15	said	[s]	[s̪]	[sʲ]	Palatalized?
16	stars	[s]	[s̪]		
17	soft	[s]	[s̪]		
18	sun	[s]	[s̪]		
	ASSORTED POSITIONS				
19	school bus	[s], [s]	[s], [s]		
20	grass	[s]	[s̪]		
21	six	[s], [s]	[s̪], [s̪]	[s]	
22	toothpaste	[s]	[s̪]		
23	smooth	[s]	[s]		
24	a zebra	[z]	[z̪]		
25	dishes	[z]	[z̪]	[z̪̥]	
26	/s/ (isolation)	[s]	[s]		Hard to tell, isn't it!

Notes: Good examples of dentalized /s/ and /z/ are nos. 15, 20, and 24. Be sure you can make the range of dentalized /s/ and /z/, from slight dentalization to almost [θ], [ð].

Clinical Phonetics CD 3, Track 4
Fricatives and Affricates Module 6: Dentalized Sibilants

TRANSCRIPTION SHEET

MODULE TIME	
TOTAL	5:16
ELAPSED	18:14–23:30

EXAMPLES			
NORMAL	[s i]	DENTALIZED	[s̪ i]
	[a͡ɪs]		[a͡ɪs̪]

	STIMULUS WORD	INTENDED	PERCEIVED	ALTERNATIVES	COMMENTS
	FINAL POSITION				
1	crayons	[z]	[ ]		
2	doghouse	[s]	[ ]		
3	fingers	[z]	[ ]		
4	potatoes	[z]	[ ]		
5	stories	[z]	[ ]		
6	glasses	[z]	[ ]		
7	nose	[z]	[ ]		
8	bus	[s]	[ ]		
9	matches	[z]	[ ]		
10	house	[s]	[ ]		
	INITIAL POSITION				
11	saw	[s]	[ ]		
12	a zebra	[z]	[ ]		
13	smooth	[s]	[ ]		
14	spoon	[s]	[ ]		
15	said	[s]	[ ]		
16	stars	[s]	[ ]		
17	soft	[s]	[ ]		
18	sun	[s]	[ ]		
	ASSORTED POSITIONS				
19	school bus	[s], [s]	[ ], [ ]		
20	grass	[s]	[ ]		
21	six	[s], [s]	[ ], [ ]		
22	toothpaste	[s]	[ ]		
23	smooth	[s]	[ ]		
24	a zebra	[z]	[ ]		
25	dishes	[z]	[ ]		
26	/s/ (isolation)	[s]	[ ]		

Clinical Phonetics CD 3, Track 5
Fricatives and Affricates Module 7:
Lateralized Sibilants

TRANSCRIPTION KEY

MODULE TIME	
TOTAL	2:39
ELAPSED	23:30–26:09

EXAMPLES			
NORMAL	[si]	LATERALIZED	[s̯i]
	[a͡ɪs]		[a͡ɪs̯]

	STIMULUS WORD	INTENDED	CONSENSUS	ALTERNATIVES	COMMENTS
1	keys	[z]	[z̥̯]		Slightly
2	glasses	[s], [z]	[s̯], [z̯]		
3	star	[s]	[s]		
4	/s/	[s]	[s̯]		Very difficult in isolation on audio sample
5	scissors	[s], [z], [z]	[s̯], [z], [z]		
6	saddle	[s]	[s̯]		
7	sack	[s]	[s̯]		
8	pencil	[s]	[s̯]		
9	fish	[ʃ]	[s̯]		
10	gates	[s]	[s]		
11	this is fireworks	[s], [z], [s]	[s̯], [z̯], [s̯]		

Note: Judges each had a "favorite" best example; item 11 appears to contain good examples of lateralized sibilants.

Clinical Phonetics CD 3, Track 5
Fricatives and Affricates Module 7: Lateralized Sibilants

TRANSCRIPTION SHEET

MODULE TIME	
TOTAL	2:39
ELAPSED	23:30–26:09

EXAMPLES

NORMAL	[si]	LATERALIZED	[s̺i]
	[aɪs]		[aɪs̺]

	STIMULUS WORD	INTENDED	PERCEIVED	ALTERNATIVES	COMMENTS
1	key<u>s</u>	[z]	[ ]		
2	gla<u>ss</u>e<u>s</u>	[s], [z]	[ ], [ ]		
3	<u>s</u>tar	[s]	[ ]		
4	/s/	[s]	[ ]		
5	<u>s</u>ci<u>ss</u>or<u>s</u>	[s], [z], [z]	[ ], [ ], [ ]		
6	<u>s</u>addle	[s]	[ ]		
7	<u>s</u>ack	[s]	[ ]		
8	pen<u>c</u>il	[s]	[ ]		
9	fi<u>sh</u>	[ʃ]	[ ]		
10	gate<u>s</u>	[s]	[ ]		
11	thi<u>s</u> i<u>s</u> firework<u>s</u>	[s], [z], [z]	[ ], [ ], [ ]		

Clinical Phonetics CD 3, Track 6
Fricatives and Affricates Module 8: Retroflexed Sibilants

TRANSCRIPTION KEY

MODULE TIME	
TOTAL	2:51
ELAPSED	26:09–29:00

	EXAMPLES		
NORMAL	[s i]	RETROFLEXED	[s̢ i]
	[a͡ɪ s]		[a͡ɪ s̢]

	STIMULUS WORD	INTENDED	CONSENSUS	ALTERNATIVES	COMMENTS
1	whistle	[s]	[s̢]		Slight
2	walking in the bus	[s]	[s̢]		
3	scissors	[s], [z], [z]	[s̢͎], [z̢͎], [z̢͎]		
4	zebra	[z]	[z̢̥͎]		Devoiced, retroflexed, and whistled!
5	Christmas tree	[s], [s]	[s], [s]		
6	ice	[s]	[s̢]		
7	base	[s]	[s̢]		
8	gas	[s]	[s̢]		
9	carrots	[s]	[s̢]	[s̪]	
10	bus	[s]	[s̢]		
11	mice	[s]	[s̢]		
12	choice	[s]	[s̢]		

Notes: These are difficult discriminations to make from audio recordings. Practice in *making* the three types of sibilant distortions—dentalized, lateralized, and retroflexed—will allow you to compare the three. Try saying the same word with a correct /s/ or /z/, then with each of the distortion types. Can someone else label correctly what you intended? How do your recorded distortions sound? Can you discriminate your own distortion types when you hear them played back on audiotape or CD?

Clinical Phonetics CD 3, Track 6
Fricatives and Affricates Module 8:
Retroflexed Sibilants

TRANSCRIPTION SHEET

MODULE TIME	
TOTAL	2:51
ELAPSED	26:09–29:00

EXAMPLES			
NORMAL	[si]	RETROFLEXED	[s̢i]
	[a͡ɪs]		[a͡ɪs̢]

	STIMULUS WORD	INTENDED	PERCEIVED	ALTERNATIVES	COMMENTS
1	whis̲tle	[s]	[ ]		
2	walking in the bus̲	[s]	[ ]		
3	s̲cis̲s̲ors̲	[s], [z], [z]	[ ], [ ], [ ]		
4	z̲ebra	[z]	[ ]		
5	Chris̲tmas̲ tree	[s], [s]	[ ], [ ]		
6	ic̲e	[s]	[ ]		
7	bas̲e	[s]	[ ]		
8	gas̲	[s]	[ ]		
9	carrots̲	[s]	[ ]		
10	bus̲	[s]	[ ]		
11	mic̲e	[s]	[ ]		
12	choic̲e	[s]	[ ]		

MODULE TIME	
TOTAL	2:54
ELAPSED	00:00–02:54

Clinical Phonetics CD 3, Track 7
Fricatives and Affricates Module 9: Sibilants Quiz

TRANSCRIPTION KEY

	STIMULUS WORD	INTENDED	CONSENSUS	ALTERNATIVES	COMMENTS
1	I lo<u>s</u>t my red <u>s</u>ock<u>s</u>	[s], [s], [s]	[s̪], [s̪], [s̪]		Slight; the first /s/ in *socks* is most dentalized.
2	i<u>c</u>y	[s]	[s̯]		
3	gla<u>ss</u>e<u>s</u>	[s], [z]	[s̪], [z̪]		
4	la<u>c</u>ing	[s]	[s̯]		
5	hou<u>s</u>e	[s]	[s̢]		
6	thi<u>s</u> Chri<u>s</u>tma<u>s</u>	[s], [s], [s]	[s], [s], [s]		
7	pla<u>c</u>emat	[s]	[s̪]		
8	whi<u>s</u>tle	[s]	[s̢]		
9	19<u>77</u>	[s], [s]	[s̯], [s̯]		
10	jui<u>c</u>y	[s]	[s]		Noise
11	bu<u>s</u>	[s]	[s̪]		
12	<u>s</u>ci<u>ss</u>or<u>s</u>	[s], [z], [z]	[s], [z], [z]		
13	balloon<u>s</u>	[z]	[z̥]		
14	minu<u>s</u>	[s]	[s̢]	[s̯]	One judge thought it sounded both retroflexed and lateralized!

Notes: One of the most difficult modules in this series. Keep in mind that in five-way scoring, all "distortions" are tallied as incorrect. If you are correctly discriminating normal from distorted but not getting the distortion category correct, you would be "reliable" in both five-way scoring and two-way scoring.

MODULE TIME	
TOTAL	2:54
ELAPSED	00:00–02:54

Clinical Phonetics CD 3, Track 7
Fricatives and Affricates Module 9:
Sibilants Quiz

TRANSCRIPTION SHEET

	STIMULUS WORD	INTENDED	PERCEIVED	ALTERNATIVES	COMMENTS
1	I lost my red socks	[s], [s], [s]	[ ], [ ], [ ]		
2	icy	[s]	[ ]		
3	glasses	[s], [z]	[ ], [ ]		
4	lacing	[s]	[ ]		
5	house	[s]	[ ]		
6	this Christmas	[s], [s], [s]	[ ], [ ], [ ]		
7	placemat	[s]	[ ]		
8	whistle	[s]	[ ]		
9	1977	[s], [s]	[ ], [ ]		
10	juicy	[s]	[ ]		
11	bus	[s]	[ ]		
12	scissors	[s], [z], [z]	[ ], [ ], [ ]		
13	balloons	[z]	[ ]		
14	minus	[s]	[ ]		

MODULE TIME	
TOTAL	5:31
ELAPSED	02:54–08:25

Clinical Phonetics CD 3, Track 8 Fricatives and Affricates Module 10: Summary Quiz

TRANSCRIPTION KEY

	STIMULUS WORD	INTENDED	CONSENSUS	ALTERNATIVES	COMMENTS
1	missing	[s]	[θ]		
2	ice cream cone	[s]	[s̯]		
3	nose	[z]	[z̥]		
4	zebra	[z]	[ð]	[ð̥]	
5	scissors	[s], [z], [z]	[s̪], [ð], [ð]	[d]	
6	this boy has a toothache	[s], [z], [θ]	[s̪], [z̪], [θ]	[θ]	
7	feather	[ð]	[d]		
8	the dog sits up	[s], [s]	[s̪], [s̪]		Second /s/ is better.
9	zipper	[z]	[z̥]	[z̪̥]	
10	shoe	[ʃ]	[s]		
11	dishes	[ʃ], [z]	[ʃ], [z]	[z̪]	
12	zipper	[z]	[d]		
13	fish	[ʃ]	[t͡s]		
14	star	[s]	[s̪]		
15	carrots	[s]	[s̪]		Possibly [θ]
16	carrots	[s]	[θ]		Contrast with no. 15
17	house	[s]	[ø]		Dubbing noise but /s/ is deleted
18	spoon	[s]	[ø]		[p⁼ũ]
19	skates	[s], [s]	[ø], [s]		[k⁼e͡ɪ t s]
20	stars	[s], [z]	[s̨], [z̨̥]		
21	fish	[ʃ]	[p]		Noisy
22	five toes	[f], [v], [z]	[f], [v], [z̥̺]		[v] is barely audible.
23	TV	[v]	[f]	[v̥]	
24	measure	[ʒ]	[z̪]	[ð]	Judges split on these two transcriptions.
25	shoe	[ʃ]	[ʃ̯]		
26	station	[s], [ʃ]	[s], [s]	[s̪]	Second /s/ may be slightly dentalized.
27	chair	[tʃ]	[t͓ʰ]		
28	placemat	[s]	[s]	[s̪]	
29	matches	[tʃ], [z]	[tʃ], [z̪]		
30	asleep	[s]	[s]		This speaker *can* say /s/ without lateralization.

MODULE TIME	
TOTAL	5:31
ELAPSED	02:54–08:25

Clinical Phonetics CD 3, Track 8 Fricatives and Affricates Module 10: Summary Quiz

TRANSCRIPTION SHEET

	STIMULUS WORD	INTENDED	PERCEIVED	ALTERNATIVES	COMMENTS
1	mi<u>ss</u>ing	[s]	[ ]		
2	i<u>c</u>e cream cone	[s]	[ ]		
3	no<u>s</u>e	[z]	[ ]		
4	<u>z</u>ebra	[z]	[ ]		
5	<u>sc</u>i<u>ss</u>or<u>s</u>	[s], [z], [z]	[ ], [ ], [ ]		
6	thi<u>s</u> boy ha<u>s</u> a too<u>th</u>ache	[s], [z], [θ]	[ ], [ ], [ ]		
7	fea<u>th</u>er	[ð]	[ ]		
8	the dog <u>s</u>it<u>s</u> up	[s], [s]	[ ], [ ]		
9	<u>z</u>ipper	[z]	[ ]		
10	<u>sh</u>oe	[ʃ]	[ ]		
11	di<u>sh</u>e<u>s</u>	[ʃ], [z]	[ ], [ ]		
12	<u>z</u>ipper	[z]	[ ]		
13	fi<u>sh</u>	[ʃ]	[ ]		
14	<u>s</u>tar	[s]	[ ]		
15	carrot<u>s</u>	[s]	[ ]		
16	carrot<u>s</u>	[s]	[ ]		
17	hou<u>s</u>e	[s]	[ ]		
18	<u>s</u>poon	[s]	[ ]		
19	<u>s</u>kate<u>s</u>	[s], [s]	[ ], [ ]		
20	<u>s</u>tar<u>s</u>	[s], [z]	[ ], [ ]		
21	fi<u>sh</u>	[ʃ]	[ ]		
22	<u>f</u>i<u>v</u>e toe<u>s</u>	[f], [v], [z]	[ ], [ ], [ ]		
23	T<u>V</u>	[v]	[ ]		
24	mea<u>s</u>ure	[ʒ]	[ ]		
25	<u>sh</u>oe	[ʃ]	[ ]		
26	<u>s</u>ta<u>t</u>ion	[s], [ʃ]	[ ], [ ]		
27	<u>ch</u>air	[tʃ]	[ ]		
28	pla<u>c</u>emat	[s]	[ ]		
29	mat<u>ch</u>e<u>s</u>	[tʃ], [z]	[ ], [ ]		
30	a<u>s</u>leep	[s]	[ ]		

MODULE TIME	
TOTAL	2:05
ELAPSED	08:25–10:30

Clinical Phonetics CD 3, Track 9
Glides and Liquids Module 1: Glide Changes

TRANSCRIPTION KEY

	STIMULUS WORD	INTENDED	CONSENSUS	ALTERNATIVES	COMMENTS
1	on<u>io</u>n	[j]	[w]		
2	flo<u>w</u>er	[w]	[w]		[w] does not always occur; i.e., [f l a͡ʊ ɚ].
3	s<u>w</u>eeping	[w]	[l]		
4	s<u>w</u>ing	[w]	[r̮]		Derhotacized /r/ See Module 4.
5	<u>y</u>es	[j]	[j]		
6	sand<u>w</u>ich	[w]	[w]		
7	flo<u>w</u>er	[w]	[l]		See comment for item 2.
8	thank <u>y</u>ou	[j]	[l]		[θ̯]
9	<u>wh</u>istle	[w]	[w]		
10	<u>y</u>es	[j]	[w]		[s̭]

MODULE TIME	
TOTAL	2:05
ELAPSED	08:25–10:30

Clinical Phonetics CD 3, Track 9
Glides and Liquids Module 1:
Glide Changes

TRANSCRIPTION SHEET

	STIMULUS WORD	INTENDED	PERCEIVED	ALTERNATIVES	COMMENTS
1	onion	[j]	[ ]		
2	flower	[w]	[ ]		
3	sweeping	[w]	[ ]		
4	swing	[w]	[ ]		
5	yes	[j]	[ ]		
6	sandwich	[w]	[ ]		
7	flower	[w]	[ ]		
8	thank you	[j]	[ ]		
9	whistle	[w]	[ ]		
10	yes	[j]	[ ]		

MODULE TIME	
TOTAL	3:22
ELAPSED	10:30–13:52

Clinical Phonetics CD 3, Track 10
Glides and Liquids Module 2:
/l/ Substitutions

TRANSCRIPTION KEY

	STIMULUS WORD	INTENDED	CONSENSUS	ALTERNATIVES	COMMENTS
1	ladder	[l]	[j]		
2	bell	[l]	[l]		
3	nail	[l]	[ne͡ɪo̥ᶻ]	[ne͡ɪʊ̥ᶻ]	
4	lion	[l]	[l]		
5	football	[l]	[fʊʔbaʊ]	[fʊbal]	
6	blocks	[l]	[w]		
7	seal	[l]	[siᵊ]		
8	that apple	[l]	[æ p ʊ]	[æ p o]	
9	whistle	[l]	[w ɪ s o]	[w ɪ s ʊ]	
10	leaf	[l]	[l]		Lengthened
11	lamp	[l]	[r]	[r̯]	
12	baseball	[l]	[be͡ɪsbɔʊ]		
13	tail	[l]	[te͡ɪo̤]		Note symbol for breathy or murmured
14	we saw a puppet lady	[l]	[j]		
15	wheel	[l]	[wio]		
16	ladder	[l]	[w]		
17	seal	[l]	[siowə]	[sɪʊwə]	Unusual

Note: Differences between [o] and [ʊ] as replacements for final [l] are unimportant.

MODULE TIME	
TOTAL	3:22
ELAPSED	10:30–13:52

Clinical Phonetics CD 3, Track 10 Glides and Liquids Module 2: /l/ Substitutions

TRANSCRIPTION SHEET

	STIMULUS WORD	INTENDED	PERCEIVED	ALTERNATIVES	COMMENTS
1	ladder	[l]	[ ]		
2	bell	[l]	[ ]		
3	nail	[l]	[ ]		
4	lion	[l]	[ ]		
5	football	[l]	[ ]		
6	blocks	[l]	[ ]		
7	seal	[l]	[ ]		
8	that apple	[l]	[ ]		
9	whistle	[l]	[ ]		
10	leaf	[l]	[ ]		
11	lamp	[l]	[ ]		
12	baseball	[l]	[ ]		
13	tail	[l]	[ ]		
14	we saw a puppet lady	[l]	[ ]		
15	wheel	[l]	[ ]		
16	ladder	[l]	[ ]		
17	seal	[l]	[ ]		

Clinical Phonetics CD 3, Track 11
Glides and Liquids Module 3:
Velarized /l/

TRANSCRIPTION KEY

MODULE TIME	
TOTAL	3:10
ELAPSED	13:52–17:02

EXAMPLES			
NORMAL	[lɔ]	VELARIZED	[l̰ɔ]
	[ɔl]		[ɔl̰]

	STIMULUS WORD	INTENDED	CONSENSUS	ALTERNATIVES	COMMENTS
1	land	[l]	[l̰]		
2	ability	[l]	[l̰]		
3	asleep	[l]	[l̰]		Slightly
4	frolic	[l]	[l]		
5	alarm	[l]	[l̰]		Slightly
6	follow	[l]	[l̰]		Slightly
7	belong	[l]	[l̰]		
8	limb	[l]	[l̰]		
9	please	[l]	[l]		
10	black	[l]	[l̰]		[bəl̰æk]
11	class	[l]	[l]		
12	glad	[l]	[l̰]		
13	I believe I belong in this village	[l], [l], [l]	[l̰], [l̰], [l̰]	[l], [l]	Slight velarization on first and last /l/
14	The lake is so still it is almost like glass	[l], [l], [l], [l], [l]	[l̰], [l̰], [l̰], [l̰], [l̰]	[l], [l]	

Notes: Comparison of nos. 11 and 12, essentially the same phonetic context for the /l/, demonstrates a normal and a velarized /l/, respectively. Items 13 and 14 are extremely difficult to transcribe. They are included here to demonstrate the effect of velarized /l/ in continuous speech.

Clinical Phonetics CD 3, Track 11
Glides and Liquids Module 3: Velarized /l/

TRANSCRIPTION SHEET

MODULE TIME	
TOTAL	3:10
ELAPSED	13:52–17:02

EXAMPLES

NORMAL	[lɔ]	VELARIZED	[ɫɔ]
	[ɔl]		[ɔɫ]

	STIMULUS WORD	INTENDED	PERCEIVED	ALTERNATIVES	COMMENTS
1	land	[l]	[ ]		
2	ability	[l]	[ ]		
3	asleep	[l]	[ ]		
4	frolic	[l]	[ ]		
5	alarm	[l]	[ ]		
6	follow	[l]	[ ]		
7	belong	[l]	[ ]		
8	limb	[l]	[ ]		
9	please	[l]	[ ]		
10	black	[l]	[ ]		
11	class	[l]	[ ]		
12	glad	[l]	[ ]		
13	I believe I belong in this village	[l], [l], [l]	[ ],[ ],[ ]		
14	The lake is so still it is almost like glass	[l], [l], [l], [l], [l]	[ ],[ ],[ ],[ ],[ ]		

Clinical Phonetics CD 3, Track 12
Glides and Liquids Module 4: Derhotacized /r/, /ɝ/, /ɚ/

TRANSCRIPTION KEY

MODULE TIME	
TOTAL	5:57
ELAPSED	17:02–22:59

EXAMPLES			
NORMAL	[ri]	DERHOTACIZED	[r̯i]
	[ir]		[ir̯]

	STIMULUS WORD	INTENDED	CONSENSUS	ALTERNATIVES	COMMENTS
1	car	[r]	[r]		Slightly devoiced
2	a zebra	[r]	[r̯]	[w]	Also labialized, i.e., [r̯ʷ]
3	/ɝ/	[ɝ]	[ɝ]		
4	they having a fire	[r]	[ʊ]	[ə]	[f a͡ɪ ʊ] or [f a͡ɪ ə]
5	/ɝ/	[ɝ]	[ʌ : ᵊ]	[ɛ : ᵊ], [ʊ° ᵊ]	Other transcriptions too!
6	chair	[r]	[ɛ ə̠]	[ɛ ɪ ə], [ɛ ɔ]	
7	raining	[r]	[r̯]		Labialized [r̯ʷ]
8	/ɝ/	[ɝ]	[ʌ̊]	[ɔ̊], [ɔ̊ᶷ]	
9	car	[r]	[r]		
10	finger	[ɚ]	[ə]	[ɚ̯], [ʊ]	Perhaps some slight *r* coloring
11	garage	[r]	[r]	[rʷ]	
12	Is the cake ready	[r]	[r̯]	[rʷ]	Slightly
13	feather	[ɚ]	[ɚ]	[ɚ̯]	Ends abruptly
14	chair	[r]	[r̯]		Almost normal
15	big brother	[r], [ɚ]	[r̯], [ɚ̯]		
16	/ɝ/	[ɝ]	[ɝ̯]		
17	orbit	[r]	[r̯]		
18	sit right here	[r], [r]	[r̯], [r]		Second /r/ slightly derhotacized?
19	read	[r]	[r]		
20	He was running to school	[r]	[r]		
21	scissors	[ɚ]	[ɚ̯]	[ə]	
22	camper	[ɚ]	[ʊ]		[k æ m pᶷ]
23	three, four, five	[r], [r]	[r̯], [ə]		[f ɔ ə]
24	cricket	[r]	[r]		
25	brush	[r]	[r̯]		
26	chair	[r]	[r]		
27	sit right here	[r], [r]	[r̯], [r̯]		Last /r/ is only slightly derhotacized.

Notes: Items 16 and 17 provide good examples of derhotacized /ɝ/ and /r/, respectively. If you are hearing *w*-like sounds in place of /r/, recall that use of this symbol indicates a phonemic substitution. The number of alternative transcriptions for the incorrect /r/ sounds brings to mind similar problems with vowel-diphthong sound modifications. These judgments are extremely demanding; specification of the central or back vowel that replaced /r/, /ɝ/, or /ɚ/ generally is not critical. The derhotacized symbols [r̯], [ɝ̯], or [ɚ̯] can be used to cover the variety of sounds that replace [r], [ɝ], or [ɚ] with only *partial r* coloring.

Clinical Phonetics CD 3, Track 12
Glides and Liquids Module 4: Derhotacized /r/, /ɝ/, /ɚ/

TRANSCRIPTION SHEET

MODULE TIME	
TOTAL	5:57
ELAPSED	17:02–22:59

EXAMPLES			
NORMAL	[ri]	DERHOTACIZED	[r̯i]
	[ir]		[ir̯]

	STIMULUS WORD	INTENDED	PERCEIVED	ALTERNATIVES	COMMENTS
1	car	[r]	[ ]		
2	a zebra	[r]	[ ]		
3	/ɝ/	[ɝ]	[ ]		
4	they having a fire	[r]	[ ]		
5	/ɝ/	[ɝ]	[ ]		
6	chair	[r]	[ ]		
7	raining	[r]	[ ]		
8	/ɝ/	[ɝ]	[ ]		
9	car	[r]	[ ]		
10	finger	[ɚ]	[ ]		
11	garage	[r]	[ ]		
12	Is the cake ready	[r]	[ ]		
13	feather	[ɚ]	[ ]		
14	chair	[r]	[ ]		
15	big brother	[r], [ɚ]	[ ], [ ]		
16	/ɝ/	[ɝ]	[ ]		
17	orbit	[r]	[ ]		
18	sit right here	[r], [r]	[ ], [ ]		
19	read	[r]	[ ]		
20	He was running to school	[r]	[ ]		
21	scissors	[ɚ]	[ ]		
22	camper	[ɚ]	[ ]		
23	three, four, five	[r], [r]	[ ], [ ]		
24	cricket	[r]	[ ]		
25	brush	[r]	[ ]		
26	chair	[r]	[ ]		
27	sit right here	[r], [r]	[ ], [ ]		

MODULE TIME	
TOTAL	4:35
ELAPSED	22:59–27:34

Clinical Phonetics CD 3, Track 13
Glides and Liquids Module 5: /r/ Quiz

TRANSCRIPTION KEY

	STIMULUS WORD	INTENDED	CONSENSUS	ALTERNATIVES	COMMENTS
1	smooth rock	[r]	[w]		
2	read	[r]	[w]	[r̮]	
3	rain	[r]	[r]		Noisy onset
4	carrots	[r]	[w]		
5	sit on the bridge	[r]	[w]		Did he say *sit?*
6	he can't run very good	[r], [r]	[r̮], [r]		
7	barn	[r]	[ɑ ɔ]	[b ɑ o n], [b a͡ʊ ːn]	
8	ring	[r]	[r̮]		Close to [w]
9	He was running to school	[r]	[r̮]		Close to [w]
10	color the map red	[ɚ], [r]	[ɚ̮], [r̮]		
11	crackers	[r], [ɚ]	[w], [ʊ̆]	[ə], [ɔ]	
12	rabbit	[r]	[r]		
13	Christmas tree	[r], [r]	[w], [r̮]		
14	parking	[r]	[r]		
15	Did the bell ring	[r]	[w]		
16	broom	[r]	[r̮]		Almost [w]
17	ice water	[ɚ]	[ɚ̮]	[ʊ], [o]	
18	He can ride a bike	[r]	[r̮]		
19	fireman	[r]	[ʊ]	[f a͡ɪ ə̫ m æ n]	
20	doorway	[r]	[r]		
21	zipper	[ɚ]	[ɚ]		

Notes: Notice some clear examples of correct /r/ and /ɚ/ and some clear examples of w/r. What falls in between these two either has *some r* coloring (derhotacized) or is transcribed as a pure vowel—usually /ə/, /ʊ/, or /ɔ/.

MODULE TIME	
TOTAL	4:35
ELAPSED	22:59–27:34

Clinical Phonetics CD 3, Track 13 Glides and Liquids Module 5: /r/ Quiz

TRANSCRIPTION SHEET

	STIMULUS WORD	INTENDED	PERCEIVED	ALTERNATIVES	COMMENTS
1	smooth rock	[r]	[ ]		
2	read	[r]	[ ]		
3	rain	[r]	[ ]		
4	carrots	[r]	[ ]		
5	sit on the bridge	[r]	[ ]		
6	he can't run very good	[r], [r]	[ ], [ ]		
7	barn	[r]	[ ]		
8	ring	[r]	[ ]		
9	He was running to school	[r]	[ ]		
10	color the map red	[ɚ], [r]	[ ], [ ]		
11	crackers	[r], [ɚ]	[ ], [ ]		
12	rabbit	[r]	[ ]		
13	Christmas tree	[r], [r]	[ ], [ ]		
14	parking	[r]	[ ]		
15	Did the bell ring	[r]	[ ]		
16	broom	[r]	[ ]		
17	ice water	[ɚ]	[ ]		
18	He can ride a bike	[r]	[ ]		
19	fireman	[r]	[ ]		
20	doorway	[r]	[ ]		
21	zipper	[ɚ]	[ ]		

MODULE TIME	
TOTAL	3:03
ELAPSED	00:00–03:03

Clinical Phonetics CD 4, Track 1
Glides and Liquids Module 6: Velarized /r/

TRANSCRIPTION KEY

	STIMULUS WORD	INTENDED	CONSENSUS	ALTERNATIVES	COMMENTS
1	chair	[r]	[r]		
2	a zebra	[r]	[r̰]		Sounds almost like a stop, i.e., [z i b g ɑ]
3	play with Brett	[r]	[r̰]		
4	rain	[r]	[r̰]		Less far back than nos. 2 and 3
5	brush	[r]	[r̰]		
6	garage	[r]	[r̰]		Slight
7	it's raining	[r]	[r]		
8	at a fire	[r]	[ʊ]		[f͡aɪ ʊ]
9	brush	[r]	[r̰]		
10	parking	[r]	[r]		
11	garage	[r]	[r̰]		
12	chair	[r]	[ʌ]	[tʃ͡eɪɔ]	
13	running	[r]	[r̰]		
14	zebra	[r]	[r]		

Notes: Can you make velarized /r/ sounds easily and rapidly? Item 9 is a good model. Recall that velarized /r/ is made and sounds exactly like velarized /l/. For example, say velarized liquids in the word pairs *light* [l̰ a͡ɪ t] and *right* [r̰ a͡ɪ t]; *lead* [l̰ ɛd] and *red* [r̰ ɛ d]; *load* [l̰ o͡ʊ d] and *road* [r̰ o͡ʊ d].

MODULE TIME	
TOTAL	3:03
ELAPSED	00:00–03:03

Clinical Phonetics CD 4, Track 1 Glides and Liquids Module 6: Velarized /r/

TRANSCRIPTION SHEET

	STIMULUS WORD	INTENDED	PERCEIVED	ALTERNATIVES	COMMENTS
1	chair	[r]	[ ]		
2	a zebra	[r]	[ ]		
3	play with Brett	[r]	[ ]		
4	rain	[r]	[ ]		
5	brush	[r]	[ ]		
6	garage	[r]	[ ]		
7	it's raining	[r]	[ ]		
8	at a fire	[r]	[ ]		
9	brush	[r]	[ ]		
10	parking	[r]	[ ]		
11	garage	[r]	[ ]		
12	chair	[r]	[ ]		
13	running	[r]	[ ]		
14	zebra	[r]	[ ]		

MODULE TIME	
TOTAL	4:56
ELAPSED	03:03–07:59

Clinical Phonetics CD 4, Track 2
Glides and Liquids Module 7: Summary Quiz

TRANSCRIPTION KEY

	STIMULUS WORD	INTENDED	CONSENSUS	ALTERNATIVES	COMMENTS
1	play	[l]	[l̰]		
2	New York	[j], [r]	[j], [ɔ^{ə}]		
3	train	[r]	[w]		[t^{ə} w e͡ɪ n]
4	brush	[r]	[l]		[b^{ə} l ʌ s]
5	balloons	[l]	[l]		
6	police car siren	[l], [r], [r]	[w], [Ø], [w]		[p^{ə}i^{s}k ɑː s a͡ɪ w ə n]
7	girl	[ɝ], [l]	[w], [ʊ]	[u]	[g ʌ w ʊ]
8	ladder	[l], [ɚ]	[m], [ɝ]		Stress change [m æ d ɝ]
9	carrot	[r]	[l]		?
10	chair	[r]	[r]		Noisy
11	apple	[l]	[ɝ]		[æ p^{h} ɝ]
12	yellow	[j], [l]	[j], [d]		[j ɛ d ə̼] or [j ɛ d ɔ]
13	sit right here	[r], [r]	[r̯], [r̯]		Second /r/ only slightly derhotacized
14	fireman	[r]	[r]		
15	yellow	[j], [l]	[^{k}j], [ð]		[^{k} j ɛ ð o ^{ʊ}]
16	tail	[l]	[o]		[t e͡ɪ o]
17	measuring cup	[ɚ]	[ɚ]		
18	nail	[l]	[ː^{ə}]	[n e͡ɪ ^{ʊ}]	
19	broom	[r]	[Ø]		[b u m]
20	feather	[ɚ]	[ə^{ɔ}]	[f ɛ ð ɔː],[f ɛ ð o^{ə}]	
21	rain	[r]	[^{ə}w]	[^{ʊ}w]	
22	the drum	[r]	[r̰]		[d^{ə} r̰ ʌ m]
23	carrots	[r]	[w]		
24	a feather	[ɚ]	[ʊ]	[ɚ̯]	
25	finger	[ɚ]	[ɚ]		

Clinical Phonetics CD 4, Track 2
Glides and Liquids Module 7:
Summary Quiz

MODULE TIME	
TOTAL	4:56
ELAPSED	03:03–07:59

TRANSCRIPTION SHEET

	STIMULUS WORD	INTENDED	PERCEIVED	ALTERNATIVES	COMMENTS
1	play	[l]	[ ]		
2	New York	[j], [r]	[ ], [ ]		
3	train	[r]	[ ]		
4	brush	[r]	[ ]		
5	balloons	[l]	[ ]		
6	police car siren	[l], [r], [r]	[ ], [ ], [ ]		
7	girl	[ɝ], [l]	[ ], [ ]		
8	ladder	[l], [ɚ]	[ ], [ ]		
9	carrot	[r]	[ ]		
10	chair	[r]	[ ]		
11	apple	[l]	[ ]		
12	yellow	[j], [l]	[ ], [ ]		
13	sit right here	[r], [r]	[ ], [ ]		
14	fireman	[r]	[ ]		
15	yellow	[j], [l]	[ ], [ ]		
16	tail	[l]	[ ]		
17	measuring cup	[ɚ]	[ ]		
18	nail	[l]	[ ]		
19	broom	[r]	[ ]		
20	feather	[ɚ]	[ ]		
21	rain	[r]	[ ]		
22	the drum	[r]	[ ]		
23	carrots	[r]	[ ]		
24	a feather	[ɚ]	[ ]		
25	finger	[ɚ]	[ ]		

MODULE TIME	
TOTAL	3:09
ELAPSED	07:59–11:08

Clinical Phonetics CD 4, Track 3
Nasals Module 1:
Nasal Deletions

TRANSCRIPTION KEY

	STIMULUS WORD	INTENDED	CONSENSUS	ALTERNATIVES	COMMENTS
1	jumping	[m], [ŋ]	[m], [ŋ]		
2	onion	[n], [n]	[ø], [n]		[e͡ɪ j ə n]
3	smooth	[m]	[m]		
4	valentine	[n], [n]	[ø], [n]	[ʔ]	
5	spoon	[n]	[n]		
6	planting	[n], [ŋ]	[ø], [ŋ]		[p l æ̃ ː t ɪ ŋ]
7	Joanne	[n]	[ø]		[ʤ o͡ʊ æ̃ ᵊ]
8	hammer	[m]	[m]		Noisy
9	can	[n]	[ə]		[k æ ː ᵊ]
10	gun	[n]	[n]		
11	lamp	[m]	[m]	[ø]	Reduced, i.e., [l æ̃ m pʰ]
12	thumb	[m]	[m]		
13	parking	[ŋ]	[ŋ]		
14	can	[n]	[n]		
15	fire hydrant	[n]	[ø]		

MODULE TIME	
TOTAL	3:09
ELAPSED	07:59–11:08

Clinical Phonetics CD 4, Track 3
Nasals Module 1:
Nasal Deletions

TRANSCRIPTION SHEET

	STIMULUS WORD	INTENDED	PERCEIVED	ALTERNATIVES	COMMENTS
1	jumping	[m], [ŋ]	[ ], [ ]		
2	onion	[n], [n]	[ ], [ ]		
3	smooth	[m]	[ ]		
4	valentine	[n], [n]	[ ], [ ]		
5	spoon	[n]	[ ]		
6	planting	[n], [ŋ]	[ ], [ ]		
7	Joanne	[n]	[ ]		
8	hammer	[m]	[ ]		
9	can	[n]	[ ]		
10	gun	[n]	[ ]		
11	lamp	[m]	[ ]		
12	thumb	[m]	[ ]		
13	parking	[ŋ]	[ ]		
14	can	[n]	[ ]		
15	fire hydrant	[n]	[ ]		

MODULE TIME	
TOTAL	3:54
ELAPSED	11:08–15:02

Clinical Phonetics CD 4, Track 4
Nasals Module 2:
Summary Quiz

TRANSCRIPTION KEY

	STIMULUS WORD	INTENDED	CONSENSUS	ALTERNATIVES	COMMENTS
1	angels	[n]	[n]		
2	jumping	[m], [ŋ]	[m], [ŋ]		
3	knife	[n]	[ᵈn]		[d ₙ a͊ɪ ə f]
4	a thumb	[m]	[m]		
5	window	[n]	[n]		
6	comb	[m]	[m͊]		[k o͊ʊ m͊]
7	some	[m]	[m͡bᵊ]	[m͊bᵊ]	[s ʌ m͊bᵊ ʔ]
8	spoon	[n]	[n]	[nᵗ]	
9	elephant	[n]	[n]	[n͊]	
10	gun	[n]	[n͊]		[g ʌ͊ n͊]
11	some	[m]	[m]	[mː]	
12	smoke	[m]	[m̥]		
13	snake	[n]	[n]		
14	hammer	[m]	[n]		
15	jumping	[m], [ŋ]	[m], [n]		
16	monkey	[m], [ŋ]	[m], [ŋ]		
17	nail	[n]	[m]		[m e͊ɪ o]
18	snowman	[n], [m], [n]	[n], [m], [n]		Extra first syllable [s ɪ m ᵊ n o ᵊ m æ̞ n]
19	knife	[n]	[n]		
20	comb	[m]	[n͊]	[n]	

Note: Notice the variety of denasalization errors, including what sounds like an *epenthetic* (added) *stop,* such as nos. 3 and 7.

MODULE TIME	
TOTAL	3:54
ELAPSED	11:08–15:02

Clinical Phonetics CD 4, Track 4
Nasals Module 2:
Summary Quiz

TRANSCRIPTION SHEET

	STIMULUS WORD	INTENDED	PERCEIVED	ALTERNATIVES	COMMENTS
1	angels	[n]	[ ]		
2	jumping	[m], [ŋ]	[ ], [ ]		
3	knife	[n]	[ ]		
4	a thumb	[m]	[ ]		
5	window	[n]	[ ]		
6	comb	[m]	[ ]		
7	some	[m]	[ ]		
8	spoon	[n]	[ ]		
9	elephant	[n]	[ ]		
10	gun	[n]	[ ]		
11	some	[m]	[ ]		
12	smoke	[m]	[ ]		
13	snake	[n]	[ ]		
14	hammer	[m]	[ ]		
15	jumping	[m], [ŋ]	[ ], [ ]		
16	monkey	[m], [ŋ]	[ ], [ ]		
17	nail	[n]	[ ]		
18	snowman	[n], [m], [n]	[ ], [ ], [ ]		
19	knife	[n]	[ ]		
20	comb	[m]	[ ]		

MODULE TIME	
TOTAL	8:36
ELAPSED	15:02–23:38

Clinical Phonetics CD 4, Track 5
Grand Quiz

TRANSCRIPTION KEY

	STIMULUS WORD	CONSENSUS		STIMULUS WORD	CONSENSUS
1	a seal	[əθil]	24	party	[pʰartʰi̝]
2	scissors	[sɪzɚz̥]	25	feather	[fɛ̠ðʊ]
3	shoe	[su]	26	bus	[bʌs̪]
4	hammer	[hæ̞̃mᵇɚ]	27	a zebra	[əzibwə]
5	lamp	[lɑ̃p]	28	yellow	[jɛ̝lo]
6	valentine	[vɛ̝wəntɑ͡ɪm]	29	arrow	[æ̞ro͡ʊ]
7	watch	[wɔt͡s̡] (palatal /s/)	30	crayons	[kre͡ɪɑ̠̃nts̪]
8	soap	[s̪̞o͡ʊp]	31	roller skates	[r̯o͡ʊlɚ̯ske͡ɪts͍]
9	bicycle	[bɑ͡ɪ̃sɪ̃kʊ̃]	32	wagon	(child was a young Republican) [əre͡ɪgən]
10	chicken	[s̪ɪkɪn]	33	bathe	[be͡ɪ̈v̥]
11	pencils	[pɛ̃ns̪o̞z̥]	34	fall	[fɔl̰]
12	garage	[gwɑᵊʤ]	35	fish	[ʧɪf]
13	banana	[p˭ɪkæ̞̃nɑ̃]	36	whistle	[brɪʔɪ]
14	spoon	[spũːn]	37	splash	[s̪plæs̪]
15	dog	[d̪ɔːg̊]	38	shoe	[tʰu]
16	skates	[k˭e͡ɪts]	39	egg	[e͡ɪg̊]
17	that apple	[dæɾæpo]	40	measure	[mæʔɪ]
18	zebra	[z̥ibrʌ]	41	blocks	[bwɑts͍]
19	cat	[kʰeᵆt]	42	string	[s̪trɪŋk]
20	teeth	[tʰif]	43	follow	[fɑl̰o͡ʊ]
21	ladder	[wæd̺ɚ] (or flap [ɾ])	44	camper	[kæ̃mpʊ]
22	pipe	[pɑ͡ɪ˃p]	45	water	[wɔdɚ̯]
23	doorway	[dɔwe͡ɪ]			

Note: You can calculate your agreement in many ways: whole word agreement, agreement for all vowels, agreement for all consonants, agreement for all fricatives, and so forth.

MODULE TIME	
TOTAL	8:36
ELAPSED	15:02–23:38

Clinical Phonetics CD 4, Track 5
Grand Quiz

TRANSCRIPTION SHEET

	STIMULUS WORD	PERCEIVED		STIMULUS WORD	PERCEIVED
1	a seal	[ ]	24	party	[ ]
2	scissors	[ ]	25	feather	[ ]
3	shoe	[ ]	26	bus	[ ]
4	hammer	[ ]	27	a zebra	[ ]
5	lamp	[ ]	28	yellow	[ ]
6	valentine	[ ]	29	arrow	[ ]
7	watch	[ ]	30	crayons	[ ]
8	soap	[ ]	31	roller skates	[ ]
9	bicycle	[ ]	32	wagon	[ ]
10	chicken	[ ]	33	bathe	[ ]
11	pencils	[ ]	34	fall	[ ]
12	garage	[ ]	35	fish	[ ]
13	banana	[ ]	36	whistle	[ ]
14	spoon	[ ]	37	splash	[ ]
15	dog	[ ]	38	shoe	[ ]
16	skates	[ ]	39	egg	[ ]
17	that apple	[ ]	40	measure	[ ]
18	zebra	[ ]	41	blocks	[ ]
19	cat	[ ]	42	string	[ ]
20	teeth	[ ]	43	follow	[ ]
21	ladder	[ ]	44	camper	[ ]
22	pipe	[ ]	45	water	[ ]
23	doorway	[ ]			

MODULE TIME	
TOTAL	4:42
ELAPSED	23:38–28:20

Clinical Phonetics CD 4, Track 6
Practice Module 1:
Single-Sound Articulation Test

DEVELOPMENTAL ARTICULATION TEST—KEY

Name ______________ Age____ Grade____ School__________ Date__________

(Score as per the following examples. Substitution: b/p; Omission: -/p; Distortion: Dist/p.
*Note: Except where otherwise noted, Developmental Age Level signifies the chronological age by which approximately 90% or more children are using the sound correctly.

Card	Dev. Age Level	Sound Tested	Check Words	1	2	3	Iso.	Comments
1	3	m	monkey, hammer, broom	+	+	O		
2	3	n	nails, penny, lion	+	+	+		
3	3	p	pig, puppy, cup	O	+	+		
4	3	h	house, dog-house, ----	+	+			
5	3	w	window, spider-web, ----	+	+			
6	4	b	boat, baby, (bib: 75%)	+	+	+		
7	4	k	cat, chicken, book	O	+	*O		*Indeterminant
8	4	g	girl, wagon, (pig: 75%)	+	O	O		
9	4	f	fork, telephone, knife	O	O	O		
10	5	y	yellow, onion, (thank-you; Alt.), --	O	O			
11	5	ng	----, fingers, ring		+	O		
12	5	d	dog, ladder, bed	+	O	+		
13	6	l	lamp, balloon, ball	O	O	O		
14	6	r	rabbit, barn, car	O	+	+		
15	6	t	table, potatoes, coat	+	O	*O		*Indeterminant
16	6	sh	shoe, dishes, fish	O	O	O		
17	6	ch	chair, matches, watch	O	O	O		
18	6	Blends	drum, clock, blocks, glasses, crayons					
19	7	v	vacuum, television, stove					
20	7	th	thumb, toothbrush, teeth					
21	7	j	jump-rope, orange-juice, orange					
22	7	s	sun, pencil, bus					
23	7	z	zebra, scissors, (rubbers: 75%)					
24	7	Blends	train, star, slide, swing, spoon					
25	8	~~th~~	this or that, feathers, ----					
26	8	Blends	scooter, snowman, desk, nest					

Notes: A strict response definition is used for this key. For example, initial unaspirated stops are scored incorrect; by a more liberal response definition, they would be correct.

MODULE TIME	
TOTAL	4:42
ELAPSED	23:38–28:20

Clinical Phonetics CD 4, Track 6
Practice Module 1:
Single-Sound Articulation Test

DEVELOPMENTAL ARTICULATION TEST—SCORING BLANK

Name ______________ Age____ Grade____ School__________ Date__________

(Score as per the following examples. Substitution: b/p; Omission: -/p; Distortion: Dist/p.
*Note: Except where otherwise noted, Developmental Age Level signifies the chronological age by which approximately 90% or more children are using the sound correctly.

Card	Dev. Age Level	Sound Tested	Check Words	1	2	3	Iso.	Comments
1	3	m	monkey, hammer, broom	+	+	0		
2	3	n	nails, penny, lion					
3	3	p	pig, puppy, cup					
4	3	h	house, dog-house, ----					
5	3	w	window, spider-web, ----					
6	4	b	boat, baby, (bib: 75%)					
7	4	k	cat, chicken, book					
8	4	g	girl, wagon, (pig: 75%)					
9	4	f	fork, telephone, knife					
10	5	y	yellow, onion, (thank-you; Alt.), --					
11	5	ng	----, fingers, ring					
12	5	d	dog, ladder, bed					
13	6	l	lamp, balloon, ball					
14	6	r	rabbit, barn, car					
15	6	t	table, potatoes, coat					
16	6	sh	shoe, dishes, fish					
17	6	ch	chair, matches, watch					
18	6	Blends	drum, clock, blocks, glasses, crayons					
19	7	v	vacuum, television, stove					
20	7	th	thumb, toothbrush, teeth					
21	7	j	jump-rope, orange-juice, orange					
22	7	s	sun, pencil, bus					
23	7	z	zebra, scissors, (rubbers: 75%)					
24	7	Blends	train, star, slide, swing, spoon					
25	8	~~th~~	this or that, feathers, ----					
26	8	Blends	scooter, snowman, desk, nest					

Notes: Clinical Phonetics Tape 4A: Practice Module 1 is based on the Hejna Developmental Articulation Test Form reproduced with permission of Robert F. Hejna.

Clinical Phonetics CD 4, Track 6
Practice Module 1:
Single-Sound Articulation Test

MODULE TIME	
TOTAL	4:42
ELAPSED	23:38–28:20

DEVELOPMENTAL ARTICULATION TEST—KEY

Name ______________ Age ____ Grade ____ School ______________ Date ______

(Score as per the following examples. Substitution: b/p; Omission: -/p; Distortion: Dist/p.
*Note: Except where otherwise noted, Developmental Age Level signifies the chronological age by which approximately 90% or more children are using the sound correctly.

Card	Dev. Age Level	Sound Tested	Check Words	1	2	3	Iso.	Comments
1	3	m	monkey, hammer, broom	+	+	–		
2	3	n	nails, penny, lion	+	+	+		
3	3	p	pig, puppy, cup	D	+	+		
4	3	h	house, dog-house, ----	+	+			
5	3	w	window, spider-web, ----	+	+			
6	4	b	boat, baby, (bib: 75%)	+	+	+		
7	4	k	cat, chicken, book	D	+	(t/k)*		*Indeterminant
8	4	g	girl, wagon, (pig: 75%)	+	D	d/g		
9	4	f	fork, telephone, knife	p/f	w/f	A		A = Addition
10	5	y	yellow, onion, (thank-you; Alt.), --	–	–			
11	5	ng	----, fingers, ring		+	D		
12	5	d	dog, ladder, bed	+	D	+		
13	6	l	lamp, balloon, ball	D	b/l	–		
14	6	r	rabbit, barn, car	w/r	+	+		
15	6	t	table, potatoes, coat	+	D	?/t		
16	6	sh	shoe, dishes, fish	h/ʃ	t/ʃ	D		
17	6	ch	chair, matches, watch	D	t/tʃ	D		
18	6	Blends	drum, clock, blocks, glasses, crayons					
19	7	v	vacuum, television, stove					
20	7	th	thumb, toothbrush, teeth					
21	7	j	jump-rope, orange-juice, orange					
22	7	s	sun, pencil, bus					
23	7	z	zebra, scissors, (rubbers: 75%)					
24	7	Blends	train, star, slide, swing, spoon					
25	8	~~th~~	this or that, feathers, ----					
26	8	Blends	scooter, snowman, desk, nest					

Notes: A strict response definition is used for this key. For example, initial unaspirated stops are scored incorrect; by a more liberal response definition, they would be correct.

MODULE TIME	
TOTAL	4:42
ELAPSED	23:38–28:20

Clinical Phonetics CD 4, Track 6
Practice Module 1:
Single-Sound Articulation Test

DEVELOPMENTAL ARTICULATION TEST—SCORING BLANK

Name ______ Age ___ Grade ___ School ______ Date ______

(Score as per the following examples. Substitution: b/p; Omission: -/p; Distortion: Dist/p.

*Note: Except where otherwise noted, Developmental Age Level signifies the chronological age by which approximately 90% or more children are using the sound correctly.

Card	Dev. Age Level	Sound Tested	Check Words	1	2	3	Iso.	Comments
1	3	m	monkey, hammer, broom	+	+	–		
2	3	n	nails, penny, lion					
3	3	p	pig, puppy, cup					
4	3	h	house, dog-house, ----					
5	3	w	window, spider-web, ----					
6	4	b	boat, baby, (bib: 75%)					
7	4	k	cat, chicken, book					
8	4	g	girl, wagon, (pig: 75%)					
9	4	f	fork, telephone, knife					
10	5	y	yellow, onion, (thank-you; Alt.), --					
11	5	ng	----, fingers, ring					
12	5	d	dog, ladder, bed					
13	6	l	lamp, balloon, ball					
14	6	r	rabbit, barn, car					
15	6	t	table, potatoes, coat					
16	6	sh	shoe, dishes, fish					
17	6	ch	chair, matches, watch					
18	6	Blends	drum, clock, blocks, glasses, crayons					
19	7	v	vacuum, television, stove					
20	7	th	thumb, toothbrush, teeth					
21	7	j	jump-rope, orange-juice, orange					
22	7	s	sun, pencil, bus					
23	7	z	zebra, scissors, (rubbers: 75%)					
24	7	Blends	train, star, slide, swing, spoon					
25	8	~~th~~	this or that, feathers, ----					
26	8	Blends	scooter, snowman, desk, nest					

MODULE TIME	
TOTAL	4:42
ELAPSED	23:38–28:20

Clinical Phonetics CD 4, Track 6
Practice Module 1:
Single-Sound Articulation Test

DEVELOPMENTAL ARTICULATION TEST—KEY

Name ________ Age___ Grade___ School________ Date______
(Score as per the following examples. Substitution: b/p; Omission: -/p; Distortion: Dist/p.
*Note: Except where otherwise noted, Developmental Age Level signifies the chronological age by which approximately 90% or more children are using the sound correctly.

Card	Dev. Age Level	Sound Tested	Check Words	1	2	3	Iso.	Comments
1	3	m	monkey, hammer, broom	m	m	ø		
2	3	n	nails, penny, lion	n	n	n		
3	3	p	pig, puppy, cup	p=	p	p		
4	3	h	house, dog-house, ----	h	h			
5	3	w	window, spider-web, ----	w	ʏw			
6	4	b	boat, baby, (bib: 75%)	b	b	b		
7	4	k	cat, chicken, book	k=	k	(t˺)* (k˺)		*Indeterminant
8	4	g	girl, wagon, (pig: 75%)	g*	g̃ OR ŋ	d		*Second time!!
9	4	f	fork, telephone, knife	p=	w̃	t͡f		
10	5	y	yellow, onion, (thank-you; Alt.), --	ø	(j̃ / ʟ)			*Indeterminant
11	5	ng	----, fingers, ring		ŋ	ŋᵏ		
12	5	d	dog, ladder, bed	d̥	d̽*	d		*Weak contact
13	6	l	lamp, balloon, ball	ɹ̡/*	b	ø		*Palatalized?
14	6	r	rabbit, barn, car	m / w	r	r		
15	6	t	table, potatoes, coat	t	t=	*ʔ		*Indeterminant: [ʔ] or [t˺] or [ø]
16	6	sh	shoe, dishes, fish	h	t / n	t͡s̡		
17	6	ch	chair, matches, watch	tθ / n	t / n	ts / n		
18	6	Blends	drum, clock, blocks, glasses, crayons					
19	7	v	vacuum, television, stove					
20	7	th	thumb, toothbrush, teeth					
21	7	j	jump-rope, orange-juice, orange					
22	7	s	sun, pencil, bus					
23	7	z	zebra, scissors, (rubbers: 75%)					
24	7	Blends	train, star, slide, swing, spoon					
25	8	~~th~~	this or that, feathers, ----					
26	8	Blends	scooter, snowman, desk, nest					

Notes: Note the problems this girl has in timing, particularly in velopharyngeal control.

MODULE TIME	
TOTAL	4:42
ELAPSED	23:38–28:20

Clinical Phonetics CD 4, Track 6
Practice Module 1:
Single-Sound Articulation Test

DEVELOPMENTAL ARTICULATION TEST—SCORING BLANK

Name ______________ Age____ Grade____ School__________ Date__________

(Score as per the following examples. Substitution: b/p; Omission: -/p; Distortion: Dist/p.
*Note: Except where otherwise noted, Developmental Age Level signifies the chronological age by which approximately 90% or more children are using the sound correctly.

Card	Dev. Age Level	Sound Tested	Check Words	1	2	3	Iso.	Comments
1	3	m	monkey, hammer, broom	m	m	ϕ		
2	3	n	nails, penny, lion					
3	3	p	pig, puppy, cup					
4	3	h	house, dog-house, ----					
5	3	w	window, spider-web, ----					
6	4	b	boat, baby, (bib: 75%)					
7	4	k	cat, chicken, book					
8	4	g	girl, wagon, (pig: 75%)					
9	4	f	fork, telephone, knife					
10	5	y	yellow, onion, (thank-you; Alt.), --					
11	5	ng	----, fingers, ring					
12	5	d	dog, ladder, bed					
13	6	l	lamp, balloon, ball					
14	6	r	rabbit, barn, car					
15	6	t	table, potatoes, coat					
16	6	sh	shoe, dishes, fish					
17	6	ch	chair, matches, watch					
18	6	Blends	drum, clock, blocks, glasses, crayons					
19	7	v	vacuum, television, stove					
20	7	th	thumb, toothbrush, teeth					
21	7	j	jump-rope, orange-juice, orange					
22	7	s	sun, pencil, bus					
23	7	z	zebra, scissors, (rubbers: 75%)					
24	7	Blends	train, star, slide, swing, spoon					
25	8	~~th~~	this or that, feathers, ----					
26	8	Blends	scooter, snowman, desk, nest					

MODULE TIME	
TOTAL	3:06
ELAPSED	00:00–03:06

Clinical Phonetics CD 4, Track 7
Practice Module 2:
Multiple-Sound Articulation Test

INDIVIDUAL RECORD SHEET FOR A SCREENING DEEP TEST OF ARTICULATION

INDIVIDUAL RECORD SHEET for A SCREENING DEEP TEST OF ARTICULATION
by Eugene T. McDonald

Name________ Birthdate________ School________ Grade________ Tester________ Date________

			[s]	[l]	[r]	[tʃ]	[θ]	[ʃ]	[k]	[f]	[t]
1 bus	fish	bʌ[s][f]ɪ[ʃ]	[+]					[o]		[+]	
2 ball	chain	bɔ[l][tʃ]en		[o]		[o]					
3 watch	lock	wɔ[tʃ][l]ɑ[k]		[o]		[o]			[+]		
4 house	flag	haʊ[s][f][l]æg	[+]	[+]						[+]	
5 ring	witch	[r]iŋwɪ[tʃ]			[o]	[o]					
6 chair	sun	[tʃ]ɛ[r][s]ʌn	[+]		[o]	[o]					
7 book	shoe	bʊ[k][ʃ]u						[+]	[o]		
8 cat	leaf	[k]æ[t][l]i[f]		[+]					[+]	[+]	[+]
9 star	thumb	[s][t]ɑ[r][θ]ʌm	[+]		[o]		[o]				[+]
10 horse	key	hɔ[r][s][k]i	[+]		[o]				[+]		
11 cat	sheep	[k]æ[t][ʃ]ip						[o]	[+]		[+]
12 ear	bell	ɪ[r]bɛ[l]		[o]	[o]						
13 tree	thumb	[t][r]i[θ]ʌm			[o]		[o]				[+]
14 teeth	lock	[t]i[θ][l]ɑ[k]		[+]			[o]		[+]		[+]
15 tooth	brush	[t]u[θ]b[r]ʌ[ʃ]			[o]		[o]	[+]			[+]
16 knife	spoon	naɪ[f][s]pun	[+]							[o]	
17 leaf	chair	[l]i[f][tʃ]ɛ[r]		[+]	[o]	[o]				[+]	
18 glove	thumb	g[l]ʌv[θ]ʌm		[+]			[o]				
19 brush	five	b[r]ʌ[ʃ][f]aɪv			[o]			[S]		[+]	
20 lock	fish	[l]ɑ[k][f]ɪ[ʃ]		[+]				[S]	[+]	[+]	
21 mouth	tie	maʊ[θ][t]aɪ					[ ]				[ ]
22 watch	fork	wɔ[tʃ][f]ɔ[r][k]			[ ]	[ ]			[ ]	[ ]	
23 fish	tooth	[f]ɪ[ʃ][t]u[θ]					[ ]	[ ]		[ ]	[ ]
24 sled	sheep	[s][l]ɛd[ʃ]ip	[ ]	[ ]				[ ]			
25 match	kite	mæ[tʃ][k]aɪ[t]				[ ]			[ ]		[ ]
26 sheep	chain	[ʃ]ip[tʃ]en				[ ]		[ ]			
27 fish	house	[f]ɪ[ʃ]haʊ[s]	[ ]					[ ]		[ ]	
28 thumb	saw	[θ]ʌm[s]ɔ	[ ]				[ ]				
29 saw	teeth	[s]ɔ[t]i[θ]	[ ]				[ ]				[ ]
30 witch	key	wɪ[tʃ][k]i				[ ]			[ ]		
31 mouth	match	maʊ[θ]mæ[tʃ]				[ ]	[ ]				

Summary of pertinent findings:

Recommendations:

No. contexts correct	[s]	[l]	[r]	[tʃ]	[θ]	[ʃ]	[k]	[f]	[t]
10	•	•	•	•	•	•	•	•	•
9	•	•	•	•	•	•	•	•	•
8	•	•	•	•	•	•	•	•	•
7	•	•	•	•	•	•	•	•	•
6	•	•	•	•	•	•	•	•	•
5	•	•	•	•	•	•	•	•	•
4	•	•	•	•	•	•	•	•	•
3	•	•	•	•	•	•	•	•	•
2	•	•	•	•	•	•	•	•	•
1	•	•	•	•	•	•	•	•	•
0	•	•	•	•	•	•	•	•	•

PHONETIC PROFILE

MODULE TIME	
TOTAL	3:06
ELAPSED	00:00–03:06

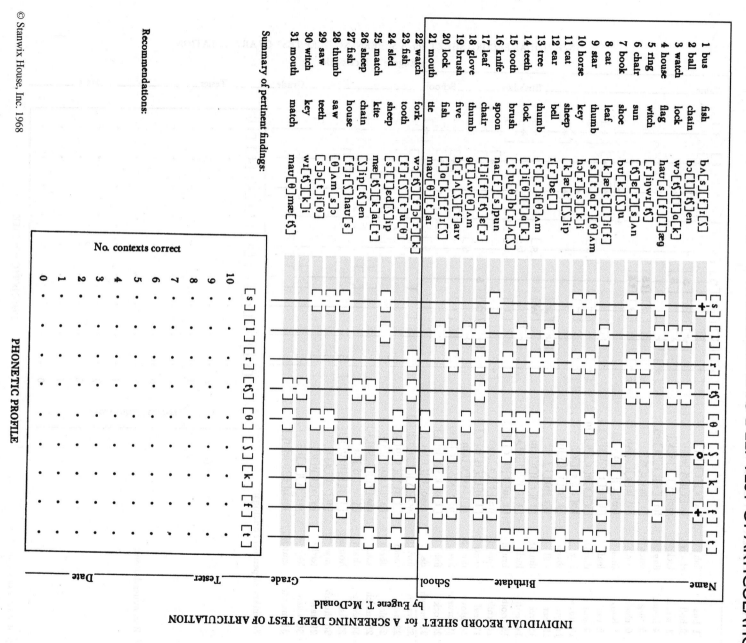

Clinical Phonetics CD 4, Track 7
Practice Module 2:
Multiple-Sound Articulation Test

INDIVIDUAL RECORD SHEET FOR A SCREENING DEEP TEST OF ARTICULATION

INDIVIDUAL RECORD SHEET for A SCREENING DEEP TEST OF ARTICULATION

by Eugene T. McDonald

Name ________ Birthdate ________ School ________ Grade ________ Tester ________ Date ________

				[s]	[l]	[r]	[tʃ]	[θ]	[ʃ]	[k]	[f]	[t]
1 bus	fish	bʌ[s][f]ɪ[ʃ]		[+]					[o]		[+]	
2 ball	chain	bɔ[l][tʃ]en										
3 watch	lock	wɔ[tʃ][l]ɑ[k]										
4 house	flag	haʊ[s][f][l]æg										
5 ring	witch	[r]iŋwɪ[tʃ]										
6 chair	sun	[tʃ]ɛ[r][s]ʌn										
7 book	shoe	bʊ[k][ʃ]u										
8 cat	leaf	[k]æ[t][l]i[f]										
9 star	thumb	[s][t]ɑ[r][θ]ʌm										
10 horse	key	hɔ[r][s][k]i										
11 cat	sheep	[k]æ[t][ʃ]ip										
12 ear	bell	ɪ[r]bɛ[l]										
13 tree	thumb	[t][r]i[θ]ʌm										
14 teeth	lock	[t]i[θ][l]ɑ[k]										
15 tooth	brush	[t]u[θ]b[r]ʌ[ʃ]										
16 knife	spoon	naɪ[f][s]pun										
17 leaf	chair	[l]i[f][tʃ]ɛ[r]										
18 glove	thumb	g[l]ʌv[θ]ʌm										
19 brush	five	b[r]ʌ[ʃ][f]aɪv										
20 lock	fish	[l]ɑ[k][f]ɪ[ʃ]										
21 mouth	tie	maʊ[θ][t]aɪ										
22 watch	fork	wɔ[tʃ][f]ɔ[r][k]										
23 fish	tooth	[f]ɪ[ʃ][t]u[θ]										
24 sled	sheep	[s][l]ɛd[ʃ]ip										
25 match	kite	mæ[tʃ][k]aɪ[t]										
26 sheep	chain	[ʃ]ip[tʃ]en										
27 fish	house	[f]ɪ[ʃ]haʊ[s]										
28 thumb	saw	[θ]ʌm[s]ɔ										
29 saw	teeth	[s]ɔ[t]i[θ]										
30 witch	key	wɪ[tʃ][k]i										
31 mouth	match	maʊ[θ]mæ[tʃ]										

Summary of pertinent findings:

Recommendations:

No. contexts correct	[s]	[l]	[r]	[tʃ]	[θ]	[ʃ]	[k]	[f]	[t]
10	•	•	•	•	•	•	•	•	•
9	•	•	•	•	•	•	•	•	•
8	•	•	•	•	•	•	•	•	•
7	•	•	•	•	•	•	•	•	•
6	•	•	•	•	•	•	•	•	•
5	•	•	•	•	•	•	•	•	•
4	•	•	•	•	•	•	•	•	•
3	•	•	•	•	•	•	•	•	•
2	•	•	•	•	•	•	•	•	•
1	•	•	•	•	•	•	•	•	•
0	•	•	•	•	•	•	•	•	•

PHONETIC PROFILE

MODULE TIME	
TOTAL	3:06
ELAPSED	00:00–03:06

Clinical Phonetics CD 4, Track 7
Practice Module 2:
Multiple-Sound Articulation Test

INDIVIDUAL RECORD SHEET FOR A SCREENING DEEP TEST OF ARTICULATION

INDIVIDUAL RECORD SHEET for A SCREENING DEEP TEST OF ARTICULATION
by Eugene T. McDonald

Name________ Birthdate________ School________ Grade________ Tester________ Date________

			[s]	[l]	[r]	[tʃ]	[θ]	[ʃ]	[k]	[f]	[t]
1 bus	fish	bʌ[s][f]ɪ[ʃ]	[+]					[s]		[+]	
2 ball	chain	bɔ[l][tʃ]en		[v]		[s]					
3 watch	lock	wɔ[tʃ][l]ɑ[k]		[A]		[s]			[+]		
4 house	flag	haʊ[s][f][l]æg	[+]	[+]						[+]	
5 ring	witch	[r]iŋwɪ[tʃ]			[D]	[ts]					
6 chair	sun	[tʃ]ɛ[r][s]ʌn	[+]		[ə]	[ts]					
7 book	shoe	bʊ[k][ʃ]u						[+]	[+]		
8 cat	leaf	[k]æ[t][l]i[f]		[+]					[+]	[+]	[+]
9 star	thumb	[s][t]ɑ[r][θ]ʌm	[+]		[-]		[s]				[+]
10 horse	key	hɔ[r][s][k]i	[+]		[-]				[+]		
11 cat	sheep	[k]æ[t][ʃ]ip						[s]	[+]		[+]
12 ear	bell	ɪ[r]bɛ[l]		[v]	[ə]						
13 tree	thumb	[t][r]i[θ]ʌm			[w]		[s]				[+]
14 teeth	lock	[t]i[θ][l]ɑ[k]		[+]			[s]		[+]		[+]
15 tooth	brush	[t]u[θ]b[r]ʌ[ʃ]			[ı]		[s]	[s]			[ ]
16 knife	spoon	naɪ[f][s]pun	[+]							[s]	
17 leaf	chair	[l]i[f][tʃ]ɛ[r]		[+]	[ʔ]	[s]				[+]	
18 glove	thumb	g[l]ʌv[θ]ʌm		[+]			[s]				
19 brush	five	b[r]ʌ[ʃ][f]aɪv			[ı]			[s]		[+]	
20 lock	fish	[l]ɑ[k][f]ɪ[ʃ]		[+]				[s]	[+]	[+]	
21 mouth	tie	maʊ[θ][t]aɪ					[s]				[+]
22 watch	fork	wɔ[tʃ][f]ɔ[r][k]			[ ]	[ ]			[ ]	[ ]	
23 fish	tooth	[f]ɪ[ʃ][t]u[θ]					[ ]	[ ]		[ ]	[ ]
24 sled	sheep	[s][l]ɛd[ʃ]ip	[ ]	[ ]				[ ]			
25 match	kite	mæ[tʃ][k]aɪ[t]				[ ]			[ ]		[ ]
26 sheep	chain	[ʃ]ip[tʃ]en				[ ]		[ ]			
27 fish	house	[f]ɪ[ʃ]haʊ[s]	[ ]					[ ]		[ ]	
28 thumb	saw	[θ]ʌm[s]ɔ	[ ]				[ ]				
29 saw	teeth	[s]ɔ[t]i[θ]	[ ]				[ ]				[ ]
30 witch	key	wɪ[tʃ][k]i				[ ]			[ ]		
31 mouth	match	maʊ[θ]mæ[tʃ]				[ ]	[ ]				

Summary of pertinent findings:

Recommendations:

No. contexts correct	[s]	[l]	[r]	[tʃ]	[θ]	[ʃ]	[k]	[f]	[t]
10	•	•	•	•	•	•	•	•	•
9	•	•	•	•	•	•	•	•	•
8	•	•	•	•	•	•	•	•	•
7	•	•	•	•	•	•	•	•	•
6	•	•	•	•	•	•	•	•	•
5	•	•	•	•	•	•	•	•	•
4	•	•	•	•	•	•	•	•	•
3	•	•	•	•	•	•	•	•	•
2	•	•	•	•	•	•	•	•	•
1	•	•	•	•	•	•	•	•	•
0	•	•	•	•	•	•	•	•	•

PHONETIC PROFILE

MODULE TIME	
TOTAL	3:06
ELAPSED	00:00–03:06

Clinical Phonetics CD 4, Track 7
Practice Module 2:
Multiple-Sound Articulation Test

INDIVIDUAL RECORD SHEET FOR A SCREENING DEEP TEST OF ARTICULATION

INDIVIDUAL RECORD SHEET for A SCREENING DEEP TEST OF ARTICULATION

by Eugene T. McDonald

Name ______ Birthdate ______ School ______ Grade ______ Tester ______ Date ______

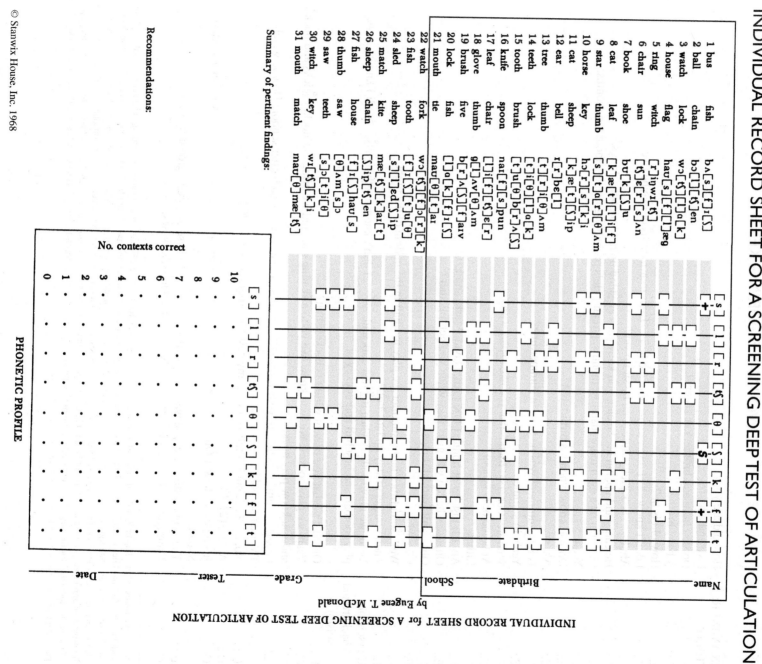

			[s]	[l]	[r]	[tʃ]	[θ]	[ʃ]	[k]	[f]	[t]
1 bus	fish	bʌ[s][f]ɪ[ʃ]	+					S		+	
2 ball	chain	bɔ[l][tʃ]en									
3 watch	lock	wɔ[tʃ][l]ɑ[k]									
4 house	flag	haʊ[s][f][l]æg									
5 ring	witch	[r]iŋwɪ[tʃ]									
6 chair	sun	[tʃ]ɛ[r][s]ʌn									
7 book	shoe	bʊ[k][ʃ]u									
8 cat	leaf	[k]æ[t][l]i[f]									
9 star	thumb	[s][t]ɑ[r][θ]ʌm									
10 horse	key	hɔ[r][s][k]i									
11 cat	sheep	[k]æ[t][ʃ]ip									
12 ear	bell	ɪ[r]bɛ[l]									
13 tree	thumb	[t][r]i[θ]ʌm									
14 teeth	lock	[t]i[θ][l]ɑ[k]									
15 tooth	brush	[t]u[θ]b[r]ʌ[ʃ]									
16 knife	spoon	naɪ[f][s]pun									
17 leaf	chair	[l]i[f][tʃ]ɛ[r]									
18 glove	thumb	g[l]ʌv[θ]ʌm									
19 brush	five	b[r]ʌ[ʃ][f]aɪv									
20 lock	fish	[l]ɑ[k][f]ɪ[ʃ]									
21 mouth	tie	maʊ[θ][t]aɪ									
22 watch	fork	wɔ[tʃ][f]ɔ[r][k]									
23 fish	tooth	[f]ɪ[ʃ][t]u[θ]									
24 sled	sheep	[s][l]ɛd[ʃ]ip									
25 match	kite	mæ[tʃ][k]aɪ[t]									
26 sheep	chain	[ʃ]ip[tʃ]en									
27 fish	house	[f]ɪ[ʃ]haʊ[s]									
28 thumb	saw	[θ]ʌm[s]ɔ									
29 saw	teeth	[s]ɔ[t]i[θ]									
30 witch	key	wɪ[tʃ][k]i									
31 mouth	match	maʊ[θ]mæ[tʃ]									

Summary of pertinent findings:

Recommendations:

No. contexts correct	[s]	[l]	[r]	[tʃ]	[θ]	[ʃ]	[k]	[f]	[t]
10	•	•	•	•	•	•	•	•	•
9	•	•	•	•	•	•	•	•	•
8	•	•	•	•	•	•	•	•	•
7	•	•	•	•	•	•	•	•	•
6	•	•	•	•	•	•	•	•	•
5	•	•	•	•	•	•	•	•	•
4	•	•	•	•	•	•	•	•	•
3	•	•	•	•	•	•	•	•	•
2	•	•	•	•	•	•	•	•	•
1	•	•	•	•	•	•	•	•	•
0	•	•	•	•	•	•	•	•	•

PHONETIC PROFILE

MODULE TIME	
TOTAL	2:39
ELAPSED	03:06–05:45

Clinical Phonetics CD 4, Track 8
Practice Module 3:
/s/ in Continuous Speech; Sample 1

TWO-WAY SCORING KEY

EXAMINER: How old are you?
CHILD: Five and a half.
E.: Do you have any brothers or sisters?
C.: A baby brother.
E.: How old is he?
C.: I don't know . . . I don't know how old he is. 'Bout four monthe̲̊ or maybe five.
E.: Ahuh . . . he's pretty little. Can he sit up yet?
C.: He can s̲̊tand up, but he, he can, you know, he can s̲̊tand up holding onto things.
E.: Oh, then he's even more than five months. [Yeah] He's probably going on about ten months.
C.: Yeah.
E.: Do you know when his birthday is?
C.: Ah, no.
E.: Is it in summer? Was he born in summertime?
C.: Yeah, in s̲̊ummer.
E.: Who are your good friends that you like to play with?
C.: At home or at s̲̊chool?
E.: Either.
C.: Ah, I'll jus̲̑t s̲̑ay at home. [OK] Ah, David, Mark, and Eric.
E.: Oh, . . . what do you guys play when you get together?
C.: Oh . . . all s̲̊ortṣ̊ of things.
E.: Like what?
C.: Well, s̲̊ometimes (?) in the s̲̊ummer (?) we play football in the middle of the night.
E.: Then you get to stay up late, huh?
C.: (school background noise) Yeah, we play football when it's̲̊ (short) real dark and, ah . . . I don't know anything els̲̊e . . . all I know . . . we play football and bas̲̊eball and hockey or
E.: Oh, that's what you play in winter is hockey, huh?
C.: Yeah, we play hockey. We, you know, we go to a s̲̊kating rink and we bring our hockey s̲̊tickṣ̊ and puckṣ̊ and you know play hockey.
E.: Great! . . . um . . . what are your favorite TV shows? What do you watch after school? Do you watch any TV after school?
C.: No, . . . I . . . but I'll tell you what my bes̲̑t TV programs are. [OK] Adam-12.
E.: Adam-12? What's that?
C.: It's̲̊ a polic̲̊e show. [Oh] And, ah, the Rookies. That's̲̊ als̲̊o a polic̲̊e show too. [Oh] And, ah, the Mod S̲̊quad.
E.: That's interesting. Do you watch any children's shows? Those are pretty grown-up shows.
C.: Umm, no . . . I like grown-up shows better than children's shows!

Notes: As discussed in Chapter 7, it is difficult and, in some situations, unwarranted to score sibilants from an audio recording. The general goals of this task and the other five modules to follow are to help you develop your discrimination skills with this type of sample. While you may not be able to discriminate subtle distinctions among target consonants, you should be able to differentiate strident from nonstrident sibilants. You should be able to discriminate a clearly incorrect /s/ when it occurs in a stressed word, and so forth. Judges agreed on approximately 85 percent of target consonants in these modules. Your item-by-item agreement with the keys may not be this high, but your percentage of correct consonants for each child should be within ± 10 percentage points of the value calculated for the key. For example, the child in this module, Practice Module 3, was 80 percent correct on /s/ as calculated from this key. Your percentage of consonants correct should be between 70 and 90 percent.

MODULE TIME	
TOTAL	2:39
ELAPSED	03:06–05:45

Clinical Phonetics CD 4, Track 8
Practice Module 3:
/s/ in Continuous Speech; Sample 1

TWO-WAY SCORING SHEET[a]

EXAMINER: How old are you?
CHILD: Five and a half.
E.: Do you have any brothers or sisters?
C.: A baby brother.
E.: How old is he?
C.: I don't know . . . I don't know how old he is. 'Bout four months or maybe five.
E.: Ahuh . . . he's pretty little. Can he sit up yet?
C.: He can stand up, but he, he can, you know, he can stand up holding onto things.
E.: Oh, then he's even more than five months. [Yeah] He's probably going on about ten months.
C.: Yeah.
E.: Do you know when his birthday is?
C.: Ah, no.
E.: Is it in summer? Was he born in summertime?
C.: Yeah, in summer.
E.: Who are your good friends that you like to play with?
C.: At home or at school?
E.: Either.
C.: Ah, I'll just say at home. [OK] Ah, David, Mark, and Eric.
E.: Oh, . . . what do you guys play when you get together?
C.: Oh . . . all sorts of things.
E.: Like what?
C.: Well, sometimes in the summer we play football in the middle of the night.
E.: Then you get to stay up late, huh?
C.: (school background noise) Yeah, we play football when it's real dark and, ah . . . I don't know anything else . . . all I know . . . we play football and baseball and hockey or . . .
E.: Oh, that's what you play in winter is hockey, huh?
C.: Yeah, we play hockey. We, you know, we go to a skating rink and we bring our hockey sticks and pucks and you know play hockey.
E.: Great! . . . um . . . what are your favorite TV shows? What do you watch after school? Do you watch any TV after school?
C.: No, . . . I . . . but I'll tell you what my best TV programs are. [OK] Adam-12.
E.: Adam-12? What's that?
C.: It's a police show. [Oh] And, ah, the Rookies. That's also a police show too. [Oh] And, ah, the Mod Squad.
E.: That's interesting. Do you watch any children's shows? Those are pretty grown-up shows.
C.: Umm, no . . . I like grown-up shows better than children's shows!

[a]Above each underlined sound, indicate if it is correct (+) or incorrect (0)

MODULE TIME	
TOTAL	3:37
ELAPSED	05:45–09:22

Clinical Phonetics CD 4, Track 9
Practice Module 4:
/s/ in Continuous Speech; Sample 2

TWO-WAY SCORING KEY

E.: Did you tell me how old you are?
C.: Yeah, six. (difficult)
E.: OK. How many brothers and sisters do you have?
C.: I have one brother and one sister.
E.: What's your sister's name?
C.: Karen.
E.: Karen . . . How old is your brother?
C.: Seven. I mean eight.
E.: He's eight. Do you and he play a lot together?
C.: Yeah.
E.: What do you do?
C.: Most of the time we play basketball.
E.: Do ya?
C.: Yeah.
E.: You both good players?
C.: He (said) alotta time he (says) I'm better'n him.
E.: How many points dya usually get?
C.: My average is about . . . 20.0
E.: Hmm . . . pretty good, pretty good. Who are your other friends that you play with?
C.: Gary.
E.: And who else . . .?
C.: At home or at school?
E.: Both.
C.: Teddy and Mark. [Uhuh] . . . and I used to play with Chad, and I play with Doug. [Uhuh] . . . and Jim and Rich.
E.: What do you like to play besides basketball?
C.: Baseball.
E.: You like sports, huh?
C.: Yeah.
E.: Do you . . . like to play any indoor games?
C.: Yeah.
E.: Like what?
C.: Trouble.
E.: Trouble . . . explain that to me.
C.: Well . . . you know, d'you know how to play Aggravation?
E.: No, I don't know how to play that either . . . so you'll have to start from the beginning.
C.: There's this little thing up here that's got a die an if that comes off . . . you just need a (?) . . . and you each have four men.

MODULE TIME	
TOTAL	3:37
ELAPSED	05:45–09:22

Clinical Phonetics CD 4, Track 9
Practice Module 4:
/s/ in Continuous Speech; Sample 2

TWO-WAY SCORING SHEET

E.: Did you tell me how old you are?
C.: Yeah, six.
E.: OK. How many brothers and sisters do you have?
C.: I have one brother and one sister.
E.: What's your sister's name?
C.: Karen.
E.: Karen . . . How old is your brother?
C.: Seven. I mean eight.
E.: He's eight. Do you and he play a lot together?
C.: Yeah.
E.: What do you do?
C.: Most of the time we play basketball.
E.: Do ya?
C.: Yeah.
E.: You both good players?
C.: He (said) alotta time he (says) I'm better'n him.
E.: How many points dya usually get?
C.: My average is about . . . 20.0
E.: Hmm . . . pretty good, pretty good. Who are your other friends that you play with?
C.: Gary.
E.: And who else . . .?
C.: At home or at school?
E.: Both.
C.: Teddy and Mark. [Uhuh] . . . and I used to play with Chad, and I play with Doug. [Uhuh] . . . and Jim and Rich.
E.: What do you like to play besides basketball?
C.: Baseball.
E.: You like sports, huh?
C.: Yeah.
E.: Do you . . . like to play any indoor games?
C.: Yeah.
E.: Like what?
C.: Trouble.
E.: Trouble . . . explain that to me.
C.: Well . . . you know, d'you know how to play Aggravation?
E.: No, I don't know how to play that either . . . so you'll have to start from the beginning.
C.: There's this little thing up here that's got a die an if that comes off . . . you just need a (?) . . . and you each have four men.

MODULE TIME	
TOTAL	3:37
ELAPSED	05:45–09:22

Clinical Phonetics CD 4, Track 9
Practice Module 4:
/s/ in Continuous Speech;
Sample 2, Continued

TWO-WAY SCORING KEY

E.: Uhuh.
C.: An ya try to . . . an there's a whole bunch of s̲̊pac̲̊es, an ya try to go around the board an then it's̲̊ got a ladder.
E.: Uhuh.
C.: Which is four spa (spac̲̊e) [not clear] an ya get each one up the ladder . . . firs̲̊t one to fill up their ladder wins.
E.: Aahhh . . .
C.: An then Aggravation . . . it's̲̊ the s̲̊ame exc̲̊ept there's, exc̲̊ept you need a s̲̊ix̲̊ or a one to get out in Aggravation . . . and als̲̊o there's a shortcut. S̲o (jus̲̊t) a little hole in the middle.
E.: Uhuh . . . who is the winner? The one who has . . .
C.: The one who gets̲̊ 'em (?) . . .
E.: Who gets 'em all up the ladder?
C.: Yeah . . . I think there's s̲̊ix̲̊ in Aggravation.
E.: Uhuh. That's interesting. How 'bout any other indoor games? Are there any other ones you like to play . . . any card games?
C.: Yeah.
E.: What?
C.: War.
E.: War . . . OK, I know how to play War, but I'd like you to explain it to me.
C.: Each pers̲on has half a deck of cards. [Mhmmm] An you take 'em and turn 'em over an' the highes̲t one wins . . .(?)
E.: The one . . . what do you mean the highest . . . the highest . . . card?
C.: Yeah.
E.: OK. Person who has the highest card takes the two that are put out [Yeah], right?
C.: And if they're both the s̲ame then puts̲̊ three down an then turn one over.
E.: Oh, . . . then that's called . . .
C.: War!

Notes: What type of distortion error on /s/ does this child have? (Hint: See "Fricatives and Affricates Module 7") Calculate his percentage of consonants correct by your two-way scoring and compare to the value derived from the key. Does your score agree within ± 10 percentage points? Notice this child's denasal and hoarse voice quality; as discussed in Chapter 7, voice quality can bias our perceptions of articulation.

MODULE TIME	
TOTAL	3:37
ELAPSED	05:45–09:22

Clinical Phonetics CD 4, Track 9
Practice Module 4:
/s/ in Continuous Speech;
Sample 2, Continued

TWO-WAY SCORING SHEET

E.: Uhuh.
C.: An ya try to . . . an there's a whole bunch of spaces, an ya try to go around the board an then it's got a ladder.
E.: Uhuh.
C.: Which is four spa (space) [not clear] an ya get each one up the ladder . . . first one to fill up their ladder wins.
E.: Aahhh . . .
C.: An then Aggravation . . . it's the same except there's, except you need a six or a one to get out in Aggravation . . . and also there's a shortcut. So (just) a little hole in the middle.
E.: Uhuh . . . who is the winner? The one who has . . .
C.: The one who gets 'em (?) . . .
E.: Who gets 'em all up the ladder?
C.: Yeah . . . I think there's six in Aggravation.
E.: Uhuh. That's interesting. How 'bout any other indoor games? Are there any other ones you like to play . . . any card games?
C.: Yeah.
E.: What?
C.: War.
E.: War . . . OK, I know how to play War, but I'd like you to explain it to me.
C.: Each person has half a deck of cards. [Mhmmm] An you take 'em and turn 'em over an' the highest one wins . . .(?)
E.: The one . . . what do you mean the highest . . . the highest . . . card?
C.: Yeah.
E.: OK. Person who has the highest card takes the two that are put out [Yeah], right?
C.: And if they're both the same then puts three down an then turn one over.
E.: Oh, . . . then that's called . . .
C.: War!

MODULE TIME	
TOTAL	3:54
ELAPSED	09:22–13:16

Clinical Phonetics CD 4, Track 10
Practice Module 5:
/s/ in Continuous Speech; Sample 3

TWO-WAY SCORING KEY

E.: What were you doing in the classroom when I took you out?
C.: I was, um, putting s̲̊ome decorations on my box̲̊.
E.: Wow, very good. What kind of box were you making?
C.: A valentine box̲̟.
E.: That's nice. What are you gonna do with the valentine box?
C.: I'm going to put cards in it to s̲̊end to people.
E.: Can you speak up a little bit?
C.: We're going to put valentine cards in it to s̲̟end to people.
E.: Very nice. Did you write your valentines out yet?
C.: No.
E.: Did you buy them yet?
C.: Uh uh.
E.: When is Valentine's day?
C.: S̲̟even more days.
E.: Seven, is that all?
C.: Yeah.
E.: Seven more school days, huh? That's great! . . . Who are your best friends? Who do you like to play with?
C.: My friend Jimmy that always s̲̊ocks̲̟ me in the belly.(!!)
E.: He socks you in the belly . . . hope he doesn't do it very hard!
C.: He does.
E.: He does? [He does] What do you and Jimmy do?
C.: We play together and we s̲̟py on girls.
E.: You spy on them. Why do you spy on them?
C.: We like to. Today my friend was running away because he didn't like me.
E.: He didn't like you today?
C.: No. S̲̟o then I told him s̲̊omething. Then he walked with me.
E.: Ah . . . sometimes friends are like that. They're changeable. One day they're real friendly and the next day they're not too friendly. . . . How many brothers and sisters do you have?
C.: Just one s̲̊is̲̊ter.
E.: Just one sister. And how old is she?
C.: Four.
E.: Do you play with her very much?
C.: No.
E.: No . . . I have a . . . couple of pictures here I'd like you to look at. What happened to all the snow?
C.: It melted.

MODULE TIME	
TOTAL	3:54
ELAPSED	09:22–13:16

Clinical Phonetics CD 4, Track 10
Practice Module 5:
/s/ in Continuous Speech; Sample 3

TWO-WAY SCORING SHEET

E.: What were you doing in the classroom when I took you out?
C.: I was, um, putting some decorations on my box.
E.: Wow, very good. What kind of box were you making?
C.: A valentine box.
E.: That's nice. What are you gonna do with the valentine box?
C.: I'm going to put cards in it to send to people.
E.: Can you speak up a little bit?
C.: We're going to put valentine cards in it to send to people.
E.: Very nice. Did you write your valentines out yet?
C.: No.
E.: Did you buy them yet?
C.: Uh uh.
E.: When is Valentine's day?
C.: Seven more days.
E.: Seven, is that all?
C.: Yeah.
E.: Seven more school days, huh? That's great! . . . Who are your best friends? Who do you like to play with?
C.: My friend Jimmy that always socks me in the belly.(!!)
E.: He socks you in the belly . . . hope he doesn't do it very hard!
C.: He does.
E.: He does? [He does] What do you and Jimmy do?
C.: We play together and we spy on girls.
E.: You spy on them. Why do you spy on them?
C.: We like to. Today my friend was running away because he didn't like me.
E.: He didn't like you today?
C.: No. So then I told him something. Then he walked with me.
E.: Ah . . . sometimes friends are like that. They're changeable. One day they're real friendly and the next day they're not too friendly. . . . How many brothers and sisters do you have?
C.: Just one sister.
E.: Just one sister. And how old is she?
C.: Four.
E.: Do you play with her very much?
C.: No.
E.: No . . . I have a . . . couple of pictures here I'd like you to look at. What happened to all the snow?
C.: It melted.

MODULE TIME	
TOTAL	3:54
ELAPSED	09:22–13:16

Clinical Phonetics CD 4, Track 10
Practice Module 5: /s/ in Continuous Speech; Sample 3, Continued

TWO-WAY SCORING KEY

E.: Doggone it. If we had some snow, what could we do outside?
C.: We can make a s̪nowman.
E.: What else could we do?
C.: Make a s̪now fort.
E.: Yeah, what else?
C.: We could s̪led.
E.: Yeah, what else?
C.: Um, we could, can't think of anything.
E.: Maybe you don't have skates, but . . .
C.: Yeah, I have s̪kates̪.
E.: Do you have skates? So, then what could you do?
C.: Ṡ̪kate.
E.: Go ice skating?
C.: Yeah.
E.: Right. This hasn't been a very good winter for ice skating, has it?
C.: Uh uh.
E.: Let's look at this little fellow here. He's lucky he's got snow outside. You tell me a little story about, I mean a sentence about each one of these pictures. By the time you're finished, we'll have a little story, OK?
C.: He's getting ready to go out and he's almos̪̊t ready. He's almos̪t ready, and he's out.
E.: What's he putting, what's he doing here?
C.: Putting on his mitten and his coat. And now he's ready to s̪̊led. He's s̪̊ledded down and he's going back up now.
E.: Here's one about a girl. It looks like a different time of year. What's your favorite time of year?
C.: S̪̊pring.
E.: Spring?
C.: Yeah.
E.: Why do you like spring?
C.: S̪̊o I can play football and get mus̪̊cles.
E.: Ah . . . what's she doing here?
C.: She's getting up, she puts̪ on her dres̪s̪. She's eating her breakfas̪̊t . . . (she catches) a s̪̊chool bus̪̊ . . . she walks̪ up to s̪̊chool and gets̪̊ ready to do her math.
E.: Ah . . . she's going to do math.

MODULE TIME	
TOTAL	3:54
ELAPSED	09:22–13:16

Clinical Phonetics CD 4, Track 10
Practice Module 5:
/s/ in Continuous Speech;
Sample 3, Continued

TWO-WAY SCORING SHEET

E.: Doggone it. If we had some snow, what could we do outside?
C.: We can make a snowman.
E.: What else could we do?
C.: Make a snow fort.
E.: Yeah, what else?
C.: We could sled.
E.: Yeah, what else?
C.: Um, we could, can't think of anything.
E.: Maybe you don't have skates, but . . .
C.: Yeah, I have skates.
E.: Do you have skates? So, then what could you do?
C.: Skate.
E.: Go ice skating?
C.: Yeah.
E.: Right. This hasn't been a very good winter for ice skating, has it?
C.: Uh uh.
E.: Let's look at this little fellow here. He's lucky he's got snow outside. You tell me a little story about, I mean a sentence about each one of these pictures. By the time you're finished, we'll have a little story, OK?
C.: He's getting ready to go out and he's almost ready. He's almost ready, and he's out.
E.: What's he putting, what's he doing here?
C.: Putting on his mitten and his coat. And now he's ready to sled. He's sledded down and he's going back up now.
E.: Here's one about a girl. It looks like a different time of year. What's your favorite time of year?
C.: Spring.
E.: Spring?
C.: Yeah.
E.: Why do you like spring?
C.: So I can play football and get muscles.
E.: Ah . . . what's she doing here?
C.: She's getting up, she puts on her dress. She's eating her breakfast . . . (she catches) a school bus . . . she walks up to school and gets ready to do her math.
E.: Ah . . . she's going to do math.

MODULE TIME	
TOTAL	4:39
ELAPSED	13:16–17:55

Clinical Phonetics CD 4, Track 11
Practice Module 6:
/r/ in Continuous Speech; Sample 1

TWO-WAY SCORING KEY

E.: Do you have any brothers or sisters?
C.: Only bṟ̊otheṟ̊s . . . two of 'em.
E.: You have two brothers?
C.: Mm hmm.
E.: What are their names?
C.: Danny and Dave.
E.: Ah . . . and what do you play with Danny and Dave?
C.: I play with, I play Old Maid . . . I play Cṟ̊azy Eights . . . I played, I play Snap . . . I play caṟ̊s, and I play . . . hmm . . . jump on Dave's bed downstaiṟ̊s. He has a double bed. [Uhuh.] And um, in the summeṟ̊ we play at the night, we play kick the can and then we play . . .
E.: That sounds like fun.
C.: Um . . . play kick the ball. Not kick the ball, but . . . mmm . . . socceṟ̊ baseball.
E.: Uh huh.
C.: And, I don't know anything else we play.
E.: Uh huh. What do you do with your friends in wintertime?
C.: Hm, we . . . we jump in the snow, and we make angels.
E.: Oh, that sounds like fun. What else?
C.: Oh, I go, I go to David's house, and pṟ̊obably sleep oveṟ̊ at his house Fṟ̊iday so I can watch caṟtoons with him. And, then with Doug . . . I play at school with him a little bit.
E.: Uh huh . . . I've a few pictures here . . . Can you tell me about this picture?
C.: Hmm . . . the boy's dṟopping the bat and he's taking a, I think it looks like a . . .
E.: It's a glove, I think.
C.: Un huh . . . took that boy's, that boy's glove. Now the police is coming.
E.: Why?
C.: Cause he took the boy's glove.
E.: What else happened?
C.: Hmmm . . . and the window bṟ̊oke.
E.: How'd that happen?
C.: Pṟ̊obably a stone.
E.: Do you think it was a stone?
C.: Oh, a bat!
E.: Did the bat break it, or what happened?
C.: He went up and bṟ̊oke it. Then he ṟan.
E.: That's a possibility. What else could he have done with the bat to break the window, besides hit it with the bat?
C.: Hmm . . . thṟ̊ow it at it.

MODULE TIME	
TOTAL	4:39
ELAPSED	13:16–17:55

Clinical Phonetics CD 4, Track 11
Practice Module 6:
/r/ in Continuous Speech; Sample 1

TWO-WAY SCORING SHEET

E.: Do you have any brothers or sisters?
C.: Only brothers . . . two of 'em.
E.: You have two brothers?
C.: Mm hmm.
E.: What are their names?
C.: Danny and Dave.
E.: Ah . . . and what do you play with Danny and Dave?
C.: I play with, I play Old Maid . . . I play Crazy Eights . . . I played, I play Snap . . . I play cars, and I play . . . hmm . . . jump on Dave's bed downstairs. He has a double bed. [Uhuh.] And um, in the summer we play at the night, we play kick the can and then we play . . .
E.: That sounds like fun.
C.: Um . . . play kick the ball. Not kick the ball, but . . . mmm . . . soccer baseball.
E.: Uh huh.
C.: And, I don't know anything else we play.
E.: Uh huh. What do you do with your friends in wintertime?
C.: Hm, we . . . we jump in the snow, and we make angels.
E.: Oh, that sounds like fun. What else?
C.: Oh, I go, I go to David's house, and probably sleep over at his house Friday so I can watch cartoons with him. And, then with Doug . . . I play at school with him a little bit.
E.: Uh huh . . . I've a few pictures here . . . Can you tell me about this picture?
C.: Hmm . . . the boy's dropping the bat and he's taking a, I think it looks like a . . .
E.: It's a glove, I think.
C.: Un huh . . . took that boy's, that boy's glove. Now the police is coming.
E.: Why?
C.: Cause he took the boy's glove.
E.: What else happened?
C.: Hmmm . . . and the window broke.
E.: How'd that happen?
C.: Probably a stone.
E.: Do you think it was a stone?
C.: Oh, a bat!
E.: Did the bat break it, or what happened?
C.: He went up and broke it. Then he ran.
E.: That's a possibility. What else could he have done with the bat to break the window, besides hit it with the bat?
C.: Hmm . . . throw it at it.

MODULE TIME	
TOTAL	4:39
ELAPSED	13:16–17:55

Clinical Phonetics CD 4, Track 11
Practice Module 6:
/r/ in Continuous Speech; Sample 1, Continued

TWO-WAY SCORING KEY

E.: Could have . . . . How do you think this lady feels? I think maybe . . .
C.: She feel(s) mad!
E.: Oh boy . . .
C.: . . . and tṟ̟ash cans, tṟ̟ash oveṟ̊ theṟ̊e foṟ̊(?) tṟ̊uck.
E.: What 'bout him?
C.: He could've bṟ̊oke the window too.
E.: What's he doing?
C.: He's going aṟ̊ound the block.
E.: Yeah, he's getting out of there, isn't he . . .
C.: Uh huh. So is he.
E.: Yeah. What would you do in that situation if you'd broken a window while you were playing baseball?
C.: I'd go ṟ̊unning . . .
E.: Would ya?
C.: Yeah . . . pṟ̊obably [go ahead] pṟ̊obably playin' baseball in the middle of the stṟ̊eet.
E.: Yeah . . . if you had broken the window, do you think you should say something?
C.: . . . soṟ̊ry!!
E.: Yeah . . . what's this man doing over here?
C.: He's getting in his caṟ̊.
E.: Looks that way.
C.: Oṟ̊, he's scṟ̟atchin' paint off his caṟ̟.
E.: Maybe a witness, huh? Watchin' it all.
C.: Yeah.

MODULE TIME	
TOTAL	4:39
ELAPSED	13:16–17:55

Clinical Phonetics CD 4, Track 11
Practice Module 6:
/r/ in Continuous Speech;
Sample 1, Continued

TWO-WAY SCORING SHEET

E.: Could have . . . . How do you think this lady feels? I think maybe . . .
C.: She feel(s) mad!
E.: Oh boy . . .
C.: . . . and trash cans, trash over there for truck.
E.: What 'bout him?
C.: He could've broke the window too.
E.: What's he doing?
C.: He's going around the block.
E.: Yeah, he's getting out of there, isn't he . . .
C.: Uh huh. So is he.
E.: Yeah. What would you do in that situation if you'd broken a window while you were playing baseball?
C.: I'd go running . . .
E.: Would ya?
C.: Yeah . . . probably [go ahead] probably playin' baseball in the middle of the street.
E.: Yeah . . . if you had broken the window, do you think you should say something?
C.: . . . sorry!!
E.: Yeah . . . what's this man doing over here?
C.: He's getting in his car.
E.: Looks that way.
C.: Or, he's scratchin' paint off his car.
E.: Maybe a witness, huh? Watchin' it all.
C.: Yeah.

MODULE TIME	
TOTAL	3:13
ELAPSED	17:55–21:08

Clinical Phonetics CD 4, Track 12
Practice Module 7:
/r/ in Continuous Speech; Sample 2

TWO-WAY SCORING KEY

E.: What did you get for Christmas?
C.: A bike . . . a helmet . . . a . . . r̲̊ace car̲̊ set . . .
E.: Hmm . . . tell me about that race car set.
C.: It's electr̲̝ic . . . you plug it into the wall . . . and ya gotta set it up anyway ya want it to [Mhmm] . . . you want it to, except ya gotta put the car̲̊ on these one little things where the electr̲̝icity comes into the car̲̊ [Mhmm] . . . and it goes ar̲̊ound the tr̲̊ack.
E.: Hmm . . . sounds neat.
C.: And sometimes you can make a br̲̊idge.
E.: Hmm, out of what?
C.: Out of the, out of the things that go like that [Mhmm] . . . and . . . and it goes up ta one hundr̲̊ed and sixty.
E.: Oh my gosh . . . hundred and sixty?
C.: First it star̲̊ts out with twenty . . . then it goes to for̲̊ty, then eighty, then one hundr̲̝ed ta sixty.
E.: Oh my gosh, that goes pretty fast, doesn't it. Do you have any pets?
C.: No.
E.: Who are your best friends?
C.: Byr̲̊on.
E.: Byron . . .
C.: . . . and R̲̊ichie.
E.: Byron and Richie. What do you, what do the three of you do together?
C.: We r̲̊ide bikes sometimes [Mhmm] . . . and we . . .
E.: What else do you do?
C.: . . . play guns [Uhuh] . . . and sometimes I push Byr̲̊on in his wagon.
E.: Oh . . . Let's look at one of these pictures . . . tell me something about this picture.
C.: A fir̲̝eman's car̲̝rying a hur̲̊t guy.
E.: How'd he get hurt?
C.: In the fir̲̊e.
E.: Well how could he get his head hurt in the fire? . . . What do you 'spose happened to him?
C.: He fell through the floor̲̊.
E.: What do you think started the fire?
C.: . . . Gasoline.
E.: How could the gasoline get started?
C.: Some guys could sneak in and star̲̊t it.
E.: Oh, you mean you think it happened on purpose, huh? What are the firemen doing here?
C.: Puttin' out the fir̲̊e.
E.: And they're . . .
C.: Climbing the ladder̲.<too weak>
E.: Are there different kinds of fire trucks, or, do you know . . .
C.: They'r̲̊e all the same except for̲̊ the chief's car̲.
E.: The chief's car . . . what is this?
C.: A fir̲̊e hydr̲̝ant . . .

MODULE TIME	
TOTAL	3:13
ELAPSED	17:55–21:08

Clinical Phonetics CD 4, Track 12
Practice Module 7:
/r/ in Continuous Speech; Sample 2

TWO-WAY SCORING SHEET

E.: What did you get for Christmas?
C.: A bike . . . a helmet . . . a . . . race car set . . .
E.: Hmm . . . tell me about that race car set.
C.: It's electric . . . you plug it into the wall . . . and ya gotta set it up anyway ya want it to [Mhmm] . . . you want it to, except ya gotta put the car on these one little things where the electricity comes into the car [Mhmm] . . . and it goes around the track.
E.: Hmm . . . sounds neat.
C.: And sometimes you can make a bridge.
E.: Hmm, out of what?
C.: Out of the, out of the things that go like that [Mhmm] . . . and . . . and it goes up ta one hundred and sixty.
E.: Oh my gosh . . . hundred and sixty?
C.: First it starts out with twenty . . . then it goes to forty, then eighty, then one hundred ta sixty.
E.: Oh my gosh, that goes pretty fast, doesn't it. Do you have any pets?
C.: No.
E.: Who are your best friends?
C.: Byron.
E.: Byron . . .
C.: . . . and Richie.
E.: Byron and Richie. What do you, what do the three of you do together?
C.: We ride bikes sometimes [Mhmm] . . . and we . . .
E.: What else do you do?
C.: . . . play guns [Uhuh] . . . and sometimes I push Byron in his wagon.
E.: Oh . . . Let's look at one of these pictures . . . tell me something about this picture.
C.: A fireman's carrying a hurt guy.
E.: How'd he get hurt?
C.: In the fire.
E.: Well how could he get his head hurt in the fire? . . . What do you 'spose happened to him?
C.: He fell through the floor.
E.: What do you think started the fire?
C.: . . . Gasoline.
E.: How could the gasoline get started?
C.: Some guys could sneak in and start it.
E.: Oh, you mean you think it happened on purpose, huh? What are the firemen doing here?
C.: Puttin' out the fire.
E.: And they're . . .
C.: Climbing the ladder.<too weak>
E.: Are there different kinds of fire trucks, or, do you know . . .
C.: They're all the same except for the chief's car.
E.: The chief's car . . . what is this?
C.: A fire hydrant . . .

MODULE TIME	
TOTAL	3:54
ELAPSED	21:08–25:02

Clinical Phonetics CD 4, Track 13
Practice Module 8:
/r/ in Continuous Speech; Sample 3

TWO-WAY SCORING KEY

E.: And who do you play with?
C.: Umm . . . my fr̲̊iend David.
E.: A friend named David. What do you and David play?
C.: Umm . . . basketball, football, baseball, and, uh, soccer̲̊.
E.: Hmm.
C.: . . . and, uh, and sometimes, ah, pool.
E.: You play pool. . . . What kind of game is it? I really don't know much about pool.
C.: You r̲̊ack 'em up on this one r̲̊ack and, and like ther̲̊e's ones with r̲̊ed, like this r̲̊ed and other̲̊s and the ones that has the str̲̊ipes, and then the one what don't haves the str̲̊ipes . . . that's the solids . . . and the other̲̊s ar̲̊e str̲̊ipes.
E.: Hmm.
C.: And then the last one who gets all the balls and shoots the eight ball in, and then they win.
E.: Mmhmm. Do you ever win?
C.: Yeah.
E.: Who do you beat?
C.: My fr̲:iend David.
E.: Mmhmm.
C.: And then I got one mor̲̊e fr̲̊iend . . . ah . . . he always comes down and play with me and, ah . . . and then I got lots of other̲̊ fr̲̊iends like ah . . . my fr̲̊iend Edgar̲̊. He always comes down and play with me. And . . . that's all the fr̲̊iends I got.
E.: Sounds like you've got a lot of friends. What'd ya get for Christmas?
C.: Umm . . . I got a Big Jim camper̲̊, a Big Jim war̲̊m-up suit and . . . umm, Big Jim basketball suit.
E.: Umhmm.
C.: And . . . got a walkie-talkie . . . and . . . I got a br̲̊and new bike, and . . . that's all.
E.: Sounds like you had a pretty good Christmas (sounds like a good Christmas). Did you ever see this picture . . . have you seen that?
C.: Umm, no.
E.: Can you tell me something about it?
C.: Ther̲̊e's a fir̲̊e and the fir̲̊eman came and pour̲̊ed it out and a guy got hur̲̊t in the fir̲̊e.
E.: How do you suppose he got hurt?
C.: In the fir̲̊e.
E.: What could have happened?
C.: He could, umm, started up the stove when his mom and dad was gone and he just . . . and the place star̲̊ted on fire.
E.: Hmm, but how would he get a hurt head from the fire?
C.: Maybe he fell against something when it star̲̊ted to fir̲̊e and then cr̲̊acked his head open.
E.: That could be. . . . What are the firemen doing here?
C.: Ah, climbing up and get some mor̲̊e people what's in the fir̲̊e.
E.: Umhmm. They're going to rescue them, I imagine. What is this called, you know?
C.: A fir̲̊e hydr̲̊ant.
E.: Mhmm. What are they for?
C.: Ah, for̲̊ fir̲̊es.
E.: Have you ever seen one used?
C.: My fr̲̊iend called up a fir̲̊eman and, and he said, umm to r̲̊un that thing out in the str̲̊eet so we had get wet, so we did and we got wet. . . .

MODULE TIME	
TOTAL	3:54
ELAPSED	21:08–25:02

Clinical Phonetics CD 4, Track 13 Practice Module 8: /r/ in Continuous Speech; Sample 3

TWO-WAY SCORING SHEET

E.: And who do you play with?
C.: Umm . . . my friend David.
E.: A friend named David. What do you and David play?
C.: Umm . . . basketball, football, baseball, and, uh, soccer.
E.: Hmm.
C.: . . . and, uh, and sometimes, ah, pool.
E.: You play pool. . . . What kind of game is it? I really don't know much about pool.
C.: You rack 'em up on this one rack and, and like there's ones with red, like this red and others and the ones that has the stripes, and then the one what don't haves the stripes . . . that's the solids . . . and the others are stripes.
E.: Hmm.
C.: And then the last one who gets all the balls and shoots the eight ball in, and then they win.
E.: Mmhmm. Do you ever win?
C.: Yeah.
E.: Who do you beat?
C.: My friend David.
E.: Mmhmm.
C.: And then I got one more friend . . . ah . . . he always comes down and play with me and, ah . . . and then I got lots of other friends like ah . . . my friend Edgar. He always comes down and play with me. And . . . that's all the friends I got.
E.: Sounds like you've got a lot of friends. What'd ya get for Christmas?
C.: Umm . . . I got a Big Jim camper, a Big Jim warm-up suit and . . . umm, Big Jim basketball suit.
E.: Umhmm.
C.: And . . . got a walkie-talkie . . . and . . . I got a brand new bike, and . . . that's all.
E.: Sounds like you had a pretty good Christmas (sounds like a good Christmas). Did you ever see this picture . . . have you seen that?
C.: Umm, no.
E.: Can you tell me something about it?
C.: There's a fire and the fireman came and poured it out and a guy got hurt in the fire.
E.: How do you suppose he got hurt?
C.: In the fire.
E.: What could have happened?
C.: He could, umm, started up the stove when his mom and dad was gone and he just . . . and the place started on fire.
E.: Hmm, but how would he get a hurt head from the fire?
C.: Maybe he fell against something when it started to fire and then cracked his head open.
E.: That could be. . . . What are the firemen doing here?
C.: Ah, climbing up and get some more people what's in the fire.
E.: Umhmm. They're going to rescue them, I imagine. What is this called, you know?
C.: A fire hydrant.
E.: Mhmm. What are they for?
C.: Ah, for fires.
E.: Have you ever seen one used?
C.: My friend called up a fireman and, and he said, umm to run that thing out in the street so we had get wet, so we did and we got wet. . . .

MODULE TIME	
TOTAL	1:29
ELAPSED	25:02–26:31

Clinical Phonetics CD 4, Track 14
Practice Module 9: All Sounds in Continuous Speech; Sample 1

TRANSCRIPTION KEY

Clinician	*Child*	*Transcription*
What kind of things do you do?	Well, well, I don't have any more school, so . . .	[w ɛ l w ɛ l a͡ɪ d õ æ ʌ ɛ n ɪ m ɔ r s u s o͡ʊ]
Now you don't have any more school so what . . .	I stay home all day.	[a͡ɪ s̯ e͡ɪ h o m ɔ d a͡ɪ]
You stay home all day.	Yeah, play.	[j ɛ a pʰ a e ː]
(What do you) Oh, and play . . . that sounds good. What kinds of things do you play?	Well, sometimes I go to . . . over to my (??) house.	[w ɛ ː ʊ s ʌ m t a͡ɪ m z a͡ɪ g o͡ʊ t̪ u h ɑ r v ɚ t ə m a͡ɪ (h a͡ɪ s̺ ã͡ɪ n z̥̚) h a͡ʊː s]
Sometimes you go over to your friend's house?	Yeah.	[j ɛ̃ᵊ]
What do you do there?	Well, I just take my Big Wheels or something.	[w ɛᵘ a͡ɪ̝ ə s t ɛ k m ɑ̝ b ɪ g w i̝ ɚ s ʌ̃ m p ɛ n]
Oh, you always take your Big Wheels or something, I see.	And, um	[a ẽ n ʌː m]
What else do you do?	Well, that's about all.	[w ɛ d̺ ɪ t s̯ b a ɔːᵘ]
That's about all?	Mhmm	[mː]
Do you ever get to play with your baby brother?	Yeah . . .	[j a ːᴵ]
Yeah, what kinds of things do you do with him?	Oh, wrestle . . .	[ã͡ɪ w ɛ̺̃ s̺õː]
Wrestle . . . oh.	I roll him over on my stomach.	[ɑ̝ w o͡ʊᴵ m h ɝ v ɚ ɔ n m ɑ s̺ ʌ̃ m ə k]
You roll him over on your stomach. Does he like that?	Yeah. He's believing it's (the) trick . . .	[j ɛ h i z b ɪ i v ɪ ŋ h ɪ z̥ z̺ ʌ t w ɪ kʰ]
He what?	He's believing it's a trick.	[ɪː t s b i̝ː v ɪ ŋ ɪ t s̯ ə t w ɪ k]
Oh, he's believing it's a trick. Yeah. Oh, so he thinks he's doing tricks with you, huh. Does he laugh a lot when you do that?	Yeah.	[j ɪ ʌ]
Yeah, does he get real silly?	Goes like this ______	[ɪ g o͡ʊ z̥ l a͡ɪ k d ɪ t k̽ k̽ k̽]
Oh . . .		

MODULE TIME	
TOTAL	1:29
ELAPSED	25:02–26:31

Clinical Phonetics CD 4, Track 14 Practice Module 9: All Sounds in Continuous Speech; Sample 1

TRANSCRIPTION SHEET

Clinician	*Child*	*Transcription*
What kind of things do you do?	Well, well, I don't have any more school, so . . .	
Now you don't have any more school so what . . .	I stay home all day.	
You stay home all day.	Yeah, play.	
(What do you) Oh, and play . . . that sounds good. What kinds of things do you play?	Well, sometimes I go to . . . over to my (??) house.	
Sometimes you go over to your friend's house?	Yeah.	
What do you do there?	Well, I just take my Big Wheels or something.	
Oh, you always take your Big Wheels or something, I see.	And, um	
What else do you do?	Well, that's about all.	
That's about all?	Mhmm	
Do you ever get to play with your baby brother?	Yeah . . .	
Yeah, what kinds of things do you do with him?	Oh, wrestle . . .	
Wrestle . . . oh.	I roll him over on my stomach.	
You roll him over on your stomach. Does he like that?	Yeah. He's believing it's (the) trick . . .	
He what?	He's believing it's a trick.	
Oh, he's believing it's a trick. Yeah. Oh, so he thinks he's doing tricks with you, huh. Does he laugh a lot when you do that?	Yeah.	
Yeah, does he get real silly?	Goes like this ______	
Oh . . .		

MODULE TIME	
TOTAL	1:31
ELAPSED	26:31–28:02

Clinical Phonetics CD 4, Track 15 Practice Module 10: All Sounds in Continuous Speech; Sample 2

TRANSCRIPTION KEY[a]

Clinician	*Child*	*Transcription*
How do you ride home?	On the buses.	[ɑ̃n də bʌsɪs]
Oh, on the buses. Tell me about the things that you do in the morning . . . that are just like the little girl.	Get up and get dressed.	[gɛʔ ʌp æ ɪ̃n gɛʔ gwɛstʰ]
(Talkover)	(??)	
And then you eat and then the school bus?	Mm, I come home.	[m̩aɪ kʌ̃ m hoʊm]
And you come home. Do you go to school in the morning . . . or in the afternoon?	No, in the morning.	[n oʊ ɪn ə̃ mɔrnɪn]
In the morning. What do you do (repeat) after you come home from school then?	Play.	[pʰ w̥ eɪ]
What kinds of things do you play?	Toys and stuff.	[tʰ ɔɪ z̥ n̩ s̪ tʌf]
Toys and stuff? Do you ever have lunch . . . when you come home?	Yeah.	[j ɛ əʰ]
What kinds of things do you have for lunch?	Sandwiches (and stuff).	[s̪ æ̃ n w ɪ t ʃ ɪ z]
Stuff like that? Do you make your own sandwiches? Or does Mom make them?	Mom makes them . . . Sometimes I make them self.	[mɑ̃ meɪ̃ks əm sʌm t ɑ̃ɪ mz ɑɪ meɪk ðəm sɛʊf]
Sometimes you make them yourself . . . Mom makes them. Yeah. What kind of sandwiches do you make yourself when you make them yourself?	Cheese . . . cheese and pickles.	[t ʃ ɪ z t ʃ i z̪ æ n pɪkʊᵊ z̥]
Ah, I'm not sure I know how to make a cheese sandwich. What would you do? How would you tell me how to make a cheese sandwich?	First put mustard on it—I mean that stuff on it and then put (ch . . .) meat and then put cheese and then close it up!	[f ɜ s̪ pʰ ɪ t m ʌ s t ɪ d ɑ̃ n ɪ t ɛ̃ min ð ɛ t s t ʌ f ɑ̃ɪʔ ɛ̃n ɛ n p ɪ t s̪ː mi t ɛ̃ n ɛ n p ʊ t t ʃ i ə n ɛ̃ n k w ɔ z̪ ɪ ɾ ʌ p]

[a]Recall that questionable segments are circled.

MODULE TIME	
TOTAL	1:31
ELAPSED	26:31–28:02

Clinical Phonetics CD 4, Track 15
Practice Module 10:
All Sounds in Continuous Speech; Sample 2

TRANSCRIPTION SHEET

Clinician	*Child*	*Transcription*
How do you ride home?	On the buses.	
Oh, on the buses. Tell me about the things that you do in the morning . . . that are just like the little girl.	Get up and get dressed.	
(Talkover)	(??)	
And then you eat and then the school bus?	Mm, I come home.	
And you come home. Do you go to school in the morning . . . or in the afternoon?	No, in the morning.	
In the morning. What do you do (repeat) after you come home from school then?	Play.	
What kinds of things do you play?	Toys and stuff.	
Toys and stuff? Do you ever have lunch . . . when you come home?	Yeah.	
What kinds of things do you have for lunch?	Sandwiches (and stuff).	
Stuff like that? Do you make your own sandwiches? Or does Mom make them?	Mom makes them . . . Sometimes I make them self.	
Sometimes you make them yourself . . . Mom makes them. Yeah. What kind of sandwiches do you make yourself when you make them yourself?	Cheese . . . cheese and pickles.	
Ah, I'm not sure I know how to make a cheese sandwich. What would you do? How would you tell me how to make a cheese sandwhich?	First put mustard on it—I mean that stuff on it and then put (ch . . .) meat and then put cheese and then close it up!	

Appendixes

Appendix A

Phonetics Symbols and Terms

At several places in the text, we have alerted the reader to the diversity of symbols and terms used to describe and classify speech sounds. The tables in this appendix should be useful for cross-referencing symbols, terms, and concepts found in a variety of sources read by students of phonetics. Table A.1 is the most recent update of the standard International Phonetic Alphabet (IPA), and A.8 includes IPA extensions for transcription of atypical speech.

CONTENTS

TABLE A.1
The International Phonetic Alphabet (revised to 1993, updated 1996). Copyright © 1996 The International Phonetic Association.

CONSONANTS (PULMONIC)

	Bilabial	Labiodental	Dental	Alveolar	Postalveolar	Retroflex	Palatal	Velar	Uvular	Pharyngeal	Glottal
Plosive	p b			t d		ʈ ɖ	c ɟ	k ɡ	q ɢ		ʔ
Nasal	m	ɱ		n		ɳ	ɲ	ŋ	ɴ		
Trill	ʙ			r					ʀ		
Tap or Flap				ɾ		ɽ					
Fricative	ɸ β	f v	θ ð	s z	ʃ ʒ	ʂ ʐ	ç ʝ	x ɣ	χ ʁ	ħ ʕ	h ɦ
Lateral fricative				ɬ ɮ							
Approximant		ʋ		ɹ		ɻ	j	ɰ			
Lateral approximant				l		ɭ	ʎ	ʟ			

Where symbols appear in pairs, the one to the right represents a voiced consonant. Shaded areas denote articulations judged impossible.

CONSONANTS (NON-PULMONIC)

Clicks		Voiced implosives		Ejectives	
ʘ	Bilabial	ɓ	Bilabial	ʼ	Examples:
ǀ	Dental	ɗ	Dental/alveolar	pʼ	Bilabial
ǃ	(Post)alveolar	ʄ	Palatal	tʼ	Dental/alveolar
ǂ	Palatoalveolar	ɠ	Velar	kʼ	Velar
ǁ	Alveolar lateral	ʛ	Uvular	sʼ	Alveolar fricative

OTHER SYMBOLS

ʍ Voiceless labial-velar fricative
w Voiced labial-velar approximant
ɥ Voiced labial-palatal approximant
ʜ Voiceless epiglottal fricative
ʢ Voiced epiglottal fricative
ʡ Epiglottal plosive

ɕ ʑ Alveolo-palatal fricatives
ɺ Alveolar lateral flap
ɧ Simultaneous ʃ and x

Affricates and double articulations can be represented by two symbols joined by a tie bar if necessary. k͡p t͜s

VOWELS

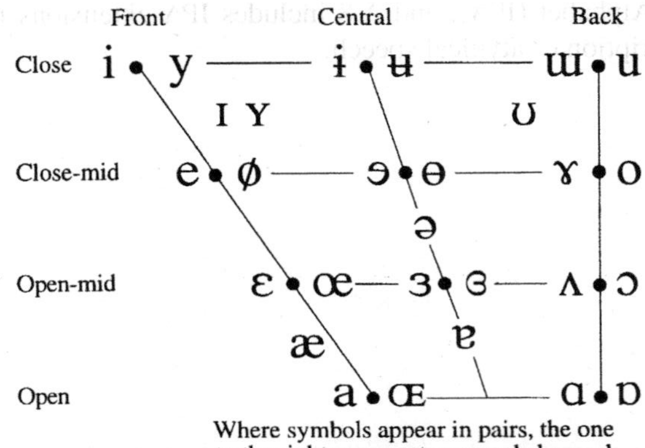

Where symbols appear in pairs, the one to the right represents a rounded vowel.

SUPRASEGMENTALS

ˈ Primary stress
ˌ Secondary stress ˌfoʊnəˈtɪʃən
ː Long eː
ˑ Half-long eˑ
˘ Extra-short ĕ
| Minor (foot) group
‖ Major (intonation) group
. Syllable break ɹi.ækt
‿ Linking (absence of a break)

DIACRITICS Diacritics may be placed above a symbol with a descender, e.g. ŋ̊

̥	Voiceless	n̥ d̥	̤	Breathy voiced	b̤ a̤	̪	Dental	t̪ d̪
̬	Voiced	s̬ t̬	̰	Creaky voiced	b̰ a̰	̺	Apical	t̺ d̺
ʰ	Aspirated	tʰ dʰ	̼	Linguolabial	t̼ d̼	̻	Laminal	t̻ d̻
̹	More rounded	ɔ̹	ʷ	Labialized	tʷ dʷ	̃	Nasalized	ẽ
̜	Less rounded	ɔ̜	ʲ	Palatalized	tʲ dʲ	ⁿ	Nasal release	dⁿ
̟	Advanced	u̟	ˠ	Velarized	tˠ dˠ	ˡ	Lateral release	dˡ
̠	Retracted	e̠	ˤ	Pharyngealized	tˤ dˤ	̚	No audible release	d̚
̈	Centralized	ë	̴	Velarized or pharyngealized	ɫ			
̽	Mid-centralized	e̽	̝	Raised	e̝ (ɹ̝ = voiced alveolar fricative)			
̩	Syllabic	n̩	̞	Lowered	e̞ (β̞ = voiced bilabial approximant)			
̯	Non-syllabic	e̯	̘	Advanced Tongue Root	e̘			
˞	Rhoticity	ɚ a˞	̙	Retracted Tongue Root	e̙			

TONES AND WORD ACCENTS

LEVEL			CONTOUR		
e̋ or	˥	Extra high	ě or	˩˥	Rising
é	˦	High	ê	˥˩	Falling
ē	˧	Mid	e᷄	˦˥	High rising
è	˨	Low	e᷅	˩˨	Low rising
ȅ	˩	Extra low	e᷈	˧˦˧	Rising-falling
↓		Downstep	↗		Global rise
↑		Upstep	↘		Global fall

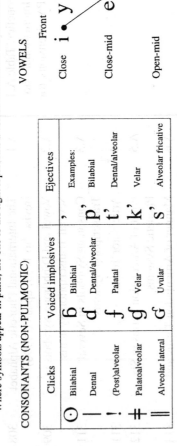

TABLE A.2
Vowel and Diphthong Symbols in Several Transcription Systems[a]

Key Word	IPA (1979)	Symbol Name[b]	Shriberg and Kent[c] (this text)	Ladefoged (1975)	Prator and Robinett (1973)	Jones[d] (1966)
beat	i		i	i	iy	iː
bit	ɪ = ɩ		ɪ	ʃ	ɪ	i
bait	e		e, e͡ɪ	e	ey	ei
bet	ɛ	"epsilon"	ɛ	ɛ	ɛ	ɛ
bat	æ	"ash"	æ	æ	æ	a
father	a		ɑ	ɑ	a	ɑː
bother	ɑ	"script A"	ɑ	ɒ	a	ɔ
bought	ɔ	"open O"	ɔ	ɔ	ɔ	ɔ, ɔː
boat	o	"closed O"	o, o͡ʊ	oɷ	ow	o, ou
put	ʊ = ɷ		ʊ	ɷ	ʊ	u
boot	u		u	u	uw	uː
but	ʌ	"caret" or "wedge"	ʌ	ʌ	ə	ʌ
above	ə	"schwa"	ə	ə	ə	ə
bite	aɩ		ɑ͡ɪ	aʃ	ay	ɑi
bout	ɑɷ		ɑ͡ʊ	aɷ	aw	ɑu
boy	ɔɩ		ɔ͡ɪ	ɔʃ	ɔy	ɔi
bird	ɝ	"reversed hooked epsilon"	ɝ	ər	ər	əː
bett<u>er</u>	ɚ	"schwar" or "hooked schwa"	ɚ	ər	ər	ə

[a] The format of this table was modified from Bronstein (1960, Appendix B) and from Ladefoged (1975, Table 4.1).

[b] Symbol names are only suggestive; alternative labels may be added by the reader. "Reversed hooked epsilon" refers to the Shriberg and Kent symbol in "bird." IPA alphabet does not differentiate stressed from unstressed [ɚ].

[c] Alternative symbols within a box represent allophonic variants by which phoneticians have symbolized tense vowels and diphthongs to indicate their increased duration and glide characteristics in certain environments (stressed syllables and open syllables [CV]).

[d] These symbols were taken from Jones's *The Pronunciation of English* (1966) and may differ somewhat from those used in his other works. They represent a Southern British form of English.

TABLE A.2
Vowel and Diphthong Symbols in Several Transcription Systems (continued)

Webster's New International							
3rd Ed. (1961)	2nd Ed. (1956)	Phonics Term[e]	Thomas (1958)	Kenyon and Knott (1953)[f]	Trager and Smith[g]	Hubbell (1950)[h]	Pike (1947)
ē	ē	"long e"	i, ɪi	i	iy	iĭ	i
i	ĭ	"short i"	ɪ	ɪ	i	i	ι
ā	ā	"long a"	e, eɪ	e	ey	eĭ	e
e	ē	"short e"	ɛ	ɛ	e	e	ɛ
a	ŏ	"short a"	æ	æ	æ	æ	æ
ä	ô		ɑ, a	ɑ	a	ɑə̆	a
ä	ō	"short o"	ɑ	ɑ	a	ɑ	ɑ
ȯ	ô		ɔ	ɔ	ɔ, ɔh, ɔw	ɔə̆	ɔ
ō	ō	"long o"	o, oʊ	o	o, ow	ou	o
u̇	ŏŏ		ʊ	ʊ	u	u	ʊ
ü	o͞o	"long u"	u, ʊu	u	uw	uŭ	u
ə	ŭ	"short u"	ʌ	ʌ	ə	ʌ	ʌ
ə	ȧ		ə	ə	ə	ə	ə
ī	ī	"long i"	aɪ	aɪ	ay	aĭ	a[i]
au̇	ou		ɑʊ	aʊ	aw	aŭ	a[u]
ȯi	oi		ɔ, ɪ	ɔɪ	oy	ɔĭ	o[i]
ər	ûr		ɜ, ɝ	ɝ	əhr	ɜə̆	r̩
ər	ẽr		ə, ɚ	ɚ	ər	ə, r	r̩

[e] Phonics terms are presented as familiar referents from traditional reading instruction that relate to the common dictionary symbols in the two columns. *Phonics* refers to standard orthography only and must be kept distinct from *phonetics*.
[f] Kenyon and Knott base their system on a Midwestern dialect of American English.
[g] Trager and Smith base their system on an Eastern dialect of American English.
[h] Hubbell bases his system on a dialect of English spoken in New York City. The semicircular diacritic conveys a nonsyllabic value to the vowel below; it may also be used to indicate the weaker element of a diphthong (IPA convention).

TABLE A.3
Consonant Symbols in Several Transcription Systems

Consonant Symbol IPA (1979)	Example	Symbol Name[a]	Kenyon and Knott (1953)	Trager and Smith (1951)	Bloch and Trager (1942)	Pike (1947)	Webster[c] (1956)
θ	thing	"theta"	θ	θ	θ	θ	th "voiceless th"
ð	this	"ethe" [εð]	ð	ð	ð	đ "bar-d"	t̶h̶ "voiced th"
ʃ	she	"esh" [εʃ]	ʃ	š "s-wedge"	š	š	sh
ʒ	beige	"ezh" [εʒ]	ʒ	ž "z-wedge"	ž	ž	zh
tʃ[b]	church		tʃ	č "c-wedge"	tš	č	ch "cha"
ʤ[b]	judge		ʤ	ǰ "j-wedge"	dž	ǰ	j "ja"
ʍ	which	"voiceless w"	hw	hw	hw	hw	hw
j	you	"palatal glide"	j	y	j	y	y
ɹ[d]	red	"consonant R"	r	r	r	r	r
ŋ	sing	"eng"	ŋ	ŋ	ŋ	ŋ	ng

[a]The names in this column apply to the first column of symbols (IPA, 1979). Names for alternative symbols appear in the box with that symbol where it first appears.

[b]Variations among the affricate symbols are due to the attempt by some systems to denote the phonemic status of these two sounds as a single phoneme of English.

[c]Common dictionary symbols for most of these consonant phonemes are letter combinations known as "digraphs" (two graphemes).

[d][r] may be substituted for any retroflex sound, including the approximant [ɹ], so long as no ambiguity with the trill [r] results (*The Principles of the IPA*, 1978, p. 13).

TABLE A.4
Articulator Terms[a]

Articulator	Combining Term: Prefixal	Combining Term: Suffixal
Lips:	labio-	-labial
Tongue:	lingua-	-lingual
	glosso-	-glossal
Tip (apex)	apico-	-apical
Front (lamina or blade)	fronto-	-frontal
	lamino-	-laminal
Center	centro-	-central
Back (dorsum)	dorso-	-dorsal
Pharynx:	pharyngo-	-pharyngeal
Larynx: (glottis)	laryngo-	-laryngeal
		-glottal

[a]See Table A.5 for use of combining form with place of articulation. This table (Table A.4) was adapted from information presented in Mackay (1978, p. 116).

TABLE A.5
Point of Articulation Terms in Six Phonetic Systems

Place of Articulation	Shriberg and Kent (this text)	Catford (1977)	Peterson and Shoup (1966)	Gleason (1961)	Hockett[a] (1958)	Bloch and Trager (1942)
Lips	Bilabial	Exolabial	Bilabial	Bilabial	Bilabial	Protruded
		Endolabial			Apico-labial	Bilabial
Teeth	Labiodental	Labiodental	Unilabial	Labiodental	Labiodental	Labiodental
	Interdental	Dental	Linguadental	Dental	Apico-interdental	Dental
	Linguadental				Apico-dental	
Alveolum (alveolar ridge)	Alveolar	Alveolar	Alveolar	Alveolar	Apico-alveolar	Alveolar
		Post-alveolar	Palatal-1	Retroflex	Lamino-alveolar	Cacuminal
Palate (vault)	Palatal	Pre-palatal	Palatal-2	Alveopalatal	Apico-domal	Pre-palatal
			Palatal-3			
		Palatal	Palatal-4			Medio-palatal
			Palatal-5	Palatal	Lamino-domal	Post-palatal
			Palato-velar			
Velum (soft palate)	Velar	Velar	Velar-1	Velar	Front dorso-velar	Pre-velar
		Post-velar	Velar-2	Uvular	Back dorso-velar	Medio-velar
			Uvular		Dorso-velar	Post-velar
Laryngo-pharynx	Glottal	Pharyngeal	Pharyngeal	Glottal	Glottal	Pharyngeal
		Laryngeal	Glottal			Glottal
						Laryngeal

[a] Hockett typically describes both the part of tongue involved as well as the point of articulation.

TABLE A.6
Manner of Articulation Terms and Classification of Sounds in Twelve Phonetic Systems

1. Shriberg and Kent (this text):

Oral Closures			Oral Continuants						
Nasals	Stops	Affricates	Fricatives			Liquids		Glides	Vowels
			Nonsibilants	Sibilants		Lateral	Rhotic		
				Grooves (Blades)					
m n ŋ	p b t d k g ɾ ʔ	tʃ dʒ	f v θ ð h	s z	ʃ ʒ	l	r	w j	

2. Calvert (1980):

Stops (Aspirates)	Fricatives (Spirates)	Affricates (Stop fricatives)	Resonants				
			Orals				Nasals
			Semivowels			Vowels	
			Glides	Lateral	Retroflex		
p b t d k g	f v θ ð s z ʃ ʒ	tʃ dʒ	w j	l	r		m n ŋ

3. International Phonetics Association (1989):[a]

Plosives	Nasals	Lateral	Flap	Fricatives	Alveolar Approximant	Palatal and Velar Approximants	Vowels
p b t d k g ʔ	m n ŋ	l	ɾ	f v θ ð s z ʃ ʒ h	ɹ	j ɰ	

[a]For complete place manner chart based on the International Phonetic Alphabet (revised to 1996), see Table A.1 on p. 308.

4. Fromkin and Rodman (1978):[b]

Consonantals						Nonconsonantals	
Nonvocalics					Vocalics	Nonvocalics	Vocalics
Sonorants	Nonsonorants				Sonorants		
Continuants	Noncontinuants	Continuants					
Nasals	Nonnasals						
		Stridents		Nonstridents	Liquids	Glides	Vowels
m n ŋ	p b t d k g	tʃ dʒ	s z ʃ ʒ	f v θ ð h	l r	w j	

[b]Adaptation of a distinctive feature system.

TABLE A.6
Manner of Articulation Terms and Classification of Sounds in Twelve Phonetic Systems (continued)

5. Tiffany and Carrell (1977)

Nonsyllabics							Syllabics	
Obstruent Consonants				Sonorant Consonants			Vowels	
Stops	Fricatives			Nasals and Lateral	Glides	Syllabic Consonants	Diphthongs	Vowels
	Nonsibilants	Sibilants						
		Concentrated	Distributed					
p b t d k g tʃ ʤ ʔ	f v θ ð h	s z	ʃ ʒ	m n ŋ l	j r w hw	m̩ n̩ l̩		

6. Ladefoged (1975, 1993):[c]

(Son.)	Obstruents			Sonorants					
Stops		Continuants							
(Nasals)	Orals	Fricatives		Approximants			Syllabics		Nasals
		Nonsibilants	Sibilants	Centrals		Lateral	Nasals	Approximants	
				Glides					
(m n ŋ)	p b t d k g	f v θ ð	s z ʃ ʒ	w j	ɹ	l	m̩ n̩ ŋ̍	ɹ̩ l̩	m n ŋ

[c]Ladefoged considers nasals to be classifiable in the stop category because they entail complete obstruction of the oral cavity.

7. Malmberg (1963):

Consonants										Vowels	
Momentary		Continuous									
Stopped Passage of Air		Constricted Passage of Air								Free Passage of Air	
Stops	Nasals	Liquids			Frictionless Continuants					Frictionless Continuants	Vowels
		Lateral	Trills		Flat	Round					
			Rolled	Flapped		Sibilants	Sibilants				
p b t d k g ʔ	m n ŋ	l	r R	ɾ	f v θ ð	s z	ʃ ʒ	ɹ	h	ɹ w j	

TABLE A.6
Manner of Articulation Terms and Classification of Sounds in Twelve Phonetic Systems (continued)

8. Hockett (1958):

Contoids					Contoid-Vocoids	Vocoids			
Obstruents					Sonorants				Pure Vocoids (vowels)
Stops	Spirants				Nasal Continuants	Liquids		Glides	
	Slit	Rill	Surface			Lateral	Retroflex		
pbtdkg	fvθð	sz	ʃʒ	h	mnŋ	l	r	wj	

9. Pike (1943):

Contoids (nonvocoids)								Vocoids
Nonresonants (rarely syllabic)					Resonants (frequently syllabic) (syllabic)			
Stops			Frictionals		Nonfrictionals			
Number of Articulator Closures			Orals	Nasals	Nasal Resonants	Oral Resonants		
						Lateral	Central	
1	2	3					Glides	Vowels
p	pbt dkg	pʰtʰkʰ	fvθðszʃʒh	"snorts"	mnŋ	l	wjr	

10. Bloomfield ([1933] 1984):[d]

Noisy Sounds					Musical Sounds					
Stops	Trills	Spirants			Nasals		Lateral	Inverted	Semivowels	Vowels
Plosives	Tongue Flip	Nonsibilants	Sibilants							
			Hisses	Hushes						
						mn	l	r	wj	
pbtdkg	ɾ	hfvθð	sz	ʃʒ	ŋ	Consonatoids		Vocaloids	Nonsyllabics	
						Semiconsonants			Semivowels	Vowels
Mutes (always nonsyllabic)						Sonants (sometimes syllabic)				(syllabic)
Consonants										Vowels

[d] For phonetic terms, read down; for phonemic terms, read up.

TABLE A.6
Manner of Articulation Terms and Classification of Sounds in Twelve Phonetic Systems (continued)

11. Jesperson (1913):

Increasing Degree of Sonorancy →								
Voiceless (surd)		Voiced (sonant)						
Stops	Fricatives	Stops	Fricatives	Nasals and Lateral	Trills and Flap	Vowels		
						Closed	Semiclosed	Open
p t k	f θ s ʃ h	b d g	v ð z ʒ	m n ŋ l	r̥ ʀ ɾ			

12. Sweet (1877):

Consonants						Vowels			
Open		Divided	Shut		Nasals	Nonround		Round	
Voiceless	Voiced		Voiceless	Voiced		Wide	Narrow	Wide	Narrow
f ʍ s θ h	v w ʒ z ð r j	l	p t k	b d g	m n ŋ				

TABLE A.7
Viseme Classes of the Phonemes of American English[a]

Class 1 (bilabials): /p/ /b/ /m/

Class 2 (labiodentals): /f/ /v/

Class 3 (linguadentals): /θ/ /ð/

Class 4 (rounded sonorants): /w/ /r/

Class 5 (palatals): /tʃ/ /ʤ/ /ʃ/ /ʒ/

Class 6 (alveolars): /t/ /d/ /s/ /z/

Class 7 (velars and alveolar sonorants): /k/ /g/ /n/ /l/

Class 8 (glottal): /h/

[a] Sounds in a viseme class share visual features. Sounds from different viseme classes can be distinguished from visual cues, such as jaw opening or lip configuration.

TABLE A.8
extIPA Symbols for Disordered Speech (revised to 2002)

CONSONANTS (other than on the IPA Chart)

	bilabial	labiodental	dentolabial	labioalv.	linguolabial	interdental	bidental	alveolar	velar	velophar.
Plosive		p̪ b̪	p͆ b͆	p̪͇ b̪͇	t̼ d̼	t̪͆ d̪͆				
Nasal			m͆	m̪͇	n̼	n̪͆				
Trill					r̼	r̪͆				
Fricative median			f͆ v͆	f̪͇ v̪͇	θ̼ ð̼	θ̪͆ ð̪͆	h̪͆ ɦ̪͆			ʩ
Fricative lateral+median								ʪ ʫ		
Fricative nareal	m͋							n͋	ŋ͋	
Percussive	ʬ						ʭ			
Approximant lateral					l̼	l̪͆				

Where symbols appear in pairs, the one to the right represents a voiced consonant. Shaded areas denote articulations judged impossible.

DIACRITICS

͍	labial spreading	s͍	͈	strong articulation	f͈	͊	denasal	m͊
͆	dentolabial	v͆	͉	weak articulation	v͉	͋	nasal escape	v͋
̪͆	interdental/bidental	n̪͆	\	reiterated articulation	p\p\p	͌	velopharyngeal friction	s͌
͇	alveolar	t͇	͎	whistled articulation	s͎	↓	ingressive airflow	p↓
̼	linguolabial	d̼	→	sliding articulation	θ→s	↑	egressive airflow	!↑

CONNECTED SPEECH

(.)	short pause
(..)	medium pause
(...)	long pause
f	loud speech [{*f* laud *f*}]
ff	louder speech [{*ff* laudɚ *ff*}]
p	quiet speech [{*p* kwaɪət *p*}]
pp	quieter speech [{*pp* kwaɪətɚ *pp*}]
allegro	fast speech [{*allegro* fast *allegro*}]
lento	slow speech [{*lento* slou *lento*}]
crescendo, ralentando, etc. may also be used	

VOICING

̬	pre-voicing	̬z
̬	post-voicing	z̬
₍̥₎	partial devoicing	₍z̥₎
₍̥	initial partial devoicing	₍z̥
̥₎	final partial devoicing	z̥₎
₍̬₎	partial voicing	₍s̬₎
₍̬	initial partial voicing	₍s̬
̬₎	final partial voicing	s̬₎
⁼	unaspirated	p⁼
ʰ	pre-aspiration	ʰp

OTHERS

◯, (C̲)	indeterminate sound, consonant	(( ))	extraneous noise ((2 sylls))
(V̲), (P̲l̲.v̲l̲s̲)	indeterminate vowel, voiceless plosive, etc.	¡	sublaminal lower alveolar percussive click
(N̲), (v̲)	indeterminate nasal, probably [v], etc.	!¡	alveolar and sublaminal clicks (cluck-click)
( )	silent articulation (ʃ), (m)	*	sound with no available symbol

REFERENCES FOR PHONETIC SYMBOL SYSTEMS

All of the phonetic symbol systems described in this appendix have been widely used in some area of linguistics or communicative disorders. The following references provide additional information on phonetic symbolization, including several systems developed for special needs. The Internet resources for more information on the International Phonetic Association additional learning materials and IPA fonts were courteously provided by Thomas Powell.

Ball, M. J. (1988). The transcription of phonation types. *Clinical Linguistics and Phonetics, 2*, 253–256.

Bernhardt, B., & Ball, M. J. (1993). Characteristics of atypical speech currently not included in the Extension to the IPA. *Journal of the International Phonetic Association, 23*, 35–38.

Bronsted, K., Grunwell, P., Henningsson, G., Jansonius, K., Karling, J., Meijer, M., Ording, U., Sell, D., Vermeij-Zieverink, E., & Wyatt, R. (1994). A phonetic framework for the cross-linguistic analysis of cleft palate speech. *Clinical Linguistics and Phonetics, 8*, 109–125.

Grunwell, P., & Russell, J. (1987). Vocalisations before and after cleft palate surgery: A pilot study. *British Journal of Disorders of Communication, 22*, 1–17.

International Phonetic Association. (1999). *Handbook of the International Phonetic Association: A guide to the use of the International Phonetic Alphabet.* Cambridge, UK: Cambridge University Press.

Laver, J. (1980). *The phonetic description of voice quality.* Cambridge, UK: Cambridge University Press.

Miller, S. (2000). *Targeting pronunciation: The intonation, sounds and rhythm of American English.* Boston: Houghton Mifflin.

PRDS Working Party. (1980). The phonetic representation of disordered speech. *British Journal of Disorders of Communication 15*, 217–223.

PRDS Working Party. (1983). *The phonetic representation of disordered speech: Final report.* London: The King's Fund.

Pullum, G. K., & Ladusaw, W. A. (1996). *Phonetic symbol guide*, 2nd ed. Chicago: The University of Chicago Press.

Trost, J. E. (1981). Articulatory additions to the classical description of the speech of persons with cleft palate. *Cleft Palate Journal, 18*, 193–203.

Woodard, M. (1991). The use of diacritics for visual articulatory behaviours. *British Journal of Disorders of Communication, 26*, 125–128.

INTERNET RESOURCES

Home Page of The International Phonetic Association

http://www2.arts.gla.ac.uk/IPA/ipa.html

IPA Learning Materials

http://www2.arts.gla.ac.uk/IPA/cassettes.html
http://www.sil.org/computing/catalog/ipahelp.html
http://hctv.humnet.ucla.edu/departments/linguistics/VowelsandConsonants/

IPA Fonts

http://www2.arts.gla.ac.uk/IPA/ipafonts.html
http://www.sil.org/computing/fonts/encore-ipa.html
http://www.chass.utoronto.ca/~rogers/fonts.html

Appendix B

Distributional, Structural, and Proportional Occurrence Data for American English Sounds, Syllables, and Words

The 15 tables in this appendix provide comprehensive statistical information on English speech sounds. These data have been compiled and arranged as a handy reference source for the clinician. It is important to note that the statistical studies cited have used many different approaches; original sources should be consulted for full details of sampling, counting procedures, and other important methodological information.

CONTENTS

TABLE B.1
Some Distributional Characteristics of American English Phonemes[a, b]

Phoneme	Characteristics
/ʒ, ŋ/	These never occur in word-initial position; all other consonants do.
/h, j, w/	These never occur in word-final position; all other consonants do.
/r/	In word-final singleton position, /r/ is generally preceded only by a tense vowel, such as *near, nor.*
/ʃ, ŋ/	In word-final singleton position, /ʃ/ and /ŋ/ are generally preceded only by a lax vowel, such as *mesh, mash; ring, rung.*
/ɪ, ɛ, æ, ʊ, ʌ/	These lax vowels never occur in open syllable words; they can only occur before consonants or consonant clusters.
/i, e, ɑ, ɔ, u/	All tense vowels and all diphthongs can occur in open syllables, such as *see, saw, sew.*
/o͡ʊ, a͡ɪ, a͡ʊ, ɔ͡ɪ]/	

[a]For a complete description of the distributional characteristics of English speech sounds, see Gimson (1970). This work is based on British pronunciation; there is nothing comparable in breadth and depth for American pronunciation, but Kenyon (1964) provides background for certain dialects (Traugott & Pratt, 1980).

[b]Exceptions to distributional characteristics in English words are indicated in the text (e.g., some proper nouns).

TABLE B.2
Distributional Characteristics of Initial and Final Consonant Clusters[a]

Word-Initial Clusters[b]		Word-Final Clusters[c]		
CC-	CCC-	-CC	-CCC	
p + l, r, j	s + p + l, r, j	p + t, θ, s	p + t, θ	+ s
t + r, j, w	s + t + r, j	t + θ, s	t + θ	
k + l, r, j, w	s + k + l, r, j, w	k + t, s	k + t	
b + l, r, j		b + d, z	m + p, f	
d + r, j, w		d + z	n + t, θ	
g + l, r, j, w		g + d, z	ŋ + k	
m + j		tʃ + t	l + p, t, k, f, θ	
n + j		ʤ + d	f + t, θ	
l + j		m + p, d, f, θ, z	s + p, t, k	
f + l, r, j		n + t, tʃ, ʤ, θ, s, z		
v + j		ŋ + k, d, z	p + s	+ t
θ + r, j, w		l + p, t, k, b, d, tʃ, ʤ, m, n, f, v, θ, s, z	t + s	
s + l, j, w, p, t, k, m, n		f + t, θ, s	k + s	
ʃ + r		v + d, z	d + s	
h + j		θ + t, s	m + p	
		ð + d, z	n + s, tʃ	
		s + p, t, k	ŋ + k	
		z + d	l + s, p, k, tʃ	
		ʃ + t	s + p, k	
		ʒ + d		
			n + d	+ z
			l + b, d, m, n, v	
			n + ʤ, z	+ d
			l + ʤ, m, v	
			k + s	+ θ
			n + t	
			ŋ + k	
			l + f	

[a]Initial and final consonant clusters do not precede or follow all vowels in English. For representative information on British English, see Gimson (1970), from which the data in Table B.2 were taken.

[b]Glides and liquids are the only consonants permitted in the third position of word-initial CCC clusters.

[c]Final CCCC patterns are formed using /t/, /d/, /s/, or /z/ as a final element to represent the grammatical morpheme for past tense or plural *(glimpsed)*.

TABLE B.3
Structural Characteristics of Monosyllabic Words[a]

Syllable Type	Example	Broad Phonetic Spelling
V	a	[ə] or [ʌ]
CV	the	[ðə] or [ði]
CCV	tree	[tri]
CCCV	screw	[skru]
VC	is	[ɪz]
VCC	its	[ɪts]
VCCC	asks	[æsks]
CVC	cup	[kʌp]
CCVC	plane	[pleɪ̄n]
CCCVC	strain	[streɪ̄n]
CVCC	sits	[sɪts]
CVCCC	sixth	[sɪksθ]
CVCCCC	sixths	[sɪksθs]
CCVCC	stacks	[stæks]
CCCVCC	stripped	[strɪpt]
CCVCCC	spanked	[spæŋkt]
CCVCCCC	glimpsed	[glɪmpst]
CCCVCCC	sprints	[sprɪnts]
CCCVCCCC	strengths	[strɛŋkθs]

[a]See Moser (1969) for a thorough compendium of monosyllabic words in English. For information on the numerous structural types of polysyllabic words, see Roberts (1965).

TABLE B.4
Proportional Occurrence of Phonetic Classes in Adults' Speech[a]

Phonetic Class	Proportion of All Phonemes
Vowels/Consonants	
Vowels and diphthongs	38.10
Retroflex vowels	2.21
Consonants	58.50
Syllabic consonants	1.19
Vowels Classified	
by Place:	
Front	14.28
Centralized	13.51
Back	7.26
Back to front: [a͡ɪ] [ɔ͡ɪ]	3.05
by Height:	
High	13.87
Mid	13.70
Low	6.84
Low to high: [a͡ɪ] [a͡ʊ] [ɔ͡ɪ]	3.69
Consonants Classified	
by Voicing:	
Voiceless	20.63
Voiced	37.87
by Manner:	
Stops	18.82
Fricatives	16.47
Affricates	1.05
Nasals	10.80
Liquids and Glides	11.36
by Place:	
Labial and labiodental[b]	12.78
Dental and alveolar[c]	35.64
Palatal[d]	2.79
Velar and glottal	7.29

[a]These data are adapted from Mines et al. (1978).

[b]Includes /w/ and /ʍ/.

[c]Includes /r/ and /θ/ and /g/.

[d]Includes /j/.

TABLE B.5
Proportional Occurrence of Phonetic Classes in Children's Speech[a]

Phonetic Class	Proportion of All Phonemes		
	1st Grade	3rd Grade	5th Grade
Vowels/Consonants			
Vowels and diphthongs[b]	40.07	39.94	40.00
Consonants	59.93	60.06	60.00
Vowels Classified			
by Place:			
Front	16.11	16.27	16.14
Central	14.31	14.34	14.73
Back[c]	5.20	5.40	5.60
Back to front: [aɪ] [ɔɪ]	3.78	3.25	2.88
by Height:			
Closed (high and mid)	16.54	17.14	17.52
Open (low)	18.98	18.80	18.90
Low to high: [aɪ] [aʊ] [ɔɪ]	4.54	4.00	3.60
Consonants Classified			
by Voicing:			
Voiceless	20.45	21.02	20.65
Voiced	39.48	39.04	39.35
by Manner:			
Stops and Affricates	19.57	19.89	19.44
Fricatives	15.00	15.05	15.77
Nasals	13.29	12.58	11.64
Liquids and Glides	12.08	12.54	13.15
by Place:			
Labial and labiodental[d]	16.58	15.78	15.53
Dental and alveolar[e]	31.49	32.01	32.02
Palatal[f]	11.29	12.52	16.57
Velar and glottal	9.89	9.88	9.27

[a]These data are adapted from Carterette and Jones (1974).

[b]For separate diphthong data, see "Vowels Classified by Height: Low to High."

[c]Includes the diphthong [aʊ].

[d]Includes /θ/ and /ð/ and /w/.

[e]Includes /r/.

[f]Palatal glide [y or j] not reported in Carterette and Jones's data summary.

TABLE B.6
Proportional Occurrence of Vowels and Diphthongs Overall and in Initial, Medial, and Final Position of Words in Adults' Speech[a]

Rank Order	Vowel Phoneme	Percent of All Vowels and Diphthongs	Percent within Phoneme			
			Initial	Medial	Final	Single
1	ə	18.10	18.80	34.71	25.28	21.18
2	ɪ	12.76	31.13	67.25	1.16	0.05
3	i	9.15	2.56	36.44	60.01	0.01
4	ɛ	7.95	0.21	76.79	2.31	0.02
5	a͡ɪ	7.36	7.82	40.17	12.30	39.71
6	æ	5.59	30.65	67.72	1.50	0.01
7	o	4.58	10.64	41.08	43.27	5.01
8	e	3.90	3.85	64.36	30.07	1.72
9	ʌ	3.63	14.54	82.11	0.05	2.83
10	ɑ	3.54	22.17	74.93	1.75	1.15
11	u	2.81	0	50.77	49.06	0.02
12	ɔ	1.90	35.26	62.48	2.26	0
13	ʊ	1.88	1.40	68.91	29.06	0.06
14	a͡ʊ	1.60	17.91	65.82	16.12	0.02
15	ɔ͡ɪ	0.20	4.65	58.14	37.21	0
Alternates:						
Front		1.57	44.92	47.65	6.98	0.05
Central[b]		6.48	12.98	74.49	10.59	2.03
Back		1.70	16.27	68.72	14.87	0.01
Retroflex vowels[c]		5.49	0.01	41.13	50.91	7.48

[a]These figures combine vowel, vowel alternate, and retroflex vowel data as originally reported by Mines et al. (1978).

[b]Central alternates include both front and back vowels, which alternate with central vowels.

[c]Retroflex vowels include ɚ, ɝ, and alternates ɚ~ ɝ, ɚ~ ur, ɚ~ ər.

TABLE B.7
Proportional Occurrence of Consonants Overall and in Initial, Medial, and Final Position of Words in Adults' Speech[a]

Rank Order	Consonant Phoneme	Percent of All Consonants	Percent within Phoneme: Initial	Medial	Final
1	n	11.49	12.42	40.97	46.48
2	t	9.88	20.68	30.04	49.18
3	s	7.88	37.09	29.35	30.75
4	r	6.61	14.64	63.26	22.06
5	l	6.21	23.72	51.92	24.31
6	d	5.70	25.18	24.55	49.99
7	ð	5.37	90.23	8.46	1.26
8	k	5.30	34.38	41.76	23.77
9	m	5.11	37.87	28.02	33.91
10	w[b]	4.81	88.29	11.40	0.01
11	z	4.70	0.06	10.72	86.41
12	b	3.24	65.25	32.78	1.83
13	p	3.07	47.77	35.96	16.00
14	v	2.97	10.53	39.41	50.00
15	f	2.65	63.15	23.49	12.87
16	h	2.23	92.18	7.82	0
17	g	2.02	68.16	23.84	7.84
18	j	1.87	78.84	20.81	0
19	ŋ	1.85	0.01	30.76	69.15
20	θ	1.19	57.44	20.52	21.35
21	ʤ	0.95	49.22	31.54	19.24
22	ʃ	0.95	32.76	58.23	8.32
23	ʧ	0.85	15.71	24.39	44.19
24	ʒ	0.15	10.11	84.27	5.62
	Allophonic Alternates				
1	ɾ	1.76	7.02	56.13	36.86
2	ʔ	0.85	15.78	20.62	61.85
3	t ~ ʔ	0.21	0	52.94	47.06
4	t ~ ɾ	0.13	17.95	46.15	35.90

[a]The data presented here are adapted from Mines et al. (1978).

[b]Both /w/ and /hw/ are combined here.

TABLE B.8
Proportional Occurrence of Vowels and Diphthongs in First-Grade, Third-Grade, and Fifth-Grade Children's Speech[a]

		Proportion of All Vowels and Diphthongs		
Rank Order	Vowel or Diphthong	1st Grade	3rd Grade	5th Grade
1	ə	31.87	32.03	32.70
2	ɪ	11.13	11.46	11.40
3	i	9.51	9.94	10.34
4	a͞ɪ	9.27	7.93	6.98[b]
5	æ	8.09	7.68	7.60
6	ɛ	7.34	7.60	6.82
7	o͞ʊ	5.09	5.49	5.63
8	e	4.15	4.05	4.20
9	ɑ	3.83	3.88	4.11
10	ɔ	3.59	3.48	3.60
11	u	3.03	3.12	3.33
12	a͞ʊ	1.92	1.89	1.78
13	ʊ	1.04	1.25	1.29
14	ɔ͞ɪ	0.15	0.20	0.23

[a]The data presented here are adapted from Carterette and Jones (1974).

[b]/a͞ɪ/ is out of rank order by one place here. Otherwise, the rank orderings remain constant across the three grades sampled.

TABLE B.9
Proportional Occurrence of Consonant Phonemes in First-Grade, Third-Grade, and Fifth-Grade Children's Speech[a]

	Percent of All Consonants					
	1st Grade		3rd Grade		5th Grade	
Rank	Consonant	Percent	Consonant	Percent	Consonant	Percent
1	n	13.63	n	13.46	n	12.59
2	r	8.20	r	8.73	r	9.01
3	t	7.91	t	7.77	t	7.69
4	m	7.49	s	7.48	s	7.31
5	s	6.94	d	6.53	d	6.81
6	d	6.31	m	6.30	m	5.43
7	w	5.57	w	5.22	l	5.33
8	l	4.96	l	5.05	w	5.05
9	k	4.96	ʔ	4.92	k	4.82
10	z	4.58	k	4.76	z	4.62
11	ʔ[b]	4.49	ð	4.58	ð	4.52
12	ð	4.42	z	4.28	ʔ	3.65
13	h	3.37	b	3.13	h	3.04
14	b	3.18	h	3.07	b	2.94
15	g	2.90	g	2.52	g	2.56
16	f	2.21	p	2.34	j	2.53
17	p	2.12	f	2.18	p	2.49
18	v	1.64	j	1.88	f	2.30
19	j	1.41	v	1.58	v	2.12
20	ŋ	1.05	ŋ	1.19	ŋ	1.38
21	θ	1.03	θ	0.96	ʃ	1.33
22	ʃ	0.84	ʃ	0.94	θ	1.04
23	ʤ	0.53	tʃ	0.57	tʃ	0.74
24	tʃ	0.51	ʤ	0.57	ʤ	0.69
25	ʒ	0	ʒ	0	ʒ	0

[a]These data are adapted from Carterette and Jones (1974).

[b]/ʔ/ is included as a "phoneme" of English in the original data.

TABLE B.10
Proportional Occurrence of Consonants in Initial, Medial, and Final Position of Words in First-Grade, Second-Grade, and Third-Grade Children's Speech[a]

Rank Order	Consonant Phoneme	Percent of Consonants	Percent Initial	Percent Medial	Percent Final
1	n	13.14	7	62	31
2	t	11.74	22	22	55
3	d	10.25	15	12	73
4	r	7.83	14	46	40
5	s	6.50	50	20	30
6	ð	6.40	93	7	0
7	l	5.55	23	41	36
8	w[b]	5.33	94	6	0
9	m	4.63	35	26	39
10	k	4.25	41	29	30
11	z	3.70	0	6	94
12	h	3.33	99	1	0
13	b	2.97	76	23	1
14	p	2.73	52	23	25
15	g	2.38	77	13	10
16	v	1.91	4	36	60
17	f	1.83	64	17	19
18	ŋ	1.61	0	22	78
19	θ	0.93	45	22	33
20	ʃ	0.84	76	17	7
21	j	0.77	98	2	0
22	ʤ	0.69	78	12	10
23	tʃ	0.55	31	24	45
24	ʒ	0.01	0	100	0

[a]These data are adapted from data originally reported by Mader (1954).

[b]The percent reported for /w/ also includes the frequency of /ʍ/, as reported in the original data.

TABLE B.11
Proportional Occurrence of the 25 Most Frequent Word-Initial and Word-Final Consonant Clusters in Adults' Speech in Three Studies

	Word-Initial Clusters							Word-Final Clusters					
	Dewey[a] (1923)		French[b] et al. (1930)		Roberts (1965)			Dewey (1923)		French et al. (1930)		Roberts (1965)	
Rank	Cluster	%	Cluster	%	Cluster	%	Rank	Cluster	%	Cluster	%	Cluster	%
1	hw-	1.63	pr-	1.06	hw-	1.64	1	-nd	4.67	-nt	4.40	-nt	1.87
2	pr-	1.31	hw-	0.91	pr-	1.06	2	-nt	1.61	-nd	2.56	-st	1.68
3	tr-	1.06	st-	0.87	fr-	0.69	3	-st	1.50	-st	1.18	-nd	1.06
4	fr-	0.76	tr-	0.69	st-	0.80	4	-rd	0.66	-ts	1.11	-rz	0.80
5	st-	0.76	fr-	0.62	pl-	0.76	5	-ns	0.65	-ŋk	0.76	-nts	0.72
6	pl-	0.57	pl-	0.36	tr-	0.56	6	-nz	0.61	-ld	0.75	-rd	0.60
7	gr-	0.41	kw-	0.28	gr-	0.34	7	-ks	0.53	-rz	0.57	-ld	0.43
8	kw-	0.35	bl-	0.23	kl-	0.28	8	-kt	0.52	-ks	0.47	-rn	0.42
9	sp-	0.35	sp-	0.19	kw-	0.27	9	-ld	0.45	-kt	0.42	-kt	0.41
10	str-	0.32	kl-	0.18	gl-	0.24	10	-rt	0.42	-rd	0.37	-ŋk	0.39
11	nj-	0.27	others	1.01	sk-	0.23	11	-ts	0.39	others	3.73	-nz	0.37
12	kl-	0.26			Tr-	0.22	12	-rn	0.32			-zd	0.29
13	dr-	0.24			θr-	0.21	13	-nts	0.20			-rt	0.28
14	θr-	0.23			kr-	0.21	14	-rs	0.19			-ks	0.28
15	kr-	0.22			sp-	0.20	15	-lf	0.18			-ts	0.25
16	dj-	0.20			fj-	0.20	16	-rst	0.18			-vd	0.25
17	br-	0.18			dr-	0.15	17	-ŋk	0.17			-rk	0.20
18	bl-	0.14			str-	0.11	18	-zd	0.16			-lz	0.18
19	tw-	0.13			bl-	0.11	19	-rk	0.16			-mz	0.17
20	fj-	0.12			sm-	0.06	20	-ŋz	0.15			-rs	0.14
21	tj-	0.12			sl-	0.06	21	-rm	0.14			-rst	0.14
22	sj-	0.09			fl-	0.05	22	-ndz	0.13			-pt	0.13
23	fl-	0.09			sw-	0.05	23	-mz	0.13			-kst	0.12
24	kj-	0.08			tw-	0.04	24	-lz	0.12			-rm	0.11
25	mj-	0.07			bj-	0.04	25	-gz	0.11			-dz	0.11

[a]Dewey (1923) data are reported for prevocalic and postvocalic positions rather than word-initial and word-final positions.

[b]French, Carter, and Koenig (1930) data are reported for the top ten clusters only. The remainder are grouped under "others."

TABLE B.12

Syllable Types and Most Frequent Syllables in Adults' Speech

Syllable Types[a]			Most Frequent Syllables[b]		
Rank Order	Syllable Type	Proportional Occurrence	Syllable	Morpheme	Proportional Occurrence
1	CVC	33.5	ðə	the	7.3
2	CV	21.8	ʌv	of	4.0
3	VC	20.3	ɪn	in	3.3
4	V	9.7	ænd	and	3.3
5	CVCC	7.8	ɪ	-y	3.2
6	VCC	2.8	ə	a	3.2
7	CCVC	2.8	tu	to	3.2
8	CCV	0.8	ɪŋ	-ing	2.4
9	CCVCC	0.5	ɚ	-er	2.1
			rɪ	-ry	1.6
			ɪt	-it	1.4
			ðæt	that	1.3
			ɪz	is	1.3
			a͞ɪ	I	1.3
			lɪ	-ly	1.2
			fɔr	for	1.1
			others		<1.0

[a]French et al. (1930). C = Consonant; V = Vowel.

[b]Dewey (1923).

TABLE B.13
Word Types and Most Frequent Words in Adults' Speech

Word Types[a]				Ten Most Frequent Words in Four Studies			
Rank Order	Type	Proportional Occurrence	Number of Words of This Type	I[b]	II[c]	III[d]	IV[e]
1	VC	14.51	29				
2	CVC	9.52	307	the	I	I	I
3	CV	8.12	14	of	you	the	and
4	CVS	7.55	85	and	the	a	to
5	SVC	5.48	104	to	a	it	the
6	VS	5.07	10	a	on	to	a
7	CVSC	3.83	394	in	to	you	of
8	SVS	3.59	24	that	that	of	in
9	SV	2.94	6	it	it	and	we
10	CVCC	2.36	298	is	is	in	for
11	V	2.32	1	I	and	he	it
12	SVSC	1.40	103				
13	VSS	1.38	4				
14	CVCVC	1.12	266				
15	VSC	1.05	28				
16	CVCVS	1.04	86				
		71.28	1759				

Proportional Occurrence of One-, Two-, and Three-Syllable Words

Syllables per Word	Proportional Occurrence	Number of Words
one	76.92	2747
two	17.05	3969
three	4.55	2247
	98.52	8963

[a]Roberts (1965). C = Consonant; V = Vowel; S = Semivowel.

[b]Dewey (1923).

[c]French et al. (1930).

[d]Denes and Pinson (1963).

[e]Roberts (1965).

TABLE B.14

Most Frequent Phonemic Words in Children's and Adults' Speech[a]

Rank	1st Grade	3rd Grade	5th Grade	Adult
1	ʔ ə m	ʔ ə m	ə m	j ɛ ɑ
2	ə m	ə m	j ə n o͞ʊ	j ə n o͞ʊ
3	ə	æ n	n o͞ʊ	w ɛ l
4	n o͞ʊ	j ə n o͞ʊ	j ɛ ɑ	n o͞ʊ
5	æ n	ʔ ə	æ n	o͞ʊ
6	æ n d	w ɛ l	w ɛ l	ə^{h}
7	w ɛ l	n o͞ʊ	o͞ʊ	æ n
8	ɑ͞ɪ	ʔ æ n	ə	ə
9	o͞ʊ	o͞ʊ	j ɛ ə	ɑ͞ɪ
10	ʔ ə	s o͞ʊ	æ n d	s o͞ʊ
11	æ n ð ɛ n	ə	ə^{h}	ə n
12	j ɛ ə	j ɛ ə	ʔ ə m	j ɛ ə
13	s ə m t ɑ͞ɪ m z	ɑ͞ɪ	h i	ə h ə
14	ð ə n	j ɛ ɑ	s o͞ʊ	ɑ͞ɪ m i n
15	ə n	ʔ æ n d	ə n	ɑ͞ɪ n o͞ʊ
Types	4569	4815	5796	3447
Tokens	5528	5963	7187	4146

[a]Carterette and Jones (1974) define *phonemic words* in terms of a prosodical feature: a pause in the flow of sound. A phonemic word is a sound group or pattern that occurs between pauses (p. 26).

TABLE B.15
Summary of Findings on the Proportional Occurrence of Speech Sounds in Children's and Adults' Speech

Factor	Finding
Phoneme and phonetic class	(1) Four consonant sounds /n, t, s, r/ account for 25 percent of all phoneme occurrences (Dewey, 1923); ten phonemes /ə, n, t, ɪ, s, r, i, l, d, ɛ/ account for nearly half (47 percent) of all phoneme occurrences (Mines et al., 1978).
	(2) Approximately two-thirds of consonant occurrences are voiced (Mines et al., 1978).
	(3) The majority of consonant and vowel occurrences are articulated at the front of the mouth. Labial and labiodental sounds (21.6) and dental and alveolar sounds (60.9) account for over 80 percent of consonant occurrences. Front and central vowels account for nearly 75 percent of vowel occurrences (Mines et al., 1978).
	(4) The majority of vowels (over 71 percent) are articulated in the high (36.4 percent), high-mid (2.9 percent), or mid (32 percent) sections of the oral cavity (Mines et al., 1978).
	(5) Of all occurrences of syllabic consonants in adult conversational speech (1.2 percent), /n̩/ is most frequent, followed by /l̩/ and then /m̩/.
Position in word	(6) Four sounds /s, ð, w, h/ comprise more than 46 percent of the initial consonant occurrences in words said by young grade-school children; five sounds /n, d, t, r, z/ comprise more than 69 percent of the final consonant occurrences in words said by young grade-school children (Mader, 1954).
	(7) Five sounds /ð, h, w, ʍ, j/ occur in the initial position in over 90 percent of their occurrences in children's conversational speech; /z/ occurs in the final position in over 90 percent of its occurrences in children's conversational speech (Mader, 1954).
Structural forms	(8) Clusters are formed by phonemes whose distinctive features are neither very similar nor very different (Saporta, 1955). The most frequent clusters are sound pairs with the same alveolar place of articulation, but different manners of articulation (Denes & Pinson, 1963).
	(9) Simple syllable shapes—vowel syllables and those released and/or arrested by a simple consonant—comprise 87 percent of the syllables used in conversational speech (Faircloth and Faircloth, 1973).
	(10) The 16 most commonly occurring syllables and 10 words in adult speech (see Tables B.12 and B.13) make up more than 25 percent of our verbal behavior (Dewey, 1923).
Demographics	(11) Overall frequency of occurrence or positional frequency of occurrence of consonant sounds is not associated with grade in school or sex of children.
	(12) Frequency of occurrence of phonemes is only slightly related to age, sex, level of education, or early place of residence of adult speakers; moreover, ". . . frequency of occurrence of phonemes in English is primarily a function of the structure of the English language itself, and its relation to form (either spoken or written) or to style is very slight" (Mines et al., 1978, p. 223).

Glossary

Académie Française An agency of the French government, one of the duties of which is to determine the adoption of loanwords into French.

Acoustic phonetics the branch of phonetics that deals with the acoustic properties of sounds; acoustics is a subfield of physics that deals with the generation and transmission of sound.

Acoustic vowel space see *F1-F2 chart.*

Addition a speech production error in which a sound is incorrectly added (before or after) to another sound.

Advanced a sound made with a tongue in a forward or fronted position in the oral cavity.

Affricate a manner of articulation; an affricate is a consonant sound formed by a stop + fricative sequence. The only English affricates are /ʤ/ (judge) and /tʃ/ (church).

African American Vernacular English a social dialect of American English that arose as consequence of contract between speakers of English and speakers of a variety of West African languages when non-English speaking Africans were brought to the United States as slaves. It has a variety of unique patterns of speech production, word choices, and other linguistic structures.

Allograph any one alphabet letter or combination of letters that represents a particular phoneme. One phoneme may be represented (spelled) by several different allographs.

Allophone one of the sound variants within a phoneme class, often used in a specified phonetic context.

Alphabet a system of written symbols used to express a language.

Alveolar a place of articulation pertaining to the alveolar ridge, or alveolus; alveolar consonants are formed by articulation of the tongue against the alveolar ridge.

Arresting another name for syllable-final sounds; they arrest (stop) the syllable.

Articulator an anatomic structure capable of movements that form the sounds of speech. The primary articulators are the tongue, jaw, lips, and velopharynx.

Articulatory phonetics the branch of phonetics that deals with how sounds are formed; also called *physiological phonetics.*

Aspirated a sound, usually a stop consonant, made with a noise segment associated with air escaping through the glottis.

Aspiration a fricative noise generated as air escapes through partly adducted vocal folds and into the upper cavities.

Backed a sound made with a posterior place of articulation.

Back vowel a vowel produced with the tongue positioned toward the back of the mouth. The back vowel series is bounded by the high-back /u/ (*who*) and the low-back /ɑ/ (*ha*).

Bilabial a place of articulation pertaining to the two lips; bilabial consonants are produced by articulations of the lips.

Blade of tongue the portion of the tongue that is located behind the tip and in front of the dorsum. The blade is the part of the tongue used to produce the *sh* consonant in *she.*

Body of tongue the mass or bulk of the tongue.

Boundary (or edge) effects phonological or phonetic characteristics that appear at the margins of a linguistic unit, such as a phrase.

Breath group the sequence of syllables and/or words produced on a single breath.

Breath group theory a theory that holds that a declarative sentence can be divided into nonterminal and terminal parts, with variation in vocal fundamental frequency permitted only in terminal part.

Breathy a noisy voice quality caused by air escaping through the vocal folds.

Broad transcription phonetic transcription that uses phonemes exclusively and does not indicate finer variations such as those marked by diacritics in a *narrow transcription.*

Bunched /r/ an allophone of the consonant /r/ for which the tongue assumes a bunched or humped shape close to the palatal region.

Burst or frication spectra the intensity-by-frequency characteristics of the noise that is generated during a stop burst or a fricative segment.

Centralized a sound, usually a vowel, made with the tongue positioned in the central or mid region of the oral cavity.

Central vowel a vowel produced with the tongue positioned in the center of the mouth; for example, the first vowel in *upon.*

Checked (held) juncture a type of juncture used to signal an intention to continue talking or to express interest in another speaker's utterance.

Clear speech a type of speech used to ensure effective communication under difficult conditions, such as speaking over background noise. It usually is characterized by a combination of prosodic and articulatory changes.

Click a stop produced with an ingressive velaric airstream.

Clinical phonetics applications of phonetics to describe speech differences and disorders, including information about speech sounds and the perceptual skills used in clinical settings.

Closed a syllable that ends in a consonant.

Close juncture a transition between sounds that is associated with typical articulation and is not given any special mark for pause or interruption.

Coarticulation overlapping of movements for two or more sounds.

Coda the final margin of a syllable, consisting of one or more consonants.

Cognate a member of a pair of sounds that are opposed or distinguished by a particular phonetic feature. For example, /d/ (*do*) and /t/ (*to*) are voiced and voiceless cognates.

Complementary distribution a term used to describe two or more allophones of a particular phoneme that occur in mutually exclusive phonetic contexts.

Conversational speech everyday, casual speech, as contrasted with *clear speech.*

Contrastive stress a stress pattern used when a speaker wishes to depart from the usual or expected pattern of stress in an utterance, as when attention is drawn to a particular word.

Corner vowel (or point vowel) a vowel located at any one of the four points of the vowel quadrilateral: high-front /i/(*he*), low-front /æ/ (*hat*), low-back /ɑ/ (*ha*), or high-back /u/ (*who*).

Deletion a speech production error in which a sound is omitted (also termed an *omission*).

Denasalized a sound produced without nasalization or without an appropriate degree of nasalization.

Dental place of articulation pertaining to the teeth; dental consonants are formed by articulations of the lips or tongue with the upper teeth.

Dentalized a sound made with the tip of the tongue against the back of the upper teeth.

Derhotacization partial loss of *r* coloring from a normally rhotacized vowel (/ɝ/ or /ɚ/ in English).

Derhotacized a reduced or absence of r-coloring in a sound.

Diacritic mark a special symbol used to modify a phonetic symbol to indicate a particular modification of sound production.

Dialect different usage patterns within a language; speakers of one dialect may or may not easily understand speakers of another dialect of the same language.

Dictionary an inventory of the words in a language, usually together with their meaning.

Digraph a sequence of two or more alphabetic characters that represent a single sound.

Diphthong a vowel-like sound that serves as a syllable nucleus and involves a gradual transition from one vowel articulation (onglide) to another (offglide).

Diphthongization alteration of a pure vowel (or monophthong) to a dynamic articulation of changing vowel quality.

Distortion a speech production error in which a speech sound is recognizable as the correct sound but is not produced exactly correctly.

Dorsum of tongue the portion of the tongue located between the root and the blade. The dorsum is the part of the tongue used to produce the *g* consonant in *go.*

Egressive associated with outflowing air; egressive sounds are formed from an outflowing airstream.

Ejective a stop made with an egressive glottalic airstream.

F1-F2 chart or F1-F2 graph a diagram in which the frequencies of the first two formants, F1 and F2, define a space in which any vowel can be represented as a single point. This acoustic space corresponds to an articulatory vowel space defined by the dimensions of tongue height and tongue advancement.

F2 locus see *Second-formant locus.*

Final the final position or segment in a word, e.g., the *t* in the word *bat* is a final consonant.

Five-way scoring a perceptual system in which speech sounds are classified as typical versus one of four error types: an addition, a deletion (or omission), a substitution, or a distortion.

Flap a manner of articulation in which a sound is formed by a quick tapping movement of an articulator against a surface. In English, flaps are allophones of stops.

Formant a resonance of the vocal tract determined by the length and shape of the tract.

Formant frequency the center frequency of a formant.

Formant transition a change in formant frequency associated with a phonetic transition, as between a consonant and vowel.

Free variation a term used to describe allophones that may be exchanged for one another in a particular phonetic context.

Fricative a manner of articulation in which a continuous noise is generated as air is channeled through a narrow articulatory constriction.

Frictionalized a sound, usually a stop consonant, made with a fricative-like noise.

Fronted a sound made with a forward place of articulation.

Front vowel a vowel produced with the tongue positioned near the front of the mouth. The front vowel series is bounded by the high-front /i/ (*he*) and the low-front /æ/ (*hat*).

Fundamental frequency of voice the basic rate of vibration of the vocal folds; fundamental frequency is the physical correlate of vocal pitch.

Geminates sounds that occur together as a pair, such as the two *k* sounds in *bookkeeper* or the two *s* sounds in *gas supply.*

Glide a manner of articulation that involves a gliding movement from a partly constricted vocal tract to a more open vocal tract shape. Glides resemble diphthongs in their dynamics but cannot serve as syllable nuclei.

Glottal place of articulation pertaining to the glottis or the vocal folds; a glottal consonant is one formed by glottal (vocal fold) articulation.

Glottalized a creaky, or irregular voice quality associated with marked aperiodicity in vocal fold vibration.

Grapheme a unit in the writing system of a language.

Hertz the term that denotes one complete cycle of vibration; Hertz, abbreviated Hz, is the unit of frequency measurement.

High vowel a vowel produced with the tongue in a high (superior) position. Vowels /i/ (*he*) and /u/ (*who*) are high vowels.

Homorganic having the same place of articulation (*homo*= "same" and *organic* = "relating to an organ or structure"). For example, /m/ and /b/ are homorganic because they share a bilabial articulation.

Homotypic having the same manner of articulation (*homo*= "same" and *typic* = "relating to type or manner"). For example, /m/ and /n/ are homotypic because they share the nasal manner.

Idiolect an individual or personal pattern of language usage. Each user of a language has an idiolect.

Infant-directed speech see *Motherese.*

Ingressive associated with inflowing air; ingressive sounds are formed from an inflowing airstream.

Initial the first position or segment in a word, e.g., the *b* in the word *bat* is an initial consonant.

Interdental a place of articulation involving insertion of the tongue tip into the space between the upper and lower incisors (the interdental space).

Internal open juncture a pause of gap typically associated with phrases.

Intonation the pattern of fundamental frequency and sound duration in speech.

Intonational unit the combined pattern of f_0 and rhythm, typically for a multisyllabic sequence.

Intonation contour the pattern of pitch changes over an utterance; also called a pitch contour.

Inverted lip a curling back of the (usually lower) lip.

Isochrony literally, equal duration; as applied to speech, isochrony refers to the impression of equalized or uniform durations of rhythmic units such as pairs of strong and weak syllables.

Labialized a sound made with a constriction at the lips.

Labiodental a place of articulation involving the lower lip and upper teeth.

Lateral a manner of articulation in which sound escapes around the sides of the tongue.

Lateralized a sound made with a release of air or energy through one or both sides of the mouth.

Laryngeal system the system of speech production identified anatomically with the larynx and functionally with control of phonation and voicing.

Larynx the "voice box" of speech; a structure made up of cartilage, muscles, and other tissues located within the neck. The larynx is located on top of the trachea and below the pharynx and serves to valve the airstream from the lungs.

Lax vowel (or short vowel) a vowel that is relatively short in duration and is assumed to be produced with a relatively relaxed vocal tract musculature. The assumption of laxness (reduced muscular tension) is difficult to verify.

Lengthened a sound that is prolonged.

Lexical stress a stress pattern that is intrinsic to a word, such as the variation between noun and verb forms of a word such as *project,* which can carry primary stress on either the first or second syllable, depending on whether it is used as a noun (*PRO-ject*) or verb (*pro-JECT*).

Lexicon an inventory of the morphemes in a language.

Linear declination theory a theory that holds that vocal fundamental frequency falls gradually and linearly throughout a sentence or clause.

Lingua pertaining to the tongue.

Lingua-alveolar a place of articulation in which the tongue completely or nearly closes against the alveolar ridge.

Linguistic complexity the context in which a sound to be transcribed is embedded, which may range from a sound in isolation to a sound occurring in conversational speech.

Liquid a cover term (manner of articulation) for the rhotic /r/ and lateral /l/, both of which have a vocal tract that is constricted only somewhat more than that for vowels. Unlike glides, which are similar, liquids do not require a movement for their auditory identification.

Loudness the perceived magnitude or strength of sound.

Lowered a sound made with the tongue in a depressed position in the oral cavity.

Low vowel a vowel produced with the tongue in a low (inferior) position. Vowels /ɑ/ (*hot*) and /æ/ (*hat*) are low vowels.

Mandible the lower jaw, the bony structure that provides skeletal support for the tongue and lower lip.

Manner of articulation an aspect of articulatory phonetics pertaining to how a sound is formed, that is, the *means* of sound generation. Whereas place of articulation describes *where* in the vocal tract a sound is formed, manner of articulation describes how the sound is made.

Medial a middle position or segment in a word (i.e., not initial or final); the *b* is medial in the words *rubber, rebut,* and *toothbrush.*

Melody see *Prosody*

Minimal contrast a sound segment distinction by which two morphemes or words differ in pronunciation. Minimal contrasts are basic to the discovery of phonemes in a language.

Monophthong a pure vowel; that is, a vowel of essentially unchanging phonetic quality throughout its duration.

Monophthongization alteration of a diphthong to a pure vowel; that is, loss of the dynamic phonetic quality of a diphthong.

Mora-timed rhythm a form of speech rhythm having a relatively constant duration of syllable types.

Morph an individual morpheme-like shape in a language sample.

Morpheme the smallest unit of language that carries a semantic interpretation (meaning).

Morphemics the study of morphemes; a subfield of linguistics.

Morphemic transcription a written account of the morphemic content of a language sample.

Morphology that part of linguistics concerned with the study of morphemes, the meaning-bearing elements of a language.

Motherese (infant-directed speech, parentese) a style of speech that adults use when speaking to infants, typically characterized by a higher pitch, exaggerated intonation, and increased repetition of words or other units.

Mutually intelligible when one language or dialect can be understood by monolingual speakers of another language or dialect, those two languages or dialects are said to be mutually intelligible.

Narrow (close) transcription includes symbols to represent both the speech sounds produced and symbols that describe slight variations in the production of those sounds.

Nasal a manner of articulation in which sound energy radiates into the nasal cavity; nasal sounds are associated with an open velopharynx.

Nasal cavity the space between the nares (nostrils) and the entrance into the pharynx.

Nasal emission the sound of noise energy released through the nose.

Nasalized a sound produced with nasal resonance, usually accomplished by an open velopharyngeal port.

Nasalized vowel a vowel produced with nasal resonances, usually because of an open velopharynx.

Nasal radiation of sound transmission of sound through the nasal cavity (rather than through the oral cavity).

New vs. given information a contrast in the type of information expressed in a verbal message, with new information being unknown to the listener and given information being already known by the listener.

Nonstandard forms in sociolinguistics, this term refers to speech production patterns, word choices, and other linguistic structures that are different from the mainstream or standard form of the language. Many of the regional and social varieties described in Chapter 10 are nonstandard forms.

Northern Cities Chain Shift a vowel pronunciation pattern characteristic of a number of dialect regions, including the Inland North, the North, the St. Louis Corridor, and Western New England. It involves the lowering of the non-low front vowels, the retraction of front-central vowels, the raising of /æ/, and the fronting of low-central and low-back vowels.

Nucleus the vowel element in a syllable.

Obstruent a sound formed with a complete or narrow constriction of the vocal tract; a stop, fricative, or affricate.

Offglide the terminal vowel or vocal tract shape of a diphthong.

One-tap trill another name for *flap*.

Onglide the initial vowel or vocal tract shape of a diphthong.

Onset the beginning of a syllable; it may take the form of no consonant (null), one consonant, or a cluster of two or more consonants.

Open a syllable that does not end in a consonant.

Open juncture a short pause or gap that separates phone boundaries in ambiguous or confusable utterances.

Oral cavity the space between the lips and the entrance to the pharynx.

Oral radiation of sound transmission of sound through the oral cavity (rather than through the nasal cavity).

Palatal a place of articulation pertaining to the palatal area, which lies behind the alveolar ridge. Palatal sounds are made with articulations of the tongue against the palate.

Palatized a sound made with the blade of the tongue approximately or touching the palatal area just behind the alveolar ridge.

Paralanguage the various nonverbal properties of speech that convey information about a speaker's emotion, attitude, and demeanor.

Parentese see *Motherese*.

Pause an interval of silence in an utterance.

Perceptual bias a tendency to identify a stimulus, such as a speech sound, as being a member of a particular category. For examples, someone who has a perceptual bias to identify fricatives as /s/ would be more likely to identify productions intermediate between /s/ and /ʃ/ as /s/ than someone without such a bias would be.

Phrasal stress phrase patterns that apply to syntactic groupings of words, such as those that occur in phrases, clauses, or sentences.

Pharyngeal cavity the space between the division of the oral and pharyngeal cavities and the entrance to the larynx; its anterior boundary is the root of the tongue, and its posterior boundary is the pharyngeal wall.

Phone a particular occurrence of a speech sound segment.

Phoneme a basic speech segment that has the linguistic function of distinguishing morphemes (the minimal units of meaning in a language).

Phonetic transcription A visual representation of speech sounds, typically accomplished with the symbols of the International Phonetic Association (IPA). The main symbols represent individual phonemes or allophones, and transcriptions also may include marks for sound modifications, stress level, and other aspects of speech. Broad transcription pertains mainly to phonemes of a language, whereas narrow transcription includes finer variations including allophonic modifications.

Phonetics study of the perception and production of speech sounds.

Radiated acoustic energy the energy that passes from the lips or nose into the atmosphere.

Raised a sound made with the tongue in an elevated position in the oral cavity.

***r* colored** a sound that carries the phonetic quality of /r/, the rhotic consonant. This quality is best described acoustically, because the articulatory correlate is complex.

Received Pronunciation [RP] a variety of English spoken in the United Kingdom, which reflects and is based on the productions of educated, upper-class people.

Reduction of a vowel generally, a shortening or unstressing of a vowel, which may be accompanied by a change in vowel quality, usually in the direction of centralization.

Regional dialect a pattern of language usage that is shared by people living in a particular geographic region. A language may have several regional dialects.

Releasing another name for syllable-initial sounds; they release (begin) the syllable.

Resonator a physical object (including air-filled tubes such as the vocal tract) that has certain natural frequencies of vibration known as the resonance frequencies (or formants in the case of the vocal tract).

Respiratory system the part of the speech production mechanism consisting of the lungs, rib cage, abdomen, and associated muscles. The respiratory system provides the major airstream of speech.

Response complexity the number of target sounds to be transcribed, which may vary from only one sound to all sounds occurring in a section of speech.

Retracted a sound made with the tongue drawn backward in the oral cavity.

Retroflex literally "turned back"; this term is used to denote sounds that carry *r* coloring, such as the vowels in the words *bird* and *further*. However, "retroflex" is a misleading and inaccurate articulatory description and is best regarded as an arbitrary label. See *Rhotacization*.

Retroflex /r/ an allophone of the consonant /r/ for which the tongue tip is turned up to point toward the palate. Although *retroflex* literally means "turned back," the tongue tip rarely can be said to assume such a shape.

Retroflexion a turning back, for example, the backward curling of the tongue sometimes used to make rhotic (r-colored) sounds.

Rhotacization a property or process related to *r* coloring. A sound that has *r* coloring, or comes to have it because of contextual influences, is called rhotacized or rhotic. A physiologic definition is complex, so an acoustic definition is preferable.

Rhotacized a sound made with r-coloring.

Rhotic a manner of articulation pertaining to *r* coloring; the rhotic consonant /r/ has several allophones and a complex and variable articulation. The two major allophones, bunched and retroflex, involve vocal tract constrictions in two or three places: labial, palatal, and pharyngeal.

Rhyme the part of a syllable that consists of the *nucleus* and an optional *coda*; for example, in a CVC syllable the V and final C constitute the rhyme.

Rhythm the distribution of events in time, such as the temporal pattern of syllables or other speech units.

Root of tongue the part of the tongue that reaches downward from the dorsum of the tongue to the epiglottis and larynx.

Rounded a sound produced with rounding or protrusion of the lips.

Rounded vowel a vowel that is produced with rounding or protrusion of the lips; for example, vowels /u/ (*who*) and /ɝ/ (*her*). Actually, either protrusion or narrowing of the mouth opening may produce the desired acoustic effects.

Schwa vowel the ultimate reduced vowel /ə/, which is described as unstressed, lax or short, and mid-central. Schwa occupies the center of the vowel quadrilateral and can achieve the minimal duration for a vowel sound.

Secondary stress a level of stress that is intermediate between primary and tertiary stress.

Second-formant locus a characteristic frequency value of the second formant associated with a consonant sound or place of articulation.

Semivowel see *Glide*.

Sentence declination an overall fall in pitch over an utterance such as a sentence.

Shortened a sound that is abbreviated or brief.

Sibilant a speech sound characterized by an intense, high-pitched noise; for example, the fricatives /s/ (*see*) and /ʃ/ (*she*).

Sign language a system of communication that uses manual symbols, such as hand positions, postures, and movements to express language.

Social dialect variation in the form of language associated with speakers who identify as members of different social groups.

Soft palate the soft-tissue structure that articulates to open or close the velopharynx.

Sonority the auditory force of a speech sound.

Source-filter theory a theory of the acoustic production of speech that states that energy from a sound source (such as the vibrating vocal folds) is modified by the resonances (formants) of the vocal tract.

Spectrogram a pattern for sound analysis showing information on energy, frequency, and time.

Spectrum (plural spectra) a graph showing the distribution of signal energy as a function of frequency.

Speech a mode of language expression based on sounds emitted through the mouth and nose.

Speech community a group of people who live within the same geographic boundaries and use the same language.

Spondee a two-syllable word having equal stress on both syllables.

Standard Language/Standard Dialect in some countries, such as France, this term *refers to* an official, government-maintained language or dialect. In other countries, such as the United States, this refers to a language or dialect whose status as "standard" is maintained through its use in national media and in educational materials.

Stop a manner of articulation in which the vocal tract is completely closed for some interval, so that airflow ceases.

Stop burst a brief explosion of air that occurs when a stop closure is released and the impounded air escapes. Stop bursts usually are about 5 to 20 milliseconds in duration.

Stop consonant a consonant that is made with complete closure at some point in the vocal tract, so that airflow is temporarily interrupted and air pressure builds up behind the point of closure.

Stop gap the acoustic interval associated with the closure period of a stop consonant; it appears on a spectrogram as an interval of silence (although a low-frequency voice bar may be evident for a voiced stop).

Stress the degree of prominence or emphasis associated with a particular syllable.

Stress-timed rhythm a form of speech rhythm having relatively constant intervals between stressed syllables.

Strident a speech sound characterized by an intense frication noise, such as that heard for /s/ (*see*) and /ʃ/ (*she*). Sibilants and stridents are similar except that some phoneticians classify the nonsibilants /f/ (*five*) and /v/ (*vine*) as stridents.

Stylistic variation variation in the form of language that is associated with the demands of the speaking task and perceptions about the person or people being spoken to.

Substitution a speech production error in which a speech sound is replaced by another speech sound.

Supralaryngeal system the system of speech production consisting of the pharyngeal, oral, and nasal structures.

Suprasegmental a phonetic effect that extends over more than one segment in an utterance.

Syllabary a phonetic writing system that uses symbols to represent syllables rather than individual sounds.

Syllabification formation of a type of reduced syllable in which a consonant serves as the syllable nucleus.

Syllable-timed rhythm a form of speech rhythm having relatively constant syllable durations.

Tap another name for *flap*.

Target sound the sound to be transcribed, as it occurs in isolation or together with other speech sounds.

Tempo the rate of an activity, such as the rate of speaking.

Temporomandibular joint the hinge joint by which the jaw, or mandible, attaches to the temporal bone of the skull.

Tense vowel (or long vowel) a vowel that is relatively long in duration and is assumed to be produced with a relatively tense or active musculature of the vocal tract.

Terminal juncture (falling and rising) juncture at the end of an utterance such as a sentence, sentence fragment, or even a single word. Falling terminal juncture is associated with declarative statements, and rising terminal juncture with interrogatives. The words falling and rising pertain to the direction of pitch change at the end of the utterance.

Tertiary stress the lowest level of stress in an utterance.

Thoracic cavity the chest cavity, containing the lungs, heart, and other organs.

Tip of tongue the forwardmost portion of the tongue, visible upon protrusion of the tongue from the mouth. The tip of the tongue is used to produce a large number of sounds, including the *th* consonant in *though* and the *t* consonant in *two*.

Tone the smallest element of a tone unit, typically with one tone for individual syllables.

Tone unit the basic unit of intonation in which pitch movements and rhythm are assigned to structures such as words, clauses, and sentences.

Tongue advancement the vowel feature or dimension pertaining to the position of the tongue body along the anterior–posterior aspect. Advancement implies anterior or frontal position.

Tongue height the vowel feature or dimension pertaining to the position of the tongue body along the superior–inferior aspect.

Tonicity (tonic placement) the selection of one syllable to stand out against all of the others in a tone unit.

Trachea the "windpipe" that connects the lungs with the larynx, or "voice box."

Trill a pulmonic consonant made with a supraglottal vibration.

Trilled a sound made with rapid, repetitive movements of alternating opening and closing.

Two-way scoring a perceptual system in which speech sound productions are dichotomized into two classes representing typical versus atypical behavior (e.g., correct vs. incorrect, right vs. wrong, etc.).

Undershoot reduced amplitude of a movement, so that it falls short of its target.

Unrounded a sound produced without rounding or protrusion of the lips.

Unrounded vowel a vowel that is produced without rounding or protrusion of the lips; for example, /i/ (*he*) and /ɑ/ (*ha*) are unrounded.

Velar a place of articulation pertaining to the undersurface of the hard and soft palate. Velar consonants are made with articulations of the dorsum of the tongue against the velar surface. Velars are also known as dorsal sounds.

Velarized a sound made with constriction of the vocal tract between the dorsum of the tongue and the posterior palate, or velum.

Velopharyngeal port the opening between the oropharynx and the nasal cavity, which can be closed to prevent the nasal transmission of sound.

Velum the soft palate, especially its muscular portion; the velum articulates to open or close the velopharynx.

Vocal differentiator a vocal expression of emotion, such as laughing or crying.

Vocal effort the amount of physiologic energy that a speaker adjusts according to the distance between the speaker and a listener.

Vocal folds the paired cushions of muscle and other tissue that vibrate within the larynx to produce the sound of voicing.

Vocal identifier a sound that is not necessarily a word but can express meaning such as agreement or disagreement.

Vocal qualifier the tone of voice that conveys emotion or attitude.

Vocal quality a characteristic phonatory pattern, such as breathy, harsh, or hoarse.

Voice bar a band of energy located on the extreme low-frequency portion of a spectrogram that represents energy associated with the fundamental frequency of voice.

Voiced associated with vocal fold vibration. A sound is said to be voiced if the vocal folds vibrate during its production.

Voiced implosive also called voiced ingressive; a stop made with an ingressive glottalic airstream.

Voiceless not associated with vocal fold vibration. A sound is said to be voiceless if the vocal folds do not vibrate during its production.

Voice onset time (VOT) the interval between an oral articulatory event (often the release of a stop) and the onset of voicing. If onset of voicing precedes the articulatory event, the sound is said to be prevoiced or to have a voicing lead (negative value of VOT), and if onset voicing follows the articulatory event, the sound is said to have a voicing lag.

Vowel a speech sound that is formed without a significant constriction of the oral and pharyngeal cavities and that serves as a syllable nucleus.

Vowel merger a pronunciation pattern in which two vowels are pronounced similarly or identically. These can occur over time (as in the *cot-caught* merger, which occurs in dialects in which the vowels /ɑ/ and /ɔ/ have come to sound like one another over time), or in a particular phonetic context (as in the *pin-pen* merger, in which the vowels /ɪ/ and /ɛ/ are pronounced as /ɪ/ before nasal consonants, but not elsewhere).

Vowel quadrilateral or trapezoid a four-sided figure having the corner, or point, vowels /i u ɑ æ/ as its vertices. The quadrilateral diagram is useful for describing the tongue position for vowel articulation, as its two basic dimensions are high–low and front–back.

Waveform a graph of amplitude as a function of time.

Whistling a sound, usually a fricative, made with a sharply tuned noise resembling a whistle.

Answers to Exercises

Chapter 1: Overview of Clinical Phonetics

Linguistic Complexity	System Complexity	Response Complexity
1. word	two-way scoring	single sound
2. continuous speech	two-way scoring	multiple sounds
3. sentences	five-way scoring	single sound
4. continuous speech	phonetic transcription	multiple sounds
5. word	five-way scoring	multiple sounds

Chapter 2: Linguistic Phonetics

1.

	Number of Morphemes	Morphemic Analysis
(a)	3	light + en +ed
(b)	1	table
(c)	3	morph + em(e) + ic
(d)	3	re + cruit + ment
(e)	3	dis + mis + (s)ed
(f)	3	tele + vis(e) + ion
(g)	1	finger
(h)	3	sing + er + s
(i)	3	re + veal + ing
(j)	4	im + pos(e) + it + ion

2. Some possibilities are:

expose	oppose	repose	dispose
exposition	appose	pose	purpose
impose	compose	suppose	propose
imposition	depose	Can you think of any others?	

3.

	Number of Phonemes	Phonetic Transcription
(a)	4	/d ɔ t ɚ /
(b)	5	/l æ f t ɚ /
(c)	3	/f o͡ʊ n /
(d)	5	/k ʌ b ɚ d /
(e)	7	/s ɛ l o f e͡ɪ n /
(f)	3	/n i d /
(g)	6	/ʃ ɪ k ɔ g o /
(h)	5	/f ɪ ŋ g ɚ /
(i)	4	/s ɪ ŋ ɚ /
(j)	4	/s ɪ k s /

4. Real Words:

(a) grith (security, protection, or peace)
(b) scute (a bony plate)
(c) trave (a cross beam)
(d) skeg (naut., after part of keel)
(e) spile (a plug or spigot)
(f) knar (a knot in wood)

Note that the made-up words contain the following sequences: *fs, sr, kt, dl, shl, gv.* Can you think of any English words that start with these sound sequences?

Chapter 3: The Three Systems of Speech Production

1. See Figure 3.7 and Figure 3.13.
2. See text.
3. (a) p—lips
   (b) g—dorsum of tongue; s—tip of tongue
   (c) f—lower lip; m—lips
   (d) l—tip of tongue; k—dorsum of tongue
   (e) th—tip of tongue; ng—dorsum of tongue
   (f) ch—blade of tongue; s—tip of tongue
   (g) c—tip of tongue; ph—lower lip
   (h) b—lips; th—tip of tongue
4. Although the tongue is very important in speech articulation, there are several reports of persons who produce intelligible speech even after most of the tongue has been surgically removed (often because of cancer). Individuals sometimes compensate surprisingly well for damage to the articulators.

Chapter 4: Vowels and Diphthongs

1. See text, especially Figure 4.3.
2. (a) /u/, high-back
   (b) /ɔ/, low-mid-back
   (c) /ɛ/, low-mid-front
   (d) /ʊ/, high-mid-back
   (e) /i/, high-front
   (f) /ɑ/, low-back
   (g) /ʊ/, high-mid-back
   (h) /i/, high-front
   (i) /ɪ/, high-mid-front
   (j) /æ/, low-front
   (k) /ʊ/, high-mid-back
   (l) /o/, mid-back
   (m) /ɝ/, central
   (n) /ɪ/, high-mid-front
3. (a) /i/—/æ/: tongue moves down, mouth opening increases
   (b) /u/—/o/: tongue moves down, mouth opening increases
   (c) /i/—/o/: tongue moves back and down, lips round for /o/
   (d) /e͡ɪ/—/ɑ/: tongue moves back and down, mouth opening increases
   (e) /o/—/ɝ/: tongue moves forward
   (f) /i/—/æ/: tongue moves down, mouth opening increases
   (g) /u/—/ɑ/: tongue moves down, mouth opening increases, and lips go from rounded to unrounded
   (h) o—/ɛ/: tongue moves forward, lips go from rounded to unrounded
   (i) /e͡ɪ/—/ɑ/: tongue moves back and down, mouth opening increases
   (j) /o͡ʊ/—/i/: tongue moves forward and up, lips go from rounded to unrounded, and mouth opening may decrease
   (k) /i/—/ɪ/: tongue moves down, mouth opening may increase
   (l) o—/ɑ/: tongue moves down, lips go from rounded to unrounded
4. Vowels are early sounds to appear in a child's speech. Front vowels tend to predominate in an infant's early vowel usage. It has been suggested that an infant could produce a set of front vowels by holding the tongue near the front of the mouth and varying the amount of jaw opening. A closed jaw position would yield /i/ and an open jaw position would yield /æ/. (Note: The article a may be produced as either a front vowel [e] ([e͡ɪ]) or a central vowel [ə].)

5. (a) money — ʌ ɪ
   (b) fencepost — ɛ oʊ
   (e) suitcase — u eɪ
   (f) library — aɪ ɛ ɪ
   (g) overpower — oʊ ɚ aʊ ɚ
   (h) laundromat — ɔ (ə/o) æ
   (i) bookmark — ʊ ɑ
   (j) reinterpret — i ɪ ɝ ɛ
   (k) knowhow — oʊ aʊ
   (l) mustard — ʌ ɚ
   (m) merciless — ɝ ɪ ə
   (c) diplomat — ɪ (ə/o) æ
   (d) lamplighter — æ aɪ ɚ
   (n) boilerplate — ɔɪ ɚ eɪ
   (o) wanderlust — ɑ ɚ ʌ
   (p) rectify — ɛ ɪ aɪ
   (q) neologism — i ɑ ə ɪ
   (r) administrate — æ ɪ ɪ eɪ
   (s) luncheonette — ʌ ə ɛ
   (t) geometry — i ɑ ə ɪ
   (u) utensil — u ɛ (ə/ɪ)
   (v) misunderstood — ɪ ʌ ɚ ʊ

Chapter 5: Consonants

1. Figure 5.41 (*a*)
   (a) bilabial
   (b) labiodental
   (c) linguadental
   (d) lingua-alveolar
   (e) lingua-palatal
   (f) lingua-velar

   Figure 5.41 (*b*)
   (a) bilabial
   (b) dental
   (c) alveolar
   (d) palatal
   (e) velar

2 (a) cough
  (b) scissors
  (c) puff
  (d) manning
  (e) rabbit
  (f) valentine
  (g) thickest
  (h) writhing
  (i) phoneme
  (j) fifteen
  (k) bookmark
  (l) baseball
  (m) shuffle
  (n) fervor
  (o) snowman
  (p) ocean

3. (a) [fɪŋgɚ]
   (b) [tuθpeɪst]
   (c) correct
   (d) [ristwɔtʃ]
   (e) [kɝtnz]
   (f) correct
   (g) correct
   (h) [tɛləfoʊn]
   (i) correct
   (j) [θæŋksgɪvɪŋ]

4.

Stop	**Nasal**	**Fricative**	**Affricate**	**Liquid**	**Glide**
can	name	this	gin	red	wheel
keep	man	saw	choose	ring	wail
chorus	nose	zipper	job	lamb	wine
bed	knew	happy			yes
pot		phone			
		show			
		thigh			
		fate			

5. (a) [f θ s]
(b) [ʒ]
(c) [n d]
(d) [m p ʃ]
(e) [k t]
(f) [s k w]
(g) [n ʧ]
(h) [ʤ d]
(i) [m s]
(j) [ð]
(k) [k t]
(l) [ʃ]
(m) [s l̩]
(n) [s w]
(o) [n ʧ t]
(p) [s t]
(q) [k] or [k j]
(r) [s t r]
(s) [θ d r]
(t) [s t l]

6. (a) [g ɝ l]
(b) [m ɪ ʃ ə n]
(c) [b ɔ͡ɪ z]
(d) [w ɪ m ɪ n z]
(e) [s v ɛ l t]
(f) [k ə n s i v]
(g) [r ɛ p t ɪ l ɪ ə n]
(h) [d ɪ m o͡ʊ ə d] or [d ɪ m o͡ʊ t ə d]
(i) [ɛ n k r ɪ p ʃ ə n]
(j) [t r æ n s m ɪ ʃ ə n]

Chapter 6: Suprasegmentals and Narrow Transcription

1. (a) directly below the phonetic symbol, [x]
(b) over the phonetic symbol (above lip symbol, if any), [ẋ]
(c) under the phonetic symbol (below tongue symbol, if any), [x̣]
(d) to the upper right of the phonetic symbol, [x˙]
(e) to the right of the phonetic symbol, [x·]
(f) above the phonetic symbol (below velopharyngeal symbol, if any), [ẋ]

2. (a) [ĩ]
(b) [p˭]
(c) [ð̆]
(d) [ɑː]
(e) [ɛ̝]
(f) [ʊ̣]
(g) [t̬]
(h) [m̥]
(i) [ʃ̜]
(j) [z̪]

3. (a) [æ̃ː]
(b) [d̥˺]
(c) [s̪ː]
(d) [ɪ̝]
(e) [ũ]
(f) [l̥̃]
(g) [ʧ̜]
(h) [t̽ʰ]

4. (a) [t r æ[2] n s k r aɪ[1] b]
   (b) [s æ[1] ɾ ɪ[3] s f aɪ[2]] (or 2-3-1 stress)
   (c) [l ɛ[1] ʤ ɪ[2] s l eɪ[2] tʃ ɚ[3]]
   (d) [f ɝ[1] n ɪ[3] tʃ ɚ[3]]
   (e) [ɛ[2] r ɪ[3] z oʊ[1] n ə[3]] (sometimes 1-3-2-3)
   (f) [ʃ ɪ[3] k ɔ[1] g o[2]]
   (g) [oʊ[1] v ɚ[3] l oʊ[2] d] (or 2-3-1)
   (h) [s k aɪ[1] s k r eɪ[2] p ɚ[3]]
   (i) [t aɪ[1] p r aɪ[2] ɾ ɚ[3]]
   (j) [l ɪ[2] θ u[2] eɪ[1] n ɪ[3] ə[3]]
   (k) [m æ[1] s t ɚ[3] p i[2] s] (sometimes 2-3-1)
   (l) [m ɪ[2] s ɪ[3] s ɪ[1] p ɪ[3]]

5 (a) [e] has schwa [ə] offglide; checked or held terminal juncture
  (b) [aɪ] is nasalized; rising terminal juncture
  (c) [ɛ] is produced with breathy voice; [o] is nasalized
  (d) [l] is devoiced; [i] is lengthened; checked or held juncture
  (e) numbers represent stress pattern: 1 = highest stress, 2 = less stress, 3 = least stress
  (f) [ʊ] is lowered, [ɔ] is nasalized; [ɪ] is centralized and nasalized
  (g) [oʊ] is lengthened, [æ] has an [ɪ] offglide; [t] is unreleased

References

(see also Appendix A)

American Speech-Language-Hearing Association. (1983). *Social dialects [Position Statement]*. Available from www.asha.org/policy.

Baker, A., Mielke, J., & Archangeli, D. (2006). *Probing the big bang with ultrasound: /s/ retraction in English*. Presentation at the Annual Meeting of the Linguistic Society of America, Albuquerque, NM. Downloaded on April 1, 2011 from dingo.sbs.arizona.edu/~apilab/research/publications/Probing%2520the%2520Big%2520Bang%2520with%2520ultrasound.ppt.

Ball, M. J. (1988). The transcription of phonation types. *Clinical Linguistics and Phonetics, 2*, 253–256.

Ball, M. J. (2008). Transcribing disordered speech: By target or by production? *Clinical Linguistics and Phonetics, 22*, 864–870.

Bankson, N. W., Bernthal, J. E., & Flipsen, P. (2008). *Articulation and phonological disorders* (6th ed.). Boston: Allyn & Bacon.

Beckman, M. E., & Edwards, J. (1990). Lengthenings and shortenings and the nature of prosodic constituency. In J. Kingston & M. E. Beckman (Eds.), *Between the grammar and physics of speech* (pp. 152–214). Cambridge, England: Cambridge University Press.

Behne, D. (1989). *Acoustic effects of focus and sentence position on stress in English and French*. Ph.D. dissertation, University of Wisconsin, Madison.

Benguerel, A.-P., & Cowan, H. (1974). Coarticulation of upper lip protrusion in French. *Phonetica, 30*, 41–55.

Bernthal, J. E., & Bankson, N. W. (1993). *Articulation and phonological disorders* (3rd ed.). Englewood Cliffs, NJ: Prentice-Hall.

Bloomfield, L. ([1933] 1984). *Language*. New York: Holt, Rinehart & Winston. Reprint. Chicago: University of Chicago Press.

Bonnot, J.-F. P., & Chevrie-Muller, C. (1991). Some effects of shouted and whispered conditions on temporal organization. *Journal of Phonetics, 19*, 473–483.

Bow, C., Blamey, P., Paatsch, L., & Sarant, J. (2002). Comparison of methods in speech acquisition research. *Clinical Linguistics and Phonetics, 16*, 135–147.

Boyce, S., & Espy-Wilson, C. Y. 1997. Coarticulatory stability in American English /r/. *Journal of the Acoustical Society of America, 101*, 3741–3753.

Brewster, K. (1989). Assessment of prosody. In K. Grundy (Ed.), *Linguistics in clinical practice* (pp. 168–185). London: Taylor and Francis.

Bunta, F., Ingram, K., & Ingram, D. (2003). Bridging the digital divide: Aspects of computerized data collection and analysis for language professionals. *Clinical Linguistics and Phonetics, 17*, 217–240.

Bunton, K., Kent, R. D., Kent, J. F., & Rosenbek, J. C. (2000). Perceptuo-acoustic assessment of prosodic impairment in dysarthria. *Clinical Linguistics and Phonetics*, 14, 13–24.

Byrd, D. (1996). Influences on articulatory timing in consonant sequences. *Journal of Phonetics, 24*, 209–244.

Byrd, D., & Saltzman, E. (1998). Intragestural dynamics of multiple prosodic boundaries. *Journal of Phonetics, 26*, 173–199.

Calvert, D. (1980). *Descriptive phonetics*. New York: Thieme-Stratton.

Campbell, F., Gick, B., Wilson, I., & Vatidiotis-Bateson, E. (2010). Spatial and temporal properties of gestures in North American English /r/. *Language & Speech, 53*, 49–69.

Campbell, T. F., & Dollaghan, C. A. 1995. Phonological and speech production characteristics of children following traumatic brain injury: Principles underlying assessment and treatment. In J. Bernthal & W. Bankson (Eds.), *Phonological characteristics of special populations*. New York: Thieme Medical Publishers.

Catford, J. 1968. The articulatory possibilities of man. In B. Malmberg (Ed.), *Manual of Phonetics*. Amsterdam: North-Holland.

Chaney, C. 1988. Acoustic analysis of correct and misarticulated semivowels. *Journal of Speech and Hearing Research 31:* 275–87.

Chen, M. 1970. Vowel length variation as a function of the variety of the consonant environment. *Phonetica, 22*, 129–159.

Chomsky, N., & Halle, M. 1968. *The sound pattern of English*. New York: Harper & Row.

Christman, S. S. 1992. Abstruse neologism formation: Parallel processing revisited. *Clinical Linguistics and Phonetics, 6*, 65–76.

Clements, G. N. 1990. The role of the sonority cycle in core syllabification. In J. Kingston & M. Beckman (Eds.), *Papers in laboratory phonology 1: Between the grammar and the physics of speech*. Cambridge, England: Cambridge University Press.

Clopper, C. G., Pisoni, D. B., & de Jong, K. (2005). Acoustic characteristics of the vowel systems of six regional varieties of American English. *Journal of the Acoustical Society of America, 118*, 1661–1676.

Costely, M., & Broen, P. (1976, November). *The nature of listener disagreement in judging misarticulated speech*. Paper presented at the American Speech and Hearing Association National Convention, Houston.

Craig, H., & Washington, J. (2005). *Malik goes to school: Examining the language skills of African American students from preschool-5th grade*. Mahwah, NJ: Lawrence Erlbaum.

Crystal, D. 1982. *Profiling linguistic disability*. London: Whurr Publishers.

De Jong, K. J. (1991). *The oral articulation of English stress accent*. Doctoral dissertation, Ohio State University.

Delattre, P., & Freeman, D. (1968). A dialect study of American *r*'s by X-ray motion picture. *Linguistics, 44*, 29–68.

Denes, P. (1955). The effect of duration on the perception of voicing. *Journal of the Acoustical Society of America, 27*, 761–64.

Denes, P., & Pinson, E. (1973; 1963). *The speech chain.* Garden City, New York: Anchor Press (1973) and Bell Telephone Laboratories, Inc. (1963).

De Pijper, J. R., & Sanderman, A. A. (1994). On the perceptual strength of prosodic boundaries and its relation to suprasegmental cues. *Journal of the Acoustical Society of America, 96,* 2037–2047.

Dewey, G. (1923). *Relative frequency of English speech sounds.* Cambridge, MA: Harvard University Press.

Diedrich, W., & Bangert, J. (1981). *Articulation learning.* Houston: College-Hill Press.

Dilley, L., Shattuck-Hufnagel, S., & Ostendorf, M. (1996). Glottalization of word-initial vowels as a function of prosodic structure. *Journal of Phonetics, 24,* 423–444.

Dodsworth, R. (2005). *Linguistic variation and sociological consciousness.* Ph.D. dissertation, Department of Linguistics. Columbus, OH: Ohio State University. Downloaded on April 1, 2011 from http://linguistics.osu.edu/files/linguistics/dissertations/dodsworth2005.pdf.

Doherty, C., Fitzsimons, M., Asenbauer, B., & Staunton, H. (2007). Discrimination of prosody and music by normal children. *European Journal of Neurology, 6,* 221–226.

Drager, K. (2008). *Language, stance, and identity at Selwyn Girls' High.* Paper presented at the 5th International Gender and Language Association Conference. Wellington, July 2008. Downloaded on April 1, 2011 from http://www.katiedrager.com/papers/Drager_IGALA.pdf.

Drager, K. (2011). Speaker age and vowel perception. *Language and Speech, 54,* 99–121.

DuBois, E., & Bernthal, J. 1978. A comparison of three methods for obtaining articulatory responses. *Journal of Speech and Hearing Disorders, 43,* 295–305.

Duckworth, M., Allen, G., Hardcastle, W., & Ball, M. (1990). Extensions to the International Phonetic Alphabet for the transcription of atypical speech. *Clinical Linguistics and Phonetics, 4,* 273–280.

Edwards, J., & Beckman, M. E. (1988). Articulatory timing and the prosodic interpretation of syllable duration. *Phonetica, 45,* 156–174.

Fonagy, I., & Fonagy, J. 1966. Sound pressure level and duration. *Phonetica, 15,* 14–21.

Fougeron, C., & Keating, P. A. (1997). Articulatory strengthening at edges of prosodic domains. *Journal of the Acoustical Society of America, 101,* 3728–3740.

Fowler, C. A., & Brancazio, L. 2000. Coarticulation resistance of American English consonants and its effects on transconsonantal vowel-to-vowel coarticulation. *Language and Speech, 43,* 1–41.

French, P., & Local, J. 1986. Prosodic features and the management of interruptions. In C. Johns-Lewis (Ed.), *Intonation in Discourse* (pp. 157–180). London: Croon Helm.

Fry, D. (1955). Duration and intensity as physical correlates of linguistic stress. *Journal of the Acoustical Society of America, 27,* 765–768.

Fry, D. B. (1958). Experiments in the perception of stress. *Language and Speech, 1,* 126–152.

Fudge, E. C. (1969). Syllables. *Journal of Linguistics, 5,* 193–320.

Gargesh, R. (2008). Indian English: Phonology. In R. Mesthrie (Ed.), *Varieties of English: Africa, South and Southeast Asia* (pp. 231–243). Berlin: Mouton de Gruyter.

Gerken, L., & McGregor, K. (1998). An overview of prosody and its role in normal and disordered child language. *American Journal of Speech-Language Pathology, 7,* 38–48.

Giles, S. B. (1971). *A study of articulatory characteristics of /l/ allophones in English.* Ph.D. dissertation, University of Iowa.

Goldsmith, J. A. (1990). *Autosegmental and metrical phonology.* Oxford, England: Basil Blackwell.

Gordon, M. (2000). Phonological correlates of ethnic identity: Evidence of divergence? *American Speech, 75,* 115–136.

Guirao, M., & Jurado, M. A. G. (1990). Frequency of occurrence of phonemes in American Spanish. *Revue Québécoise de Linguistique, 19,* 135–149.

Green, L. (2002). *African American English: A linguistic introduction.* Cambridge, England: Cambridge University Press.

Hall-Lew, L. Coppock, E., & Starr, R. (2010). Indexing political persuasion: Variation in the *Iraq* vowels. *American Speech, 85,* 91–102.

Hejna, R. (1955). *Hejna developmental articulation test.* Madison: Wisconsin College of Typing.

Hillenbrand, J.M., Getty, L.A., Clark, M.J., & Wheeler, K. (1995). Acoustic characteristics of American English vowels. *Journal of the Acoustical Society of America, 97,* 3099–3111.

Hinton, L., & Pollock, K. (2000). Regional variations in the phonological characteristics of African-American Vernacular English. *World Englishes, 19,* 59–71.

Hooper, J. B. (1972). The syllable in linguistic theory. *Language, 48,* 525–540.

Huber, J. E., Stathopoulos, E. T., Curione, G. M., Ash, T. A., & Johnson, K. (1999). Formants of children, women, and men: The effects of vocal intensity variation. *Journal of the Acoustical Society of America, 106,* 1532–1542.

Hyman, L. (1975). *Phonology: Theory and analysis.* New York: Holt, Rinehart & Winston.

Ingram, D. (1989). *Phonological disability in children* (2nd ed.). San Diego: Singular Publishing Group.

Ingle, J. K., Wright, R. A., & Wassink, A. B. (2005). *Pacific Northwest vowels: A Seattle Neighborhood dialect study.* Poster presented at the annual meeting of the Acoustical Society of America, Vancouver, BC. See also *Journal of the Acoustical Society of America, 117,* 2459.

Irwin, J., Weston, A., Griffith, F., & Rocconi, C. (1976). Phoneme acquisition using the paired-stimuli technique in the public school setting. *Language, Speech and Hearing Services in Schools, 7,* 220–229.

Jacewicz, E., Fox, R. A., & Salmons, J. (2007). Vowel duration in three American English dialects. *American Speech, 82,* 367–385.

Jacewicz, E., Fox, R., & Salmons, J. (2011). Regional dialectal variation in the vowel systems of typically developing children. *Journal of Speech, Language, and Hearing Research, 54,* 448–470.

Jones, D. (1917). *An English pronouncing dictionary.* London: Dent.

Junqua, J.-C. (1993). The Lombard reflex and its role on human listeners and automatic speech recognizers. *Journal of the Acoustical Society of America, 93,* 510–524.

Kahn, D. 1980. *Syllable-based generalizations in English phonology.* Doctoral dissertation, Massachusetts Institute of Technology. New York: Garland Press.

Kantner, C., & West, R. (1941). *Phonetics.* New York: Harper & Row.

Keating, P. (1983). Comments on the jaw and syllable structure. *Journal of Phonetics, 11,* 401–406.

Keating, P. A. (1990). The window model of coarticulation: Articulatory evidence. In J. Kingston & M. E. Beckman (Eds.), *Papers in laboratory phonology I. Between the grammar and physics of speech* (pp. 451–470). Cambridge, England: Cambridge University Press.

Kent, R. (1976). Anatomical and neuromuscular maturation of the speech mechanism: Evidence from acoustic studies. *Journal of Speech and Hearing Research, 19,* 421–447.

Kent, R., & Moll, K. (1972). Cinefluorographic analyses of selected lingual consonants. *Journal of Speech and Hearing Research, 15,* 453–473.

Kent, R. D. (1970). *A cinefluorographic investigation of the component gestures in lingual articulation.* Unpublished doctoral dissertation, University of Iowa, Iowa City, IA.

Kent, R. D. (1982). Contextual facilitation of correct sound production. *Language, Speech, and Hearing Services in Schools, 13,* 66–76.

Kent R. D., Mitchell, P. R., & Sancier, M. (1991). Evidence and role of rhythmic organization in early vocal development in human infants. In J. Fagard & P. Wolff (Eds.), *The development of timing control and temporal organization in coordinated action* (pp. 135–149). Amsterdam: Elsevier.

Kent, R. D., & Netsell, R. (1971). Effects of stress contrasts on certain articulatory parameters. *Phonetica, 24,* 23–44.

Kent, R. D., Pagan, L., Hustad, K. C., & Wertzner, H. F. (2009). Children's speech sound disorders: An acoustic perspective. In R. Paul & P. Flipsen (Eds.), *Child speech sound disorders: Essays in honor of Lawrence D. Shriberg* (pp. 93–114). San Diego: Plural Publishing.

Kent, R. D., & Read, W. C. (2002). *The acoustic analysis of speech,* Albany, NY: Singular/Thomson Learning.

Kenyon, J., & Knott, T. (1953). *A pronouncing dictionary of American English.* Springfield, MA: Merriam.

Kerek, A. (1976). The phonological relevance of spelling pronunciation. *Visible Language, 10,* 323–338.

Klatt, D. (1968). Structure of confusions in short-term memory between English consonants. *Journal of the Acoustical Society of America, 44,* 401–407.

Klatt, D. (1976). Linguistic uses of segmental duration in English: Acoustic and perceptual evidence. *Journal of the Acoustical Society of America, 59,* 1208–1221.

Klatt, D. H. (1975). Vowel lengthening is syntactically determined in a connected discourse. *Journal of Phonetics, 3,* 129–140.

Knight, R.-A. (2010). Transcribing nonsense words: The effect of numbers of voices and repetitions. *Clinical Linguistics and Phonetics, 24,* 473–484.

Ko, E.-S. (2007): Acquisition of vowel duration in children speaking American English. In *INTERSPEECH-2007,* 1881–1884.

Kohnert, K. (2007). *Language disorders in bilingual children and adults.* San Diego, CA: Plural Publishing.

Labov, W. (2001). *Principles of linguistic change, social factors (Volume II).* Malden, MA: Wiley-Blackwell.

Labov, W., Ash, S., & Boberg, C. (2006). *The atlas of North American English.* Berlin: Mouton de Gruyter.

Labov, W. Cohen, P., Robins, C., & Lewis, J. (1968). *A study of the non-standard English of Negro and Puerto Rican speakers in New York City. Volume I: Phonological and grammatical analysis.* Cooperative Research Report 3288. Philadelphia: U.S. Regional Survey.

Ladefoged, P. (1971). *Preliminaries to linguistic phonetics.* Chicago: University of Chicago Press.

Ladefoged, P. (1975). *A course in phonetics.* New York: Harcourt Brace Jovanovich.

Ladefoged, P. (1993). *A course in phonetics* (3rd ed.). Fort Worth: Harcourt Brace Jovanovich.

Ladefoged, P., DeClerk, J., Lindau, M., & Papcun, G. (1972). An auditory-motor theory of speech production. *UCLA Working Papers in Phonetics,* No. 22, 48–75. Department of Linguistics, UCLA.

Lakoff, R. (2000). *The language war.* Berkeley: University of California Press.

Landahl, K. H. (1980). Language-universal aspects of intonation to children's first sentences. *Journal of the Acoustical Society of America 67,* Suppl. 1, S63.

Lawrence, W. (2000). /str/->/str:/ assimilation at a distance? *American Speech, 75,* 82–87.

Levelt, W. J. M., Roelofs, A., & Meyer, A. S. (1999). A theory of lexical access in speech production. *Behavioral and Brain Sciences, 22,* 1–75.

Lieberman, P. (1967). *Intonation, perception, and language.* Cambridge, MA: M.I.T. Press.

Lieberman, P., Katz, W., Jongman, A., Zimmerman, R., & Miller, M. (1985). Measures of the sentence intonation of read and spontaneous speech in American English. *Journal of the Acoustical Society of America, 77,* 649–657.

Lieberman, P., & Tseng, C. Y. 1981. On the fall of the declination theory: Breath-group versus "declination" as the base form for intonation. *Journal of the Acoustical Society of America,* Suppl. *67,* S63.

Lienard, J. S., & Di Benedetto, M. G. (1999). Effect of vocal effort on spectral properties of vowels. *Journal of the Acoustical Society of America, 106,* 411–422.

Lindblom, B., & Sundberg, B. (1969). A quantitative model of vowel production and the distinctive features of Swedish vowels. *Quarterly Progress and Status Report,* No. 1, 14–32. Speech Transmission Laboratory, Royal Institute of Technology, Stockholm.

Mackay, I. (1978). *Introducing practical phonetics.* Boston: Little, Brown.

Maddieson, I. (1984). *Patterns of sounds.* Cambridge, England: Cambridge University Press.

Maddieson, I., & Precoda, K. (1990). Updating UPSID. *UCLA Working Papers in Phonetics, 74,* 104–111.

Maeda, S. (1976). *A characterization of American English intonation.* Cambridge, MA: M.I.T. Press.

Malmberg, B. (1963). *Phonetics.* New York: Dover.

McDonald, E. (1964). *Articulation testing and treatment: A sensory-motor approach.* Pittsburgh: Stanwix House.

McDonald, E. (1968). *A screening deep test of articulation.* Pittsburgh: Stanwix House.

McSweeny, J. L., & Shriberg, L. D. (2001). Clinical research with the prosody-voice screening profile. *Clinical Linguistics and Phonetics, 15,* 505–528.

Mendoza-Denton, N. (2008). *Homegirls: Language and cultural practice among Latina youth gangs.* Malden, MA: Wiley-Blackwell.

Mines, M., Hanson, B., & Shoup, J. (1978). Frequency of occurrence of phonemes in conversational English. *Language and Speech, 21,* 221–241.

Mitchell, P. (1988). *Phonetic variation and final syllable lengthening in multisyllable babbling*. Doctoral dissertation, University of Wisconsin, Madison.

Moll, K. L., & Daniloff, R. G. (1971). Investigation of the timing of velar movements during speech. *Journal of the Acoustical Society of America, 50,* 678–684.

Morrison, J. A., & Shriberg, L. D. (1992). Articulation testing versus conversational speech sampling. *Journal of Speech and Hearing Research, 35,* 259–273.

Mowrer, D., Baker, R., & Schutz, R. (1970). *Modification of the frontal lisp: Programmed articulation control kit.* Palos Verdes Estates, CA: Educational Psychological Research Associates.

Munson, B. (2009). *Gender biases in fricative identification revisited.* Oral presentation at the annual meeting of the Linguistic Society of America, San Francisco, CA. Downloaded on April 1, 2011 from http://www.tc.umn.edu/~munso005/LSA2009_Munson.pdf

Munson, B., Edwards, J., Schellinger, S.K., Beckman, M.E., & Meyer, M.K. (2010). Deconstructing phonetic transcription: Covert contrast, perceptual bias, and an extraterrestrial view of Vox Humana. *Clinical Linguistics and Phonetics, 24,* 245-260.

Nearey, T. (1978). *Phonetic feature systems for vowels.* Ph.D. dissertation, University of Connecticut, 1977. Reproduced by Indiana University Linguistics Club.

Niedzielski, N. (1999). The effect of social information on the perception of sociolinguistic variables. *Journal of Social Psychology, 18,* 62–85.

Ogilvie, M., & Rees, N. (1969). *Communication skills: Voice and pronunciation.* New York: McGraw-Hill.

Oller, D., & Eilers, R. (1975). Phonetic expectation and transcription validity. *Phonetica 31:* 288–304.

Orwin, M. (1990). *Aspects of Somali phonology.* Dissertation, Department of Linguistics, University of London.

Otomo, K., & Stoel-Gammon, C. (1992). The acquisition of unrounded vowels in English. *Journal of Speech and Hearing Research, 35,* 604–616.

Paynter, E., Ermey, J., Green, J., & Draper, D. (1978, November). *Articulation development of English consonants in Mexican-American children.* Paper presented at the American Speech and Hearing Association National Convention, San Francisco.

Peppé, S. J. E. (2009). Why is prosody in speech-language pathology so difficult? *International Journal of Speech-Language Pathology, 11,* 258–271.

Peppé, S., & McCann, J. (2003). Assessing intonation and prosody in children with atypical language development: The PEPS-C test and the revised version. *Clinical Linguistics and Phonetics, 17,* 345–354.

Peppé, S., McCann, J., Gibbon, G., & Rutherford, M. (2007). Receptive and expressive prosodic ability in children with high-functioning autism. *Journal of Speech, Language and Hearing Research, 50,* 1015–1028.

Peterson, G. E., & Barney, H. L. (1952). Control methods used in a study of the vowels. *Journal of the Acoustical Society of America, 24,* 175–184.

Perkell, J. (1969). *Physiology of speech sound production: Results and implications of a quantitative cineradiographic study.* Cambridge, MA: M.I.T. Press.

Perkell, J. (1971). Physiology of speech production: A preliminary study of two suggested revisions of the features specifying vowels. *Quarterly Progress Report,* No. 102. Cambridge, MA: M.I.T. Research Laboratory of Electronics.

Pike, K. (1943). *Phonetics.* Ann Arbor: University of Michigan Press.

Plichta, B., & Preston, D. (2005). The /ay/s have it: The perception of /ay/ as a north-south stereotype in United States English. *Acta Linguistica, 37,* 107–130.

Pollock, K. E. (1991). The identification of vowel errors using traditional articulation or phonological process test stimuli. *Language, Speech, and Hearing Services in Schools, 22,* 39–50.

Pollock, K. E., & Keiser, N. J. (1990). An examination of vowel errors in phonologically disordered children. *Clinical Linguistics and Phonetics, 4,* 161–178.

Preston, D. (1989). *Perceptual dialectology: Nonlinguists' view of areal features.* Providence, RI: Foris.

Price, P. J. (1980). Sonority and syllabicity: Acoustic correlates of perception. *Phonetica, 37,* 327–343.

Proctor, M. I. Shadle, C. H., & Iskarous, K. (2010). Pharyngeal articulation in the production of voiced and voiceless fricatives. *Journal of the Acoustical Society of America, 127,* 1507–1518.

Purnell, T., Idsardi, W., & Baugh, J. (1999). Perceptual and phonetic experiments on American English Dialect identification. *Journal of Language and Social Psychology, 18,* 10–30.

Ramig, L. 1975. *Examiner bias in perceptual ratings of nasality in cleft palate speakers.* Masters thesis, University of Wisconsin–Madison.

Ramsdell, H. L., Oller, D. K., & Ethington, C. A. (2007). Predicting phonetic transcription agreement: insights from research in infant vocalizations. *Clinical Linguistics and Phonetics, 21,* 793–831.

Raphael, L., & Bell-Berti, F. (1975). Tongue musculature and the feature of tension in English vowels. *Phonetica 32:* 61–63.

Recasens, D. (1985). Coarticulatory patterns and degrees of coarticulatory resistance in Catalan CV sequences. *Language and Speech, 28,* 97–114.

Recasens, D., Pallares, M. D., & Fontdevila, J. (1997). A model of lingual coarticulation based on articulatory constraints. *Journal of the Acoustical Society of America, 102,* 544–561.

Renfrew, C. (1966). Persistence of the open syllable in defective articulation. *Journal of Speech and Hearing Disorders 31,* 370–373.

Reuvers, M., & Hargrove, P. M. (1994). A profile of speech-language pathologists' prosody during language therapy. *Child Language Teaching and Therapy, 10,* 139–152.

Rickford, J. (1999). *African American Vernacular English: Features, evolution, educational implications.* Malden, MA: Wiley-Blackwell.

Rostolland, D. (1982). Acoustic features of shouted voice. *Acustica, 51,* 80–89.

Russell, G. (1928). *The vowel.* Columbus: Ohio State University Press.

Santa Ana, O., & Bayley, R., (2004). Chicano English phonology. In E. W. Schneider, B. Kortmann, K. Burridge, R. Mesthrie, & C. Upton (Eds.), *A handbook of varieties of English: Phonology* (V. 1, pp. 407–424). Berlin: Mouton de Gruyter.

Sapir, E. (1921). *Language: An introduction to the study of speech.* New York: Harcourt Brace Jovanovich.

Schulman, R. (1989). Articulatory dynamics of loud and normal speech. *Journal of the Acoustical Society of America, 85,* 295–312.

Schwartz, J. L., Boe, L. J., Vallee, N., & Abry, C. (1997). Major trends in vowel system inventories. *Journal of Phonetics, 25,* 233–253.

Shriberg, L. (1972). Articulation judgments. Some perceptual considerations. *Journal of Speech and Hearing Research, 15,* 876–882.

Shriberg, L. (1975). A response evocation program for /ɝ/. *Journal of Speech and Hearing Disorders, 40,* 92–105.

Shriberg, L. D. (1980). An intervention procedure for children with persistent /r/ errors. *Language, Speech, and Hearing Services in Schools, 11,* 102–110.

Shriberg, L. D. (1993). Four new speech and prosody-voice measures for genetics research and other studies in developmental phonological disorders. *Journal of Speech and Hearing Research, 36,* 105–140.

Shriberg, L. D., Allen, C. T., McSweeny, J. L., & Wilson, D. L. (2001). PEPPER: Programs to examine phonetic and phonologic evaluation records [Computer software]. Madison, WI: Waisman Center, University of Wisconsin.

Shriberg, L. D., Ballard, K. J., Tomblin, J. B., Duffy, J. R., Odell, K. H., & Williams, C. A. (2006). Speech, prosody, and voice characteristics of a mother and daughter with a 7;13 translocation affecting FOXP2. *Journal of Speech, Language, and Hearing Research, 49,* 500–525.

Shriberg, L. D., Fourakis, M., Hall, Karlsson, H. K., Lohmeier, H. L. McSweeny, J., Potter, N. L., et al. (2010a). Extensions to the Speech Disorders Classification system (SDCS). *Clinical Linguistics and Phonetics, 24,* 795–824.

Shriberg, L. D., Fourakis, M., Hall, S., Karlsson, H. K., Lohmeier, H. L, McSweeny, J., Potter, N. L., Scheer-Cohen, A. R., Strand, E. A., Tilkens, C. M., & Wilson, D. L. (2010b). Perceptual and acoustic reliability estimates for the Speech Disorders Classification System (SDCS). *Clinical Linguistics and Phonetics, 24,* 825–846.

Shriberg, L. D., Hinke, R., & Trost-Steffen, C. (1987). A procedure to select and train persons for narrow phonetic transcription by consensus. *Clinical Linguistics and Phonetics, 1,* 171–189.

Shriberg, L. D., Jakielski, K. J., & El-Shanti, H. (2008). Breakpoint localization using array-CGH in three siblings with an unbalanced 4q:16q translocation and childhood apraxia of speech (CAS). *American Journal of Medical Genetics: Part A, 146A,* 2227–2233.

Shriberg, L., & Kwiatkowski, J. (1980). *Natural process analyses (NPA): A procedure for phonological analyses of continuous speech samples.* New York: John Wiley.

Shriberg, L. D., & Kwiatkowski, J. (1985). Continuous speech sampling for phonologic analyses of speech-delayed children. *Journal of Speech and Hearing Disorders, 50,* 323–334.

Shriberg, L. D., & Kwiatkowski, J. (1994). Developmental phonological disorders. I.: A clinical profile. *Journal of Speech and Hearing Research, 37,* 1100–1126.

Shriberg, L. D., Kwiatkowski, J., & Rassmussen, C. (1990). *Prosody-voice screening profile (PVSP).* Tucson, AZ: Communication Skill Builders.

Shriberg, L. D., McSweeny, J. L., Anderson, B. E., Campbell, T. F., Chial, M. R., Green, J. R., Hauner, K. K., Moore, C. A., Rusiewicz, H. L., & Wilson, D. L. (2005). Transitioning from analog to digital audio recording in childhood speech sound disorders. *Clinical Linguistics and Phonetics, 19,* 335–359.

Shriberg, L. D., Paul, R., McSweeny, J. L., Klin, A., Volkmar, F. R., & Cohen, D. J. (2001). Speech and prosody characteristics of adolescents and adults with high functioning autism and Asperger syndrome. *Journal of Speech, Language, and Hearing Research, 44,* 1097–1115.

Shriberg, L. D., Paul, R., Black, L. M., & van Santen, J. P. (2011). The hypothesis of apraxia of speech in children with Autism Spectrum Disorder. *Journal of Autism and Developmental Disorders, 41,* 405–426.

Shriberg, L. D., Potter, N. L., & Strand, E. A. (2011). Prevalence and phenotype of childhood apraxia of speech in youth with galactosemia. *Journal of Speech, Language, and Hearing Research, 54,* 487–519.

Shriberg, L., & Swisher, W. (1972, November). *Development of an articulation scoring training program (ASTP).* Paper presented at the American Speech and Hearing Association National Convention, San Francisco.

Shriberg, L. D., & Widder, C. J. (1990). Speech and prosody characteristics of adults with mental retardation. *Journal of Speech and Hearing Research, 33,* 627–653.

Silverman, K., & Pierrehumbert, J. B. (1990). The timing of prenuclear high accents in English. In J. Kingston & M. E. Beckman (Eds.), *Papers in laboratory phonology I: Between the grammar and the physics of speech.* Cambridge, England: Cambridge University Press.

Smit, A. B., & Bernthal, J. E. (1983). Voicing contrasts and their phonological implications in the speech of articulation-disordered children. *Journal of Speech and Hearing Research, 26,* 486–500.

Sorensen, J. M., & Cooper, W. E. (1980). Syntactic coding of fundamental frequency in speech production. In R. A. Cole (Ed.), *Perception and production of fluent speech* (pp. 399–440). Hillsdale, NJ: Lawrence Erlbaum.

Staum Casasanto, L. 2008. *Experimental investigations of sociolinguistic knowledge.* Ph.D. Dissertation, Department of Linguistics. Palo Alto, CA: Stanford University.

Stephens, I., & Daniloff, R. (1974, November). *Trouble with /s/.* Paper presented to the American Speech and Hearing Association National Convention, Las Vegas.

Stevens, K. N. (2000). Diverse acoustic cues at consonantal landmarks. *Phonetica,* 57, 139–151.

Strand, E., & Johnson, K. (1996). Gradient and visual speaker normalization in the perception of fricatives. In D. Gibbon (Ed.), *Natural language processing and speech technology: Results of the 3rd KONVENS Conference, Bielfelt, October 1996* (pp. 14-26). Berlin: Mouton de Gruyter.

Stoel-Gammon, C., & Harrington, P. B. (1990). Vowel systems of normally developing and phonologically disordered children. *Clinical Linguistics and Phonetics, 4,* 145–160.

Stojanovik, R. (2010). Prosodic deficits in children with Down syndrome. *Journal of Neurolinguistics*; doi: 10.1016/j.neuroling.2010.01.004.

Tabain, M. (2001). Variability in fricative production and spectra: Implications for the hyper- and hypo- and quantal theories of speech production. *Language and Speech, 44,* 57–94.

Thomas, E. (2007). Phonological and phonetic characteristics of African-American Vernacular English. *Language and Linguistics Compass, 1,* 450–475.

Thorsen, N. G. (1985). Intonation and text in standard Danish. *Journal of the Acoustical Society of America, 77,* 1205–1016.

Tiffany, W., & Carrell, J. (1977). *Phonetics: Theory and application* (2nd ed.). New York: McGraw-Hill.

Traunmuller, H., & Eriksson, A. (2000). Acoustic effects of variation in vocal effort by men, women, and children. *Journal of the Acoustical Society of America, 107,* 3438–3451.

Trim, J. (1953). Some suggestions for the phonetic notation of sounds in defective speech. *Speech, 17,* 21–24.

Trost, J. E. (1981). Articulatory additions to the classic description of the speech of persons with cleft palate. *Cleft Palate Journal, 18,* 193–203.

Van den Heuvel, H., Cranen, B., & Rietveld, T. (1996). Speaker variability in the coarticulation of / a , i , u /. *Speech Communication, 18,* 113–130.

Venneman, T. (1972). On the theory of syllabic phonology. *Linguistische Berichte, 18,* 1–18.

Vorperian, H.K., & Kent, R.D. (2007). Vowel acoustic space development in children: a synthesis of acoustic and anatomic data. *Journal of Speech, Language and Hearing Research, 50,* 1510–1545.

Watson, P., & Munson, B. (2007). The influence of phonological neighborhood density and word frequency on vowel-space dispersion in older and younger adults. In J. Trouvain & W. Barry (Eds.), *Proceedings of the International Congress on Phonetic Sciences* (pp. 561–564). Saarbrucken, Germany: University of Saarland.

Wells, J. C. (2000). Orthographic diacritics and multilingual computing. *Language Problems and Language Planning, 24,* 249–272.

Wells, J. C., Peppé, S., & Goulandris, N. (2004). Intonation development from five to thirteen. *Journal of Child Language, 31,* 749–778.

Wightman, C. W., Shuttuck-Hufnagel, S., Ostendorf, M., & Price, P. J. (1992). Segmental durations in the vicinity of prosodic phrase boundaries. *Journal of the Acoustical Society of America, 91,* 1707–1717.

Wise, C. (1957a). *Applied phonetics.* Englewood Cliffs, NJ: Prentice-Hall.

Wise, C. (1957b). *Introduction to phonetics.* Englewood Cliffs, NJ: Prentice-Hall.

Wolfram, W., & Thomas, E. (2002). *The development of African American English.* Malden MA: Blackwell.

Woodard, M. (1991). The use of diacritics for visual articulatory behaviours. *British Journal of Disorders of Communication, 26,* 125–128.

Zawadzki, P., & Kuehn, D. (1980). A cineradiographic study of static and dynamic aspects of American English /r/. *Phonetica, 37,* 253–266.

Index

C

D

N

O

P

T